Released 1995

MEDICAL HOLOCAUSTS I
EXTERMINATIVE MEDICINE IN NAZI GERMANY AND CONTEMPORARY AMERICA

MEDICAL HOLOCAUSTS I
Exterminative Medicine in Nazi Germany and Contemporary America

by

WILLIAM BRENNAN

VOLUME I
in
THE NORDLAND SERIES IN CONTEMPORARY
AMERICAN SOCIAL PROBLEMS

General Editors
DR. RICHARD S. HAUGH
DR. EVA M. HIRSCH

1980

NORDLAND PUBLISHING INTERNATIONAL, INC.
BOSTON   NEW YORK   HOUSTON

Library of Congress Catalog Card Number 80-82305

ISBN 0-913124-39-7

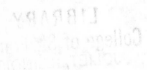

PRINTED IN THE UNITED STATES OF AMERICA

This book is dedicated to all those unwanted human beings, born and unborn, whose lives have been proficiently snuffed out by prestigious medical executioners under the cloak of sophisticated technology in a spineless and deplorable regression back to the dark ages of pre-Hippocratic medicine, when the physician functioned in the schizophrenic role of killer-healer.

About the Author

William Brennan has a bachelor's degree in history, a master's in social work, and a doctorate in sociology. Currently, he is a professor in the School of Social Service at St. Louis University. Dr. Brennan is the recipient of several fellowships and academic honors and is a member of the American Sociological Association and the American Historical Association. In addition to authoring numerous articles in professional journals and magazines, he has spoken extensively on the subject of medical holocausts in many parts of the United States.

Foreword

BY

MARVIN I. WEINBERGER *

Those who read for ethereal enjoyment should delve no further, for Dr. Brennan has not written a "pleasant" book. This volume, and its companion—*Medical Holocausts II: The Language of Exterminative Medicine in Nazi Germany and Contemporary America*—are only for those willing to confront the dark side of America, perhaps the somber twilight of American social justice.

Until the spring of 1977, I was largely oblivious to the dark parallels of which Dr. Brennan so pointedly writes. I caught a first glimpse of them in the law library of Boston University while reading news accounts of the trial of a California obstetrician who had performed a saline abortion on a woman *seven and a half months pregnant*. A few hours later, according to an eyewitness, he strangled to death the child who unexpectedly survived this abortion and was being cared for in the hospital nursery. Charged with murder, the obstetrician protested roundly. His reasoning provided a grim enlightenment. Why, the doctor insisted, should he be prosecuted for killing an *unwanted newborn*, if *unwanted unborn*

*Marvin I. Weinberger, J.D., a graduate of Boston University Law School, received his A.B. from the University of Michigan, where he graduated Magna cum Laude and was elected Phi Beta Kappa. He lectures nationally on the topics of abortion, euthanasia, and the "art of citizen advocacy," and has appeared on a number of national television programs. Mr. Weinberger is the founder and president of a professional consulting firm, MIW Associates, and is one of the consultants for the Nordland Series in Contemporary American Social Problems.

children can be legally killed even later in pregnancy? How could the abortion he performed in the morning (a "morally meaningless act") become murder in the afternoon? Nothing, after all, had changed. The strangled child was no more or less human for having been born. And, most importantly, the child *was* unwanted.

As a Jew, I found these arguments chilling. Many of my relatives in Europe had been slaughtered because they were "unwanted." And, as Dr. Brennan points out, the German medical profession was one of the first groups to preach the crude ethical relativism that led to the later destruction of the Jews. My mother, a survivor, once told me that evil rarely bursts upon a society with guns blazing; more often it creeps unannounced, from within. As I sat in the library I wondered: could it be happening here? Was it too late to protect the sanctity-of-life ethic? Little did I realize then how close we in America might be to losing this cherished ethical tradition.

There is a Yiddish proverb: The truth can walk around naked, only lies must be clothed in euphemism. As Dr. Brennan explains, pro-abortionists lust for euphemisms to disguise their utilitarian bent. This was made plain in an editorial appearing in *California Medicine* entitled "A New Ethic for Medicine and Society." The editorial asserts that the "old ethic" of intrinsic and equal value for every human life (regardless of condition or status) is being replaced by a "new ethic" that measures life relativistically. The problem: since the old ethic has not yet been *fully* displaced, it has become necessary to separate the idea of abortion from the concept of killing a human being. The result: "a curious avoidance of the scientific fact" that human life begins at conception and is a continuum until death. The authors conclude that "this schizophrenic sort of subterfuge" would continue to be necessary until the public had completely accepted the new ethic. ("A New Ethic for Medicine and Society," *California Medicine* 113 [September 1970]: 67-68.)

What is most troubling is that the "new ethicists" (whose views are neither "new" nor "ethical") are increasingly wont to publicly say exactly what they mean. Consider the official editorial that appeared in the influential *New Republic* magazine. There, the authors admit that "metaphysical arguments" about life's beginnings are of no avail; that there is "no logical or moral distinction" between an unborn and a newborn baby; that "abortion cannot be reasonably distinguished from euthanasia." Having said this about abortion, the authors, with clear conscience, conclude: "Nevertheless we are for it." *Why?* Because: "It is too facile to say that human life always is sacred; obviously it is not . . . ." ("The Unborn and the Born Again," *The New Republic*, July 2, 1977, pp. 5-6.)

Writing in the Washington Post, noted liberal commentator Nicholas von Hoffman admits with chilling clarity that "the case for abortion is terribly weak." Consequently, pro-abortionists are forced to retreat to euphemisms when speaking in public. "Interrupting a pregnancy" sounds better than saying "killing an unborn child"; it is an even better euphemism than "terminating a pregnancy," because that sounds too irreversible. Sardonically, von Hoffman points out that the Nazi Minister of Propaganda Joseph Goebbels would have done well to characterize the Nazi atrocities as the " 'interruption' of the Jewish Question." Nevertheless, von Hoffman concludes that abortion should be legal, that there are "other classes of murders which should be stopped first." But, in any event, "we might recognize abortion for what it is and not fool ourselves by calling it a medical procedure." (Nicholas von Hoffman, "In the Eye of the Beholder," *Washington Post*, March 17, 1975, p. B1.)

Perhaps the most forthright admission of abortion as exterminative medicine was made in 1978 by Dr. Warren Hern. In a paper delivered before the Association of Planned Parenthood Physicians, Hern points out that the challenges of late abortion are not in the "technical questions of medical treatment" but rather in how doctors *feel* about performing these procedures. "Some part of our cultural and perhaps even biological heritage recoils at a destructive operation on a *form similar to our own*" (emphasis added). He concludes that "We have reached a point in this particular technology where there is no possibility of denial of an act of destruction by the operator." (Warren M. Hern and Billie Corrigan, "What

About Us? Staff Reactions to the D & E Procedure," a paper presented at the annual meeting of the Association of Planned Parenthood Physicians, San Diego, California, October 26, 1978.)

Why have the abortionists become so bold? Because, of course, they seem to be winning. In 1977 (the last year for which full statistics are available) there were *1.3 million* abortions performed in the United States. Under the guise of social justice, *8 million innocent children* have been killed since the legalization of abortion in 1973. In the ten minutes it takes to read this foreword, another forty children will have died by abortion in America.

Whatever happened to the California obstetrician who first prompted my awakening? The criminal charges against him were ultimately dropped and he was exonerated by the medical establishment. As is evident from this and many other cases, abortion *has* become infanticide. Will it stop there? I fear not, for life is a continuum from conception onwards, and if we can allow the slaughter of helpless unwanted babies, why not eliminate the sick and elderly as well? This, Dr. Brennan points out, is already beginning to happen.

The killing habit is so hard to break. The Germans, for all their intellectual prowess, could not keep their logic on a leash. Can we? It has been said that the greatness of a society is measured by the dignity it affords the least of its members. America at this moment is failing this test of greatness; our vaunted reputation for compassion is presently being obfuscated by operations of near flawlessness on unseen victims.

I pray that the dissemination of Dr. Brennan's findings will help guide us from evil's way. I pray that those who cherish life's sanctity may resurrect the true ideals of social justice which swathed America in her infancy. But the darkness is fast upon us; for many, the light is gone forever. Whether our efforts shall be but a forlorn flicker in the stormy night, I know not.

I cry for the children; I fear for America.

Boston
July 25, 1980

Contents

Part Two THE TECHNOLOGY OF DESTRUCTION

Acknowledgments

Acknowledgment is made to the following for permission to quote from the publications listed:

Leo Alexander, "Medical Science Under Dictatorship," Reprinted by permission from *The New England Journal of Medicine*, Vol. 241, pp. 39-41, 1949.

Gila Berkowitz, "Desperate Measures," *Medical Dimensions*, October 1974, p. 9. Copyright © 1975, MBA Communications, Inc. Used by permission.

"Between Guilt and Gratification: Abortion Doctors Reveal Their Feelings," by Norma Rosen, April 17, 1977. Mag. © 1977 by The New York Times Company. Reprinted by permission.

Karl Binding and Alfred Hoche, *The Release of the Destruction of Life Devoid of Value* (Leipzig, Germany: Felix Meiner, 1920), comp. Robert L. Sassone, 900 N. Broadway, Santa Ana, Calif., 92701, A Life Quality Paperback, 1975. Reprinted by permission of Robert L. Sassone.

From Jerome S. Bates and Edward S. Zawadzki, *Criminal Abortion: A Study in Medical Sociology*, 1965. Courtesy of Charles C. Thomas, Publisher, Springfield, Illinois.

Sally Kilby-Kelberg, "The Abortion," *Medical Dimensions*, May 1974, p. 36. Reprinted by permission of author.

Preface

Of all the terms ever invoked to characterize destruction, the most ominous is the word "holocaust." Its most frequent application has been to the killing of millions of Jews during the Nazi era. Since then its scope has expanded to civilization itself, as indicated in the terrifying expression "nuclear holocaust." At the most fundamental level, holocaust means a great slaughter or massacre; destruction of a large number of people.

The methods of killing employed in a holocaust — whether they involve shooting, gassing, burning, mutilation, vacuuming, poisoning, or stabbing — reflect the state of exterminative technology at the time of destruction. The victims of a holocaust also vary depending upon which individuals or groups are considered dangerous, subhuman, or unworthy of existence. Frequently, the unborn have been declared appropriate products for destructive consumption. At other times the expendables include defective newborns, the terminally ill, the nonfunctional aged, mongoloids, Jews, Gypsies, Poles, asocials, useless eaters and those of the undesired sex. In fact, anyone who is not wanted or fails to measure up to imposed notions of acceptability becomes fair game.

Such words as kill, destroy, annihilate, exterminate, medical killer, executioner, perpetrator, scientific butchery, mutilation, slaughter, dismember and other similar terms are employed throughout this book in order to convey the harsh but unadorned truth of destruction at the hands of medical practitioners. These expressions are perfectly valid ways for describing the various facets of past and present holocausts. It should be kept uppermost in mind that at the time of the Nazi atrocities, they were blanketed with a huge volume of abstract,

3

euphemistic phrases manufactured by medical and non-medical bureaucrats.

When blunt language is used to characterize the modern-day abortion and euthanasia movements, controversy erupts. It is somehow considered offensive or a matter of poor taste to mention in these contexts any words associated with the idea of killing. Today's American society, like that of Nazi Germany, is dominated by language that portrays killing as something other than killing and the victims as something other than human.

Beyond the rhetoric, however, abortion constitutes nothing less than the intentional killing (putting to death), destruction (depriving of existence), or extermination (utter destruction) of unique human beings at the prenatal phase of the human life cycle. When the destructive act is performed by a physician, he then in fact becomes a medical killer (one who deprives another of life), executioner (one who puts another to death), or perpetrator (one who commits a destructive act). It is equally appropriate to employ the designations butchery (bloody slaughter), mutilation (cutting off or otherwise destroying limbs or organs), and dismember (tear into pieces) to describe what happens in D & C and D & E abortions: sharp instruments called curettes literally slice, cut, tear, rip apart, and obliterate the tiny bodies of living, growing, developing human beings inside the womb.

Furthermore, dramatic breakthroughs in microbiology, genetics, fetology, and allied sciences indicate beyond a shadow of a doubt that what exists during pregnancy is not a piece of protoplasm, a form of animal existence or a potential life, but an actual human life with potential. Those who still cling to the tissue theory of prenatal development as a rationalization of abortion might well ponder the revelations of Dr. Bernard N. Nathanson, who openly acknowledged being "deeply troubled" by the "increasing certainty" that he had "in fact presided over 60,000 deaths" during his tenure as director of a large abortion clinic in the early 1970s:

> There is no longer serious doubt in my mind that
> human life exists within the womb from the very

onset of pregnancy, despite the fact that the nature
of the intrauterine life has been the subject of considerable dispute in the past. Electrocardiographic evidence
of heart function has been established in embryos as
early as six weeks. Electroencephalographic recordings
of human brain activity have been noted in embryos
at eight weeks. Our capacity to measure signs of life
is daily becoming more sophisticated, and as time goes
by, we will doubtless be able to isolate life signs at
earlier and earlier stages in fetal development.

Life is an interdependent phenomenon for us all.
It is a continuous spectrum that begins in utero and
ends at death — the bands of the spectrum are designated by words such as fetus, infant, child, adolescent,
and adult.

We must courageously face the fact — finally —
that human life of a special order is being taken. . . .
Denial of this reality is the crassest kind of moral
evasiveness.[1]

Nathanson resigned as clinic head and took a new position.
Currently, one of his major tasks consists of bringing difficult pregnancies to term and helping prematurely born infants survive. This has prompted him to cut through the de-
ceptive semantics and reflect more fully on the reality of life
before birth. "All that propaganda you've been spewing out
about abortion not involving the taking of human life is nonsense," he admitted. "If that thing in the uterus is *nothing,*
why are we spending all this time and money on it?"

When I first began researching this topic seven years ago,
I did so with the utmost caution. The climate then, as now,
was not favorable to drawing parallels between the Nazi
atrocities and those of the present, let alone probing them in
depth. Anyone who dared summon the specter of the holocaust in these comparisons was trodding on sacred ground and
risked being labeled a monger of unabashed sensationalism
bent on distorting history for political ends. Considerable
concern exists in some quarters that using the "Nazi experience" to understand what is happening today will lead to a

situation of linguistic overkill, in which every violent outburst will be called a holocaust. This would then dilute and detract from the enormous and unspeakable suffering of those who perished in the death camps. Others, particularly contemporary medical executioners of the unborn, are quite defensive whenever the issue of the Nazi holocaust is raised. Such a reaction is hardly surprising, especially since their destructive activities amount to a replay of what doctors did to their victims during the Nazi regime.

Immersing oneself in the literature of past and current atrocities is a sobering as well as eye-opening experience replete with profoundly disturbing revelations. The image often conveyed of the Nazi holocaust as a totally unique, unrepeatable historical episode with little or no contemporary relevance does not square with the facts examined. What emerges from the material with striking clarity and persistence are the numerous similarities between killing in Nazi Germany and killing in contemporary American society. Not only is the term "holocaust" a perfectly legitimate one to use in this context, but perhaps the only one that captures fully the scope and horror of massive annihilation while providing an indispensable perspective for exploring the many continuities involved.

Among the similarities found, the most pervasive and distressing of all is the extensive role played by physicians in the destruction processes of both countries. The horrendous practices highlighted in this book are not the handiwork of incompetent butchers who *accidentally* kill their patients because of surgical errors or inappropriate treatment procedures. They are, rather, the creation of highly skilled practitioners who *deliberately* and *proficiently* destroy unwanted human beings before and after birth. Hitler's Germany spawned a new branch of medical science, exterminative medicine, and a new breed of physicians, specialists in perverting medical skills for destructive purposes. An increasing number of doctors today, within the antiseptic settings of hospitals, university medical centers, and abortion clinic chambers, are continuing the legacy of exterminative medicine pioneered in the hospitals, euthanasia institutions, and concentration camps of the Third Reich. Bolstered by advanced killing techniques, contemporary medical killers are responsible for a far greater toll of human lives than their German counterparts.

The following chapters will examine the assembly-line killing of pre- and postnatal discards by the medical technocrats of Nazi Germany and contemporary America. They will focus on the historical factors leading up to mass extermination and the stages of technological destruction, including death selection, processing of the victims, killing methods, body disposal procedures, management of breakdowns in destructive techniques, and death statistics.

This book provides a chilling account of the utter contempt with which the medical perpetrators view their victims. Many of the incidents described are closely akin to horror stories straight out of Aldous Huxley's science fiction classic, *Brave New World*, and George Orwell's negative utopia, *1984*. What appears here, however, is all too true, and thoroughly documented. It is based on information drawn from the correspondence, memoranda, and conference notes compiled by the perpetrators; war crimes trials testimony; medical and legal journals; concentration camp survivors' accounts; medical policy statements; historical records and documents; books on various facets of past and present destructive actions, and many other sources.

Since the findings of this book are confined largely to published materials, they represent only the tip of the reprehensible iceberg of medical assaults against those who cannot protect themselves. Some of the Nazi victims lived to testify against their persecutors. Most did not survive to bear witness regarding the barbarities of genocide. Horrible as the extant accounts are, they still provide only an inkling of the vast magnitude and malevolence of the atrocities. Lost forever with the dead are countless stories of untold human tragedies. So too for the modern medical war on the unborn. There are no survivors to reveal the brutalities of extermination inside the womb. The handful of reports portraying abortion as a destructive act usually come from those few medical abortionists bothered by the sight of bodies or body parts being sucked, cut, or ejected from the uterus. They are more than offset, nonetheless, by the huge bulk of medical journal articles on abortion saturated with euphemistic terminology and self-serving ideology.

It has taken humankind a long time to evolve the principle that all human beings, despite their stage of development or degree of perfection, are of inestimable value and deserve equal protection under the law. During the Nazi era doctors played a significant part in subverting this principle at the core, as well as flagrantly violating the sanctity-of-life ethic embodied in the more than 2,000 year-old Hippocratic Oath for physicians. Today the Hippocratic tradition, together with its modern version, the Geneva Code of 1948, is again coming apart at the seams. An alarming number of doctors show no qualms about destroying, manipulating, and mutilating human castoffs under the banner of science, legality, and humanity in an orgy of raw medical power that has long since surpassed the most virulent excesses of Nazi medicine. The prospects of survival for the defective, imperfect, and unwanted will become increasingly precarious. Above all, the material contained herein demonstrates with frightening tenacity the extreme manifestations of science without ethics, the triumph of technology over humanity, the brutalization of medical science, and the severe erosion of empathy for the least visible and most vulnerable members of the human race.

Introduction

Not since the end of World War II has there been a comparable outpouring of interest in the holocaust of the Third Reich as during the late 1970s. A monstrous episode that had been forgotten or evaded for decades suddenly became an "in" topic. Everyone, it seems, was either discovering again or learning for the first time the horrendous and unbelievable details about one of the darkest chapters in human history. Holocaust studies have been introduced on the high school level and a 9½ hour television dramatization of the Nazi holocaust was watched by 120 million Americans in April 1978.

And not a moment too soon. The fear that current and future generations would distort, never know, or forget altogether one of the worst evils ever to befall mankind began to materialize in an alarming number of instances. A professor at an American university has written a book called *The Hoax of the Twentieth Century*, in which he claims that the Nazi extermination of six million Jews was a complete fabrication. A study conducted in 1977 of West German students revealed that many held positive notions about the Nazi era, had only the most fragmentary knowledge of the annihilation of the Jews, and viewed Hitler as a great leader. A significant portion of students surveyed in the Seattle area thought the holocaust was a Jewish holiday. All the more reason that such urgency exists about setting the historical record straight.

The major motivation behind keeping the memory of the holocaust alive is not to inflame passions or resurrect ancient hostilities. Neither is it to satisfy a sadistic craving for the most extreme examples of violence. Nor is it to point the finger of blame at an endless list of perpetrators and ac-

9

complices. The real thrust underlying the current emphasis on learning more about the extermination of six million Jews and others relates to an understanding of the past, application of the past to the present, and hope for the future.

On the first count, there is a compelling obligation to the truth to demonstrate with unmistakable clarity that, no matter how incredible they seem, heinous acts were actually perpetrated against millions. Secondly, it is imperative to examine carefully how the barbarities of Nazi Germany compare with present day atrocities. Whatever similarities exist must be identified and communicated. Finally, and most importantly, confrontation with the horrors of the Third Reich provides indispensable insurance against them ever happening again. If civilized society allows itself to become informed about as many aspects of the Nazi holocaust as possible, it will be better equipped to recognize the danger signs leading up to genocide and therefore be in a strategic position to prevent its recurrence. Therein lies the hope for the future.

It was concern for the future that prompted the philosopher George Santayana's famous statement: "Those who do not remember the past are condemned to relive it." Thus, a knowledge of the past is intended to help us stop repeating the errors of the past. Even many of those most severely devastated — the survivors — have been able to go beyond the universe of their own indescribable sufferings and courageously summon the strength to warn the world that a holocaust is not so unique that it cannot or will not happen again. Their most priceless legacy to civilization is to raise and sustain the level of consciousness high enough so the lessons of history are heeded.

Although every holocaust ever perpetrated is an unprecedented event in its own right, this should not detract from what all holocausts share in common. The central element of any holocaust — whether it involves the extermination of Jews by the Nazis, the annihilation of Russians by the Soviet regime, or the slaughter of Cambodians by the Khmer Rouge — is the systematic and widespread destruction of millions looked upon as indiscriminate masses of subhuman expendables. The basic ingredients for a holocaust exist whenever any society can be misled into defining individuals as less than human and therefore devoid of value and respect. This is all the fuel necessary to ignite destruction on the level of a holocaust. Once one group of individuals is deemed unworthy of the designation human, the precedent is established for defining ever growing numbers of people and groups out of the human race and along with that, denying their most fundamental right, the right to life itself. When the rights of some are extinguished, the rights of all are in jeopardy. As callousness to the value of human life increases, so does the likelihood of a monumental holocaust.

As the holocaust of Hitler, Goering, Himmler, and other Nazi butchers receives greater attention, relatively unexamined aspects of destruction before and during the Nazi era are bound to open up. The major one uncovered is the role of medical doctors in the destruction process. One of the main theses of this book is that *the involvement of German doctors in promoting, planning, and implementing the killing of unwanted and defective human beings before as well as after birth was so great as to constitute a medical holocaust.*

During the 1920s, German physicians were violating the strict abortion law then in effect and simultaneously agitating for legalizing abortion for an expanding list of indications. Their efforts bore fruit by the 1930s, when the Nazi government passed a permissive law that allowed abortions on the grounds of health, eugenics, or when the mother's life was at stake. Doctors thus became the first legal killers of the Third Reich, by inaugurating a systematic program of eliminating unwanted unborn German children suspected of not being up to par with the Aryan concept of perfection. Later this form of medical killing moved beyond the borders of Germany to engulf the unborn offspring of women in captive European nations and concentration camps of the Eastern territories.

Medical participation was predominant in the euthanasia program directed against defective or allegedly defective Germans. Decades before Hitler came to power, physicians and like-minded elitists waged a relentless campaign to rid Germany of the unfit by portraying them as overburdening the economy and threatening the purity of the German race. The propaganda intensified during the Nazi regime and had a profound influence on Hitler's euthanasia order of 1939, granting doctors the authority to accord a mercy death to incurables. Relying upon superficial information and the most cursory examinations, psychiatrists played the leading role in deciding who merited the benefits of a "merciful release." How blatantly this power was abused is revealed in the statistics: from 1939 until the fall of the Third Reich doctors, in collaboration with nurses and medical attendants, were responsible for putting to death approximately 275,000 German patients in euthanasia hospitals and institutions. The totals would have surely mounted much higher if the thousand-year Reich had not come to a premature and ignominious end after only twelve years of existence.

Medical involvement in destruction was not confined to abortion and euthanasia. In 1941, when Hitler was faced with elaborating a final solution to the Jewish question, he could not help but be impressed by the efficient models of destruction pioneered by physicians in hospitals and euthanasia centers. Only several years earlier psychiatrists from leading medical schools and others had gathered to test the first gas chamber. The locale was one of the euthanasia hospitals and the subjects were mental patients. Some of the doctors and technicians of these institutions were transferred to the concentration camps, where their talents could be employed for the more enormous task of racial genocide. The ultimate test of their training and its effectiveness is disclosed in Nazi hunter Simon Wiesenthal's observation that "machines broke down, but the people handling them never did . . . the people operating the gas chambers and ovens were more reliable than the machines."

The medical role in the massive killing operations of the death camps was absolutely immense. Physicians were far and away the most active death selectors. In an egregious display of raw medical power, they perverted the task of professional diagnosis at the very core by sending huge numbers to the gas chambers on the basis of their unfitness to perform slave labor for the Nazi war effort. Doctors chose victims upon arrival, inside the camp compound and in the camp hospital. Commissions of physicians also toured the death camps in a search-and-destroy mission aimed at rooting out the physically and mentally defective who had escaped the initial screening processes.

Inside the camps, medical doctors performed a wide range of other destructive activities. Their typical answer to frequent outbreaks of epidemics was extermination of the afflicted with lethal injections or consignment to the crematorium. They conducted an orgy of experimental atrocities on the inmates before, during, and after destruction. They arrogantly used the victims' condemnation to death as an excuse for exploiting their bodies and remains for scientific, pseudoscientific, and commercial purposes.

The presence of physicians in every phase of the killing endowed destruction with an incomparable aura of respectability. How psychologically consoling it must have been for the non-medical perpetrators to have such a dedicated group of medical people to plan, lead, and help implement the machinery of destruction!

Who were these doctors of infamy? How representative were they of German medicine as a whole? From the vantage point of many people, their brand of medical violence can only be understood as the handiwork of psychopathic butchers on the fringes of professional medicine. While on the surface this explanation seems persuasive, it did not ring true for many doctors involved in the destruction process. Most were not simply Nazi fanatics or puppets. Many had established impeccable professional reputations and had made important contributions to science and humanity long before Hitler became a powerful political force. Yet even they made a mockery of medical science and flagrantly violated the more than 2,000 year-old Hippocratic tradition: *primum non nocere* — first of all, do no harm.

The tragic failure of German medicine to speak out against colleagues who participated in the euthanasia program and the implication for the more massive destruction unleashed in the concentration camps is nowhere more forthrightly expressed than by American medical science consultant to the

Nuremberg Doctors' Trial, Dr. Andrew C. Ivy. "Had the profession taken a strong stand against the mass killing of sick Germans before the war, it is conceivable that the entire idea and technique of death factories for genocide would not have materialized," he declared. "Far from opposing the Nazi state militantly, part of the German medical profession cooperated consciously and even willingly, while the remainder acquiesced in silence."

The highly significant role of doctors in the overall holocaust of Germany remains a disturbing fact unknown to most of the public. The eminence of many of the medical executioners is another alarming fact that many people are totally unaware of. The time has come to face such disquieting but truthful realities.

The overriding question resulting from a greater understanding of the Nazi holocaust is, "Can it happen again here or any other place?" Holocausts have flourished in the Soviet Union and Cambodia and will continue to thrive in any country where some group asserts its power through the denial of human rights to others.

When the destruction of human lives is viewed from the perspective of the medical holocaust perpetrated during the Third Reich, then the question "Can it happen again?" is hopelessly outdated. This leads to the other major thesis of this book: *another medical holocaust is already upon us and has been around for a number of years.*

A disturbingly large number of respectable American doctors have been or are currently involved in the same destructive activities as their German counterparts: massive violations of laws protective of human life, agitation for legalized destruction of the unborn and born, selection of candidates for extermination, implementation of killing procedures, and experimental exploitation of those destined for extinction. Today's victims are largely unwanted unborn expendables. Unwanted postnatal defectives and the nonfunctional aged are increasingly being endangered by the authority of an amoral, utilitarian medical ethic.

The time is long overdue for the spotlight to shift onto the medical holocausts of Nazi Germany and today's America.

The comparisons and parallels already outlined and others to follow will be drawn with a degree of depth and documentation never before undertaken.

Part One

HISTORICAL PERSPECTIVES

Part One

HISTORICAL PERSPECTIVES

CHAPTER 1

Physicians as Healers

Throughout history, the predominant role of the doctor has been to save, preserve, and heal human lives. It is this humanitarian orientation that has attracted so many idealistic and gifted individuals to the profession of medicine. It is also responsible for the incomparable esteem in which physicians have been held by the public. The image of the selfless doctor totally committed to the welfare of the patient and humanity is a pervasive one in most cultures. Even in the past, when physicians had been responsible for killing more individuals than they cured, their professional image remained untainted. Their involvement in killing was unintentional; it was due to inadequate knowledge or therapies.

The killing perpetrated by German physicians during the time of the Third Reich was unique insofar as it was intentional and not accidental; it was perceived as being part of the doctor's professional role rather than a radical departure from it. So too for the destruction of unborn children by today's physicians in America and other countries; it is defined as a valid medical procedure.

What were the historical traditions of medicine out of which these medical atrocities erupted? Did they proceed from an atmosphere of corruption and decay in the medical profession as a whole, or did they arise during a time of unprecedented medical progress and enlightenment? Paradoxically, the involvement of doctors in programs of mass extermination began to take hold in Nazi Germany and contemporary America after decades of outstanding contributions to society and humanity by the medical professions of both countries. This is a historical reality that must be understood more fully before attempting to comprehend the radical disruptions that followed.

The Golden Age of German Medicine

The healing, curing thrust of German medicine was well established by the time of Hitler's ascendance to power. During the last half of the nineteenth and first quarter of the twentieth century the contributions of German physicians to alleviating the diseases and ravages of mankind could not be matched by any other country in the world. German medicine was head and shoulders above everyone in terms of fundamental scientific discoveries and therapeutic advances. This was truly the golden age of German medicine, a period of growth and development that may be difficult to ever again fully duplicate.

A brief historical sketch will provide some comprehension of the unparalleled developments and personages in German medicine prior to the Nazi period.[1]

Much of the scientific foundation of medicine can be attributed to Johannes Müller, professor of anatomy, physiology, and pathology at the University of Berlin until his death in 1848. Not only was he considered the greatest pathologist of his time, but he also had an enormous influence on his pupils, who were to pioneer some of the most important discoveries in the history of medicine. Among them were Theodor Schwann, co-founder of the cell-theory in 1838—one of the greatest biological discoveries of all time; Jacob Henle, creator of the science of histology and one of the outstanding anatomists in history; Hermann von Helmholtz, formulator of the principle of the conservation of energy and inventor of the ophthalmoscope in 1851; and Rudolf Virchow, the outstanding physician of his generation and creator of the modern science of pathology.

Other giants of German medicine had worldwide impact.

Robert Koch demonstrated in 1876 the bacterial origin of many diseases and the techniques for finding this out. Koch is rated one of the greatest bacteriologists who ever lived. Wilhelm Konrad Röntgen, professor at the University of Würzburg, discovered x-rays in 1895. Paul Ehrlich laid the foundation of modern hematology, created the new science of chemotherapy, did pioneer work in infectious diseases, and in 1910 discovered salvarsan, a widely used drug for the treatment of syphilis. Hans Berger developed the electroencephalograph in 1929, while Gerhard Domagk received the Nobel Prize in 1939 for his work on the therapeutic value of sulfonamides.

The dominance of German medicine did not stop at discoveries in the basic sciences of chemistry, physics, bacteriology, anatomy, and pharmacology. German doctors also led the way in applying their discoveries to combatting diseases. This was particularly the case in the area of bacteriology:

> The development of bacteriology, the demonstration of the bacterial and parasitic cause of many diseases, pointed the way to their control or eventual elimination. The demonstration that typhoid fever was the result, in great measure, of a contaminated water supply, that cholera commonly was caused by infected food, that many epidemics were caused by infected milk, that tuberculosis was disseminated by dried sputum, that malaria and yellow fever were carried by mosquitoes, that sleeping sickness was transmitted by the bite of a fly, and that the common house fly was a carrier of typhoid and other diseases — all these discoveries called for the application of measures that were obviously outside and beyond the field of private medical practice. The ancient principle of prevention of diseases now acquired a new meaning and a new force since the means of prevention were clearly understood.[2]

Germany's medical and surgical clinics were the best in the world. They served as models for other countries to follow. In the field of public health Max von Pettenkofer directed the first institute of hygiene, was influential in the development of pure water supplies for cities and towns and in the passage of regulations for food inspection.

German medical universities were also far and away the finest in the world. The high quality of the financially poor German universities compared with their well-financed British counterparts was acknowledged by the prominent English scientist Thomas H. Huxley as early as 1870: "as for works of profound research on any subject, a third-rate, poverty-stricken German university turns out more produce of that kind in one year than our fine and wealthy foundations elaborate in ten." [3] It is not surprising, then, that doctors from other countries chose to study at these superb centers of medical education. From 1870 until 1914, some 15,000 American doctors were trained in German speaking universities at the post-graduate level. [4] Johns Hopkins University Hospital and School of Medicine, founded during the closing years of the nineteenth century in Baltimore, Maryland, was directly patterned after the German universities. Up until this time American universities were primarily overgrown colleges. Johns Hopkins, with its emphasis on graduate studies, superior students, and distinguished faculty, opened up a new chapter in American medicine.

German medicine retained its position of predominance until the First World War. The war had a devastating effect on the moral, political, and economic institutions of the Rhineland. Also hard hit were the universities and medical schools. Surprisingly, however, in 1924, only six years after the war's end, Abraham Flexner gave a highly laudatory assessment of medical education in Germany compared with America, England, and France:

> There the German universities stand — still as a
> group the best organized, the best equipped, and the
> most soundly conceived that exist. Neither teaching
> nor research has stopped. With a tenacity that shows
> how deeply rooted in the national consciousness is the

respect for learning, scientists, young as well as old, are struggling to produce.[5]

All this prodigious activity by German physicians not only indicated an unyielding commitment to advancing the frontiers of knowledge, but also revealed a deep concern for human life. Many of these men devoted their entire careers to ridding mankind of plagues and diseases that had from ancient times taken countless human lives. Their investigations and their discoveries were intended for all human beings, not just the superior or the strong. German physicians were healers in the best sense of the word. They were more than healers, they were scientific healers. They were not content with the superstitions and unfounded speculations of the past. They waged a relentless battle against ignorance and thus furnished their healing skills with an incomparable ally: science.

The role played by German psychiatry in caring for mental patients provides another example of how doctors viewed the most defenseless human lives. As far back as the closing decades of the sixteenth century, the University of Würzburg hospital was admitting and humanely treating the mentally ill.[6] In the nineteenth century, psychiatric institutions in Germany came to realize more fully their therapeutic capabilities. This meant not only liberating the insane from their chains, but also providing individualized treatment in an institutional setting.[7] By the twentieth century German public psychiatric hospitals were among the best and most humane in the world.

The Ascent of American Medicine

Eighteenth and nineteenth-century American medicine was not nearly as advanced as German medicine. American doctors did not have the facilities, training, or firmly established scientific tradition to compete with German physicians. By the middle of the twentieth century, however, American medicine found itself in a position of world leadership similar to the past golden age of medicine in Germany. Since then, American medical scientists have continued to make far-reaching contributions to the alleviation of illness and the restoration of health.

For purposes of this book, only some of the phenomenal accomplishments of American medicine, especially during the twentieth century, can be touched upon.[8]

Continuing efforts of the American Medical Association to upgrade the quality of medical education, plus the financing of medical research by such private sources as the Carnegie and Rockefeller Foundations and more recently by such governmental agencies as the National Institutes of Health and the Department of Health, Education and Welfare, have helped to stimulate much significant research activity on the part of American medical scientists. Significantly, the types of research activities pursued have had dramatic therapeutic payoffs.

American medicine has been in the forefront of developing and employing sulfa drugs, antibiotics, and hormones for therapeutic purposes. Surgical advances have been equally impressive: open heart surgery, organ transplants and intensive care of infants. The continuing development of sophisticated diagnostic procedures augurs well for identifying and combatting those afflictions yet to be conquered. The great names of American medicine — Benjamin Rush, Charles and William Mayo, Oliver Wendell Holmes, William Osler, Harvey Cushing, Karl Menninger, Jonas Salk — have been individuals of vision and compassion. One further measure of how far American medicine has progressed is indicated by the Nobel Prizes awarded in the field of medicine. Before 1930 not one native-born American doctor had ever won a Nobel Prize; after the early 1930s American physicians began to lead all others in this international recognition of scientific achievement.[9]

In addition to the modern emphasis on science, research, and technology, a strong strain of humanitarianism and impeccable ethical conduct has always characterized American medical thought and practice. The role of the doctor as the wise, kindly, totally devoted servant of the sick and weak is an inherent part of the American experience. This is particularly fitting, since America is a country founded by individuals willing to band together and help each other in building a new civilization out of an often hostile environment. The frontier doctor, the horse and buggy doctor, and the family doctor represent ideal types, whose sole purpose was to render unselfish care to patients. The thrust was in the direction of going out to the patient at all hours of the day or night. Although doctors of eighteenth and nineteenth-century America may have been short on scientific sophistication and knowhow, they were long on tireless energy channeled in behalf of their patients.

In Defense of Human Life

In addition to their unremitting battle against diseases in the face of overwhelming odds, the uncompromising commitment of American medicine toward all human life was clearly enunciated in the American Medical Association's policy statement on abortion of 1859. After two years of studying the problems of criminal abortions, an AMA committee unequivocally condemned the practice of induced abortion at all stages of pregnancy, with the sole exception being when the mother's life was at stake.[10]

At several points in the report the committee clarified its reason for opposing abortion: "[it is] no mere misdemeanor, no attempt upon the life of the mother, but the wanton and murderous destruction of her child; the slaughter of countless children now steadily perpetrated in our midst; such unwarrantable destruction of human life." From these descriptions of the nature of abortion, it is obvious that the AMA opposed abortion not because it was a hazardous surgical procedure for the woman but because it was a fatal one for the unborn child.

Why was the AMA so insistent on condemning abortions at all phases of gestation? Why was it so sure that even abortions performed early in pregnancy constituted the destruction of human life? After all, a long-accepted theory in medical and legal circles held that actual human life does not begin until quickening, when the woman first feels the movement of the child in her womb at about the sixteenth to eighteenth week of pregnancy. Before quickening the assumption was that there is no life present. For centuries the laws of many countries reflected this theory. This was also true for most laws in mid-nineteenth century America: "statutes dealt severely with abortions performed after quickening, but were relatively quite lenient as to abortions at an earlier stage." [11]

The AMA in 1859 chose to speak out against abortion in every phase of intrauterine development because of some commonly held misconceptions about the facts of prenatal life and what abortion does to that life: "a wide-spread popular ignorance of the true character of the crime — a belief, even among mothers themselves, that the foetus is not alive till after the period of quickening." The report labeled such a contention as an error "based, and only based, upon mistaken and exploded medical dogmas." [12]

The whole issue of when human life begins and whether life in the womb is really human even early in gestation had been scientifically answered by the mid 1850s.[13] Cognizant of this, American medicine felt obliged to set the record straight, especially since many of the unfounded assumptions and misconceptions about human life before birth had been perpetuated by physicians:

> If, as is also true, these great, fundamental, and fatal faults of the law are owing to doctrinal errors of the profession in a former age, it devolves upon us, by every bond we hold sacred, by our reverence for the fathers in medicine, by our love for our race, and by our responsibility as accountable beings, to see these errors removed and their grievous results abated.[14]

The AMA committee on abortion was not merely content to challenge well-entrenched and unscientific theories about the nature of life before birth, but also wanted to expose abortion for what it really was — "the slaughter of countless children." Its resolutions, passed unanimously, also called upon physicians as an important part of their professional responsibility to condemn abortion and persuade state legislatures to pass restrictive abortion laws protective of human life at all stages of development:

Resolved, That while physicians have long been united in condemning the act of producing abortion at every period of gestation, except as necessary for preserving the life of either mother or child, it has become the duty of this Association, in view of the prevalence and increasing frequency of the crime, publicly to enter an earnest and solemn protest against such unwarrantable destruction of human life.

Resolved, That in pursuance of the grand and noble calling we profess, the saving of human lives, and of the sacred responsibilities thereby devolving upon us, the Association present this subject to the attention of the several legislative assemblies of the Union, with the prayer that the laws by which the crime of procuring abortion is attempted to be controlled may be revised, and that such other action may be taken in the premises as they in their wisdom may deem necessary.

Resolved, That the Association request the zealous cooperation of the various State Medical Societies in pressing this subject upon the legislatures of their respective States; and that the President and Secretaries of the Association are hereby authorized to carry out, by memorial, these resolutions.[15]

In 1871 the AMA again felt compelled to issue another public pronouncement against abortion. The Association continued to refute the false contention "that life does not exist in the foetus because no motion is felt" with a quote from *Archbold's Criminal Practice and Pleadings:*

It was generally supposed that the foetus becomes animated at the period of quickening; but this idea is exploded. Physiology considers the foetus as much a living being immediately after conception as at any other time before delivery, and its future progress but as the development and increase of those constituent principles which it then received. It considers quickening as a mere adventitious event, and looks upon life as entirely consistent with the most profound foetal repose and consequent inaction. Long before quickening takes place, motion, the pulsation of the heart, and other signs of vitality, have been distinctly perceived, and, according to approved authority, the foetus enjoys life long before the sensation of quickening is felt by the mother. Indeed, no other doctrine appears to be consonant with reason or physiology but that which admits the embryo to possess vitality from the very moment of conception.[16]

Significantly, much of the Association's severest criticism was directed not against abortionists in general but *physician abortionists* in particular:

There we shall discover an enemy in the camp; there we shall witness as hideous a view of moral deformity as the evil spirit could present. There we shall find a class of men in every respect the opposite of the former; men who cling to a noble profession only to dishonor it; men who seek not to save, but to destroy; men known not only to the profession, but to the public, as abortionists. . . . Yes, it is false brethren we have most to fear; men who are false to their profession, false to principle, false to honor, false to humanity, false to God.

"Thou shalt not kill." This commandment is given to all, and applies to all without exception. . . . notwithstanding all this, we see in our midst a class of men, regardless of all laws, human and divine, regardless of all principle, regardless of all honor, who daily destroy that fair fabric of God's creation; who daily pull down what he has built up; who act in antagonism to that profession of which they claim to be members.

These modern Herods, like their prototype, have a summary mode of dealing with their victims. They perform the triple office of Legislative, Judiciary, and Executive, and, to crown the tragedy, they become the executioners. They seem impatient for the sacrifice; the "fiat" goes forth, and those innocent and helpless victims are not permitted ever to breathe that vital air which God in His providence has destined for their use in common with the rest of the human family. Their resting-place is rudely invaded, and that which would grow and ripen into manhood is cut off from existence by the hand of an educated assassin. Mark the monster as he approaches his work! . . . he stands by the bedside of his victim, with poisoned cup or instrument in hand, ready to proceed to the work of destruction. Does any compunction assail his corrupt soul, as he gazes on the field of his labors? Does he measure the extent of the foul deed he is about to commit? Or does he not fear that the uplifted hand of an avenging God will suddenly fall on his guilty head? No; Judas-like, he solaces himself with the prospect of thirty pieces of silver, and this forms the climax of his aspirations!

But, as is found in many other cases of murder, there is no extenuating circumstance here that can change or modify the character of his guilt. As in ordinary cases of murder, there is no anger to prompt him to the deed, no wrongs to be avenged, no jealousies to be appeased. These he cannot point to as extenuating circumstances, and it matters not at what stage of development his victim may have arrived — it matters not how small or how apparently insignificant it may be — it is a murder, a foul, unprovoked murder; and its blood, like the blood of Abel, will cry from earth to Heaven for vengeance.

We have no foreign enemy to contend with, but we have a domestic enemy, and that enemy is in our midst; it surrounds us; yes, we have an unprincipled, an insidious, an unmitigated foe to deal with, an enemy to the human family, as dark and as malignant as the spirit that sent it, and it now becomes us to do our part faithfully towards God in this matter, to crush the monster, and to place the profession right before the public. For it is at this late date in the nineteenth century a doubtful question whether or not the profession of medicine, with all its boasted intelligence, with all the aids and appliances which science and art can bestow — it is doubtful, with such a disgusting caudal appendage as the abortionist attached to it, whether that profession is an advantage or a disadvantage, whether it is a blessing or a curse, to the human family. . . . The abortionists are more destructive to human life than ten British armies.

Yet these monsters of iniquity are permitted to stalk abroad in open day, carrying worse than contagion with them, poisoning wherever they are permitted to touch, invading the very sources of life, and fattening on the blood of their victims. And yet the profession of medicine remains inactive — that profession which is styled an honorable one; that profession so far-famed for its charity and benevolence, whose mission on earth is to do as much good and as little evil as possible to the human family — that profession, in the face of these evils, tolerates in its midst these men, who, with corrupt hearts and blood-stained hands, destroy what they cannot reinstate, corrupt souls, and destroy the fairest fabric that God has ever created, and yet all is done under the aegis, under the cloak, of that profession.[17]

Highly significant also is the harsh manner in which the Association recommended dealing with physician-abortionists:

Every practicing physician in the land (as well as every good man) has a certain amount of interest at stake in this matter. Every physician, as far as his practice extends, should feel that in his professional department he is the shepherd of his flock, and it becomes his duty to see that these wolves in sheep's clothing not make any inroads among them. The members of the profession should form themselves into a special police to watch, and to detect, and bring to justice these characters. They should shrink with horror from all intercourse with them, professionally or otherwise. These men should be marked as Cain was marked; they should be made the outcasts of society.

It is time that the seal of reprobation were placed on these characters by all honest men; it is time that respectable men should cease to consult with them, should cease to speak to them, should cease to notice them except with contempt.[18]

At the end of this remarkably vivid and strongly worded document six equally forceful resolutions directed at the medical, educational, clerical, and legal professions were passed:

> *Resolved*, That we repudiate and denounce the conduct of abortionists, and that we will hold no intercourse with them either professionally or otherwise, and that we will, whenever an opportunity presents, guard and protect the public against the machinations of these characters by pointing out the physical and moral ruin which follows in their wake.

> *Resolved*, That in the opinion of this Convention, it will be unlawful and unprofessional for any physician to induce abortion or premature labor, without the concurrent opinion of at least one respectable consulting physician, and then always with a view to the safety of the child — if that be possible.

> *Resolved*, That we respectfully and earnestly suggest to private teachers and professors in public institutions the propriety of adopting, according to their judgment, the means best suited for preserving their

pupils, and those who may hereafter come under their care, from the degrading crime of abortion.

Resolved, That we respectfully call the attention of the clergy of all denominations to the perverted views of morality entertained by a large class of females — aye, and men also — on this important question, and the ruin which has resulted and continues to result daily to the human family from such views.

Resolved, That we respectfully solicit the different medical societies, both State and local, to send delegates to the clergymen in their respective districts to request their aid in so important an undertaking.

Resolved, That it becomes the duty of every physician in the United States, of fair standing in his profession, to resort to every honorable and legal means in his power to crush out from among us this pest of society; and, in doing so, he but elevates himself and his profession to that eminence and moral standard for which God has designed it, and which an honorable and high-toned public sentiment must expect at the hands of its members.[19]

Of all the many words ever written on the subject of abortion, none have condemned the destruction of unborn children more passionately, frankly, and completely than the AMA reports of 1859 and 1871. Not even the most avid contemporary right-to-life proponents have surpassed the severity with which these denunciations were expressed. The rationale for the use of such blunt language is clearly set forth in the report of 1871:

If in the foregoing report our language has appeared to some strong and severe, or even intemperate, let the gentlemen pause for a moment and reflect on the importance and gravity of our subject, and believe that to do justice to the undertaking, free from all improper feeling or selfish considerations, was the end and aim of our efforts. We had to deal with human life. In a matter of less importance we could entertain no compromise. An honest judge on the bench would call things by their proper names. We could do no less.[20]

By taking an unequivocal stand in defense of the most vulnerable human lives in the strongest possible terms, the AMA solidified the physician's role as a healer par excellence. This served notice that educated assassins of the unborn would no longer be tolerated as a part of legitimate American medical practice. Practically speaking, the resolutions of 1859 and 1871 had a profound impact. The medical profession led the way in getting the permissive abortion laws of the mid 1800s changed to restrictive ones by the late 1800s. In fact, the part played by doctors in getting laws protective of human life at all stages of pregnancy enacted in the states was so significant that historian James C. Mohr dubbed the period 1857-1880 as a veritable "physicians' crusade against abortion."

Mohr compiled a list of the many state and local medical societies that memorialized their state legislatures on the topic of abortion. The anti-abortion activity began in 1857 with statements passed by the Atlanta Medical Society and ended in 1878 with pronouncements of the Medical Society of the State of California. Others involved in anti-abortion action between 1857 and 1878 included medical societies from the states of Indiana, Illinois, Iowa, Maine, Maryland, Massachusetts, Michigan, Missouri, New York, Ohio, Pennsylvania, Vermont, and Virginia.[21]

He also delineates just how successful the anti-abortion efforts of the regular doctors (those with formal medical education and credentials) actually were:

Between 1860 and 1880 the regular physicians' campaign against abortion in the United States produced the most important burst of anti-abortion legislation in the nation's history. At least 40 anti-abortion statutes of various kinds were placed upon state and territorial lawbooks during that period; over 30 in the years from 1866 through 1877 alone. Some 13 jurisdictions formally outlawed abortion for the first time, and at least 21 states revised their already existing statutes on the subject. More significantly, most of the legislation passed between 1860 and 1880 explicitly accepted the regulars' assertions that the interruption of gestation at any point in a pregnancy should be a crime and that the state itself should try actively to restrict the practice of abortion. The anti-abortion policies sustained in the United States through the first two-thirds of the twentieth century had their formal legislative origins, for the most part, in the wave of tough laws passed in the wake of the doctors' crusade and the public response their campaign evoked.[22]

It seems inconceivable that the rich and humanitarian soil of medical progress exemplified by Germany and America could spawn a group of physicians willing to participate in programs of mass annihilation.

At a time when Germany's leading role in medical science had been established for decades, some 300 or more of its practitioners deviated from this tradition on a scale never before thought possible. In just a few short years these doctors of infamy made a mockery of everything German medicine had stood for. They destroyed hundreds of thousands of human beings. They experimented on them before and after destruction. While some of these doctors were sadists and hacks, a great many more were highly skilled physicians with long careers of humane service. A number had established their impeccable reputations long before Hitler had ever been heard from. All the more reason why it is so hard to believe what they ended up doing.

In a parallel fashion, American physicians are showing the same arrogant disregard for a firmly embedded tradition of caring for the most seriously afflicted and defenseless of human lives. In the last quarter of the twentieth century, a period when American medicine had reached a position of world leadership, thousands, not hundreds, of American doctors are destroying millions of unborn children. These unwanted expendables are also being experimented upon before and after destruction. Many of today's leading killers of the unborn are eminent physicians affiliated with prestigious universities and medical centers. Some have even carved out brilliant careers developing advanced techniques for saving the lives of prematurely born children who would otherwise succumb to the hazards of extrauterine existence. All the more reason why it is so difficult to understand their involvement in contemporary destructive activities.

A possible key to comprehending such severe discontinuities with a history of progress and service could be the overemphasis of science at the expense of humanity. Perhaps medical science in Germany advanced to such a high level of development that it quickly became an end in itself by the time Hitler came to power. This may be why German physicians expressed so few qualms about killing and experimenting on concentration camp inmates: as long as they were done in the name of science, it was all right.

Similarly, American medical science and technology have progressed so rapidly and have made so many valuable contributions to humanity that it would be considered almost un-American to offer any criticism or challenge. In an achievement-oriented American society a disproportionately high value is placed on science. Even when it comes to killing or experimenting on the unborn, as long as these activities are carried out in a safe, sanitary, and scientific manner by a credentialed executioner, they are acceptable.

The irrevocable bond between science and humanity that had helped German medicine flourish was perverted at its very core. Science somehow became disconnected from humanity, resulting in an unparalleled era of exterminative medicine. This identical science-without-humanity mentality makes it possible for today's American doctors to end the lives of countless human beings inside the womb with little or no compunction.

CHAPTER 2

The Illegal Killers

The long traditions of scientific and humanitarian medicine in Germany and America would seem to have presented almost foolproof bulwarks against physician involvement in any kind of killing operation, whether the victims be unwanted, defective Germans and Jews or the expendable, deficient unborn or born. At first glance, it appears like all of the killing in Nazi Germany was perpetrated by hoodlums, sadists, or power-hungry maniacs. A closer look, however, reveals that reputable doctors played a far greater role in destruction than is generally acknowledged. A similar conclusion holds for contemporary American society, but even more so. It is still believed by much of the public that most underground killing of the unborn was perpetrated by corrupt, punitive, and nonmedical perverts. Those doctors involved in this horrendous business are commonly perceived to be only a tiny minority of incompetent, money-mad butchers, unrepresentative of the rest of American medicine. Actually, respectable physicians did the bulk of illegal abortions long before the law was changed.

It is time to provide a long overdue historical perspective on the highly significant role of licensed physicians as illegal killers, both in Germany during the period of the Third Reich and in America from the 1930s through the early 1970s. The assumption of this role represents the most radical departure from medical ethics, the laws of both countries, and the laws of humanity.

Nazi Sadists

It is difficult to comprehend the Nazi holocaust in terms other than an unimaginable orgy of unprecedented killing. How else can one begin to explain the destruction of millions of innocent victims in such a short time-span. It is equally difficult to visualize the perpetrators except as sadistic madmen giving unlimited vent to overpowering aggression.

Because what happened in Nazi Germany is so hard to believe, all the more reason for some of the many horrible incidents to be retold. While words are not up to the task of fully conveying the utter brutality with which some human beings treated their fellow humans, they can at least capture some of the horrors. It must be established as fact that they did occur, no matter how unbelievable they seem. To depict them as something less than barbaric would be a great injustice to the truth as well as to those victims who suffered so ago-nizingly.

The SS is the group most frequently credited with com-mitting the worst crimes. Under Heinrich Himmler it grew into a powerful organization of troops fanatically loyal to Hitler and the aims of the Nazi party. SS members played a major role in implementing the final solution to the Jewish question in the death camps and elsewhere. A glimpse into some of their training methods and activities provides a grim reminder of Nazi bestiality.

Although some members of the SS had long-standing his-tories of sadism, others had to go through intense indoctri-nation in order to develop the proper qualities for experi-encing both joy in and emotional detachment from killing. A preparatory step in this direction was the "hardening" process through which SS candidates had to pass. Its purpose was "to let the novices taste the primitive satisfactions ob-tained from regression to infantile-sadistic patterns and to keep the taste alive in the initiated." The beginning of the brutalization course involved a "hardening experiment" toward animals:

The young SS woman who told the story stated that

at one point during her training she and every other member of her group of novices were given a young puppy for a pet. After a few weeks, time enough for each to grow fond of her pet, they were suddenly given an order for each of them to kill her dog with her own knife; those who could not do it were supposed to be dismissed from SS training. They all complied, since none wanted to leave in disgrace. It was on this basis that people ... were quite systematically conditioned to sadistic patterns.[1]

The theory underlying the attainment of this type of mentality is what Dr. Leo Alexander, former psychiatric consultant to the Nuremberg War Crimes Trials, refers to as *thanatolatry*, the "idolatrous delight in death." He provides an explanation of this theory, as a way of better understanding how destruction characterized by delight and detachment is possible:

The re-awakening of this destructive drive in the leaders and followers of Nazism and its symbolic expression, the thanatolatrous concept, made it easier and more desirable for SS men to kill by facilitating a greater and unhampered emotional satisfaction to be derived from the act of killing. Killing also became further removed from reality because of the distortion of reality by the thanatolatrous concept; and conversely, dying likewise became more removed from reality also. At the same time, however, by its removal from reality death also was deprived of its real meaning and cheapened in the process. Thus, the thanatolatrous concept, which started with a perverted exaltation of death, at the same time debased the value of life and thereby deprived death of its tragedy and dignity.[2]

An indication that this perverted level had been reached was when an individual could, as Himmler himself expressed it, "derive strength and joy not only from the act of killing but also from the process of gazing upon heaps of 100, 500, or 1,000 freshly killed corpses with frank enjoyment or with a veneer of rationalization." [3] Another example was the festive atmosphere at Auschwitz surrounding the burning of live prisoners, especially children, in pits on piles of gasoline-soaked wood. Many came to view these ghastly spectacles as if they were attending a picnic, party, or public celebration. They experienced the events with a "peculiar mixture of enjoyment and detachment." According to Leo Alexander:

> The enjoyment in most cases was of an infantile sadistic sort not actually connected with any sexual sadism. In the main these atrocities provided a feast of that irrelevant excitement of which Santayana speaks — of a peculiar impersonal and unreal sort which of course entails complete coldness and pitilessness of which only people without proper ego functions could be capable. [4]

Just how brutal the SS and other Nazi terrorists acted toward their victims can be gleaned from the accounts of concentration camp survivors. Dr. Gisella Pearl lived to tell the terrible truth about the fate of pregnant women at Auschwitz:

> They were surrounded by a group of S.S. men and women, who amused themselves by giving these help-less creatures a taste of hell, after which death was a welcome friend. They were beaten with clubs and whips, torn by dogs, dragged around by their hair and kicked in the stomach with heavy German boots. Then, when they collapsed, they were thrown into the crematory — alive. [5]

The cruelty imposed on children in the death camps defies even the wildest imagination. Pearl provides a stark picture of how children were dealt with upon arrival at Auschwitz.

> The children . . . did not go with their mothers into the gas chambers. They were taken away, crying and screaming, with wild terror in their eyes, to be un-dressed, thrown into the waiting graves, drenched with

some inflammable material and burned alive. Hundreds of thousands of little children ... all died to satisfy the sadistic instincts of these perverts.[6]

Existing literature on concentration camp atrocities mainly focuses on killings carried out by sadistic guards and low-level functionaries. There is evidence, however, that doctors also took part in these brutal killings. The euthanasia institutions and death camps seemed to attract, like an irresistible magnet, the most unscrupulous and demented members of the medical profession. The extermination centers served as sites for them to act out their severe psychological problems and express their sadistic impulses at the expense of defenseless human victims.

Those physicians who subjected concentration camp inmates to painful and death-dealing experiments probably best epitomize the type of crazed individuals involved. Dr. Sigmund Rascher, who was responsible for forcing inmates to undergo agonizing deaths in freezing and high-altitude experiments, was a mediocre, ambitious, and corrupt pseudo-scientist.[7] Another sadistic physician, Dr. Erwin Ding, kept a diary of death caused by murderous experiments in which subjects were infected with typhus.[8] Dr. Herta Oberhauser specialized in cruel post-operative treatment of Polish women whose arms, shoulder blades, or legs had been amputated in the horrendous bone, muscle, and nerve regeneration and bone transplantation experiments conducted at the Ravensbrück concentration camp.[9]

A sampling of experiments carried out by these and other doctors of infamy reveals unbelievable savagery at work. In one mad experiment, hundreds of sick prisoners were laid out in the blazing sun for the purpose of learning "how long it would take a sick person to die under the sun without water." [10] Another sick experiment involved finding out the effect of bad news on women's menstrual flows. The bad news communicated to women inmates during their periods was, "You will be shot in two days." This even resulted in an article being published in a German scientific journal by a professor of histology in Berlin regarding "his observation on hemorrhages provoked in women by such bad news." [11]

Among concentration camp doctors, few could match Auschwitz physician Dr. Josef Mengele for sheer sadism. A favorite pastime of his was to go about selecting victims for the gas chambers while whistling operatic tunes from Puccini or Wagner.[12] When one woman pleaded for her father's life, Dr. Mengele replied, "Your father is seventy years old. Don't you think he has lived long enough?" [13] Mengele's capacity for outright brutality was nowhere more evident than in his violent outburst against a female inmate who tried to escape:

> Dr. Mengele left the head of the column and with a few, easy strides, caught up with her. He grabbed her by the neck and proceeded to beat her head into a bloody pulp. He hit her, slapped her, boxed her, always her head, only her head — screaming at the top of his voice. "You want to escape, don't you ... You can't escape now ... This is no truck, you can't jump ... You are going to croak, you dirty Jew." And he went on hitting the poor, unprotected head. ...
>
> Half an hour later Dr. Mengele returned to the hospital. He took a piece of perfumed soap out of his bag and whistling gaily, with a smile of deep satisfaction on his face, he began to wash his hands.[14]

Mengele also possessed an active interest in pregnancy and childbirth. During delivery he took every correct medical precaution, "watching to see that all aseptic principles were rigorously observed and that the umbilical cord was cut with care. Half an hour later he sent the mother and child to the crematory oven." [15] At other times he issued new orders: Jewish women would no longer be killed because of pregnancy, but their children would still have to die. Inmate doctor Gisella Pearl was somewhat relieved — at least the lives of the mothers would be spared. This, however, was only a temporary reprieve, as Dr. Pearl was soon to find out. "I had two hundred ninety-two expectant mothers in my ward when Dr. Mengele changed his mind. He came roaring into the hospital, whip and revolver in hand, and had all the two hundred and ninety-two women loaded on a single truck and tossed — alive — into the flames of the crematory." [16]

Backstreet Butchers

Long before the Supreme Court of the United States affixed its seal of legal respectability on the destruction of the unborn, illegal abortions were persistently portrayed as constituting an epidemic of law-breaking resulting in the death, maiming, and mutilation of thousands of women. A figure in excess of one million was commonly cited as the number of abortions being performed outside the law each year. In 1933 Dr. Abraham Rongy, a fellow of the American College of Surgeons, reported that almost two million illegal abortions were performed annually in the United States.[17] By 1936, Washington University obstetrics professor Dr. Frederick J. Taussig said he knew of "no other instance in history in which there has been such frank and universal disregard for a criminal law." [18] Researchers Jerome E. Bates and Edward S. Zawadzki became impatient with what they referred to as a futile "acrimonious scholarly debate over the exact annual incidence." In a 1964 sociological study of criminal abortions, they expressed their discontent in the following terms: "One might as well dispute whether 2,000,000 persons were gassed at Auschwitz or perhaps only 1,849,372. Suffice it to say that experts agree the number of illegal abortions performed annually in this country is substantial." [19] Their allusion to Auschwitz is far closer than intended.

The number of maternal deaths due to unlawful, bungled, clandestine abortions was put at five thousand to ten thousand per year. Although this is a highly inflated range, based on projections derived from data collected at a birth control clinic between 1925 and 1929,[20] it was adopted as gospel by many pro-abortion doctors. A brochure put out by the California Committee on Therapeutic Abortions in 1966, entitled "The Truth About Abortion: Must 10,000 Women Die This

Year?" is just one example of the greatly exaggerated figures that were employed.

All this was simply a prelude. The stage was set for placing the burden of responsibility for such a horrendous flouting of the law on the shoulders of the most despicable character in American history and folklore, the backstreet butcher. He is overwhelmingly depicted as a technically incompetent, unsavory, unscrupulous individual who exploits desperate women by subjecting them to dangerous, unsanitary operations for the sake of making a fast buck or giving vent to sadistic or perverted inclinations.

Pro-abortion journalist Lawrence Lader provides a collection of thumbnail portraits highlighting the horrors frequently associated with backalley butchery:

> I was pushed into an underworld I never imagined. I had to crawl through the filth of a system society had forced on me. For weeks I called doctors, nurses, friends — anyone who could offer the slightest clue to an abortionist, and got on my knees to beg for help. Finally I was given a phone number in a Long Island suburb, and made an evening appointment. It was a decrepit, decaying house. An old man opened the door. His shirt was stained. He spoke almost incoherently. Everything about him and his house disgusted me. "You'll stay and rest overnight after the operation," he explained, starting to paw my arm. I knew I couldn't stand it another second. I turned and ran. . . .
>
> It was the last Christmas Eve for Jacqueline Smith, a twenty-year-old fashion designer. . . . Miss Smith had been taken to a cut-rate abortionist — a Brooklyn hospital attendant with no medical training who offered a bargain price of $100. When she died on the operating table on December 24, 1955, the attendant and his helper dismembered her body and disposed of the wrapped pieces in trash cans along Broadway. Both eventually received long prison sentences. . . .
>
> When a Los Angeles girl, sixteen-year-old Brenda B., was brought by her mother to an abortionist, a

real-estate salesman by occupation, the girl died on
the table from almost four times the correct dose of
anesthesia.[21]

One of the case histories included in the study of criminal
abortion by Bates and Zawadzki gives a revealing picture of
the personality of a female abortionist responsible for four
maternal deaths. Of particular note here is the blend of
greed, aggressiveness, and sadism motivating this particular
woman:

> Her dominant traits are her acquisitiveness, which
> amounts to greed, and her almost masculine aggressive-
> ness. It appears that she has allowed few inhibitions to
> impede her conduct or interfere with her desires during
> a long period of her life. She has shown a marked
> determination and ruthlessness in attaining her ob-
> jectives. . . .
> She has a cold, almost sadistic outlook on life and
> has little regard for the patients who were made ill or
> crippled by her forceful ministrations. When asked to
> comment on their predicament, she replied, "They had
> their fun — now let them pay for it." [22]

The definite impression left by these and many other
equally sordid stories was that no ethical physician would
become involved in the unsavory business of clandestine baby-
killing. Those doctors who did were commonly portrayed as
hacks, as the dregs of the medical profession, as mentally
demented individuals unable to succeed in legitimate medical
practice. Several case studies of convicted physician-abortionists compiled by Bates and Zawadzki serve to reinforce this
image. They conclude that "almost without exception, the
physician-abortionist is a deviate in some manner." [23]

The following two cases illustrate the prevalence of alcoholism among doctors performing illegal abortions:

> "Dr. Milligan," as we will call him, reached a
> point when at the age of thirty he had a rather com-

pulsive need to be intoxicated during the greater portion of every day. At times he would drink as much as
two fifths of whiskey daily. His modest but growing
practice began to diminish rapidly. His wife divorced
him and he was forced to remove his practice to a
shabby neighborhood in an interstitial area. Finally,
as he admitted to a probation officer, "I did an abortion
or two a week to keep myself in whiskey." As one
might almost expect, Dr. Milligan was arrested as a
result of a deathbed statement by one of his patients
who suffered a punctured uterus at his somewhat shaky
hands and died of a resultant septic condition. . . .

Several years ago a girl was brought to the medical
examiner's office. Autopsy proved she died as a result
of a particularly brutal abortion. The physician had
tried to empty the pregnant uterus with a curette. He
was so drunk that he could not find the cervical os and
perforated the vagina entering the peritoneal cavity
and tearing loops of bowel with the curette. His practical nurse was so sickened that she, along with the
girl's boy friend, volunteered testimony against him.
Alcohol had so robbed this man of his skills that he
degenerated to the practice of criminal abortion and
even this he could not perform with any greater skill
than the most ignorant midwife.[24]

Greed, sadism, perversion, and alcoholism are the dominant themes in another case history of a physician-abortionist
cited by Bates and Zawadzki:

The defendant, George Braunstein, had been an
abortionist for twenty-five years and had operated a
mill from which he derived a lucrative income. . . .
The County Physician . . . states that Braunstein apparently has recently attempted to stimulate his failing
sexual powers by indulging in practices involving cun-
nilingus and mutual masturbation. One of the complaining witnesses, Susan Cohen, was aborted "for
half-price" ($200) as she allowed him to spank her

lightly and thereafter, at his direction, walked back and forth in a pair of old shoes he kept in his desk. . . . Another woman, Frieda Wojtulewicz, declared that as Braunstein approached her with a curette, he paused and drank a half glass of whiskey, stating that he "needed it to steady his hands." The sadistic tendencies of the defendant are obvious.

In view of his advanced age, the steadily growing danger he presents to society, his lifelong history of medical malpractice involving at least two homicides, and his almost compulsive need to continue in illegal practice which now involves the satisfaction of neurotic needs with sadistic overtones, it is recommended that Braunstein be confined in a closed, controlled institution where society may be protected.[25]

All these factors — the figure of one million or more illegal abortions per year, the horror stories of underworld abortions, and the range of five thousand to ten thousand maternal deaths annually as a result — coalesced to present a grim picture for public and professional consumption. The image projected was unmistakably clear: huge numbers of women were being exploited, injured, butchered, and killed by unscrupulous, sadistic, and dangerous psychopaths. The purportedly few doctors implicated were portrayed as representing the scum of the medical profession — inept, perverted, and money-hungry hacks.

The Respectable Medical Executioners of Nazi Germany

The perpetration of unimaginable acts of brutality by mad fiends, sadistic guards, and a few outcasts from the medical profession is a believable portrait. But it is far from the whole story. Another facet, often overshadowed by the abundance of horrifying incidents, is the destruction of many more lives not by maniacs but by ordinary, perfectly sane, and even idealistic individuals. Raul Hilberg, in his definitive study on the destruction of European Jewry, indicated the broad scope of citizen involvement in the holocaust: "The machinery of destruction was a remarkable cross-section of the German population. Every profession, every skill, and every social status was represented in it." [26]

The inhumanity of ordinary people is a difficult reality to grasp. It seems much more logical to blame horrendous atrocities on hoodlums or madmen than on normal individuals. This is precisely the reasoning behind the prosecution attempts to depict Adolf Eichmann as a sadistic monster during his trial in 1963 in Jerusalem. It is as if "the monstrous deeds carried out by Eichmann required a brutal, twisted, and sadistic personality, evil incarnate." [27]

What came out of the trial regarding Eichmann's personality was quite different than expected. What emerged was not a devil with horns but an average, somewhat colorless technician who did his duty in a meticulous, efficient, and rational manner — the task being the dispatching of millions to their deaths. On the basis of psychiatric examinations, Eichmann was declared normal. One psychiatrist described him as "more normal, at any rate, than I am after having examined him." Another psychiatrist found that "his whole psychological outlook, his attitude toward his wife and children, mother and father, brothers, sisters, and friends, was 'not only normal but most desirable.' " Furthermore, Eichmann's case was not one of "insane hatred of Jews, of fanatical anti-Semitism or indoctrination of any kind. He 'personally' never had anything whatever against Jews; on the contrary, he had plenty of private reasons for not being a Jew-hater." [28]

Thus, the disturbing truth of the holocaust was laid bare for all the world to see: far more destruction was perpetrated at the hands of dispassionate civil servants like Eichmann than by half-crazed concentration camp guards. Never has evil been so clearly divested of its revulsion and reduced to such an utterly banal and commonplace phenomenon!

The same kind of conclusion holds for those doctors involved in the massive destructive activities. Although such sadistic individuals as Drs. Rascher, Ding, and Mengele are generally believed to be the dominant types of physicians in the Nazi program of extermination, this is actually not so. Most physicians who planned and carried out the killing were not perverted butchers, but psychologically normal and highly skilled doctors in good professional standing. The inclusion of highly trained medical scientists and practitioners in the holocaust gave it a level of expertise and credibility it would not have otherwise possessed.

One of the first indications that doctors had been heavily involved in destruction came during the Nuremberg War Crimes Trials, when twenty physicians, many of whom were prominent members of the medical profession in Germany, were tried and most were convicted of war crimes and crimes against humanity. The types of physicians responsible and the precise roles they played were clearly delineated in the opening statement of the prosecution on the 9th of December 1946:

> The defendants in the dock are charged with murder, but this is no mere murder trial.... These defendants did not kill in hot blood, nor for personal enrichment.... Most of them are trained physicians and some of them are distinguished scientists. Yet these defendants, all of whom were fully able to comprehend the nature of their acts, and most of whom were exceptionally qualified to form a moral and professional judgment in this respect, are responsible for wholesale murder and unspeakably cruel tortures....
>
> The 20 physicians in the dock range from leaders of German scientific medicine, with excellent international reputations, down to the dregs of the German medical profession. All of them have in common a callous lack of consideration and human regard for, and an unprincipled willingness to abuse their power over the poor, unfortunate, defenseless creatures who had been deprived of their rights by a ruthless and criminal government. All of them violated the Hippocratic commandments which they had solemnly sworn to uphold and abide by, including the funda-

mental principle never to do harm — "primum non nocere."

Outstanding men of science, distinguished for their scientific ability in Germany and abroad, are the defendants Rostock and Rose. Both exemplify, in their training and practice alike, the highest traditions of German medicine. Rostock headed the Department of Surgery at the University of Berlin and served as dean of its medical school. Rose studied under the famous surgeon, Enderlen, at Heidelberg and then became a distinguished specialist in the fields of public health and tropical diseases. Handloser and Schroeder are outstanding medical administrators. Both of them made their careers in military medicine and reached the peak of their profession. Five more defendants are much younger men who are nevertheless already known as the possessors of considerable scientific ability or capacity in medical administration. These include the defendants Karl Brandt, Ruff, Beiglboeck, Schaefer, and Becker-Freyseng.

A number of the others such as Romberg and Fischer are well trained, and several of them attained high professional position. . . .

This case is one of the simplest and clearest of those that will be tried in this building. It is also one of the most important. It is true that the defendants in the box were not among the highest leaders of the Third Reich. They are not the war lords who assembled and drove the German military machine, nor the industrial barons who made the parts, nor the Nazi politicians who debased and brutalized the minds of the German people. But this case, perhaps more than any other we will try, epitomizes Nazi thought and the Nazi way of life, because these defendants pursue the savage premises of Nazi thought so far. The things that these defendants did, like so many other things that happened under the Third Reich, were the result of the noxious merger of German militarism and the Nazi racial objectives. We will see the results of this merger in many other fields of German life; we see it here in the field of medicine. . . .

Guilt for the oppressions and crimes of the Third Reich is widespread, but it is the guilt of the leaders that is deepest and most culpable. Who could German medicine look to to keep the profession true to its traditions and protect it from the ravaging inroads of Nazi pseudo-science? This was the supreme responsibility of the leaders of German medicine — men like Rostock and Rose and Schroeder and Handloser. That is why their guilt is greater than that of any of the other defendants in the dock. They are the men who utterly failed their country and their profession, who showed neither courage nor wisdom nor the vestiges of moral character.[29]

It cannot be emphasized enough that these doctors were not bloodthirsty hacks who killed, maimed, or experimented on their victims because of sadism or inability to contain violent impulses. They killed for scientific, pseudo-scientific or ideological purposes. They went about their tasks of destruction not in an impulsive, enraged fashion but in a highly rational, systematic manner.

The highly significant role of reputable doctors in the overall destruction process was also very evident in the euthanasia program. By the late 1930s, doctors were holding conferences for the purpose of implementing the destruction of German defectives. In attendance at these meetings were several eminent professors from the leading German medical schools. Before Hitler inaugurated the final solution to the Jewish question in 1941, doctors had already become the most experienced killers in Germany. From 1939 until 1945 physicians were almost exclusively responsible for putting to death around 275,000 German adults and children in mental hospitals and euthanasia institutions.[30]

Psychiatrist Dr. Fredric Wertham's research reveals startling details and conclusions about the massive scope of euthanasia in Nazi Germany and the prominence of those doctors who participated:

The mass killing of mental patients was a large project. It was organized as well as any modern community psychiatric project, and better than most. It began with a careful preparatory and planning stage. Then came the detailed working out of methods, the formation of agencies for transporting patients, their registration and similar tasks (there were three main agencies with impressive bureaucratic names), the installing of crematory furnaces at the psychiatric institutions, and finally the action. It all went like clockwork, the clock being the hourglass of death. The organization comprised a whole chain of mental hospitals and institutions, university professors of psychiatry, and directors and staff members of mental hospitals. Psychiatrists completely reversed their historical role and passed death sentences. It became a matter of routine. . . .

In July, 1939 . . . a conference took place in Berlin in which the program to kill mental patients in the whole of Germany was outlined in concrete, final form. Present and ready to participate were the regular professors of psychiatry and chairmen of the departments of psychiatry of the leading universities and medical schools of Germany: Berlin, Heidelberg, Bonn, Würzburg. . . . At a conference in Dresden in March 1940, Professor de Crinis, of Berlin University, talked over the program with the chief psychiatrists of large public mental hospitals (state hospitals). The classification of mental disorders on which devoted physicians in all countries had worked for centuries was reduced to a simple formula: patients "not worthy to live" and patients "worthy to be helped." There was no opposition on the part of the physicians, every one of whom held a responsible position in the state-hospital system. Questions of ethics or the juridical aspects were not even mentioned. The only questions raised by the participants at the conference were how the project could be carried through most "practically and cheaply." . . .

For several years during the time of the program,

psychiatrists held meetings every three months in Heidelberg under the chairmanship of the professor of psychiatry at the University of Heidelberg. At these conferences the ways to conduct the extermination action were studied, and suitable measures were suggested to assure its efficacy.[31]

The caliber of doctors responsible for planning and implementing euthanasia was on a level with many of those eminent physicians involved in the murderous experiments carried out in the concentration camps. Wertham furnishes profiles of their contributions to science, scholarship, and humanity before embarking on careers heavily devoted to extermination:

> The backbone of the whole project was the experts. It was their decision which sealed the fate of every victim. Who were these men? That is the most remarkable part of the story — and the most important one for the future of violence and, I believe, of mankind. They were not nonentities or outsiders. Most of them had all the hallmarks of civic and scientific respectability. They were not Nazi puppets, but had made their careers and reputations as psychiatrists long before Hitler came to power. Among them were more than twelve full professors at universities. Most of their names read like a roster of prominent psychiatrists. They have made valuable contributions to scientific psychiatry. They are still quoted in international psychiatric literature. . . .
>
> One of the most distinguished (and most unexpected) members of the team of experts which was the heart of the whole killing operation was Werner Villinger, who at the time was professor of psychiatry at the University of Breslau. Prior to that he was head of the department of child psychiatry at Tuebingen and psychiatric director at Bethel, a world-famous institution for epileptics and mentally and physically disabled persons. . . . He wrote especially on

the psychological and social difficulties of children and youths, on child guidance, group therapy, juvenile delinquency, and similar subjects.

His name alone, quite apart from his activity in it, gave a great boost to the "euthanasia" project. For his name suggested to others, especially younger psychiatrists, that there could be nothing wrong with the "action." It is difficult to understand how a man with concern for youths could not only consent to but actively participate in projects of killing them.

To find Dr. Carl Schneider as a leading member of a wholesale murder project is also unexpected. For twelve years he was professor of psychiatry at the University of Heidelberg. As such he held the same important position as Emil Kraepelin a generation ago. And Kraepelin was the founder of modern clinical psychiatry. . . . He studied epilepsy . . . and his research on that subject is still quoted. He wrote two books on schizophrenia. The first, *The Psychology of Schizophrenia*, is considered a landmark of this type of clinical study.

Carl Schneider was very active in all phases of the program. He served as expert for the processing of death questionnaires, participated in the frequent conferences, and regularly instructed younger psychiatrists in the methods and procedures of the project. Perhaps the most extraordinary part of this story is that before going to Heidelberg, he, like Werner Villinger, had held the highly respected position of chief physician at the universally recognized institution Bethel. Ten years later, when he was professor at Heidelberg, he appeared with an SS commission at Bethel, went over the questionnaires, ordered the personnel to present patients to him, and personally selected the candidates for extermination. When, after the defeat of the Nazi regime, Dr. Schneider was to be put on trial, he committed suicide. . . .

Perhaps the greatest break with the humane traditions of psychiatry is connected with the name of Dr.

Werner Heyde. Heyde was professor of psychiatry at the University of Würzburg and director of the psychiatric clinic there. Few places in the world can look back on such a long history of successful care of mental patients. . . . in the same place where mental patients were treated most humanely in 1583, they were doomed to be killed in 1940. . . .

Dr. Heyde's reputation as a scientific psychiatrist was excellent. He worked for several years in the clinic, became director of the out-patient department, and began his teaching there in 1932. . . .

Heyde was a key figure in the program. When carbon monoxide was suggested as a method for killing, this proposal had to be submitted first to him for evaluation. He approved the method and directed the idea into the proper administrative channels for its practical realization. . . . He played the leading role in the preparatory and organizing conferences . . . helped in working out the questionnaires, functioned as chief expert, and selected the younger psychiatrists for the program and instructed them in their task.

From the beginning, he personally inspected the death institutions and the installation of the gas chambers, to make sure that everything functioned expeditiously. . . .

His trial at Limburg was delayed for four years for preliminary investigation. . . . When he was left unguarded in his cell five days before the trial was due to start, he committed suicide.[32]

It is hard to imagine a group of executioners with more impressive backgrounds and impeccable credentials!

The speed and efficiency with which doctors administered euthanasia did not go unnoticed by Hitler when he was confronted with resolving the Jewish question. The euthanasia program stood as a highly successful model of destruction worthy of emulation for the more formidable task of racial genocide.[33] Although doctors' involvement in racial genocide was not as total as in euthanasia, their participation looms as being much more important than generally admitted. Actually, euthanasia served as a precursor for the massive destruction unleashed on the Jews, and physicians played the crucial pivotal role linking both programs. Doctors first tested out the gas chambers and crematoriums on German patients in psychiatric hospitals before they were used on Jews and others in concentration camps. Physicians also selected death candidates in psychiatric institutions, a function that they repeated in a number of concentration camps.

Like the physician-induced concentration camp experiments and killings, the physician-led euthanasia program constituted a blatant violation of medical ethics, the laws of Germany, and the laws of humanity. Because eminent doctors were so totally involved in euthanasia, they tried to give the impression that their destructive activities were sanctioned by law. The few doctors brought to trial for euthanasia killings said they were simply obeying a law signed by Hitler ordering them to grant a mercy death to mentally and incurably ill patients. At the Hadamar trial in 1945, Alfons Klein, director of the Hadamar euthanasia institution, justified the killing of several hundred allegedly tubercular Russian and Polish patients on the basis that "these sick people were covered by the same law as covered the German mentally diseased." [34]

What was the so-called law that Klein and other defendants so often referred to? Actually it was not a law at all. It was simply a cautiously worded note written on Hitler's private stationery, dated October 1939, and predated September 1, 1939, granting authority for the mercy killing of the incurably ill. Its exact contents are as follows:

> Reichsleiter Bouhler and Dr. Brandt, M.D., are charged with the responsibility of enlarging the authority of certain physicians to be designated by name in such a manner that persons who, according to human judgment, are incurable can, upon a most careful diagnosis of their condition of sickness, be accorded a mercy death.
>
> [Signed] A. Hitler [35]

As can be seen from this note, there is no mention of mentally ill patients or those with tuberculosis. Despite the pretense of legality, there was no duly enacted law allowing doctors to put so many individuals to death under the guise of mercy. This would also be true even if the substance of Hitler's note had been enacted into law, which it was not. Wertham's comments on this are especially pertinent:

> The note does not give the order to kill, but the *power* to kill. That is something very different. The physicians made use of this power extensively, ruthlessly, cruelly. The note is not a command but an assignment of authority and responsibility to a particular group of persons, namely, physicians, psychiatrists, and pediatricians. This assignment, far from ordering it, did not even give psychiatrists official permission to do what they did on a grand scale, *i.e.*, kill all kinds of people who were not at all incurable or even mentally ill, making no attempt even to examine them first.[36]

The rampant lawlessness of the entire euthanasia operation was its most common characteristic. Doctors did not need a law or an order, they became a law unto themselves. Again, as so pungently pointed out by Wertham:

> The tragedy is that the psychiatrists did not have to have an order. They acted on their own. They were not carrying out a death sentence pronounced by somebody else. They were the legislators who laid down the rules for deciding who was to die; they were the administrators who worked out the procedures, provided the patients and places, and decided the methods of killing; they pronounced a sentence of life or death in every individual case; they were the executioners who carried the sentences out or — without being coerced to do so — surrendered their patients to be killed in other institutions; they supervised and often watched the slow deaths.
>
> The evidence is very clear on this. The psychiatrists

did not have to work in these hospitals; they did so voluntarily, were able to resign if they wished, and could refuse to do special tasks. For example, the psychiatrist Dr. F. Hoelzel was asked by the psychiatric director of the mental institution Eglfing-Haar to head a children's division in which many handicapped and disturbed children were killed (right up to 1945). He refused in a pathetic letter saying that his "temperament was not suited to this task," that he was "too soft." [37]

The Respectable Medical Executioners of America

Although most of the public and a large segment of the medical profession have been led to believe that thousands of women were being butchered to death each year in the United States by greedy and sadistic non-medical perpetrators, the truth of the matter is just the opposite. Most illegal abortions performed in the first two-thirds of the twentieth century resulted in few maternal deaths because a large majority of them were done not by incompetent butchers but by highly skilled physicians of excellent professional standing. All along the backstreet butchers were in fact credentialed medical executioners. These are astounding revelations that the medical profession as a whole and the public have not yet come to grips with.

Contrary to popular belief, such sadistic and inept individuals as Drs. Milligan and Braunstein are not the kinds of physicians who dominated the illicit abortion scene. An overwhelming majority of doctors who blatantly violated the law by exterminating the unborn were frequently normal, technically competent, prominent members of the medical profession. In this sense they are not that much different from those eminent German doctors responsible for the illegal destruction of human lives in the euthanasia hospitals and concentration camps of the Third Reich. The heavy involvement of reputable American doctors in the lawless holocaust perpetrated against human beings before birth endowed the killing with an incomparable aura of respectability. This, more than anything else, paved the way for public approval.

One of the first public indications that the bulk of illegal abortions was performed by credentialed physician-executioners came during the early 1930s. By the mid 1950s, into the 1960s, and up to the 1970s this fact began to be increasingly acknowledged.

In 1933, Dr. Abraham J. Rongy estimated that there were "thousands of medical practitioners and many more thousands of nurses and assistants" involved in performing abortions in violation of the law.[38] He described the physician as "the chief agent of abortion," as the one who "flouts the law and enables the community to continue its disregard of the dictates of religion." [39] Several years later Dr. Frederick J. Taussig characterized criminal abortion statutes as the most universally disregarded laws in history. And who were the main American violators? "To put it more crudely," admitted Taussig, "we are the official 'boot-leggers' of abortion." [40]

At a conference on abortion problems sponsored by the National Committee on Maternal Health that took place in New York City on June 19 and 20, 1942, Dr. Howard C. Taylor, Jr. revealed that "although the performing of abortions has been forbidden to physicians since the time of Hippocrates, nevertheless the abortionist is drawn principally from the ranks of this profession." [41]

A study conducted by the Alfred C. Kinsey Institute in 1958 found that physicians accounted for between 84 and 87 percent of all illegal abortions. Many were described as "reputable physicians, in good standing in their local medical associations, who performed abortions on their wives, other relatives, friends, or other patients out of sympathy." As doctors were doing most of the abortions, it is not surprising that the Kinsey group was "impressed with their technical ability and the low number of deaths and ill effects resulting from their operations." One of the physician-abortionists they interviewed claimed that he had performed "thirty thousand abortions without a single death in the course of his medical practice." [42]

In 1960, Dr. Mary S. Calderone, then medical director of

the Planned Parenthood Federation of America, presented an identical portrayal of how heavily illegal abortions were dominated by respectable physicians:

> 90 percent of all illegal abortions are presently being done by physicians. Call them what you will, abortionists or anything else, they are still physicians, trained as such; and many of them are in good standing in their communities. They must do a pretty good job if the death rate is as low as it is. . . . Another corollary fact: physicians of impeccable standing are referring their patients for these illegal abortions to the colleagues whom they know are willing to perform them.[43]

A survey of 180 obstetricians in North Carolina regarding their attitudes toward the permissive North Carolina Abortion Act of 1967 clearly demonstrates how blatantly physicians took the law into their own hands long before the legalization process set in. A large majority acknowledged that the new law had little effect on the performance of abortions "other than to legalize long-established practices." This theme was repeated by many respondents. As one obstetrician put it, "Most obstetrician-gynecologists consider this law to have simply legalized something that we had been doing for many years." Another portrayed it as "not affecting my practice at all. It only legalizes what I have been doing all the time." The authors of this study conclude that the law helped doctors feel more secure since "what they were doing as a matter of course for years has now been sanctified by the legislature."[44]

In October 1970, psychiatrist Jerome M. Kummer summed up the whole matter of physician involvement in illegal abortion thusly: "While few physicians are believed to be engaged in the performance of illegal abortions, it has been shown that most illegal abortions have been performed by physicians, many physicians refer patients to illegal abortionists indirectly and some directly, even in writing."[45]

Widespread flouting of abortion laws by physicians was not confined to the front or back rooms of doctors' offices;

they also took place inside the walls of prestigious hospitals and medical centers under the guise of so-called therapeutic abortions.

Dr. Alan Guttmacher reported that 85 percent of the abortion operations done at Mount Sinai Hospital in New York from 1952 to 1956 "at least *bent* the law, if they did not fracture it." [46] In an article appropriately titled, "The Law That Doctors Often Break," which appeared in the August 1959 issue of *Redbook*, Guttmacher gave a fuller account of how physicians went about fracturing the law:

> The law of New York permits abortion only to preserve the life of the mother. In the six years 1953-1958 my own obstetrical service at Mount Sinai Hospital performed 147 therapeutic abortions. Let us examine them to see whether or not we actually preserved the lives of 147 women.
>
> Thirty-nine per cent of these abortions were performed for psychiatric reasons. Most of these patients had, it is true, threatened suicide, but it is known that pregnant women threatening suicide rarely carry out their threats. . . .
>
> Thirty-one per cent of the abortions were performed for eugenic reasons, to forestall the birth of children likely to be born with severe abnormalities. No mother's life is threatened by such a birth, so no mother's life in this group could have been saved by abortion.
>
> By the strictest interpretation of the law, then, more than 90 per cent of these 147 abortions were illegal.[47]

Another breach in the law occurred at Johns Hopkins Hospital. From 1964 to 1968 doctors there had been performing abortions not in compliance with the abortion law then in effect. Instead of breaking the law, the process was referred to as "gradually liberalizing the indications for abortion under the former Maryland law." [48]

Unlawful baby-killing in the womb induced by physicians

was not an atypical phenomenon concentrated in only a few illustrious hospitals. Findings released by the Committee on Human Reproduction to the House of Delegates of the AMA in June 1967 indicated this was a widespread practice in many hospitals throughout the United States:

> Today, with modern prenatal, obstetrical, and post-partum care, it is an unusual pregnancy which cannot safely be carried to term. Yet, each year in the United States approximately 10,000 pregnancies are terminated by licensed physicians in accredited hospitals with the knowledge and concurrence of consulting colleagues. Few of these are necessary to save the mother's life. American medicine is therefore confronted with a situation whereby conscientious practitioners performing therapeutic abortions for reasons other than those posing a direct threat to the life of the mother are acting contrary to existing laws.[49]

One of the first in-depth portraits of the respectable medical executioners of the unborn in defiance of the law came at the conference on abortion sponsored by the Planned Parenthood Federation of America and the New York Academy of Medicine at Arden House in 1955. Dr. G. Loutrell Timanus, an abortionist since the late 1920s, was introduced to the conference participants in glowing terms by Dr. Alan Guttmacher:

> Our next speaker, Dr. Timanus, has been very gracious in coming here to give us a frank exposition of the work as it was carried on by, in my estimation, an extremely competent abortionist.
> Dr. Timanus has been known to me for almost three decades, and I value his friendship.
> He was graduated from the University of Maryland Medical School around 1915, and had a residency in nose and throat work. Then because of his interest in youth, he became Assistant Director and chief physician for the Public Athletic League of the State of Maryland.

For reasons which, perhaps, are not germane to our discussion, Dr. Timanus drifted into the task of carrying out abortions, which most of us feel were illegal abortions. This was done very skillfully by him during a period of some twenty years or more in the City of Baltimore, and he has always had a genuine social interest in the problem. He kept records of practically all the cases he served, and has given great thought to the whole problem of abortion and to his role in it.

Dr. Timanus some years ago fell into disagreement with the law, and is no longer in practice, but is retired.[50]

Here was a man personally responsible for taking over five thousand unborn lives. He had intentionally violated the most fundamental and ancient ethic of the physician — do no harm — an ethic unequivocally supported by the American Medical Association's policy statements of 1859 and 1871 condemning abortion as the "unwarrantable destruction of human life." [51] On at least five thousand different occasions he also broke the law that allowed abortion only when the mother's life was at stake. Despite such a horrendous record of death and destruction, he was treated like visiting royalty, like some venerable sage willing to at last impart the wisdom of the ages to his eager disciples. One can hardly conjure up a more ludicrous tragicomedy. Dr. Timanus and his rapt audience, however, were deadly serious.

Many things divulged by Timanus about his abortion experiences reflect themes repeated over and over again by almost every respected physician who has ever committed mayhem on the unborn. For one thing, he began by denying that his abortion participation was motivated by financial considerations: "Mr. Chairman, I *am* retired, but I would like it understood that my financial requirements for this were not met through the performance of abortions, but through fortunate purchase of some Florida real estate." [52]

Also highlighted was a full discussion of Timanus' techniques of abortion. Apparently, his equipment and technical skills were formidable: just two maternal deaths out of 5,210 abortions performed. Regarding these, he was quick to point out, "Whether these two deaths were attributable to my negligence or whether they were incidental, I would find it hard to say." [53] Timanus claimed that none of his patients suffered any physical complications either. He believed this all indicated an admirable safety record, particularly because it was achieved at a time when antibiotics were not in general use. [54]

In order to endow his particular "specialty" with further respectability, Timanus emphasized that his patients came to him on referral from 353 prominent physicians in Maryland, the District of Columbia, and adjacent locales. Moreover, he enjoyed a unique position as the abortionist for needy individuals closely associated with the medical profession. At least 10 percent of his caseload included woman physicians, medical students, nurses, and wives, relatives, or sexual partners of doctors. [55]

Dr. Timanus' referral sources, if nothing else, illustrate how fully implicated many members of the medical profession had become in abortions long before the legalization process set in. Even those doctors who refused to kill unborn children themselves were not adverse to sending them elsewhere to be destroyed. One is reminded of a similar situation in the psychiatric institutions of the Third Reich. Many physicians tried to minimize their responsibility for euthanasia by stating that they never killed a single patient. They showed no reluctance, nevertheless, to send patients to institutions where they were exterminated by other doctors. As Wertham so aptly put it, "That is participating in murder too." [56]

Another physician-abortionist, Dr. Robert D. Spencer, was eulogized in the February 17, 1969 issue of *Newsweek* under the caption, "King of the Abortionists," one week after his death at the age of 79. [57] This title seemed particularly apropos, since in a career spanning some forty years Dr. Spencer claimed credit for performing more than thirty thousand abortions with only one maternal death. Next to this record, Dr. Timanus is a mere pretender to the throne.

Newsweek also attempted to single out Spencer as many

cuts above most underground abortionists: "Certainly Spencer was an antiseptic contrast to the typical criminal — often not an M.D. at all — who practices furtively in dingy walk-ups and sleazy hotel rooms, and charges as much as $1,500 for his hastily performed and often botched services." [58]

This portrait is considerably distorted. Spencer is not really a contrast to the run-of-the-mill criminal abortionists, but a highly typical representative of the credentialed breed of antiseptic scientific killers who dominated the illegal abortion scene for decades.

Like many other criminal abortionists with medical degrees, Dr. Spencer is portrayed by the media as a kind of devout, freethinking folk hero, a courageous rebel who battled against an antiquated law to bring one more vital medical service to the women of a small mining town. Pro-abortion writer Lawrence Lader is an even more ardent defender and glorifier of Spencer's accomplishments. His descriptions of Spencer are particularly noteworthy: the leading family doctor in town, noted for his philosophic and humanitarian motives, a legend in his state, one of the most popular members of the Rotary Club, an individual characterized by a frugal and modest style of life ("His home, a simple seven-room frame house, indistinguishable from dozens of others, on an unimpressive street" and "neither his home furnishings nor his clothes indicate great wealth. His one luxury is a Cadillac, with which he and his wife indulge their hobby of travel"), and a man loved by his patients ("His files are filled with letters of appreciation, one Catholic calling him 'one of the most beautiful humans that ever lived.' ").[59]

Of special interest is Lader's account of Spencer as a radical philosopher:

> Both his home library and his office study, hidden away on the floor above his operating room, are crammed with books on economics, political science, and population problems. His desk holds a statue of Thomas Paine. His walls are crowded with pictures ranging from Lincoln and Franklin (under whose

great-great-grandson he studied) to Joseph Lewis, president of the Free Thinkers of America.[60]

Dr. Spencer emerges as larger than life, a man before his time, a rare mixture combining the common sense of Tom Paine, the sagacity and wit of Ben Franklin, and the foresight, courage, and homespun ways of Abe Lincoln.

What unadulterated praise is showered on the illegal physician-abortionists, Timanus and Spencer, in these mini biographies! How radically different they are from the 1871 AMA document condemning physician-abortionists as "men who cling to a noble profession only to dishonor it. . . . men who seek not to save but to destroy. . . . false brethren, modern Herods, educated assassins. . . . an unprincipled, an insidious, an unmitigated foe. . . . a disgusting caudal appendage attached to the medical profession." [61]

Rarely have such contradictory portraits ever been so clearly drawn!

Although Dr. Alan Guttmacher could not claim credit for personally extinguishing the lives of as many unborn children as Drs. Timanus and Spencer, he did pioneer therapeutic abortion committees in the 1950s as a major device for death selection. He even admitted that 90 percent of the abortions approved by the committee he headed were illegal. At that time he mentioned what a frustrating problem therapeutic abortion presented for "the doctor with liberal, humanitarian instincts." [62]

In another sense, Dr. Guttmacher's influence in the destruction of the unborn was far more pervasive than that of either Drs. Timanus or Spencer, due to the fact that he operated in the most elite circles of organized medicine. Like many of the euthanasia experts of Nazi Germany, Guttmacher was no ordinary everyday family practitioner. During his entire career he was affiliated with the most prestigious universities and medical schools in America. He received his M.D. from Johns Hopkins University Medical School and became a professor there. He also served as chief of obstetrics at the Sinai Hospital in Baltimore, director of the department of obstetrics and gynecology, Mount Sinai Hospital, New York, clinical professor of obstetrics and gynecology at Columbia University, and a special lecturer in maternal and child health at Harvard University. Dr. Guttmacher also wrote extensively on the subjects of pregnancy, birth control, and abortion. His numerous writings appeared in books, medical journals, and popular magazines. In addition, as president of the Planned Parenthood Federation of America, Guttmacher had another vehicle with which to espouse unborn baby killing as a private matter between physician and mother, despite what the law said.

Guttmacher's long and vigorous career, devoted to repealing the abortion laws, influenced generations of younger doctors to take up this cause. If a man of Dr. Guttmacher's prestige and stature did not think abortion was wrong, it stands to reason that other doctors of equal or lesser repute could not help but be swayed to the same belief. This is not unlike the situation in Nazi Germany, where young doctors had few qualms about becoming involved in euthanasia because so many of the leaders were eminent physicians affiliated with prestigious universities.

Soon after his death in 1974 at the age of 75, Guttmacher was lavishly praised in the *New England Journal of Medicine* for his "tremendous energy and unswerving devotion" to abortion as being a matter "solely for the woman and her physician to decide, and completely removed from legislative restrictions." Because Dr. Guttmacher "lived to see most of his beliefs accepted by society," the author of this eulogy fittingly titled it "Alan Guttmacher, M.D.— A Life Fulfilled." [63] Tragically, the fulfillment of Dr. Guttmacher's life and the lives of other credentialed executioners has meant the destruction of the lives of untold millions of unborn children.

Among psychiatrists, one of the most prominent and persistent defenders of abortion has been Dr. Harold Rosen, a professor of psychiatry at the Johns Hopkins University School of Medicine. Rosen not only has an M.D. but also a Ph.D. in philology from the University of Pennsylvania. He has authored a number of important scientific papers, especially in the field of hypnosis. In 1951 and 1952, Dr. Rosen and a group of eminent psychiatrists, obstetricians, gynecologists, and representatives of allied disciplines played an important role in helping to advance the campaign against laws protective of human life before birth through a series of papers and discussions. These were published in 1954 by the Julian Press, under the title *Therapeutic Abortion: Medical, Psychiatric, Legal, Anthropological and Religious Considerations*, with Dr. Rosen as editor. The popularity and influence of this book is attested to by the fact that it was reissued by the Beacon Press in 1967 under a new title, *Abortion in America.*

Another prominent psychiatrist, Dr. John F. McDermott, professor and chairman of the department of psychiatry at the University of Hawaii, reflects the type of schizophrenic thinking prevalent among so many prestigious modern-day psychiatrists when it comes to the subject of killing unborn children. In the *American Journal of Psychiatry* of November 1973, McDermott emphasized the importance of the concept of *child advocacy*, "the idea that every child is *entitled* to the basic care and assistance he needs for optimum growth and development" and the "recognition by society that the developmental needs of its children are of such importance that they must be ensured as rights to be promoted and protected by societal structures." [64] These are excellent principles, reflecting humanitarian psychiatry at its best.

Several years before, however, Dr. McDermott, together with Dr. Walter F. Char, was called into Hawaiian hospitals to help nurses psychologically disturbed by their abortion work. Through the ventilation of feelings in group sessions the nurses were enabled to redefine "the role, philosophy, and ethics of nursing and medicine" in order to incorporate abortion as a valid medical procedure. [65] Apparently, Dr. McDermott had no qualms about aiding the nurses to continue their involvement in such destructive procedures.

Where is his concept of child advocacy in this situation? Does not the child in the womb also need care and assistance for optimum growth and development? Are not the needs of unborn children also of such crucial importance that they too "must be ensured as rights to be promoted and protected by societal structures"? As a minimal starting point, should not their lives also be protected by law?

The United Nations thinks so, and even goes much further. In the Preamble to the Declaration of the Rights of the Child, proclaimed by the General Assembly of the United Nations on November 20, 1959, it states that "the child, by reason of his physical and mental immaturity, needs special safeguards and care, including appropriate legal protection, before as well as after birth." Furthermore, the fourth principle of this declaration specifies that "special care and protection shall be provided to [the child] and to his mother, including adequate prenatal and post-natal care." [66]

Next to these principles, Dr. McDermott's ideas of child advocacy are severely constricted and elitist notions not intended to cover unwanted children before birth, currently the most vulnerable and endangered members of the human community. This kind of blindly inconsistent and schizophrenic mode of thought, deplorably, is not just a malady afflicting eminent physicians of the Third Reich.

Thus, long before respected doctors were given the legal power to destroy unborn lives for non-medical reasons, they had already become well-established as the most experienced killers of the unborn in America. Like the Nazi physicians, American doctors did not need a law in order to kill; they took the law into their own hands, they became a law unto themselves. It is not the Nazi sadists or backstreet butchers that the expendables of Nazi Germany and contemporary America have had to fear the most. Far more destruction has been accomplished at the hands of credentialed medical executioners. The holocaust in both countries did not really get rolling until reputable, technically proficient killers from organized medicine set the pace.

CHAPTER 3

Medical Agitation for Legal
Destruction

The next step, and the one that really propelled the killing to the status of a monumental holocaust, was for doctors to propagandize for legalizing their acts of unlawful destruction.

German physicians played a significant role in agitating for legalized destruction of human lives long before the legal machinery of Nazi Germany stripped away the laws that had previously provided protection for many vulnerable segments of German society. The propaganda groundwork for euthanasia was laid in the latter half of the nineteenth century, grew with increased ferocity during the 1920s, and continued unabated into the late 1930s and early 1940s. It was also during the 1920s and early 1930s that many physicians were busy mounting an intensified campaign directed toward legalizing the killing of unborn human lives for medicosocial and eugenic reasons. Publications and meetings provided channels for the dissemination of destructive propaganda to both the medical profession and the public. Several polls reveal how fully wedded to legal destruction an alarming proportion of medical opinion had already become before the Nazi government embarked on its massive program of extermination under the guise of bureaucracy and law.

The US Supreme Court's devastating blow dealt to laws protective of unborn human life did not result from an impulsive, overnight revolution, but was the culmination of a

prolonged evolutionary process of medical killing and agitation for legalization of destruction. Many American physicians were killing unborn babies in defiance of the law and
simultaneously building a legal case for their destructive activities long before legalization actually took hold. Evidence
of this propaganda can be found in medical publications and
meetings from as far back as the early 1930s. Polls taken of
physicians' attitudes toward abortion in the 1960s and early
1970s indicate the dramatic inroads the agitation for the
killing of the unborn has made among a large segment of the
American medical community. An identical historical pattern
of pushing for the legal sanctification of what is being done
in violation of the law also characterizes the contemporary
medical effort to legalize euthanasia for increasing numbers
of victims.

An excerpt from a speech of Abraham Lincoln to the US
Congress in 1862 — "The dogmas of the quiet past are inadequate to the stormy present. . . . As our case is new, so
must we think anew and act anew" — is not the kind of insight one would expect to be put at the service of propagandizing for legalization of killing. Yet these very words were
cited to support both Nazi and American medical attacks
against laws protective of human life. During the Doctors'
Trial at Nuremberg in 1946, this quotation from Lincoln
formed part of the rationale employed by the defense to
justify the horrendous experiments conducted on concentration camp inmates by German physicians.[1] Dr. Nicholson
J. Eastman, in a speech presented at the University of North
Carolina in 1966, also resorted to this same quotation from
Lincoln after praising abortion as a "practical utilitarian approach" for resolving the "countless social problems met by
obstetricians."[2] It was used by Dr. Robert B. Benjamin, too,
in the March 1969 issue of *Minnesota Medicine*, as an introduction to an article calling for repeal of "Minnesota's
antiquated abortion law" of 1886.[3]

What a blatant abuse of historical wisdom! Lincoln's remarks were intended to challenge the slavery laws so destructive of human life and dignity. Some doctors have distorted
them for the opposite purpose: to tear down laws protective

of human life. Those bent on destruction can hardly be expected to exercise scruples in their use of historical citations.

The Lincoln quote serves as a prelude to the many ways in which German and American doctors have utilized publications, meetings, and opinion polls to push for the legal killing of the deformed, inferior, defective, and unwanted.

Documents for Destruction

1. German Publications

The impetus for legal killing of those considered unfit did not suddenly emerge with the ascendance of Hitler and National Socialism to power in 1933. The pernicious ideas that led to the destruction of millions predated Hitler by many decades. They were not the product of the uneducated masses, but originated with the educated elite.

The scientific roots underlying the rise of Nazi racist thought can be traced back to Dr. Ernst Haeckel, a physician who also became one of the most famous biologists of nineteenth-century Germany. Haeckel received his medical degree in 1858, after having studied at Würzburg and Berlin. He spent a brief time in medical practice, pursued graduate studies in zoology, and then accepted a position at the University of Jena, where he pursued a distinguished career of university teaching and research.

In addition to his strictly scientific activities, Haeckel turned out to be an ardent supporter of such racist-infected ideas as the inequality of the races, the relative value of human life, the Aryan concept of racial supremacy, the survival of the fittest, and radical eugenics. Through his numerous books and other writings, he infused national racism with considerable scientific authority and academic respectability.[4]

One of Haeckel's most persistent themes was advocacy of artificial selection as a means of facilitating survival of the biologically fit. In the first volume of *The History of Creation*, published in 1876, and an English translation of the eighth German edition published in 1892, he expressed unbounded admiration for the manner in which the ancient Spartans practiced artificial biological selection to insure the survival of their fittest members:

> All newly-born children were subject to a careful examination and selection. All those that were weak, sickly, or affected with any bodily infirmity, were killed. Only the perfectly healthy and strong children were allowed to live, and they alone afterwards propagated the race. By this means, the Spartan race was not only continually preserved in excellent strength and vigour, but the perfection of their bodies increased with every generation. No doubt the Spartans owed their rare degree of masculine strength and rough heroic valour (for which they are eminent in ancient history) in a great measure to this artificial selection.[5]

In *The Wonders of Life* (1904), Haeckel used the example of the Spartans as a rationale for discrediting laws against infanticide: "The destruction of abnormal newborn infants — as the Spartans practised it, for instance, in selecting the bravest — cannot rationally be classified as 'murder,' as is done in even modern legal works." [6]

Haeckel also reduced "the widespread belief that man is bound under all circumstances to maintain and prolong life, even when it has become utterly useless" to the insignificant status of a traditional dogma. He was especially unhappy because of the "hundreds of thousands of incurables — lunatics, lepers, people with cancer, etc.," who were being "artificially kept alive . . . without the slightest profit to themselves or the general body." His prescription for dealing with them consisted of elimination by "a dose of some painless and rapid poison." [7] He favored leaving this "act of kindness" or "redemption from evil" in the hands of "a commission of competent and conscientious medical men." [8]

In addition to the chronically ill and deformed, Dr. Haeckel agitated for disposing of those he referred to as "incorrigible and degraded criminals" through retention of laws permitting capital punishment. His rationale, as stated in *The History of Creation*, was a predominantly eugenic one:

> And yet capital punishment... is not only just, but also a benefit to the better portion of mankind. The same benefit is accomplished by destroying luxuriant weeds, for the prosperity of a well-cultivated garden.
>
> In the same way as by a careful rooting out of weeds, light, air, and ground is gained for good and useful plants, in like manner, by the indiscriminate destruction of all incorrigible criminals, not only would the struggle for life among the better portion of mankind be made easier, but also an advantageous artificial process of selection would be set in practice, since the possibility of transmitting their injurious qualities by inheritance would be taken from those degenerate outcasts.[9]

Haeckel's writings had an enormous impact on the educated sector of society, particularly doctors and scientists. Dr. Wilhelm Schallmayer, a leading German eugenicist, subscribed to the theory that the cultural and social superstructure of a nation was primarily determined not by social and economic forces but by the germ plasm of its members. He too favored biological selection as a means of preventing the "biological decay" of German civilization.[10] Another follower of Haeckel's, Dr. Heinrich Ziegler, conjured up ominous images of "a veritable army of the feeble-minded who committed most of the crimes"[11] as fuel for propaganda aimed at eliminating the unfit.

Another important outlet for transmission of Haeckel's racist and eugenic ideology was the Monist League, formed in 1906. The Monists, an organization of intellectual elites devoted to spreading the tenets of Social Darwinism, believed in literally refashioning Germany according to the laws of biological evolution. Taking their lead from Haeckel, they called for elimination of diseased members of society. Largely through numerous books and pamphlets, they decried the fact that civilization was becoming too humane and, like Haeckel, argued against efforts to keep the weak and sick alive through artificial means: "Our humanitarianism one sidedly considers the well-being and complaints of unfortunate individuals who are alive at present and is extremely indifferent or blind to the suffering which they inflict by their complacency on the next or on later generations." The Monists also favored denying care to the weak and crippled over the practice of "always increasing healing and nursing asylums for the spiritually and mentally ill, homes for cripples, etc." [12]

In *The Riddle of the Universe* (1899), Haeckel expended considerable energy attacking Christianity and its sanctity-of-life ethic. He blamed the Christian doctrines of equality, submission, and weakness for inverting the natural hierarchy of the world and leading the German people to the brink of biological collapse. He accused the Catholic Church of being opposed to everything modern and characterized the history of the papacy as "an unscrupulous tissue of lying and deceit, a reckless pursuit of absolute mental despotism and secular power," and portrayed the great majority of popes as "pitiful imposters, many of them utterly worthless and vicious." [13]

Besides the ventilation of considerable personal hatred, Haeckel's unrestrained campaign of vilification against Christianity served a much broader and more important purpose: it was far easier to legitimize placing a relative value on human life if it could be demonstrated that the laws protective of all human lives, especially the most useless, were simply the product of an unnatural, oppressive, and superstition-laden religion led by the rankest imposters. Thus, the more Christianity could be maligned, the greater the possibility of justifying the establishment of a social structure that permitted elimination of the unfit according to natural and contrived laws of biological hegemony.

This pernicious propaganda was transmitted to a vast audience; *The Riddle of the Universe* sold more than a hundred thousand copies in its first year of publication. By 1919 it had gone through ten editions, and by 1933 almost half a million copies had been bought in Germany alone. [14] The atrocities of the Third Reich attest to the ultimate impact of this and other horrendous diatribes churned out by Haeckel and his disciples.

The campaign of propaganda supporting legalized destruction of the weak and unfit received a further boost in 1920 with the publication of a highly influential book, *The Release of the Destruction of Life Devoid of Value*.[15] The authors were Karl Binding, professor of jurisprudence at the University of Leipzig, and Dr. Alfred Hoche, professor of psychiatry and director of the psychiatric clinic at Freiburg. The book's major thrust consisted of persistent appeals for changing the laws in Germany to allow the killing of persons considered "devoid of value."

Early in the book, mention is made of how enlightened the ancient Romans were for not punishing the killing of persons who gave their consent to be killed. Compared to this, the German law of the 1900s was "backward," because it failed to make a distinction between the "destruction of life worth living or not worth living." The authors then made a strong plea to enshrine such a distinction into law, on the assumption that the terminally ill or mortally injured do not need "the full protection of law," and the desire for their destruction "should legally find much more consideration than the desire for destruction of a strong healthy life." [16]

Carrying forward a theme developed previously by Dr. Haeckel and his followers, Binding posed his most urgent question, "Is there any human life that has to such a degree lost its legal rights, that its continuation is of no value for itself or to society?" Answering in the affirmative, he declared:

> Realizing that there is indeed human life whose continuation is of no interest to any reasonably thinking person, then it is up to the legislature to ask this fateful question: "Is it our duty to continually defend this unsocial life by giving it full protection of the law or is it our duty to release it for euthanasia?" You could also pose this question from a legal point of view: Shall we prefer to see the continued support for this kind of life as an example of the sacredness of

life or shall we consider the legalization of the mercy killing, so relieving for all those involved, as the smaller evil.

If we use sound reasoning, there is no doubt about the answer to this question.[17]

Dr. Hoche focused on the status of the mentally dead — those who have "no clear conception, feeling or will power. They cannot conceive a word picture of what is going on in life. They have no sensitivity to the environment." Other qualities of the mentally dead were also highlighted: "a parasite . . . on modern society; the absence of any productivity; a condition of complete helplessness." "One of these days," said Hoche, "maybe we will come to the conclusion that elimination of the mentally dead is no crime, nor an immoral act, and no unfeeling cruelty, but a permissible and necessary act." His portrayal of destruction as non-invasive to their rights is the height of medical arrogance: "Because the condition of the mentally dead person prevents him from making a demand for life, if you take away his life you are not invading any of his rights." [18]

In the interim, Hoche saw his task as countering "the modern effort to keep alive all kinds of weaklings and to care for all of those who are perhaps not mentally retarded, but are still a large burden." Like Dr. Haeckel, he blamed Christianity for the deplorable attempts "to preserve life without dignity by all means." From the vantage point of "a higher state morality," Hoche reached an opposing view: "We doctors know that in the interest of the whole human organism, single, less valuable members have to be abandoned and pushed out." [19]

Again the question was posed, this time by Dr. Hoche, "Is there any human life which has lost so many human characteristics the continuation of the life for the person as well as society has lost all its value?"

Hoche acknowledged that "a long time of rethinking and readjustment" plus a change in the "general opinion of society" would be necessary "in order to answer this question correctly." He identified the current state of affairs as one in which "the support of every existence — no matter how worth-less — has become the highest moral norm." Nevertheless, he predicted that "a new time will come when we no longer in the name of higher morality will carry out this demand that has its origin in an exaggerated idea of humanity." [20] His role was to fulfill this prediction, and this he did with tenacity.

Like the writings of Dr. Haeckel, and others before them, Binding and Hoche's small book made a significant contribu-tion to the ideological foundations of the Third Reich. Some of the doctors tried for crimes against humanity at Nurem-berg even based part of their defense on *The Release of the Destruction of Life Devoid of Value* and the ideas contained therein.[21]

By the early 1930s, articles and books authored by physi-cians and scientists advocating extermination of the unfit ap-peared with increasing regularity. At first, the main thrust of the propaganda was on getting rid of the weak and in-ferior through so-called programs of prevention — com-pulsory sterilization and abortion. This soon gave way to heightened agitation for outright extermination of those already born.

Hans Löhr, in an article entitled "The Physician Must Come to Terms with the Irrational," published in 1935, speci-fied that the physician's "holy obligation" to the state meant "not merely to induce patients with congenital diseases to un-dergo voluntary sterilization but also to report such cases to the authorities." This Löhr saw as being mandated by the racial and eugenics sterilization law of 1934, which he characterized as "a pillar of the National Socialist state." [22]

Destruction in the name of racial hygiene also encom-passed abortion of the defective. In 1934, the Hamburg Eugenics Court approved of abortions in cases where "either parent has been legally declared to present hereditary and transmissible defects." The eugenic rationale for this decision was unmistakably clear: "For the sake of the continued ex-istence and health of the German people, an unborn child that is likely to present hereditary and transmissible defects may be destroyed." [23] According to the *Journal of the Amer-*

ican Medical Association's Berlin correspondent, "these questions are now being eagerly discussed in the special medical journals bearing on these problems." [24]

From the mid 1930s on, agitation for euthanasia began to appear more frequently in the writings of medical doctors. In 1935 the anti-Christian, racist foundation for killing was advanced by public health director Dr. Arthur Guest, in his book, *The Structure of Public Health in the Third Reich:*

> The ill-conceived "love of thy neighbor" has to disappear, especially in relation to inferior or asocial creatures. It is the supreme duty of a national state to grant life and livelihood only to the healthy and hereditarily sound portion of the people in order to secure the maintenance of a hereditarily sound and racially pure folk for all eternity. The life of an individual has meaning only in the light of that ultimate aim, that is, in the light of his meaning to his family and to his national state. [25]

Dr. Leo Alexander, American medical-science consultant to the Nuremberg War Crimes Trials, pointed out that by 1936 "extermination of the physically or socially unfit was so openly accepted that its practice was mentioned incidentally in an article published in an official German medical journal." [26] The specific article highlighted the importance of keeping the morale of patients in public tuberculosis sanitariums up as they were being sent to concentration camps. [27]

A book, *Mission and Conscience* (1936), written by Berlin ophthalmologist Dr. Helmut Unger, paved the way for further acceptance of euthanasia. Its subject was mercy killing; a doctor puts an end to his wife's suffering at her request. The principal justification given was salvation from incurable suffering. [28] This message received wider circulation in 1941, when a movie based on the book was produced. In the film version, *I Accuse*, the doctor kills his wife "to the accompaniment of soft piano music rendered by a sympathetic colleague in an adjoining room." [29]

Propaganda for legal destruction of the inferior and those

deemed worthless continued at an intensified pace before and during the euthanasia program that officially began in the fall of 1939. Particularly notable here were the writings of Dr. H. W. Kranz, professor of eugenics at Giessen University and regional leader of the Office for Racial Politics. His main ideas were set forth in the April 1940 issue of *NS Volksdienst*, in an article entitled "The Problem Posed by the People who are Incapable of Social Interaction in the Upgrading Process of Our Nation." Kranz called for the "weeding-out" of one million psychopaths and numerous "clans of asocials," who stood in the way of the "most enormous upgrading process which, so far, a nation has ever begun on this earth." [30]

The implementation of his proposals by physicians, nurses, and attendants was already well under way in the psychiatric and euthanasia institutions of the Third Reich.

2. American Publications

One of the earliest American medical attempts to discredit the laws protective of unborn human life was launched by Dr. Abraham J. Rongy in a book entitled *Abortion: Legal or Illegal?*, published by Vanguard Press in 1933. This must rate as one of the most unabashedly pro-abortion tracts ever written. In a highly distorted historical overview of abortion laws, Rongy's main goal was to depict them as just one more illustration of the individual's behavior being dictated by "religion and mystical taboos." [31] His attack was a two-pronged one: the linking of abortion laws with Christianity, and the equation of Christianity with superstition. Viewed from this perspective, the power of abortion statutes to induce compliance is rendered impotent because they are reduced to nothing more than the irrational product of centuries-old superstitions.

Of more than passing interest is the reason Dr. Rongy gave to account for "the extreme antagonism of Christian civilization to the practice of abortion." Foremost was the almost obsessive desire of a minority and militant religion interested in increasing its ranks with "man and woman power to wage the battle of the Lord." Then Rongy proceeded to highlight one of his favorite themes: the Church as a kind of hostile military force intent on an unlimited expansion of power. "The Church almost from its earliest days," he said, "was a militant organization; and militancy needs large hordes from which it can draw its fighting strength." [32]

Dr. Rongy's diatribes were not just confined to Christianity in general or Roman Catholicism in particular. Pope Pius IX became the target for much of his ire. It seems that the pope committed the unpardonable offense of issuing an encyclical, *On Christian Marriage* (1931), that in one part strongly condemned abortion. Needless to say, this did not set too well with Dr. Rongy. He lost no time in unleashing a barrage of ridicule against both the contents of the encyclical and the pope. In what is possibly meant to be a burst of poetic vigor, one section of the papal statement is called "the platitudes of a brief and pious papal paragraph." An outpouring of pedestrian verse continued to be the chosen vehicle for lampooning the pontiff's pronouncements: "The theological cloud is thick with its taboos and imprecations — and its utter remoteness from contact with the realistic implications of childbearing and child-rearing. The religious imagination ... contents itself by conjuring up a Heavenly court with fiats and regulations and penalities." [33] What Dr. Rongy was really getting at was a portrayal of legal restrictions on abortion as a prime example of the state in "the role of errand boy for the papal instructions." [34]

After linking abortion laws with a papal plot to impose one brand of sectarian morality on the rest of society, Rongy moved on to another major theme: impugning the integrity of legal restraints on abortion because of their widespread violation by upstanding physicians. His emphasis was not on questioning the ethics of doctors who broke the law, but on questioning the ethics of the law itself. Why? Simply because it was not in accord with the abortion practices of so many reputable doctors, who, Rongy estimated, numbered in the thousands. His portrayal of the doctor who "conspires against the law and who helps a woman escape from the visitation of an unwelcome pregnancy" is that of a "sort of benign Robin Hood who defies the law to help the needy." [35]

Few readers possess the stamina required to wade through the many pages of religious bigotry parading under the guise of enlightened analysis according to "the ideals of liberalism," so fervently proclaimed by Dr. Rongy. On the final page of the book he had the gall to describe his effort as "an examination of the facts." Immediately after this absurd statement, he could not resist delivering what was intended to be a final, lethal blow that would free abortion laws from the shackles of religious domination: "once the subject has been stripped of the supernatural taboos with which it has been surrounded, the way will be indicated for dealing with it rationally in accordance with the needs of an intelligent and a happier society." [36]

Not since the writings of Germany's Dr. Ernst Haeckel in the late nineteenth and early twentieth centuries has there been such a ferocious assault against Christianity for the purpose of legalizing destruction.

In 1936 a comprehensive volume on abortion, *Abortion Spontaneous and Induced*, authored by Dr. Frederick J. Taussig, was published. It was an ambitious endeavor, full of facts and data on almost every facet of abortion, including medical and technical information as well as material on historical, anthropological, economic, theological, ethical, and legal aspects. Also included were chapters on legal abortion in Russia and recommendations for control of abortion, backed up by a summary of abortion statutes in every state of the union, plus an extensive bibliography. [37]

The book's purpose, according to Taussig, was "to give without bias or exaggeration all the essential information on this subject that is at present available." Information for the sake of information is not the only thing Taussig was after; he had bigger things in mind: "It is my hope therefore that by presenting the subject from its wider medical and social aspects this monograph may prove of some value in stimulating thought and furnishing data that may serve as a basis for a program of revision." [38]

For a book whose stated purpose is an objective and comprehensive presentation of facts and information, an inordinate amount of space is devoted to attacking anti-abortion laws. What Taussig did was employ the respectable auspices of university scholarship as a base from which to launch a persistent campaign of vilification against laws restricting the practice of abortion.

The assault began early. In the very first chapter, Dr. Taussig refers to "the ridiculous and contradictory laws at present on our statute books." Further on, he levels another broadside: "Our present laws are certainly antiquated.... Let us first of all clear our law books of those mid-Victorian regulations." References are also made to the "unjust, unenforceable laws" and the "ridiculous, ofttimes incomprehensible, and harsh statutes on our books." [39]

The only alternatives left for the ethical doctor, according to Taussig, are to either break these harsh, unjust laws, or get them changed. He justified both approaches in the same breath: "Thus by common consent we have become lawbreakers, until a slow-moving world will make the law conform to us instead of having us conform to the law." [40] His strategy of first discrediting the existing abortion laws and then urging that they either be changed or done away with established a model that was persistently followed by many advocates of permissive abortion.

The number of publications containing physician-led attacks on the laws protective of human life in the womb and recommendations that they be liberalized or repealed has proliferated since the mid-1930s. How frequently the pages of illustrious medical journals and books have served as forums for intensified propaganda in support of legal killing at the hands of respectable physicians! How often pro-abortion doctors have been able to have their views disseminated through the printed word! How infrequently one finds any medical opinions in the published literature in defense of unborn human life!

From the early 1960s on, prestigious medical journals became major vehicles for much of the campaign against anti-abortion statutes.

Psychiatrist Dr. Jerome M. Kummer's pro-abortion views

have been granted a more than generous airing by a number of medical journals. In a 1961 issue of *California Medicine,* Kummer discussed the need for "modification of the present unenforceable laws." [41] In the December 1969 issue of *Obstetrics and Gynecology,* he pointed to the "updated therapeutic abortion laws" passed in California and two other states since 1967 as evidence of things "advancing at a geometric progressive rate" toward "imminent complete legalization of abortion." He closed with a strong plea for "leaving the decision to abort, as with any other medical procedure, up to the woman and her physician." [42] A similar theme is found in the *Journal of Reproductive Medicine* of October 1970. After declaring "that existing restrictions or prohibitions on abortion have become meaningless and unrealistic" and admitting that the liberal interpretation of abortion laws by psychiatrists "can virtually accommodate any and every woman wishing to terminate her pregnancy," Kummer again concluded with the same old refrain: "The decision to abort, as with any other medical procedure, should be left to the woman and her physician." [43]

In a 1965 issue of the *Western Reserve Law Review,* Dr. Harold Rosen blamed abortion laws for keeping women at the level of chattel. "Mature legal consideration of mother, family, children, and society," according to Rosen, "would lead legislatures not to pass more liberalized abortion laws but to abolish such laws altogether." His prescription for change was to grant women "the right to decide whether or not they wish to carry a specific pregnancy to term" because of their status "as mature human beings with all the respect and dignity to be accorded mature human beings." [44] According to Rosen's scale of values, immature human beings before birth count for nothing; they exist at a level even lower than that of chattel.

Dr. Robert E. Hall of the department of obstetrics and gynecology at Columbia University used the *American Journal of Public Health* of March 1971 as an outlet for advocating a noteworthy brand of coercion: "Hospitals should be forced, by law if necessary, to assume full responsibility for the performance of every abortion in this country." This is a peculiar stance, indeed, for a physician with such impeccably liberal credentials. According to Hall's calculations, if only ten thousand out of the more than twenty thousand obstetricians in the United States performed "an average of two abortions a week," more than one million abortions a year could "easily be handled on a semiambulatory basis." This could be accomplished by persuading the hospitals "to open their doors and the doctors to open their hearts." [45]

The abortion-on-demand mentality of psychiatrist Dr. Natalie Shainess is found in many publications. One of her favorite pastimes is to demolish abortion laws by depicting them as devices to keep "women in sexual bondage to men."

A form of this appeared in the *New York State Journal of Medicine* of December 1, 1968, where restrictive abortion laws were blamed on the inability of men "to empathize with or to understand the feelings of a woman under these circumstances." Dr. Shainess followed this up by urging that "an unwelcome pregnancy" be considered a valid justification for abortion.[46] The May 1970 issue of *Psychology Today* gave her another chance to reduce abortion to a power struggle between oblivious men, and women kept in a state of servitude: "Men have borne up well while forcing women to bear down in unwelcome labor and to bow down in lifetime subservience to the unwanted fruits of sex." On this occasion she also recommended the repeal of all abortion laws as being "the only decent answer to the problem," on the faulty premise that abortion laws "were adopted to protect women at a time when abortion meant almost certain death." [47] This statement reflects a woeful lack of acquaintance with historical facts. The reason for the passage of abortion laws in the nineteenth century was to protect the unborn child from the onslaughts of physician and non-physician abortionists alike.

Dr. Shainess' antipathy toward men because of their alleged motivation to dominate women through the imposition of strict abortion laws received a much fuller airing on July 1, 1972, in the *New York State Journal of Medicine*. She began by proclaiming her indignation "at the uncaring, casual, insensitive way that men have legislated women's reproductive lives." She then portrayed men as being "deaf and perhaps also blind to the complex issues involved in unwelcome pregnancy for women," and complained about how men have "espoused the playboy philosophy" while denying abortion to the woman.[48]

Dr. Shainess is again way off the mark. Those who espouse the playboy philosophy are overwhelmingly in favor of abortion. One need only glance at the editorials in *Playboy* magazine to know that. Furthermore, hard core pro-abortion groups such as the National Association for the Repeal of Abortion Laws have received financial grants from the Playboy Foundation headed by Hugh Hefner.[49]

Shainess also managed to include the pope's decisions on abortion as a prime example of male dominance and female subservience. She even claimed to have the lowdown on the pope's motives: "The subterranean reasons for the Pope's decisions are based on power... the power in numbers."[50] Shainess then tried to discredit abortion laws on the basis of their presumed religious sectarian affiliation by resurrecting an old stereotype employed by Dr. Haeckel in the late nineteenth and early twentieth centuries, Dr. Rongy in 1933, and many others ever since: "Catholics and Orthodox Jews are entitled to their theologic position but have no right, in my opinion, to legislate that view against the best interests of society."[51]

At the very core of Dr. Shainess's 1972 article is an incredible re-interpretation of the Declaration of Independence. "The right to life, liberty and the pursuit of happiness," she asserted, is possible only when the woman is granted another inalienable right: the right to abort her unborn child.[52] The irreconcilable contradiction between the right to life and the right to destroy life seems to have escaped Dr. Shainess altogether.

The Group for the Advancement of Psychiatry, an organization of prominent psychiatrists dedicated to studying the application of psychiatric knowledge to the fields of mental health and human relations, brought the full brunt of their prestige behind the movement to totally repeal all abortion laws with the 1969 publication of a book entitled, *The Right to Abortion: A Psychiatric View*. In a typical display of pro-abortion rhetoric, they characterized the abortion laws as standing "foursquare" against the women's right "to control her own reproductive life" because they denied a woman "the right to rectify error through the process of abortion." Laws enacted on behalf of the unborn were also portrayed as if they required all women "to carry the fetus to term and as a consequence in many instances to serve a lifetime sentence."[53]

This group of illustrious psychiatrists concluded their assaults against legal protection of human life before birth with a recommendation for outright repeal of all abortion laws, followed by an astounding statement equating abortion rights with marital rights: "We recommend that abortion, when performed by a licensed physician, be entirely removed from the domain of criminal law. We believe that a woman should have the right to abort or not, just as she has the right to marry or not."[54]

Dr. Zigmond Lebensohn, chairman of the committee responsible for this destructive pronouncement, did not end his literary career here. In a 1972 issue of the *American Journal of Psychiatry*, he stressed the "grave psychological consequences" created by the "forced arrival of an unwanted, unloved child" because of "cruel, archaic abortion laws." Dr. Lebensohn called upon physicians to take the lead in making it possible "for women, regardless of socioeconomic status, to terminate unwanted pregnancies with medical safety, dignity, and privacy — and without public stigma."[55]

Comprehensive Psychiatry (March/April 1973) furnished another opportunity for Lebensohn to blame the "forced arrival" of unwanted children on "cruel, archaic abortion laws, and antiquated medical practices." From here it was just a short step toward reiterating a time-worn but persistently employed proposal: "All special and punitive laws governing abortion should be repealed. Abortion would then become a matter between the woman and her physician just as it is in any medical procedure."[56]

One of the most influential statements in favor of legalizing the destruction of the unborn on demand was published in the April 1, 1972 issue of the *American Journal of Obstetrics and Gynecology*. It was signed by one hundred professors

of obstetrics and chairmen of the obstetrics-gynecology departments of the leading medical schools in America. Their names,
professorial ranks, and prestigious university affiliations are
prominently displayed at the end of the statement.[57]

The esteemed professors opened their campaign against
legal restraints on killing the unborn with what was supposed
to reflect an accurate assessment of the relationship between
abortion practices and the law:

> In view of the impending change in abortion prac-
> tices generated by new state legislation and federal
> court decisions, we, the undersigned professors and
> chairmen of the obstetric-gynecologic services, believe
> that it will be helpful to the medical profession at
> large to enunciate our position with regard to this in-
> creasingly liberal course of events.[58]

This is a serious misstatement of the facts. Abortion practices did not follow new state legislation and federal court
decisions; they led the way. If it hadn't been for the massive,
illegal killing of the unborn perpetrated by so many notable
physicians, the permissive abortion laws would never have
been enacted in the first place. As previously indicated, it was
doctors who were largely responsible for violating the law or
molding it to conform to their destructive activities, rather
than the other way around.

Why, then, did this distinguished array of medical professors persist in perpetuating such a myth? Why didn't they
just come forward and admit that they wanted the law
changed, in order to sanction what they had already been
doing in violation of the law for many years? There was a risk
in being too blunt. An identification of physicians as one of the
most active law-violating groups in society might not set too
well with a public nurtured on the proposition that doctors
are endowed with close to God-like qualities. The pedestal
could not be shaken too severely. It would be far more tactful
for physicians to present themselves as concerned professionals in the forefront of obeying enlightened directives emanating from prestigious legal and judicial auspices.

This is precisely the route they decided to pursue. Their strategy was clearly evident from the outset:

> In order to comply with the new laws and court decisions, however, it will be necessary for physicians to realize that abortion has become a predominantly social as well as medical responsibility. For the first time, except perhaps for cosmetic surgery, doctors will be expected to do an operation simply because the patient asks that it be done. Granted, this changes the physician's traditional role, but it will be necessary to make this change if we are to serve the new society in which we live.[59]

The doctor's traditional role was indeed altered, and radically so, to encompass extermination of the most unwanted and vulnerable of human lives! Dr. Herbert Ratner's comments on the concept of exterminative medicine inherent in this abortion statement are right on target:

> The notion of a fourth end of medicine, exterminative medicine, in which the physician serves as killer is as monstrous as expecting the learned profession of law to serve injustice, or of the ministry to serve vice and sin, and to promote hell as well as heaven.[60]

Further along, the medical professors make what seems to be a broadminded concession to doctors who refuse to perform abortions: "The doctor with conscientious objections must, of course, be excused, but he will be expected to refer his patients elsewhere."[61] How generous of them to tolerate the existence of dissent within the ranks! A careful scrutiny reveals that their generosity is more apparent than real. By and large, physicians who object to doing abortions take this position because they recognize abortion for what it is: the destruction of an innocent human being. Those holding such convictions can hardly be expected to comply with a policy which says in effect that they must send potential victims to doctors who are willing to kill them. Besides making them accessories in a system of mass medical extermination, it would also constitute a serious breach of their consciences. Yet this is the very thing they are expected to do, according to the dictates fashioned by the illustrious professors of medicine.

The remainder of the statement is given over to repeated expressions of confidence that American obstetricians, with the help of "careful planning, conscientious effort, and modern techniques," are capable of handling an anticipated "load" of one million abortions per year.[62]

At the time this statement was released for professional consumption in 1972, permissive abortion had not yet been incorporated into the legal fabric of most states. In fact, after a flurry of successful assaults against the abortion statutes of several states in the latter 1960s and early in 1970, the momentum had begun to swing in the opposite direction. A growing number of state legislatures began to resist the pro-abortion onslaught and refused to change their abortion laws. In an unprecedented move, both houses of the 1972 New York State Assembly even voted to overturn the permissive abortion law enacted in 1970.

There was still time left to stem the tide of physician-led agitation for legal destruction of unborn children and to insist that the only appropriate role for a doctor in a civilized society is to protect and heal human lives. Unfortunately, this stellar aggregate of obstetrics professors lacked the moral courage and leadership required to withstand the insidious barrage of physician-initiated pro-abortion propaganda. Rather than oppose a trend that reduced the physician to the unconscionable status of technical executioner, they took the path of least resistance with a disastrous capitulation to the tyranny of technology and the ideology of the anti-life forces within the medical profession.

Propaganda for legalized killing is not directed against the unborn alone. Now that their destruction has become a legal reality, the spotlight has shifted with increasing intensity towards the defective newborn. The physician-abortionist pattern of agitating for what was already being done illegally is also being duplicated by contemporary advocates of euthanasia.

In a 1973 edition of *Prism*, a magazine published by the American Medical Association, Nobel laureate Dr. James D. Watson expressed displeasure with a situation where medicine has been able to "keep sick people alive longer," thereby producing "more people living wretched lives." He acknowledged some uncertainty as to "how you get society to change on such a basic issue; infanticide isn't regarded lightly by anyone." Watson was particularly concerned about the limitations of prenatal diagnostic techniques for detecting abnormalities in children during pregnancy: "Most birth defects are not discovered until birth." [63]

He did, however, have a remedy in mind: "If a child were not declared alive until three days after birth, then . . . the doctor could allow the child to die if the parents so choose and save a lot of misery and suffering." Dr. Watson does not see his approach as one of several alternatives either, but as "the only rational, compassionate attitude to have." This, of course, would necessitate changing the law to accord with what Watson refers to as a re-evaluation of "our basic assumptions about the meaning of life." [64]

Dr. Watson's suggestions have long since moved beyond the realm of theory. A number of doctors, sometimes on their own and sometimes in collaboration with parents and other staff members, decide to withhold treatment from defective, deformed, or retarded infants, thereby resulting in their deaths. Many of these practices are clearly in violation of the law, but still they persist, and increase with each passing year. The Johns Hopkins Hospital case, in which a mongoloid baby was allowed to starve to death over a fifteen-day period in one of the most prestigious medical centers in America, is only one of the many instances of what is being done. [65]

Another much-publicized example of medical involvement in the destruction of defective infants together with justification for legalization was revealed in an article written by Drs. Raymond S. Duff and A. G. M. Campbell in the *New England Journal of Medicine* of October 25, 1973. During a thirty-month period, forty-three impaired infants at the Yale

University intensive-care nursery were denied vital life-sustaining treatment because "parents and physicians in a group decision concluded that prognosis for meaningful life was extremely poor or hopeless." [66] Duff and Campbell recommended permitting considerable latitude in decision-making regarding the future of such children, with death as an appropriate management option. They recognize the legal implications of the actions described in their paper, but then conclude on a very familiar note: "If working out these dilemmas in ways such as those we suggest is in violation of the law, we believe the law should be changed." [67]

The strategy here is identical to that employed by pro-abortion doctors: agitation for changes in the law in order to legitimize practices in violation of it.

An intense campaign of propaganda is also being currently waged to legalize the "mercy" killing of the terminally ill and those elderly who are incompetent or even depressed about living a meaningless existence. Much of this can be subsumed under the beneficient sounding "death-with-dignity" label.

One essential element in the contemporary euthanasia lobby's arsenal of propaganda involves heartrending cases of terminally ill patients with excruciating pain being kept alive against their wills, senselessly hooked up to artificial respirators. Thumbnail sketches from Marya Mannes's book, *Last Rights: A Case for the Good Death* (1973), provide some examples:

> My own dear wife is 76 years of age and recently . . . suffered a severe stroke, resulting in partial paralysis, loss of speech. She is unable to swallow any solid foods and has difficulty swallowing liquids. Partial loss of memory and the failure of other body organs which usually accompany a severe stroke. It's breaking my heart even to watch her.

> My mother was 88 and deaf and blind. She suffered a lesion of the brain in June and quickly became bed-ridden. Pneumonia was expected to carry her off but huge quantities of drugs prevented this, causing her

to linger on in a pitiful physical condition and mental
torment. . . . It made me afraid to go on living knowing
that anything so terrible could happen at the end of
one's life.

The most hideous aspect of it all was that I actually
wondered whether she was exhibiting signs of drug
addiction. . . . she had frequent spells of incessant
talking. . . . she had delusions. . . . she kept saying she
was going mad and repeatedly asked for "my pill."

A change in the law cannot come soon enough to
prevent such prolonging of the act of dying. . . . the
dead themselves would be its strongest supporters.[68]

It is not always clear how many of these stories are contrived for propaganda purposes. Some of them do accurately
reveal the agony and inhumanity associated with prolongation
of dying in the impersonal, antiseptic atmosphere of hospital
intensive-care units and nursing homes. The impression intended and conveyed, however, is that this particular use of technology is completely out of hand and that the only way to
contain it is through legislation, so that the doctor will feel
free to pull the plug and release the dying patient from the
shackles of mindless machines.

Such stories recall the tales of backalley butchery so persistently circulated by pro-abortion physicians. They also
bring to mind the horror stories of veritable armies of the
feeble-minded and incompetent being kept alive unnecessarily
in the hospitals and institutions of Germany before and during
the Nazi regime.

Contrary to euthanasia propaganda, many elderly patients
on respirators fear that their lives will be cut short rather than
prolonged unnecessarily. According to Gila Berkowitz, former
editor of *Medical Dimensions*, this is especially so because of
the overwhelming emphasis on the quality of life for those
considered worthwhile at the expense of life for those deemed
of little worth:

One of our readers reported a disturbing new phenomenon recently. As a physician who treats many

elderly patients, he often admits people for serious surgery and the care of degenerative and terminal diseases. Lately, he's been faced with a growing number of patients who have been begging him tearfully not to "pull the plug" if treatment does not go well. These patients are convinced that if they lose the power of speech or become disabled in some other way, their lives may be unceremoniously extinguished by whoever holds the switch to the respirator.

At first our correspondent thought that paranoia was spreading wildly among his emotionally vulnerable patients. But further conversations convinced him that these elderly people were being terrified by a growing fashionable humanism expressed by many eminent physicians and other authorities, who would "relieve" the dying of the burden of a life that, in the opinion of the healthy doctors, is not worth living.

At first glance, the right to die is a kind of ultimate liberty appropriate to the most advanced democratic societies. But looking beneath the slick surface of rhetoric, we suspect that it is at worst a manipulative means to a fascist end. At best it is a foolish superstition.

One frail, arthritic 86-year-old man being hospitalized for pneumonia, pleaded quietly that his doctor make heroic efforts to save his life. "I know I'm not much good to anybody anymore, but I want to live. I want to live no matter what." Clearly, the man understood one of the major reasons that "the right to die" has gained popularity among so many medical, political, social, and even religious leaders. He also grasped the corollary to the right to death: if death is to be made a right, life will become, de facto, a privilege — to be extended by the powerful to those who are useful to the rest of society.

Then there are those who, in advocating euthanasia, appeal to compassion. They present to their audience patients dying in horrible pain in order to convince that death would be a relief to so wretched

an existence. We believe, however, that what the terminally ill really desire is freedom from pain, and
freedom from becoming embittering financial burdens
to their families.[69]

Current euthanasia literature is saturated by portrayals
of doctors opposed to legalized euthanasia as unfeeling technicians obsessed with preserving life at all costs, as individuals who see each death as both a personal and professional
defeat. In contrast, doctors in favor of legalizing death with
dignity come across as humane, sensitive individuals compassionately concerned with respecting the deteriorating patient's wish to be freed from the tyranny of technology, as
individuals who view death as an integral and inevitable part
of the human life cycle.

A number of physicians have come forward with confessions about how many patients they have allowed to die or
even actually put to death by a painless dose of some lethal
drug. It is more than coincidental that most of them have
surfaced after the legalization of unborn baby killing began
to take hold in the late 1960s. It is also significant to note
that such revelations are intended to justify breaking the law,
in order to get the law changed. This is a strategy identical to
that employed by such physician abortionists as Drs. G. Loutrell Timanus, Robert D. Spencer, and many others who have
publicly acknowledged flouting the abortion laws with the
aim of getting them liberalized or repealed.

In the April 2, 1973 issue of *Medical Economics*, perennial
euthanasia proponent, physician-state legislator Dr. Walter
W. Sackett, Jr. of Florida, is described as an MD crusader who
"tells how he avoids legal and other obstacles." The title of
the article tells it all — "I've let hundreds of patients die.
Shouldn't you?" He is quite proud of his record and entreats
other physicians to follow his lead and push for legislation
to enshrine such activities into law. [70]

In 1974 Dr. George Mair, a sixty-year-old retired English
doctor, admitted deliberately killing many patients in a long
career that began in 1939. These mercy-killing disclosures were
made in his autobiography, *Confessions of a Surgeon*. Mair

acknowledged "it was, of course, completely illegal and totally unethical," but defended these practices on humanitarian grounds: "It was merciful to the people concerned. It saved them weeks and months of pain, worry and possibly even fear." [71]

The fact that death-with-dignity bills have been introduced in most states attests to the significant inroads made by the euthanasia propagandists. In what may well prove to be an opening wedge for complete legalization of mercy killing, a death-with-dignity type bill was actually signed into law on September 30, 1976 by Governor Jerry Brown of California. Since then a number of other states have followed suit.

Forums for Extermination

1. German Meetings

In addition to promoting their destructive cause in articles, books, and other types of publications, doctors in Germany also pushed for public and legal acceptance of killing in meetings of medical organizations and at professional conventions. The sequence of propaganda covered abortion, sterilization, and then euthanasia.

From 1920 through the early 1930s, many intense debates took place at meetings of medical societies over the issue of whether Germany's strict abortion law (passed in 1871) should be changed. Many doctors favored expanded indications for performing abortions and a diminution in the severity of punishment meted out to those who violated the abortion law.

In September 1925, at a session of the League of German Medical Societies in Leipzig, Dr. Vollmann, a prominent gynecologist and editor of a medical journal, cited statistics that indicated that induced abortion had reached epidemic proportions. His approach toward ameliorating this problem was to modify the abortion law to allow physicians more leeway in performing abortions, especially in situations where pregnancy constituted a danger to the woman. On this occasion, Dr. Vollmann did not come out in favor of abortion on eugenic grounds (to prevent the birth of physically and mentally inferior children). His lack of support for this measure was not due to personal revulsion against destruction of the unfit, but simply because the state of eugenic knowledge was based on considerations too unsettled to provide a reliable diagnostic guide for physicians.[72]

Berlin gynecologist Dr. Max Hirsch, speaking in the auditorium of the Langenbeck-Virchow-Haus in 1926, recommended revising the German abortion law by the insertion of the following provision: "The interruption of pregnancy shall be exempt from punishment provided it is performed by a physician in accordance with the teachings of medical science." [73] According to Dr. Hirsch, the teachings of medical science were broad enough to incorporate eugenic indications as a valid basis for getting rid of offspring that would probably be defective before birth.

At a meeting held in January 1929, the prestigious Berlin Chamber of Physicians passed resolutions supporting abortion for reasons of health as well as eugenics:

> The Chamber of Physicians is of the opinion that a physician must have the right to interrupt a pregnancy if the pregnancy or the expected birth will seriously endanger the health of the mother. The following eugenic indications may be regarded as of equal weight with the foregoing indication concerning the life of the mother: cases of mental disease, epilepsy, cases of severe, and especially, asocial psychopathy and proved incest. [74]

Before a large assembly of physicians and lawyers in Berlin in 1931, Dr. Friedrich Wolf dealt a devastating blow to the abortion law by calling for its complete abolition. This he saw as the only way to legitimize both medical and social indications for interruption of pregnancy. Dr. Wolf ended with a quote from George Bernard Shaw: "A country that cannot feed its children has no right to demand children." [75]

Another important component in the German doctors'

campaign to legalize abortion was the contention that legalization would cut down on the number of unsafe, illicit abortions performed by incompetent non-medical hacks. It appears, however, that physicians performed many of the illegal abortions. In his address to the League of German Medical Societies in September 1925, gynecologist Dr. Vollmann employed the word "epidemic" to describe the number of abortions induced. He also indicated that 89 percent of abortions at the Berlin University Women's Hospital in 1916 were artificially induced. Rather than criticize doctors for their illicit assaults on the unborn, Dr. Vollmann called for modifying the law to allow physicians more discretion in performing abortions.[76] In 1931, a small-town physician revealed that he had performed 426 artificial abortions in one year, most of which were clearly against the law — being done on very slight pretexts.[77]

This all bears a striking resemblance to those American doctors who sought legal sanctification for their unlawful destructive activities against human lives in the womb.

Medical agitation for legalized killing of the unborn bore fruit by 1933, under the government of Adolf Hitler. According to the new laws that were enacted, abortion based on "genuine medical indications" was not subject to punishment when demanded and performed by legally qualified physicians.[78] Genuine medical indications were interpreted to encompass a pregnancy that threatened the life or health of the mother, plus eugenic considerations. Health was interpreted as a broad concept covering a variety of social and economic considerations.

Thus, the Nazi regime initiated one of its first phases of legal destruction by drawing upon a decade or more of intense, unrelenting assaults on Germany's law protective of human life before birth. The fact that so many leading doctors and organizations of physicians were in the forefront of this movement facilitated Hitler's initial thrust to get rid of the unwanted and defective members of German society. Although Hitler is often portrayed as an impulsive psychopath, which he no doubt was, some of the most destructive decisions enacted by his government were preceded by a considerable amount of backing from influential segments of the medical establishment, as well as other professional groups.

At a number of meetings held in the 1920s, dire warnings about the degeneration of the German people from an over-abundance of inferior individuals emanated from physicians and scientists. Their eventual purpose was to pave the way for changing the law to permit sterilization on eugenic grounds, in order to purge Germany of its impure elements.

A meeting of the Berlin Society for Public Health Culture in 1921 gave Professor H. Poll an opportunity to call for application of the laws of heredity to counter the threatening signs of degeneration among the German people. He outlined a strategy of "education," with far-reaching implications for the legalization of sterilization, as well as abortion and euthanasia:

> If by a process of education it should prove possible to develop a sense of the responsibility of the individual toward the people as a whole, so that public health as the highest and most valuable possession of the nation might be protected against the destructive attacks of individuals; if physicians should be able to fix in the public mind the conviction that it is a crime to bring sick children into the world, then eugenic ordinances and laws that today are looked on as baleful interferences with personal freedom would come to be accepted as a matter of course.[79]

In 1921, Professor Erwin Baur, director of the Biological Institute in Potsdam, addressed the Eugenics Society of Berlin on the topic of hereditary transmission and natural selection. He took this occasion to lament the decline of natural selection, in which nature helped preserve the species by eliminating the most unfit members of society. Dr. Baur looked with disfavor upon "the large number of mental inferiors, whose lives are not only preserved, but who are also allowed every opportunity to propagate." He ended by advocating "eugenic selection as a substitute for natural selection, which has been lost. We must endeavor to prevent propagation among hereditary inferiors." [80]

By the 1930s, sterilization of those defined as unfit began to come of age. Meetings of professional groups, especially physicians, provided a continuing forum from which to facilitate and reinforce the legalization of sterilization for growing numbers of expendables.

A meeting of the Prussian Council on Health was convened on July 2, 1932, with the goal of relating eugenics to the area of public welfare. In attendance were many experts from the fields of hereditary science, psychiatry, medicine, jurisprudence, and public welfare. The tone of the proceedings was considered moderate. According to the members present, "the legal approval of a strict eugenic sterilization (not castration), under suitable controls, is demanded, although no general compulsory legislation is proposed." Special assurances were given that the destruction of seriously defective living human beings was not being contemplated. [81]

The propaganda had a telling impact by July 14, 1933, with the enactment of the "Law for the Prevention of Hereditary Disease in Posterity." This was a radical law, which in effect legalized sterilization, both voluntary and enforced, for individuals with a wide range of afflictions. Justification for its passage was based on the highly distorted images conjured up of a population explosion of fertile defectives who would soon outnumber and overrun the normal segments of Germany. The following formed part of the rationale accompanying the sterilization law:

> Countless individuals of inferior type and possessing serious hereditary defects are propagating unchecked, with the result that their diseased progeny becomes a burden to society and is threatening, within three generations, to overwhelm completely the valuable strata. . . . sterilization is the only sure means of preventing the further hereditary transmission of mental disease and serious defects. [82]

Additional support for the sterilization law came from

the gynecologists of Germany, at their annual congress held in October 1933. Participants involved in a discussion of the topic "Operations Based on Eugenic Indications" expressed "absolute approval of the new law pertaining to sterilization." [83]

In 1935, the Berlin Medical Society devoted its session to the theme, "A Year of the Sterilization Law." A jurist informed the group that the eugenics courts often rendered sterilization decisions "without the person affected appearing, which saves the patient the pain of an unpleasant hearing." No one in this august body protested against the compulsory nature of most sterilization decisions and the flagrant denial of human rights associated with them. Instead, most of the session degenerated to the level of reports by physicians on the results of the surgical techniques employed in implementing the sterilization law. [84]

In late August 1938, the German Committee for Mental Hygiene, a branch of the Society of German Neurologists, sponsored the Congress of the European Society of Mental Hygiene. By this time all pretenses about a so-called voluntary sterilization program had just about disappeared. A major focus of the Congress was to enhance racial purity by discouraging marriages and even interaction among defectives and between the fit and unfit members of society. Psychiatrist Dr. Ernst Rüdin emphasized that the first duty of a family physician trained in eugenics is "to try to prevent all genetically and nationally undesirable mesalliances." Former Hamburg psychiatrist Dr. Weygandt stated that "the improvement and purification of hereditary characters cannot be attained without the use of force." [85]

In spite of periodic assurances that no law was being considered to destroy seriously defective human beings after birth, it was commonly recognized in medical circles that the laws of hereditary transmission were not perfected enough to weed out all the defectives. Aborting the probably defective and sterilizing or castrating those with blemished genetic backgrounds were not foolproof solutions to the problem of ridding the super race of all its impurities. The Nazi government still had to contend with the hundreds of thousands of defectives already born and those unfit individuals who defied the laws of hereditary transmission by being born of parents with untainted hereditary histories. One final link — destruction of the deficient after birth — remained to be forged before the Nazi dream of complete racial purity could be fulfilled.

It was within this climate that advocacy of euthanasia began to flourish. The seeds of euthanasia propaganda had been planted firmly by Dr. Ernst Haeckel as far back as the latter half of the nineteenth century, and had been continually sown by medical and biological scientists ever since then. By the 1930s, the momentum picked up and references to doing away with the unfit were increasingly heard at meetings of medical and other professional groups.

Sterilization and euthanasia of individuals with chronic mental illnesses was a topic of discussion among psychiatrists at a meeting in Bavaria in 1931.[86]

In 1933, Professor W. Schultze, State Commissioner for Public Health of the Bavarian Ministry of the Interior and a euthanasia proponent, spoke at the opening ceremonies of the second state-medical academy's meeting in Munich. He emphasized that care for the weak had to end immediately, to be replaced by "care for the health of the racially intact and the hereditarily able." After equating psychopaths with the mentally retarded, Schultze advocated "weeding-out" inferior people for whom sterilization alone was not enough.[87]

In the same year, Dr. Ernst Rüdin of the German Research Institute for Psychiatry addressed a session of the Kaiser Wilhelm Society for the Advancement of Science on the subject of hereditary prognosis. He identified the basis of all race hygiene as "preservation of the healthy hereditary elements and eradication of the pathological elements." With the aid of statistical data, Rüdin indicated that "persons with hereditary disorders must be detected, and in their progeny the percentages of the same or similar disorders must be determined and compared with the percentages found, on the average, in the general population." The main purpose of this ambitious endeavor was to assign "every person, whether presenting healthy or pathologic hereditary antecedents, to a characteristic hereditary type." This would then provide a diagnostic rationale "to eliminate the elements with undesirable hereditary traits." [88]

The propaganda meetings quickly degenerated into final-solution type conferences, where the insidious ideas began to be put into practical application.

Dr. Ludwig Sprauer, medical officer of Baden from 1934 through 1944, testified during the Nuremberg trials that he had taken part in discussions and conferences in the Reich Ministry of the Interior every two or three months. It was at these meetings that the participants were informed of the plans to introduce a law on euthanasia. [89]

According to information uncovered by psychiatrist Dr. Fredric Wertham, a conference took place in Berlin in July 1939 at which the program to exterminate mental patients throughout all of Germany "was outlined in concrete, final form." The cooperation demonstrated by eminent psychiatrists was nothing short of astounding: "Present and ready to participate were the regular professors of psychiatry and chairmen of the departments of psychiatry of leading universities and medical schools of Germany." [90]

Hitler's note of September 1, 1939, giving doctors power to kill for so-called reasons of mercy, like many of his other decisions, did not arise out of a vacuum. There is evidence that the many decades of propaganda cranked out under medical auspices in support of eliminating the unfit after birth had a significant impact on this authorization. Joseph C. Harsch, an American journalist in Berlin, indicates in his book *Pattern of Conquest* that medical proponents of euthanasia not only composed the contents of the note, but also influenced Hitler to sign it:

> So far as can be learned, the plan originated in the medical sections of the Gestapo and SS. . . . Those who proposed it are understood to have asked Hitler for a written edict, or law, which would officially authorize them to proceed with the "mercy killings." Hitler is represented as having hesitated for several weeks. Finally, doubting that Hitler would ever sign

the official order, the proponents of the project drafted a letter for him to sign which merely expressed his, Hitler's, general approval of the theory of euthanasia as a means of relieving incompetents of the burden of life. While this letter did not have the character of law, it was adequate in Nazi Germany. The Fuhrer had expressed approval of the practice. It went ahead.[91]

What came to be known as the "Fuhrer-order" resulted from a discussion involving leading Reich physicians Drs. Karl Brandt and Leonardo Conti, together with non-medical euthanasia administrator Philipp Bouhler.[92]

2. American Meetings

Conferences and meetings dominated by pro-abortion physicians and likeminded allied professionals have frequently served as occasions for discrediting laws protective of human life in the womb and propagandizing for their relaxation and eventual removal altogether. The typical pattern consisted of inviting experts to deliver papers on various facets of abortion. This would then be followed by discussions of the presentations by conference participants. By and large, the stated purpose of most of these meetings was to explore and more fully understand the problem of induced abortions, particularly those performed outside the law, with a view toward prevention, control, and reduction of abortions. Most meetings, however, actually provided a forum for abortion advocates to push for legally sanctioned destruction of the unborn. Doctors with impressive professional and university affiliations were the prime initiators and leaders at these get-togethers. Sociologists, attorneys, psychologists, demographers, anthropologists, radical feminists, and others readily cooperated.

One of the first conferences to broach the topic of abortion was held on July 19 and 20, 1942, at the New York Academy of Medicine, sponsored by the National Committee on Maternal Health, an organization "founded in 1923 in New York

City by a group of progressive physicians who felt that medicine should play a larger part in studying the general field of sex and reproduction."[93] Of the forty-six participants, thirty-three were medical doctors, and among them were Dr. Robert Dickinson, a prominent birth control advocate, Dr. John Rock, father of the birth-control pill, Dr. Sophia Kleegman, an early proponent of liberalized abortion, and Dr. Frederick J. Taussig, famous for his 1936 book on abortion. Some of the non-medical attendees included the well-known family sociologist Ernest W. Burgess, John H. Amen, Assistant Attorney General of New York State, and New York City magistrate Judge Anna Kross.

While Chairman Dr. Howard C. Taylor believed the conference had been called "in the hope that suggestions may be made either for investigation of the problem or of actual measures for abortion control," a number of participants entertained far more ambitious goals. Dr. Taussig referred to the "illogical character of the wording" of the abortion laws in the forty-eight states and indicated that "the purpose of this Conference should be primarily directed to drafting a model abortion law which could be accepted by all the states of this country." [94] His idea of uniformity meant considerable liberalization of abortion laws on socioeconomic and other grounds.

Dr. Sophia Kleegman began her assault on restrictive abortion by posing a question, "Hasn't the time come for a re-evaluation of the indications for abortion?" What she was pointing to here was broadening them to encompass far more than saving the mother's life or health. Like many other abortion proponents, she blamed the restrictive legal situation on the Catholic Church: "Is it right for one particular church to enforce its tenets on members of other churches?" [95] Following along similar lines, Dr. Robert Dickinson characterized legal restraints on abortion as being "formulated largely by theological dogma." In what amounted to advocacy of abortion on demand, he recommended granting the ultimate decision-making authority for going through the "serious condition" of pregnancy to the pregnant woman rather than to doctors "who never had labors." [96]

The only concrete resolution passed by the conference was a commitment to the "establishment of free and open public discussion of human reproduction and the problems of abortion." [97] The pattern was set for the development of future forums where physicians, in league with other sympathetic professionals, could continue to sharpen their attacks on abortion statutes and agitate for medical killing of the unborn without fear of legal reprisals.

In April 1955 at Arden House in New York City, the Planned Parenthood Federation of America sponsored a major conference on abortion attended by forty-three experts from the fields of medicine, law, and demography. Two months later most of the participants returned for a full-day session at the New York Academy of Medicine. Like the 1942 conference, physicians constituted an overwhelming majority: thirty-three of the forty-three participants were medical doctors. Some of those who took part in the 1942 conference were also on hand, including the familiar faces of Drs. John Rock, Sophia Kleegman, Abraham Stone, and Howard C. Taylor. They were joined by some of the most ardent leaders of the pro-abortion movement in America: Dr. Alan F. Guttmacher, director of the department of obstetrics and gynecology at Mount Sinai Hospital; Dr. Robert W. Laidlaw, chief, division of psychiatry at Roosevelt Hospital; Dr. Theodore Lidz, professor of psychiatry at Yale University; Dr. Harold Rosen, a psychiatrist affiliated with the Johns Hopkins Hospital; Dr. Christopher Tietze, abortion statistician; Dr. Mary S. Calderone, medical director of the Planned Parenthood Federation; Dr. Louis M. Hellman, professor of obstetrics and gynecology at the State University of New York and later a prominent official in the Department of Health, Education and Welfare; and Dr. Lawrence C. Kolb, director of the New York State Psychiatric Institute and a professor at Columbia University. [98]

Among the non-medical participants were famous sex researcher Dr. Alfred C. Kinsey; Irene B. Taeuber, demographer in the Office of Population Research at Princeton University; and Yale University law student Edwin M. Schur, who later authored a book that placed abortion in the category of "crimes without victims."

The attacks on the anti-abortion laws by the Arden House participants were far more vigorous, numerous, and relentless than was the case at the 1942 conference. The entire tenor and thrust of the proceedings was accurately captured in introductory comments by anthropologist M. F. Ashley Montagu.

> The laws need to be brought up to date. It is through conferences and publications such as this one, organized and brought into being by the Planned Parenthood Federation of America, that legislation will eventually be developed to deal with the social problem of abortion in a manner rather more appropriate than is the case at the present time.[99]

Continuing on with a theme she developed at the 1942 conference, Dr. Sophia Kleegman pointed to the need for enlarging the legal indications for therapeutic abortions so that ethical physicians would no longer "resort to referring some of their patients to abortionists." Her idea of enlargement included "room for more consideration of humanitarian reasons as an additional indication for abortion for all women," plus "the eugenic aspect," which was seen as crucial for protecting and enriching "future generations in regard to our most precious resource — the human race."[100]

Dr. Alan Guttmacher's approach was to first of all declare abortion laws "inoperable" and emphasize the "harm that accrues therefrom" and then to "suggest changes in the laws so that they become workable." Just what changes did Dr. Guttmacher have in mind? In his own words, "I should like to see a more permissive law, so that those of us who do carry out what we honestly consider to be needed therapeutic abortions would not be doing so with a haunting feeling that our acts are half-legal, or pseudo-legal."[101]

Like many pro-abortion physicians before and since, psychiatrist Theodore Lidz couldn't resist capping his attack on antiabortion laws by linking them with the Catholic Church: "We should take the stand, in a democratic way, that no religious group should seek to maintain the religious and ethical standards of its own members by the imposition of laws applied to the general population." [102]

Again, the Catholic Church is thrust into the role of a sinister, oppressive force trying to impose its peculiar brand of sectarian morality on everyone else. What Lidz and other medical proponents of easy abortion always fail to mention is that the restrictive abortion laws under attack were enacted at a time (mid to late-1800s) when the state legislatures were dominated by those of the Protestant and not the Catholic faith. Besides, the AMA policy statements on abortion of 1859 and 1871 clearly show that it was physicians who led the way toward changing the permissive abortion laws then in effect. Their logical rationale for tighter abortion laws was not based on the Catholic theological position that the human soul is infused at conception, but on the scientific fact that a unique human life begins at conception. Their moral rationale for strict abortion laws was not based on a commandment unique to Catholicism, but one that transcends all religions and creeds — "Thou shalt not kill." [103]

Dr. Robert Laidlaw called for a change in the law that would allow the doctor to perform abortions just as it permits him to perform any legitimate medical procedure. Apparently, Laidlaw saw no significant difference between killing an unborn baby and removing a ruptured appendix:

> We can most certainly take the point of view that we deplore the necessity for abortion. . . . We can regret a ruptured appendix — but if we had a law which said that under certain circumstances you might operate on a ruptured appendix and in other circumstances you might not, we would feel shackled in the exercise of our medical judgment there, just as we now feel shackled in connection with the abortion problem. [104]

Arch-abortionist Dr. G. Loutrell Timanus' sentiments about the abortion laws would not be difficult to predict. An individual with such a long career devoted to destroying the unborn in violation of the laws would hardly be inclined to keep them on the books. What better way could there be to vindicate such persevering dedication than by legalizing what Timanus and many credentialed executioners had been doing all along! It is not surprising that he chose to characterize the abortion laws as being "unenforceable" and "generally violated everywhere." His forging of a bond between the abortion and prohibition laws is particularly noteworthy: "Few of us have forgotten the prohibition law which, because it was not enforceable, was finally repealed." [105] This is precisely what Timanus felt the fate of abortion laws should be.

The question dominating the conference was not whether the abortion laws should or should not be changed; change was already a given. The question was how radical the changes should be. While a number of participants were obviously pushing for outright repeal, most at least agreed that socioeconomic and so-called humanitarian factors constituted valid indicators for doctors to use in justifying the performance of abortions.

Amidst an atmosphere so heavily laden with pro-abortion rhetoric was one breath of fresh air. It came in the person of Dr. Joseph P. Donnelly, medical director of the Margaret Hague Maternity Hospital in Jersey City, New Jersey. Dr. Donnelly had the courage to cut through the dense fog of propaganda and expose the proceedings for what they were. He presented constructive alternatives to destruction and supplied disturbing but essential historical perspectives for understanding what the eminent medical participants were really up to — promoting the legalization of killing for increasingly wider indications. His comments are well worth quoting, not only because of their rarity and the eloquence with which they were expressed, but also because of how incisively they cut to the truth:

> As medical men, I believe we should definitely confine our indications for therapeutic abortion to strictly medical reasons. Therefore, I would like to say a few words on the so-called socioeconomic reasons for therapeutic abortion. Can the patient afford to have

another child? Will the older children have sufficient educational opportunities if their parents have another child? Aren't two, three or four children enough? I am afraid such statements are frequently made in the discussion of a proposed therapeutic abortion. It seems from other discussion that psychiatrists are the ones who are most frequently asked to consider socioeconomic reasons in recommending an abortion. We should be doctors of medicine, not socioeconomic prophets. How many students in medical schools today, who were born in the depths of a depression in 1932, were good economic risks at the time of their birth? If we go back three or four generations in any of our families and eliminate all the poor economic risks among our antecedents, this conference today might never have convened.

Slums and delinquency exist. It may seem very easy to sit around here and say that certain cases will be aborted and that will solve the problem, but I am afraid it is going to take public housing, good health care, high minimum wages, family allowances, and the general raising of the standards of the American people to solve these problems. It looks very easy to eliminate the unfit and the poor socioeconomic risks from our civilization with the curette and thereby to build a better society, but I think it is simply a distinction without a difference between this type of reasoning and the reasoning of a man of unhappy memory who thought he could raise the standards of society by eliminating the so-called unfit with the gas chambers of Buchenwald.[106]

Here was a unique opportunity for those in attendance to confront the truth. Here was a chance for the participants to tackle the problem of illegal unborn baby killing head on by insisting that doctors obey the law and stop the illicit and unethical destruction of unborn lives. Here was an occasion for doctors to publicly disavow the role of executioner and rededicate themselves to saving, healing, curing, and protecting the most vulnerable of human lives.

Tragically, Dr. Donnelly's remarks caused little more than a ripple, a fleeting moment of unease. Whether it was a matter of arrogance, intellectual pride, amorality, personal blindness, or what have you, a vast majority of those in attendance were already too far bent on justifying and providing legal sanctions for the horrendous bloodbath perpetrated primarily by respectable physicians.

The most far-reaching resolution adopted by the Arden House conference was a strong plea for legalizing abortions according to a greatly expanded series of indications:

> Authoritative bodies such as the National Conference of Commissioners on Uniform State Laws, the American Law Institute, and the Council of State Governments should study the abortion laws in the various states and frame a model law that could, perhaps jointly, be presented to the states for their consideration to replace existing statutes.... Such commissions should recognize that, when current statutes are interpreted exactly as written, almost no therapeutic abortions performed today are legal, since with the improvement of modern medicine it rarely becomes necessary to perform an abortion to save life. They should also recognize the mounting approval of psychiatric, humanitarian, and eugenic indications for the legal termination of pregnancy; the propriety of such indications merits extensive study and appraisal, and the commissions should engage in such study in order to be able to give careful consideration to the advisability of so modifying abortion statutes as to give to physicians latitude to include these indications in their recommendations for therapeutic abortion.[107]

This resolution shows clearly the direction in which the influence flowed. It was not a matter of prominent attorneys telling doctors what the law should be, but just the other way around. Legal bodies, such as the American Law Institute, were to reflect what certain influential physicians desired or insisted upon; the initiative and leadership came from the ranks of organized medicine. This was a prophetic design for how medical propaganda was to be transmitted through professional organizations and eventually to the public at large.

The movement for even greater relaxation of legal restrictions on killing of the unborn was provided with an additional boost at one of the largest and most prestigious meetings ever held on abortion, convened by the Association for the Study of Abortion at Hot Springs, Virginia on November 17 and 18, 1968. Like the previous abortion conferences, this one was also dominated by medical doctors. Out of eighty-seven participants from nineteen different countries, fifty-four had medical degrees.[108]

Also like the other meetings, it was stacked with the most eminent and adamant pro-abortionists. In their book on the abortion controversy, researchers Betty Sarvis and Hyman Rodman aptly describe the roster of attendees as reading like a "Who's Who of the abortion world — all the U.S. veterans of the abortion controversy and most of the international ones." [109] Even a cursory glance at the list of participants reveals the accuracy of this portrayal: Drs. Mary S. Calderone, Alan F. Guttmacher, Robert E. Hall, Louis M. Hellman, Kurt Hirschborn, Sophia J. Kleegman, Jerome M. Kummer, Robert W. Laidlaw, Theodore Lidz, Harold Rosen, Natalie Shainess, Christopher Tietze, and others.

The non-medical participants were also among the most vociferous pro-abortionists in the world: Protestant theologian and situation ethicist Joseph F. Fletcher, biologist and abortion semanticist Garrett Hardin, author Lawrence Lader, sociologist Alice S. Rossi, and attorneys active in attacking laws protective of unborn human life — Roy Lucas, Cyril C. Means, Harriet F. Pilpel, Ruth Roemer, and Edwin M. Schur.

Only three individuals, none of them physicians, could be described as being genuinely against legalizing the destruction of unborn humans — Jesuit theologian Thomas J. O'Donnell and lawyers Eugene Quay and David Granfield. Although each did an excellent job of articulating the legal and moral case for the unborn, they were hopelessly outnumbered by the huge contingent of pro-abortion zealots. In most instances, their comments fell on deaf ears.

Dr. Robert E. Hall began by identifying what he called the primary objective of the conference:

> The primary purpose of the conference was not to debate or promote abortion law reform, not to incite controversy or achieve consensus, but rather to explore the field of abortion, to exchange knowledge about abortion, and to expose this knowledge to public view.[110]

This statement, more than most, highlights the severe discrepancy between stated and actual goals. No longer were a majority of participants talking about liberalizing abortion laws along the American Law Institute's Model Penal Code lines. They gathered together for much bigger stakes: complete removal of all abortion laws, thus allowing the destruction of unborn children to be either a strictly private matter between the physician and the woman or entirely the right of the woman.

At one of the conference panels, "Abortion and Psychiatry," several individuals came out strongly for abortion law repeal. Dr. Natalie Shainess declared that the woman "should have ready access to abortion and this should be a matter between the woman and her physician or the clinic" during the period before quickening, because this is the time when "the fetus is not a reality, not a child, to the woman." [111] Dr. Jerome M. Kummer used this occasion to launch a tirade against abortion laws: "Rigid laws, rigid restrictions against people following natural instincts for self-preservation and preservation of the family, rigid restrictions against physicians who practice their profession to the best of their ability in the best interests of their patients." From this he proceeded to his usual conclusion that "any woman wanting an abortion should be entitled to it after she has had a chance to discuss and explore it more fully with trusted counsel." [112]

Another variation of this was expressed by Dr. Leona Baumgartner, visiting professor of social medicine at Harvard. During a panel on "Abortion and Public Health," she presented the American Public Health's policy stand on abortion for conference consideration: "Abortion is an important means of securing the right to spacing and choosing the number of children wanted. . . . Safe legal abortion should be available to all women." She followed this up with a reference to the Planned Parenthood-World Population's suggestion that "all criminal laws regarding abortion should be abolished." [113]

The panel on "Abortion and Obstetrics" produced a noteworthy exchange between attorney Roy Lucas and Dr. Alan Guttmacher:

> LUCAS: I want to ask Dr. Guttmacher about a statement that he made in his most recent book to the effect that the public in the United States would not be able to accept a freedom-of-choice plan in which the woman had the right to decide herself. If the courts, in particular the Supreme Court, ultimately decide that a woman has a private right to determine whether she wants to have an abortion, do you think that the medical profession would sabotage this right, through committees and through interposing itself between a woman and her gynecologist?
>
> GUTTMACHER: My statement was based on repeated polls. . . . I would say the American public is not willing to have abortion on demand. They would be willing for themselves, but not for their neighbors. The physician follows the public, he does not lead the public. If 70 per cent of the public says Yes, then we will have abortion on demand. The doctors are not going to lead the public into that attitude, that is all I am trying to say. [114]

Guttmacher's response has to be the understatement of at least several decades. It stands in direct contradiction to the overwhelming evidence that physicians, through their massive violations of abortion laws and propaganda efforts, have been largely responsible for leading the public to accept abortion as a valid medical procedure for non-medical or no reasons at all. This is the very thing that Guttmacher devoted such a significant part of his long career to. Why he replied the way he did is difficult to fathom. Perhaps it was another way of trying to displace responsibility for approval of abortion on demand from the medical profession to the public.

Despite Dr. Guttmacher's disclaimer, just about every doctor who attended the meeting willingly jumped on the abortion-on-demand bandwagon. Perennial conference partic
ipant Dr. Sophia Kleegman, carrying through on a theme begun at the 1942 Abortion Conference, sponsored by the National Committee on Maternal Health, stated that the only way to provide "honest, just health services to all our women is to have all legal restrictions removed entirely to allow physicians to take care of their patients within the framework of sound medical judgment and practice." [115] Psychiatrist Dr. Ruth Lidz expressed her basic agreement with this view-point, saying, "I would like very much to have all restrictive abortion laws removed." [116] For Dr. Leon Eisenberg the prob-lem would not be solved by "any of the so-called liberalized laws," but by posing the crucial question, "Do the parents want the child or not?" From this he concluded, "Abortion is a question of the rights of mothers and of human dignity and happiness." [117]

A distinctive feature of the Hot Springs conference, be-sides the overwhelming medical consensus regarding the necessity for repeal of all abortion laws, was the presence of so many experienced lawyers to show the doctors various paths toward accomplishing such a goal. Harriet Pilpel set the stage by stressing the value of mounting constitutional attacks against abortion laws:

> The fact that just bringing test cases, and the dia-logue and debate which result, may be extremely helpful. And experience, I think, has proven that chal-lenging the constitutionality of laws, even if the cases are lost, tends to have a public educational effect, and often induces the legislature to do something which otherwise it might not do.

The fact that attacks are mounted and the public is educated as to the infirmities in the laws will become, I think, extremely useful.[118]

Attorney Roy Lucas focused on two lines of attack: (1) "that the typical state abortion laws violate some freedom of association," particularly between husband and wife and between doctor and patient; (2) "that the laws regulating abortion are laws respecting an establishment of religion." Elaborating on this latter point, Lucas explained, "The quickest way to sum this up is to show that the abortion restrictions arise out of a metaphysical theory that the fertilized ovum is a human being entitled to the protection of ultimate birth and life." Pilpel found time to toss one more possibility in the hopper: "That the abortion laws represent the infliction of cruel and unusual punishment in violation of the Ninth Amendment." [119]

Thus, lawyers supplied the legal semantics necessary to get physicians off the hook for perpetrating unborn baby killing by endowing their destructive activities with legal respectability. Never has there been such an unholy alliance entered into by two professional groups!

Pressures for the approval of legal destruction of human lives before birth for reasons other than saving the life of the mother finally reached the top rungs of organized medicine on June 21, 1967, at the annual meeting of the American Medical Association. The House of Delegates, the AMA's 242 member policy-making body, adopted a statement favoring the performance of abortion along lines similar to the American Law Institute's Model Penal Code proposals:

The American Medical Association is opposed to induced abortion except when:
(1) There is documented medical evidence that continuance of the pregnancy may threaten the health or life of the mother, or
(2) There is documented medical evidence that the infant may be born with incapacitating physical deformity or mental deficiency, or

(3) There is documented medical evidence that continuance of a pregnancy, resulting from legally established statutory or forcible rape or incest may constitute a threat to the mental or physical health of the patient;

(4) Two other physicians chosen because of their recognized professional competence have examined the patient and have concurred in writing; and

(5) The procedure is performed in a hospital accredited by the Joint Commission on Accreditation of Hospitals.[120]

This was not just some lone, atypical backstreet butcher using the pages of a prestigious medical journal in order to gain acceptance of his assaults on prenatal life. Neither was it a small nonrepresentative group of elitist, credentialed executioners gathered together for the purpose of attacking and discrediting laws protective of human life before birth under the guise of a comprehensive and objective assessment of abortion. Nor was it the opinion of only a few medical societies trying to cover up massive physician violations of statutes by pushing for legalization within the borders of their respective states.

This was the AMA, far and away the largest (216,000 members in 1967) and most influential medical body, speaking through its delegates for all of organized medicine in America. While all physicians are not members of the association and do not always subscribe to every policy adopted, the assumption was that, in the case of abortion, the policy passed truly reflected the sentiments of a vast majority of American doctors. This assumption was clearly evident in the various conclusions accompanying the policy statement. One of them indicated "the majority of physicians believe that, in the light of recent advances in scientific medical knowledge, there may be substantial medical evidence ... which would warrant the institution of therapeutic abortion either to safeguard the health or life of the patient, or to prevent the birth of a severely crippled, deformed or abnormal infant." Another emphasized that "all points of view were expressed" regarding the abortion policy recommendation with the "preponderance of testimony" favoring adoption.[121]

Other data was given to bolster the claim of widespread medical support for liberalized abortion laws, in particular, resolutions — all highly favorable — issued by numerous county and state medical societies and such medical groups as the American College of Obstetricians and Gynecologists, the American Psychiatric Association, the American Public Health Association, and the New York Academy of Medicine.[122]

The AMA House of Delegates would never have recommended such radical departures from past policy on abortion if they had not been firmly convinced that a substantial majority of doctors supported such changes. Their suppositions regarding medical opinion on the subject, unfortunately, were only too true.

Thus, for the first time in its history, the American Medical Association in 1967 went on record in favor of exterminative medicine, so long as the extermination was safely carried out in a scientific manner by credentialed executioners in the antiseptic setting of an accredited hospital. This is similar to a stance taken by a number of German doctors before and during the time of the Third Reich. A far greater proportion of American doctors, however, have willingly taken on the role of scientific killer than did their German counterparts. The German medical profession as a whole never did reach the point where destruction became official medical policy.

The abortion-on-demand mentality finally infected the AMA at its annual meeting of June 25, 1970, in Chicago, Illinois. For the first time in the 123-year history of the association, the House of Delegates, by a vote of 103 to 73, adopted resolutions that placed organized medicine in America on record in favor of the complete abolition of all abortion laws. This in effect made the decision to kill unborn children a private matter between the physician and the pregnant woman. The exact wording of the key resolution is as follows:

RESOLVED, That abortion is a medical procedure and should be performed only by a duly licensed physician and surgeon in an accredited hospital acting only after consultation with two other physicians chosen because of their professional competency and in conformance with standards of good medical practice and the Medical Practice Act of his state.[123]

The AMA statements of 1967 and 1970 catapulted doctors into the role of legal executioners. These policies profoundly reversed the previously enacted AMA stands of 1859 and 1871, which strongly condemned the practice of abortion as immoral, unethical, and despicable. It is interesting to note that no mention was made of the early policy statements, not even a footnote, in any of the publications and conferences dominated by pro-abortion propaganda. It is as if they never existed. One exception is a brief reference to the 1871 condemnation of abortion in the report submitted with the 1967 AMA recommendations to liberalize abortion.

It is a giant step backwards from the abortion as an "unwarrantable destruction of human life" stance of 1859 to the abortion as a "medical procedure" position of 1970. One is a complete reversal of the other. The early statements placed the AMA solidly and unequivocally behind the physician as a healer and preserver of human life, while the recent statements set the doctor up as a paid executioner of human life. A summary comparison of the AMA policy proposals of 1859 and 1871 with those of 1967 and 1970 demonstrates how drastically the state of medical ethics regarding the value of human life has deteriorated. (See the Appendix — "The American Medical Association on Abortion: An Anatomy of Contrasting Policy Statements.")

Various meetings of prestigious professional groups have also served as fertile ground for American doctors to push for legalization of euthanasia. Such forums were first held in the late 1930s. The propaganda spewed forth from physicians at pro-abortion gatherings, culminating in the 1973 Supreme Court decision, has provided an eminently successful model for legalizing what was once thought impossible. The number of medical and scientific meetings convened to discuss and justify getting rid of unwanted defectives after birth has been escalating enormously ever since the pro-abortion victories. Hardly a week goes by without encountering a pronouncement uttered at some influential meeting about allowing the doctor to institute a policy of benign neglect for or activate the release of individuals defined as vegetables or possessing little hope of achieving meaningful humanhood.

A meeting of the Society of Medical Jurisprudence held in February 1939 afforded Dr. Foster Kennedy, a prominent professor of neurology at Cornell University Medical School and newly elected president of the American Euthanasia Society, a chance to assault laws that prevented doctors from taking the lives of born defectives. "If the law sought to restrict euthanasia to those who could speak out for it, and thus overlooked these creatures who cannot speak," asserted Kennedy, "then, I say as Dickens did, 'The law's an ass.' It's time the law changed its mind." [124]

In 1972, a conference attended by geneticists, biologists, physicians, theologians, philosophers, and writers was held in Washington, D.C. to ponder the question of whether mongoloid infants should be allowed to live. A substantial number of individuals representing the scientific community expressed an unwillingness to grant mongoloids an undisputed right to life. Their reasoning was founded on the contention that such creatures "are an intolerable burden to their parents, to society, and to themselves." [125]

Dr. J. Alex Haller, a pediatric surgeon at Johns Hopkins University, indicated at a meeting of the American Academy of Pediatrics in October 1973 that society must give doctors the ethical option of not helping a seriously retarded or defective newborn survive. "Couldn't it be in the best interest of that life not to survive?" asked Dr. Haller. "We must at least have that option open to us." [126]

An alarmingly large majority of individuals who attended the 1975 Conference on Ethical Issues in Neonatal Intensive Care in Sonoma, California expressed support for various methods of eliminating seriously ill infants. The twenty participants, nine of whom were physicians, all answered "yes" to the questions: "Would it ever be right not to resuscitate an infant at birth?" and "Would it ever be right to withdraw life support from a clearly diagnosed, poor-prognosis infant?" Eighteen out of twenty answered "yes" to the question: "Would it ever be right to displace the poor-prognosis infant A in order to provide intensive care to the better-prognosis infant B?" A huge consensus (seventeen out of twenty) even responded affirmatively to the question: "Would it ever be right to directly intervene to kill a self-sustaining infant?" [127]

In the euthanasia decision, as in the abortion decision, the individual most drastically affected has no say in his or her survival. As agitation for medical destruction of an increasing variety of postnatal expendables becomes a more pronounced part of medical meetings, look for the American Medical Association to enact a resolution declaring that euthanasia, like abortion, should be a private matter to be resolved by the physician, parents, or legal guardians of the affected individual. Lawmaking bodies, acutely sensitive to what doctors desire or are already doing in violation of the law, are ever ready to revise or repeal the laws against killing when medical consensus for disposing of the unwanted unfit is perceived as sufficiently strong. Medicine will lead the way and the law, like a sheep, will follow blindly.

Consensus on Killing

1. German Surveys

Information on surveys taken of German physicians regarding their attitudes toward abortion and euthanasia is sparse indeed. Much of this is probably due to the fact that opinion surveys were not nearly such a prominent part of German society in the 1930s as they are today.

Nevertheless, in 1931 the Hamburg Chamber of Physicians sent out a questionnaire to 1,266 doctors with the purpose of assessing their attitudes toward Germany's abortion law. Based on a 70 percent return rate (880 respondents sent back completed questionnaires), three-fourths favored changing the law to allow abortions for medicosocial indications. [128]

This trend was even more pronounced in the results of a

mailed questionnaire circulated among all graduate women physicians early in 1930. Only 6 percent of the 1,352 women doctors queried favored retention of the abortion law then in effect. An overwhelming majority supported legal abortion on general health and medicosocial grounds. A large number, 559, were even in favor of purely social indications as a sufficient rationale for abortion.[129]

Since agitation for abortion had been going on in medical circles many years before these polls were conducted, it shows that a consensus on killing the unborn had already crystallized among various segments of German medicine before the early stages of the Nazi regime. The growing medical acceptance of abortion for expanded indications undoubtedly played an important role in the passage of the eugenic abortion laws of the early to mid-1930s.

Although German physicians' attitudes toward euthanasia had not been formally surveyed, it likewise can be safely assumed that quite a few doctors favored this practice for the weak, the defective and the terminally ill. The intense propaganda for their elimination had persisted at least from the time of Dr. Haeckel in the latter half of the nineteenth century. It was bound to make considerable headway by the 1930s.

While there are no precise figures available on the extent of medical acceptance of euthanasia, enough physicians became actively involved to accomplish the eradication of huge numbers of weak, deformed, or defenseless Germans, Jews and others. This reflected a disturbingly high degree of acceptance regarding the medical extermination of lives considered devoid of value. In addition, there was another segment of the German medical community that, while not actively pursuing exterminative medicine, can be said to have been favorably disposed because of their silence, because of their refusal to speak out against the destructive activities of their colleagues.

2. American Polls

Most polls taken of American physicians' attitudes toward

abortion before the US Supreme Court decision of 1973 lead to one unmistakable conclusion: An overwhelming majority of the doctors questioned favored abortions for reasons other than saving the life of the mother. An astonishing proportion even approved of abolishing all legal restrictions on abortion. These conclusions hold for general practitioners as well as specialists. The results of opinion polls reflect how profoundly a large segment of the medical profession was influenced by the intense propaganda campaign mounted on behalf of legalized killing by eminent colleagues.

The polls indicate that psychiatry has proven to be the field of medical specialization most susceptible to pro-abortion sentiment.

In December 1965, the Association for the Study of Abortion conducted a mailed questionnaire survey of members of the American Psychiatric Association. It found that 5,289 psychiatrists "overwhelmingly favor liberalization of criteria for legal interruption of pregnancy. Percentages in favor varied from 86 to 97 percent of psychiatrists who replied." In addition, almost one-quarter (23.5 percent) favored abortion on request.[130]

In 1967 the magazine *Modern Medicine* asked 40,089 physicians about their attitudes regarding liberalizing the laws on therapeutic abortion. On the whole, 86.9 percent answered in the affirmative. At the top of the list were psychiatrists: 94.6 percent expressed support for liberalization.[131] Another poll published in *Modern Medicine* in 1969 revealed that 63 percent of the 27,741 physicians questioned favored abortion on request. Again, psychiatrists led the pack: 80 percent of the 2,041 psychiatrists who replied were in favor of abortion on request.[132]

Why, out of all the specialized fields in medicine, has psychiatry been so positively disposed to permitting abortion on demand? A plausible explanation is that psychiatrists are rarely involved in actually performing abortions. They do not see unborn victims being sucked, scraped, poisoned, burned, or cut out of the womb. They are therefore far removed from the unpleasantries and horrors associated with abortion procedures. They perceive the entire matter from a highly abstract vantage point with little or no interest in the plight of the unborn child. Their efforts are focused exclusively on the needs and wishes of the woman carrying an unwanted child.

While psychiatric blindness to the fate of human beings slated for abortion is close to being a professional imperative, it is incomprehensible how a similar mentality could prevail among those doctors, namely obstetricians, responsible for delivering babies into the extrauterine world in the most trauma-free manner possible. It would seem like such an impossible contradiction to ask the obstetrician to assume responsibility for both saving and destroying human lives. How difficult it must be to reconcile the roles of protector and executioner!

Despite this, the polls also show that a large percentage of baby doctors favor relaxed abortion laws, or no laws at all.

In 1967, the American College of Obstetricians and Gynecologists and the American Public Health Association sponsored a study of contraception, sterilization, and therapeutic abortion carried out in conjunction with hospital teaching and services programs. Part of this survey involved assessing medical attitudes toward the abortion laws then in effect. Replies received from chiefs of obstetrics departments of 372 hospitals throughout the United States and Canada indicated that a huge majority of 78.6 percent favored "abolition or liberalization of the law." [133]

Among the 40,089 doctors polled by *Modern Medicine* in 1967, 83.7 percent of the obstetrician-gynecologists who replied expressed support for liberalizing the laws on therapeutic abortion.[134] The other *Modern Medicine* poll conducted in 1969 revealed that 50.6 percent of 2,651 ob-gyns went even further by favoring abortion on request.[135]

In July 1970, 50 percent of all ob-gyns in the state of New York were asked about their attitudes toward New York's abortion-on-request law. Field interviews disclosed that seven out of ten respondents favored the law and 92 percent were either willing to perform an abortion or to refer the woman elsewhere for one.[136] A follow-up study indicated that the percentage of obstetricians in favor of the new law rose from 73 percent in July 1970 to 76 percent in January 1971.[137]

The acceptability-of-killing mentality has made even more phenomenal inroads among younger obstetricians in training. According to the findings of a questionnaire sent to sixty-seven full-time, attending, and housestaff members of the Johns Hopkins Hospital department of gynecology and obstetrics, "more recently educated physicians held more liberal attitudes toward performing abortion on request." The precise statistical breakdown is startling as well as depressing: "Nearly 90% of the full-time, attending, and housestaff would perform an abortion on request for pregnancies 12 weeks or less, and over 80% for pregnancies 12 to 20 weeks." [138]

A study of attitudes among forty-eight obstetric and gynecologic residents in the San Francisco Bay area toward abortion resulted in similar conclusions. Of this group, 98 percent admitted performing therapeutic abortions and 83 percent expressed willingness to provide abortion on request. This percentage rose to eighty-eight when the abortion was to be done in the first trimester of pregnancy. [139]

In light of the above findings, it would do well to reexamine Dr. Arthur Peck's observations regarding abortion on request, made in 1968:

> Medical education, emphasizing the physician's role in aiding life and health and postponing death, gives rise to serious conflicts within the physician who is confronted with a woman's request to be aborted. That an obstetrician, having chosen to specialize in helping babies to be born, should be the very physician expected to perform abortions is a situation in which serious conflict is unavoidable.
>
> Abortion on request is so foreign to attitudes fostered in physicians during their medical training that conflicts arise not only between physicians and those pressing for widespread legal abortion but also within the physicians most directly involved in the abortion process. [140]

How quickly something so foreign as destruction on request has become an increasingly routine component of obstetrical practice! The shift is as dramatic as it is substantive. How speedily the conflict between two inherent irreconcilables has been resolved! The ease with which those trained to bring forth new human life snuff out new human life is absolutely incredible, as well as frightening!

There are signs that the barriers against medical involvement in the destruction of human life after birth are also being irreparably eroded. Polls conducted of American doctors indicate that growing proportions favor the legalization of positive as well as negative euthanasia.

In the late 1960s, Dr. Robert H. Williams of the University of Washington Medical School sent questionnaires on a range of human life issues to the total membership of the Association of Professors of Medicine and the Association of American Physicians. In all, his return rate was 97 percent (333 out of 344 individuals queried responded). The main finding was that 87 percent expressed support for negative euthanasia while 80 percent admitted having practiced this form of doing away with patients. Although only 15 percent favored positive euthanasia, Dr. Williams implies that this percentage will increase with changes in the law and public opinion.[141]

Around the same time, 418 physicians from two hospitals in the Seattle, Washington area replied to a questionnaire formulated by Dr. Norman K. Brown and a group of medical researchers associated with the University of Washington Medical School. A large majority (72 percent) said they would "exercise negative euthanasia by not performing dialysis on all patients with chronic uremia." Also of significance were the good-sized minorities favoring positive euthanasia: 31 percent supported a "change in social attitudes which would allow positive euthanasia to be carried out in selected patients," and 28 percent related that "they would practice positive euthanasia in selected patients if the evolution of social attitudes permitted."[142]

A possible indication of the shape of medical opinion on euthanasia in the future can be gleaned from a 1969 survey of 163 medical students at the University of Washington. The responses in the area of positive euthanasia are especially startling: "About 50 percent of students favored changes permitting positive euthanasia" and "almost twice as high a proportion of medical students (46 percent) as of attending physicians (27 percent) felt they would practice positive euthanasia if changes occurred in social attitudes." [143]

Similarities between the American medical consensus on abortion and the one fast developing on euthanasia are uncomfortably close. They are inextricably bound together; they are integral components of an anti-life mentality glutting influential sectors of American medicine. Polls conducted of doctors regarding their attitudes toward both abortion and euthanasia led Dr. Norman K. Brown and colleagues to place the whole abortion-euthanasia package under the highly positive label of the physician as a change agent:

> Thus, the most change-oriented physician as defined by us would (1) carry out negative euthanasia after having a statement signed by the patient or his relatives; (2) favor changes in social mores which would allow for positive euthanasia; (3) carry out positive euthanasia if society were to sanction it; and (4) favor abortion for medical, social, and economic reasons and for convenience. [144]

Euphemisms aside, the pattern of medical violations of laws against euthanasia as a means of getting the laws changed to accord with the illegal practices has been established. Along with it, surveys of physicians reflecting the acceptability of euthanasia by omission and commission will undoubtedly be employed as another device for altering the legal climate to allow doctors to expand their power over the fates of increasing numbers of human discards.

A brief pause at this point will allow an opportunity to reflect on the distressing findings thus far uncovered, the main one being the highly significant role physicians have played in destruction and agitation for legalizing destruction both in Nazi Germany and in contemporary America.

In Germany, the long-standing campaign mounted by doctors against the defective and the unwanted could not help but have an impact on Hitler and other leaders of the Third Reich. The speed and efficiency with which physicians almost single-handedly administered euthanasia did not go unnoticed when the National Socialist regime was confronted with resolving the Jewish question. The euthanasia program stood as a highly successful model of destruction worthy of emulation for the more massive task of racial genocide. And doctors played the pivotal role in linking the euthanasia and racial genocide programs.

The words of Dr. Andrew C. Ivy, American medical-science consultant to the Nuremberg War Crimes Trials, go to the very heart of the matter:

> Had the profession taken a strong stand against the mass killing of sick Germans before the war, it is conceivable that the entire idea and technique of death factories for genocide would not have materialized. . . . far from opposing the Nazi state militantly, part of the German medical profession cooperated consciously and even willingly, while the remainder acquiesced in silence. Therefore, our regretful but inevitable judgment must be that responsibility for the inhumane perpetrations of Doctors Brandt, Handloser, and Conti, rests in large measure also upon the bulk of the German medical profession, because the profession without vigorous protest permitted itself to be ruled by such men.[145]

In contemporary American society physicians have assumed an even more active role in agitating for destruction and destroying the defective and unwanted unborn as well as expanding their destructive propaganda and technology to engulf retarded infants and others in the postnatal phase of the human life cycle. When the Supreme Court was faced with the question of what to do with unwanted unborn children, it was acutely aware of the exceptional skill demonstrated by doctors in disposing of them in the antiseptic atmospheres

of hospitals and abortion chambers. The justices were especially impressed by the oft repeated contention that abortion
in the hands of the licensed physician is safer than bringing the
child to term.[146] Thus, skill in technological extermination has
come to be a predominant criterion for the acceptability of
destruction.

If the American Medical Association and other prestigious
groups of physicians had taken a strong stand against killing
in the womb in the 1960s, it is quite likely that most doctors
would have ceased their destructive activities. Furthermore,
the Supreme Court would never have sanctioned the legalized
killing of the unborn if it had not already been convinced
that this is what most doctors wished or were already doing
in violation of the laws. Evidence from publications, meetings,
and surveys indicates an overwhelming medical consensus in
favor of abortion law liberalization or repeal. Even if these
sources are not entirely representative, most physicians have
been apathetic at best with regard to protecting the legal
right to life of the unborn. Medical killing today closely parallels medical killing in the Third Reich, but goes even further: a considerably greater part of organized medicine in
America cooperates consciously and even willingly in the destruction of unborn lives, while the remainder, for the most
part, acquiesces in silence. This same pattern of involvement
in and apathy toward killing on the part of American medicine
also threatens the existence of many human beings after
birth.

Part Two

THE TECHNOLOGY OF
DESTRUCTION

CHAPTER 4

Death Selection

A death-selection process that culminates in the destruction of millions cannot be a random, disorganized, or personalized undertaking. It must be a systematic, bureaucratic
endeavor that allows little room for personal initiative. It
must be a technical, abstract and impersonal enterprise, with
much of the decision making entrusted to committees of experts. In Nazi Germany physicians were among the most
active death selectors; in contemporary American society
doctors, parents, and others have played major roles in the
task of choosing candidates for oblivion. A fuller grasp of
how the mechanics of death selection operated in the Third
Reich and how they function today provides insight into how
it is possible to kill so many individuals with so much facility.

Death Selection in Nazi Germany

During the 1920s in Germany the choice of which unborn
human lives should be destroyed was often simply a matter
between the woman who desired the abortion and the doctor
who was willing to carry out her wishes. The process amounted to abortion-on-demand, with the physician in the role of
technical executioner.

As doctors began to clamor for changing the strict abortion law to legitimate what in effect many physicians were
already doing illegally, they also recommended the institution

of formalized procedures for choosing unborn expendables. Most of them included provisions for groups of medical specialists to determine whether bringing a pregnancy to term constituted a threat to the woman's life or health. While presented under the banner of moderation, the concept of health was elastic enough to provide doctors with considerable leeway in certifying unborn candidates for extermination through abortion.

In 1927, the Chamber of Physicians for the province of East Prussia published criteria for abortion emphasizing that "the decision for interruption of pregnancy must be reached unanimously, following a consultation of at least two physicians, one of whom is a member of the commission appointed for that purpose by the executive committee of the Chamber of Physicians — in certain instances, at the suggestion of the medical societies." [1] The 1933 law permitting legalized destruction of the unborn by licensed physicians included a provision for decision making by a system of consulting physicians. It also specified that abortions were to be performed only in approved public hospitals and private clinics. [2] By 1935 the Nazi government had created "expert centers" to approve simultaneous sterilization and abortion "so long as the child is not viable; that is, before the end of the sixth month of pregnancy." Only Aryan doctors were allowed to serve as experts. [3]

Abortion was also exported beyond the borders of Germany to encompass the unwanted and subpar unborn of the captive eastern territories. The usual decision-making apparatus, designed to give a semblance of a reputable, thoroughly deliberated process, was dispensed with altogether. Selection for extinction was reduced to the desires of the woman pregnant with an unwanted child. The decree granting approval for abortion-on-request for female Eastern workers was issued on April 5, 1943 by Reich Health Leader Dr. Leonardo Conti:

> Subject: Interruption of pregnancy of female Eastern workers.
>
>   In agreement with the Reich Commissioner for the

Strengthening of Germanism, basing myself on the
authority delegated to me by the Plenipotentiary General for Labor Allocation on 12 May 1942, I herewith
order that in the case of female Eastern workers the
"Directions for Interruption of Pregnancy and Sterilization for Health Reasons" ... may be departed from
and that the pregnancy may be interrupted if the
pregnant woman so desires.[4]

Not all pregnant female Eastern laborers were fully indoctrinated. Some resisted being aborted. If the so-called
"racial examinations" conducted on the pregnant woman and
the suspected father revealed that the unborn child possessed
the probability of an impure hereditary endowment, the doctors decided on abortion against her wishes. According to
one of the documents entered in evidence at the trial of the
Race and Settlement Main Office: "It is known that racially
inferior offspring of Eastern workers and Poles is to be avoided
if at all possible. Although pregnancy interruptions ought
to be carried out on a voluntary basis only, pressure is to be
applied in each of these cases."[5]

The medical selection of postnatal expendables for extermination began in the fall of 1939, when questions drafted
by medical experts in the Reich Ministry of the Interior were
sent to the heads of German mental hospitals. Information
on each patient, including the type and degree of illness and
disability, had to be filled out and the completed forms returned to the Ministry of the Interior. Photostats were made
of the forms and sent to four psychiatric experts in the medical
section of the Euthanasia Program, headed by Dr. Karl
Brandt. After a cursory glance at the documents, they made
a determination of life or death. When all four psychiatrists
or a majority of them decided upon euthanasia for the patient,
a top senior medical expert gave the final authorization for
implementation of this decision.[6]

The selection apparatus, the many committees and individuals involved at various levels of decision making, conveyed
the impression that decisions of life and death were being
made only after careful deliberation and consultation. In

actual practice, death selection turned out to be a wholly arbitrary and indiscriminate process that consumed countless victims for a wide range of reasons. The 'incurable" designation became a convenient diagnostic catchall encompassing many categories of patients, including the mentally ill, defectives, epileptics, deaf mutes, and others. The psychiatric experts showed little reluctance about certifying candidates for death at a staggering rate. Hundreds of thousands of patients were sentenced to death on the basis of forms inaccurately, incompletely, and ambiguously filled out.

In those psychiatric institutions where doctors were in short supply the carefully designed medical-bureaucratic charade crumbled entirely. The power of death selection was frequently delegated to nurses and attendants. How flagrantly they abused this awesome authority was revealed by a German physician to Nuremberg War Crimes psychiatric consultant Dr. Leo Alexander:

> Whoever looked sick or was otherwise a problem was put on a list and was transported to the killing center. The worst thing about this business was that it produced a certain brutalization of the nursing personnel. They got to simply picking out those whom they did not like, and the doctors had so many patients that they did not even know them, and put their names on the list.[7]

A medical-bureaucratic procedure was also at the center of the selection of children for destruction. A special agency, the Reich Committee for Research on Hereditary and Constitutional Severe Diseases, coordinated this phase of the destruction process. Questionnaires this time were filled out by health departments, chiefs of children's hospitals, midwives, and various children's institutions. Another committee of experts, composed primarily of pediatricians and psychiatrists, decreed euthanasia for children on the basis of these questionnaires. The recipients included defective, retarded, handicapped, and mentally ill children, as well as bed wetters and delinquents.[8]

Sometime in 1941 commissions of physicians were choosing death candidates in the concentration camps. Under the code name "14 f 13," medical commissions made numerous visits to concentration camps for the purpose of selecting mentally and physically deficient inmates for the gas chambers. They examined candidates and filled out forms. The examinations involved only a cursory study of personal records in the presence of the inmates.[9]

Dachau camp physician Dr. Julius Muthig testified as to the speed and superficiality of the physician-conducted selections:

> We four doctors sat at four tables placed between two huts, and several hundred prisoners had to file in front of us. The prisoners were divided according to their fitness for work and their political record. Since this commission stayed at Dachau only a few days, it was impossible for it to examine so many prisoners in so short a time. The examinations consisted solely of a rapid study of the documents in the prisoner's presence.[10]

In many instances the medical commissions did not even bother to go through the motions of looking at the camp inhabitants. A letter from Dr. Fritz Mennecke to his wife on November 25, 1941, provided information on how this procedure was carried out at the Buchenwald camp:

> As a second group a total of 1,200 Jews followed, all of whom do not need to be "examined," but where it is sufficient to take the reasons for their arrest from the files (often very voluminous!) and to transfer them to the reports. Therefore, it is merely theoretical work which will certainly keep us busy.... Exactly as the day I described above, the following days will pass — with exactly the same program and the same work. After the Jews, another 300 Aryans follow as a third group who will again have to be "examined." [11]

Besides the selections carried out by visiting medical commissions, each camp evolved its own method of choosing who would live and who would die. Concentration camp doctors assumed considerable responsibility for carrying out this particular task.

The first selections in the camps usually occurred just after the victims got off the trains onto the unloading platforms. The immediate purpose was to weed out all those deemed unfit to work because of age, disability, pregnancy, and illnesses of various kinds. Rudolph Höss described how the process of medical selections worked at Auschwitz:

> We had two SS doctors on duty at Auschwitz to examine the incoming transports of prisoners. The prisoners would be marched by one of the doctors who would make spot decisions as they walked by. Those who were fit for work were sent into the camp. Others were sent immediately to the extermination plants. Children of tender years were invariably exterminated since by reason of their youth they were unable to work.[12]

The major role played by doctors in selecting millions for extermination unfolded with conspicuous clarity at the Belsen trial, held in Lüneburg from September 17 through November 17, 1945. On this occasion, Josef Kramer and forty-four others were tried for war crimes and crimes against humanity conducted in the death camps of Auschwitz and Belsen. Although the survivors and the accused often presented conflicting testimony about what went on in the camps, they generally agreed that the bulk of the selections was carried out by physicians.

Defendant Franz Hoessler told the court about the physician-conducted death-selection process at Auschwitz:

> Whilst I was there selection of prisoners for the gas chamber was done by Dr. Klein, Dr. Mengele and other young doctors whose names I do not know. I have attended these parades, but my job was merely

to keep order. Often women were paraded naked in front of the doctors and persons selected by the doctors were sent to the gas chamber. I learnt this through conversation with the doctors. I think those selected were mostly those who were not in good health and could not work. When transports of prisoners arrived the prisoners were taken from the train and marched to the camp. On arrival they were paraded in front of the doctors I have mentioned, and persons were selected for the gas chamber.... Train-loads of 2000 and 3000 arrived at the camp and often as many as 800 went to the gas chamber. The doctors were always responsible for these selections.[13]

Prosecution witness Dr. Ada Bimko, a Jewish doctor from Poland who survived Auschwitz, gave attorney Colonel T. M. Backhouse a comprehensive picture of how physicians chose victims in three locations: on arrival, within the camp, and in the camp hospital.

When we got to Auschwitz Station we left the train and were lined up, men on one side and women on the other. Women and children were loaded on trucks and sent away. An S.S. doctor pointed with his fingers and said "Right" and "Left," looking at the women and children, and we, the younger women, were treated in the same way. Part of these people selected were loaded on to trucks and later I was told they were sent into the crematorium and gassed.

After that date did you attend any other selections of this kind? — Yes. I was working as a doctor in the hospital and was present at seven selections. The first of these happened on the day of the greatest feast of the Jews, the Day of Atonement. There were three methods of selection. The first one immediately on the arrival of the prisoners; the second in the camp among the healthy prisoners; and the third in the hospital amongst the sick. The camp doctor was always present and other S.S. men and S.S. women.

At the selections that you attended or saw in the hospitals, how were people chosen there? — All the sick Jews were ordered to parade quite naked in front of the doctor. The seemingly weak people were put aside at once, but other times the doctor looked also at the hands or at the arms and any small sort of thing which caught his attention was sufficient for him.... The S.S. doctors who took part in the selections were Dr. Rohde, Dr. Tilot, Dr. Klein, Dr. König and Dr. Mengele.[14]

Even one of the most prominent death selectors, defendant Dr. Fritz Klein, indicated before the Belsen tribunal that he and his colleagues assumed a large share of the responsibility for dispatching death candidates to the gas chambers. The following series of questions and responses between defense attorney Major T. C. M. Winwood and Dr. Klein provides the kind of frank details about death selection largely absent from the testimony of most medical perpetrators brought to trial:

Will you tell us what happened on selections? — Dr. Wirtz, when the first transport arrived, gave me orders to divide it into two parts, those who were fit to work and those who were not fit, that is those who because of their age, could not work, who were too weak, whose health was not very good, and also children up to the age of fifteen. The selecting was done exclusively by doctors. One looked at the person and, if she looked ill, asked a few questions, but if the person was healthy then it was decided immediately.

What happened to those people who were selected as capable of work? — The doctor had only to make the decision. What happened to them afterwards was nothing to do with him.

What happened to those people whom the doctors selected as unfit for work? — The doctor had to make a selection but had no influence on what was going to happen. I have heard, and I know, that part of them were sent to the gas chambers and the crematoria.[15]

In a statement submitted to the court, Dr. Klein included additional information about the prominence of medical involvement in death selection:

> There were several doctors in that camp, the chief one being Dr. Wirtz; others whose names I can remember are Dr. Fischer, Dr. Kitt, Dr. Lucas, Dr. Mengele, Dr. Thilo, Dr. Rohde and Dr. König. When transports arrived at Auschwitz it was the doctor's job to pick out those who were unfit or unable to work. These included children, old people and the sick. I have seen the gas chambers and crematoria at Auschwitz, and I knew that those I selected were to go to the gas chamber. . . . All the doctors whom I have previously mentioned have taken part in these selections, and although S.S. guards were on parade they took no active part in choosing those who were unfit to work. . . . It was not a pleasure to take part in these parades, as I knew the persons selected would go to the gas chamber. Persons who became pregnant whilst in the camp and therefore unfit for work were also selected on later parades.[16]

Most doctors involved in the death selection process performed their tasks in a perfunctory, robot-like fashion. There were those, nonetheless, who seemed to relish exercising power over life and death. This was particularly the case for Auschwitz physician Dr. Josef Mengele. He had a habit of making selections almost any time of day or night while whistling operatic tunes:

> He did not waste too much time. He made the internees disrobe to the skin. Then they had to march before him with their arms in the air while he continued to whistle his Wagner. As the frightened women came forward he pointed out with his thumb: to the left; to the right!

No medical considerations governed his decisions. They seemed to be entirely arbitrary.[17]

On other occasions Dr. Mengele dispensed with the pretense of selection altogether and "stood there like a statue, his arm always pointing in the same direction: to the left. Thus whole trainloads were expedited to the gas chambers and pyres."[18]

The entire selection process, whether implemented by committees of physicians or camp doctors, was nothing less than a mockery of medical science. The diagnostic function was severely perverted and turned into an instrument for sending huge numbers to their deaths. The arbitrary and promiscuous manner in which physicians wielded power over life and death was unprecedented. There seemed to be no end to the numbers and types of candidates suitable for extermination.

The medical death selectors did not ordinarily view the horrible consequences of their decisions. They could therefore go on indefinitely without being bothered. Their involvement remained at the psychologically safe and abstract level of shuffling papers and placing marks on documents.

Death Selection American Style

The decision regarding which unborn children would live and which would be killed by abortion had, like the Nazi death-selection process, fairly modest beginnings, and then blossomed into a full-scale bureaucratic endeavor, routinely implemented by committees of experts.

When hospital therapeutic abortion committees were first formed in the late 1940s, those who served on them assumed that the medical destruction of unborn children was to be a highly restricted practice, a last-resort alternative allowed only in situations where bringing the child to term would surely kill the mother or severely threaten her life. In fact, one of the major reasons for the establishment of therapeutic

abortion committees was to "serve as a deterrent to the indiscriminate use of therapeutic abortion." [19]

Committee members were acutely aware of what was at
stake. It was a truly monumental moral dilemma they faced,
sometimes boiling down to the stark reality of the mother's
life versus the life of her unborn child. The margin for error
in decision making had to be cut to the bare bone. There
was no glossing over the fact that a decision in favor of therapeutic abortion meant that one human life would be sacrificed
to save another human life. The committees did not attempt
to minimize the gravity of the conflict, as is so often done
today, by portraying it in terms of the woman's privacy versus an unwanted and expendable piece of tissue.

With such awesome and irreversible consequences to
ponder, it is understandable why these committees moved
with the utmost caution. They worked out procedures, rules,
and levels for assessments and selections. Typically, the decision-making process was initiated by the woman's physician,
because he believed her life was endangered by the pregnancy.
He was required to specify in writing the reasons for recommending abortion and to supply supporting documentation.
The independent opinion of another physician was also generally required. In addition, the signed consent of both the
woman and her husband was needed before any decisions
could be made. All the documents were submitted to the
therapeutic abortion committee, which had the final authority
over life and death.

The committee membership usually consisted of three and
not more than ten individuals. Obstetricians and gynecologists
made up the bulk of the members while the inclusion of psychiatrists became a frequent practice once psychiatric reasons
began to dominate the death-selection process in the 1960s.
A unanimous decision of the committee was often necessary
before an unborn child could be condemned to death. Sometimes a majority of three-fourths or some other figure was
sufficient. Whatever the differences in the procedures adopted,
each committee tried to obtain a comprehensive and objective
picture before making a choice. Most committees were very

reluctant to grant approval for an abortion request unless the supporting documentation was clear and compelling.

If the procedures developed seemed overly cumbersome they at least held the number of abortions and abortion requests down to a minimum. Just how effective·therapeutic abortion committees were in counteracting unrestrained abortion can be gleaned from the records of various hospitals. During the ten-year period from July 1952 through July 1962, the therapeutic abortion committee at the Marin General Hospital in San Rafael, California received only eighteen applications for abortion, and out of these, twelve were approved and six denied.[20] Statistics compiled at the Santa Monica Hospital from 1958 through 1962 indicated a rejection rate of 60 percent; only six of fifteen abortion requests were granted.[21]

The original restrictive intent underlying therapeutic abortion committees was swept away in the 1960s and 1970s, when the reasons justifying abortion frantically increased with neither moral nor legal restraint. The committees quickly degenerated into instruments for certifying unprecedented numbers of unborn children for destruction. They became handy bureaucratic mechanisms for processing hundreds of thousands of victims to oblivion.

A lion's share of the credit for this irresponsible display of raw medical power must be laid on the shoulders of psychiatrists. As long as a psychiatrist could be found to authorize that continuation of the pregnancy would prove psychologically harmful for the woman, the committees simply served as rubber stamps to legitimize such an assessment. Because the supply of psychiatrists willing to stand behind such a Godlike diagnosis proved more than ample, the door to massive indiscriminate destruction was swung wide open.

Psychiatrists often resorted to invoking the increased-risk-of-suicide-during-pregnancy canard as a convenient device for justifying the decision to abort. Research studies, by contrast, have indicated that suicide among pregnant women is so rare as to be almost nonexistent. A study conducted in Sweden in the late 1940s revealed that 62 out of 344 women whose requests for therapeutic abortion were refused threatened to commit suicide, but none of them carried out their threats.[22]

After reviewing the records of suicides from 1950 to 1956, the coroner of Birmingham, England concluded: "We have no record of any woman known to be pregnant having committed suicide." [23] While the incidence of suicide for all women of childbearing years, age 14 through 50, in New York City in 1953 was 5.5 per 100,000, it was 0.55 per 100,000 for pregnant women. Thus, the suicide rate among pregnant women was only one-tenth that of non-pregnant women. [24] Psychiatric duplicity notwithstanding, pregnancy is far more likely to be a protection against rather than a precipitant of self-destruction.

Almost overnight, huge majorities of 85 to 90 percent of abortions were performed on mental health grounds. In the first year of California's "liberal" abortion law, for example, 88 percent of abortions were performed for psychiatric reasons. Such false widespread certification of susceptibility to mental illness of pregnant women in order to rationalize abortion on psychiatric grounds shows how far psychiatrists went in prostituting the task of professional diagnosis.

At an abortion conference held in 1955 in New York City, Yale psychiatrist Dr. Theodore Lidz gave his assessment of what was really going on:

> Let us be frank about this. When the psychiatrist says that there is a suicidal risk, in many instances he does not mean that at all, but feels that there are strong socioeconomic grounds for a therapeutic abortion. Since the only ground for abortion in many states is if it is felt there is threat of death, suicidal risk is thus established as the only legal way out of the situation. [25]

By 1969, even the illustrious Group for the Advancement of Psychiatry had to admit that "most abortions now performed legally by licensed physicians were performed by stretching the concept of 'psychiatric grounds' to the breaking point." [26]

Another account reflecting the rank hypocrisy of psychiatric involvement in the death-selection process was provided in the early 1970s by a medical staff member of a New York abortion hospital:

> For a hundred dollars the patient went to the psychiatrist and he would say, "You're going to kill yourself if you don't have this abortion?" "Yes," "Okay, goodbye." Then he dictates a nice long letter she's suicidal. So. Two psychiatrists, two hundred dollars. It was a farce.[27]

It should be recalled that among the medical specialities responsible for choosing German expendables for euthanasia, psychiatry was predominant. The psychiatric role in choosing unwanted postnatal individuals for destruction during the late 1930s and 1940s in Nazi Germany was a blatant abuse of power and a perversion of psychiatry. An identical conclusion holds regarding psychiatric participation in authorizing unwanted prenatal lives for extinction during the 1960s and early 1970s in the United States.

Gone from the American therapeutic abortion committee system was any semblance of balance, objectivity, and careful weighing of factors. Decision making was reduced to the perfunctory task of shuffling papers, checking signatures, and routinely authorizing destruction for great numbers of victims for an almost unlimited range of reasons. These committees came to closely resemble the committees of Nazi experts who so easily chose an untold number of candidates for destruction in an equally cursory manner.

For the most part, it became exceedingly rare for the therapeutic abortion committees of the 1960s and 1970s to refuse any requests for abortion. However, there were some recalcitrant committees that refused to play the game; against overwhelming odds, they tried to maintain some semblance of a valid decision-making process. This angered the pro-death forces to no end; such committees were not producing their share of death candidates. A campaign of vilification was mounted against these renegades; they were called rigid and reactionary (common designations used by pro-abortionists against any group that disagrees with their so-called enlightened and liberal posture). This led to intensified attacks leveled against all therapeutic abortion committees, even those that cranked out impressive numbers of death sentences. The strategy was to portray the committees as worthless bureaucratic relics that had outlived their usefulness. The next logical step was to get rid of them altogether. A paper presented to the Ontario Hospital Convention on October 25, 1971 by Dr. Edward Wilson incorporates this tactic: "The only practical solution is to eliminate the administrative encumbrances imposed on medical staffs and hospital administration by ... deleting the necessity of therapeutic abortion committees." [28]

What abortion proponents fail to mention is that it was often their ideas in the first place that led to the creation of what they characterized as bureaucratic monstrosities. It is almost as if they were formed on purpose in order to more fully discredit them and thus pave the way for what many abortion zealots were really after: repeal and not liberalization of abortion laws. What repeal does in effect is remove the necessity for therapeutic abortion committees, since the decision to destroy becomes strictly a matter between the woman and her doctor and no one else.

The drive for repeal won out with the US Supreme Court decision on abortion of January 22, 1973. The power to kill was suddenly de-bureaucratized. All mediating structures and hope for even moderate restraints vanished. The Court declared that "abortion in all its aspects is inherently, and primarily, a medical decision, and basic responsibility for it must rest with the physician." [29] How very similar this is to the power granted to Nazi physicians by Adolf Hitler for implementing the euthanasia program in 1939! [30]

The Supreme Court's bestowal of authority to kill the unborn is even more far-reaching than that granted by Hitler to eliminate those already born. While only certain doctors in Nazi Germany were given the power to decide who would be killed, all American physicians can exercise this power if they so choose. Furthermore, while there is some controversy over the question of how legally binding a pronouncement written on Hitler's personal stationery was, there is no doubt whatsoever about the Supreme Court declaration being the law of the land in all fifty states of the union. Despite these differences, both statements not only give the authority to kill to doctors, but also allow them considerable latitude in setting up structures and procedures for carrying out this authority.

Further parallels are evident in the matter of practical application. As we have seen, the "careful diagnosis" imperative of Hitler's pronouncement was abused beyond imagination. Nazi physicians had no qualms about exercising the power of death selection ruthlessly and indiscriminately. The same holds true for contemporary American physicians. The prodigious number of unborn children destroyed by doctors since the Supreme Court decision stands in stark contradiction to Chief Justice Warren Burger's statements that "the vast majority of physicians observe the standards of their profession, and act only on the basis of carefully deliberated medical judgments relating to life and health" and "the Court today rejects any claim that the Constitution requires abortions on demand." [31] While the Constitution as interpreted by the Supreme Court may not require abortion-on-demand, it certainly allows it. Despite disclaimers to the contrary, abortion-on-demand is in fact the law of the land in present-day America, and there is no letup in sight.

Although many physicians view their involvement in death selection as a routine matter, some feel very uncomfortable in this kind of role. Their reservations are not due, unfortunately, to any personal or professional opposition to killing unborn babies per se. Their reluctance stems rather from the fact that a huge proportion of abortions are done for reasons having no relation to medicine whatsoever. They therefore favor leaving the decision-making responsibility entirely in the hands of the woman pregnant with an unwanted child. Their only concern is a technological one: to make sure that a decision already made by someone else is implemented efficiently and safely. This in essence constitutes a handy denial of responsibility for destruction. It is closely akin to the higher orders concoction manufactured by Nazi physicians. Doctors in the Third Reich justified medical killing on the basis of law (Hitler's euthanasia directive) and decisions made by other authorities (committees of experts).

Today's doctors also place the liability for destruction elsewhere: on the law (the Supreme Court abortion decision) and on other authorities (therapeutic abortion committees, and more recently, the pregnant woman).

On the other hand, those who actually make the decision to kill unborn babies likewise do not feel culpable, since their involvement is primarily on an abstract level. This is especially true for death selection by committees. Committee members participate in a sometimes philosophical but mainly arbitrary, routine activity. The most crucial element of death-selection committees is that they are composed of bureaucratic paper handlers who stay personally removed from the harsh consequences of their decisions. When pregnant women assume the major burden for choosing abortion, many of them see the matter only in terms of availing themselves of a constitutional right. They go to a hospital or clinic as recipients of what is defined as respectable medical treatment. As long as they do not have to perform the destructive act or see it in operation, their consciences can remain undisturbed.

The entire gist of this is: nobody feels responsible for anything. It is an incredibly effective system for allaying scruples by shifting responsibility onto someone or something else. Its kinship with the medical death-selection process of Nazi Germany is striking and uncomfortably close.

The unbridled killing of unborn children has gotten so out of hand that even some pro-abortion doctors have begun to demonstrate concern. There is even talk about returning to some type of committee arrangement for deciding who should live and who should be aborted. Foremost among advocates of this position is Dr. Bernard N. Nathanson. After presiding over what he finally admitted were "60,000 deaths" as director of the Center for Reproductive and Sexual Health, "the largest — abortion clinic in the Western world," Dr. Nathanson exhibited dismay over the fact that "the most serious responsibility a woman can experience in her lifetime" was taken so lightly. The profound sense of loss normally associated with the taking of human life had gotten completely squelched in the assembly-line dispatching of victims through this facility. Nathanson recognizes the emptiness of the phrase "between a woman and her physician," because it invariably means death for the unborn child. He believes that genuine decision making would be better served by the addition of a consultative body of new types of specialists — "a psychohistorian, a human ecologist, a medical philosopher, an urbanologist-clergyman." Such a group could, according to Nathanson, bring to the pregnant woman "the whole sweep of human experience to bear on the decision — not just the narrow partisanship of committed young women who have had abortions and who typically staff the counselor ranks of hospitals and clinics now." [32]

Even though unborn children constitute by far the largest category of individuals selected for destruction, there are others besides the unborn who are considered fair game. Physicians, parents, relatives or groups composed of both physicians and family members are starting to take on an expanded role in deciding whether defective newborn children should live or be allowed to die by withholding treatment or directly hastening death. In the fall of 1963, doctors at the Johns Hopkins Hospital Center in Baltimore, Maryland decided not to perform a routine operation on a newborn mongoloid child with an intestinal obstruction because his parents did not want him. The failure to operate resulted in the child's death fifteen days later. [33] In this case the parents were granted the decision-making authority over life and death while the doctors submitted to and implemented this decision. What happened at Johns Hopkins, unfortunately, is not that unique. It was also disclosed that three other mongoloid children at Johns Hopkins had previously suffered the same fate as this child: "Placed in a corner to die of starvation and dehydration." [34] Who knows in how many other hospitals before and since the Johns Hopkins case have parents sentenced their postnatal children to death because of defects of one sort or another! An educated guess is that such a practice occurs far more often than the public is aware of.

Group death selection was the mode responsible for the deaths of forty-three critically ill and congenitally deformed infants at the Yale University intensive-care nursery during the period January 1, 1970 through June 30, 1972. This disclosure reflects a growing tendency for doctors, parents, nurses, and other hospital personnel to join forces in reaching decisions of such "awesome finality." The death-selection process at Yale is described as taking place in a small closely-knit community of parents and hospital staff members "in which a concerted attempt is made to ensure that each member may participate in and know about the major decisions that concern him or her." Final decision making, however, resides with the doctor, "so that the family will not have to bear that heavy burden alone." [35]

After a review and discussion of these forty-three deaths, Drs. Raymond S. Duff and A. G. M. Campbell came up with their own conclusions regarding the burdens of death selection. While disavowing any "allocation of death" policy according to the extreme excesses of Hegelian "rational utility" under a dictatorship, they are all for a policy that allows "much latitude" in decision making: "Society and the health professions should provide only general guidelines," but the "burdens of decision making must be borne by families and their professional advisors because they are most familiar with the respective situations." [36] What this boils down to is: as long as the doctor gives a full and honest presentation of "all management options and their expected consequences," the parents should have the authority to decide if the child should live or die.

The debate will continue to rage over which individual, group, or system can best make life-and-death decisions for unborn children and deficient infants. The tragedy here is that so few doctors bother to even question the assumption of death selection as an acceptable management option.

A group of doctors at the Maryland Institute for Emergency Medicine took it upon themselves to select and kill accident victims whose spinal cords had been severed just below the base of the skull. The procedure followed was revealed to the *Washington Post* on March 10, 1974:

> When these patients arrive at the shock trauma
> unit, physicians insert breathing tubes and hook them

up to respirators. After a few weeks of treatment and study, and after the doctors are sure there is no chance for improvement, the quadraplegics are killed. Without a patient's knowledge or consent, he is drugged so that he will not know what is happening and will not feel the terror of dying. Then he is unplugged. These doctors feel it would be "inhumane" to ask the patient if he wants to live or die since, as one doctor puts it, "everyone dearly loves life." [37]

In September 1967, it was learned that Dr. William McMath, superintendent of a London hospital, posted a notice on the bulletin board instructing the staff not to resuscitate certain elderly patients. The instructions read in part:

> The following patients are not to be resuscitated: very elderly, over 65; malignant disease. Chronic chest disease. Chronic renal disease . . . Top of yellow treatment card to be marked NTBR (i.e., not to be resuscitated). [38]

Public protests notwithstanding, Dr. McMath's actions were upheld by the Regional Hospital Board. He was criticized not for the resuscitation orders, but for their wording and the indiscreet manner in which they were displayed. It was considered more appropriate to convey this type of guidance in a less public, more confidential way.

One of the greatest similarities between the approaches employed to choose candidates for destruction in Nazi Germany and in today's society is that those selected for death are usually the very ones left out of the decision-making process. Someone else decides their fate. They are considered incapable of making such a determination because of age, incapacity and other reasons; or they are declared ineligible because of being unwanted. The legal right to choose the destruction of others, whether born or unborn, and the license to carry out their death sentences represent the ultimate forms of oppression. For their ultra-efficient role in routinely consigning massive numbers of victims to oblivion, physicians surely rank among the most prominent oppressors in history.

CHAPTER 5

Assembly-Line Processing at the Killing Sites

It is no insignificant feat to kill millions; it is a task bound to be fraught with innumerable problems. It cannot be done alone. It must be a cooperative venture requiring meticulous planning, special equipment, and buildings, personnel, and operational procedures. Above all, it must be a highly organized undertaking that integrates all these ingredients into a smoothly functioning operation. The modern industrial factory with its assembly line provides the ideal model for the enormous task of dispatching so many to their deaths.

In Nazi Germany, the euthanasia institutions and concentration camps served as the death factories where the victims were systematically processed out of existence. The key to their success was the presence of individuals and groups of specialists at crucial points all along the assembly line of death. Doctors played the leading role in the euthanasia hospitals, and had a significant part in the concentration camps as well. Able assistance came from various professional and technical specialists, such as nurses, attendants, administrators, gassing technicians, body-disposal squads, statisticians, and others.

Assembly-line extermination of the unborn takes place in two types of modern-day death factories: hospitals and abortion clinics. The array of specialists employed in these facilities is vast and impressive. It includes psychiatrists, obstetricians, pediatricians, surgeons, nurses, anesthesiologists, attendants, pathologists, scientists, researchers, counselors, receptionists, clerks, statisticians, and others.

The employment of so many specialists is necessary in order to insure the success of such gigantic projects of destruction. The involvement of doctors and nurses is an especially consoling sight and helps sustain the myth of a valid medical undertaking rather than a horrendous atrocity. The utilization of different individuals for the performance of diverse tasks throughout the various phases of destruction has had the effect of so dispersing the responsibility for killing that no one feels personally accountable. Each individual is merely a technician busily preoccupied with his or her specialized task. Thus, the doctor who helps select the victims does not kill them; the doctor who administers the lethal substance or wields the sharp instrument is only "medically" implementing a decision made by someone else; the nurse generally neither selects nor kills but simply assists the doctor in carrying out a medical procedure; the body disposers merely remove dead bodies already selected and killed by others. What a convenient division of labor!

Euthanasia Hospitals

One of the most significant but least publicized findings to come out of the Nazi holocaust is that those physicians and non-physician technicians who were responsible for so efficiently destroying individuals in the concentration camps did not become proficient death specialists overnight. Many of them first learned to kill in hospitals. Several years before Hitler gave approval for the final solution to the Jewish question, doctors had already begun to practice and perfect their destructive skills on the mentally ill and retarded, the chronically and incurably ill, the unproductive aged, and other unwanted Germans in the euthanasia hospitals of the Third Reich. Six institutions — Grafeneck, Brandenburg, Hartheim, Sonnenstein, Hadamar, and Bernburg — were set aside for the purpose of exterminating adults, while four

others — Eichberg, Idstein, Kantenhof, and Gorden — specialized in killing children.[1]

Simon Wiesenthal, an individual who has spent his life
hunting down Nazi war criminals still at large, came upon
documentation that revealed a major function of euthanasia
centers in addition to killing lives considered not worth
living: as schools for mass murder. Typical among them was
Hartheim, which "was organized like a medical school —
except that the 'students' were not taught to save human life
but to destroy it as efficiently as possible."[2]

Graduates of such places learned their lessons well. When
called upon to take charge of the more monumental job of
exterminating millions in the gas champers of Belzec, Sobibor,
Treblinka, Auschwitz, and Dachau, they succeeded admirably.
Their success can be attributed, in large part, to the superior
technical and psychological training they received in the
euthanasia institutions. The following facts cannot be reiter-
ated enough: physicians directed the entire euthanasia program; killing was supervised and often done by doctors; the
gas chambers were first developed and tested in euthanasia
hospitals; the technical excellence displayed by doctors in
perfecting hospital assembly-line destruction provided a model
worthy of emulation for the more massive program of racial
genocide carried out in the concentration camps; the presence
of doctors in the camps gave a legitimacy to the destruction
process it would not have otherwise possessed. Although far
more lives were destroyed in the concentration camps than in
the euthanasia institutions, what went on in these hospitals
set a standard of technological destruction that spread to other
destructive projects.

Euthanasia institutions, to repeat, specialized in killing
Germans not up to par with the Aryan ideal of perfection.
Although the main victims were Germans, Jews and others
were later included. It is important to gain a more specific
grasp of how the destruction process operated in the euthanasia centers before analyzing the concentration camps.

The process of killing German defectives and later those
not so defective was a major undertaking. It was the first time
a medical bureaucracy had ever been given the task of remov-

ing a considerable number of individuals from society and
various institutions with the intent of putting them to death
within the confines of hospital settings. The euthanasia program contained elaborate procedures for selecting victims and
sending them to the appropriate institutions, where they were
killed in specially constructed gas chambers and burned in
furnaces. Later, when the chambers were dismantled and
transferred to the camps, the method of destruction changed
to lethal injections, and body disposal was by burying in community graves.

Destruction was helped along by the physical layout of
the euthanasia institutions, which was designed to conceal
the killing behind a facade of immaculate hospital-type surroundings. The victims felt consoled up to the very end as
they were injected with lethal substances and tucked into
comfortable hospital beds. The situation at the Hartheim institution typified how important the setting was for relieving
inmate fears. The first glimpse that those sent there received
was a reassuring one: a secluded Renaissance castle with a
beautiful colonnade. The interior resembled a medical school
where the victims thought they would be getting superior
care while making contributions to scientific knowledge.[3]
Instead, they were dispatched to extinction within the confines of a medically-clad and orchestrated setting.

Another feature of decor pioneered in the euthanasia institutions was the idea of disguising gas chambers as shower
rooms. The patients were deceived into believing they were
simply going to take a shower. They went to their deaths
calmly and peacefully. Victor Brack's testimony to the Nuremberg tribunal revealed how smoothly this worked out in practical application: "The patient did not realize that he was
about to be killed. There were benches and chairs in the
chamber. A few minutes after the gas was let in, the patient
became sleepy and tired and died after a few minutes. They
simply went to sleep without even knowing that they were
going to sleep."[4] This was considered such a masterful means
of hiding destructive intentions from the victims that it was
imported to the concentration camps for adoption on a massive scale.

The series of phases through which those slated for extermination passed were models of deception and efficiency of operation. Throughout the journey the victims were handled with care and compassion, as if they were bona fide patients. The transfer of individuals from old age homes, general hospitals, and children's institutions to the euthanasia hospitals was accomplished with the help of many built-in reassurances. Patients with ability to comprehend what was going on were told the transfers would help them get well. Disturbed patients were given sedatives to ease their journey. They were allowed to wear their own clothing and their personal possessions were carefully packed and sent along with them.[5] The reason for this was to give credence to the myth of proper medical care. It also proved comforting for the victims, because although they were being transferred to a new institution, their private identities as persons associated with clothing and possessions would be respected and kept intact. They could not help but perceive this as an example of thoughtfulness on the part of their caretakers. With this kind of attention paid to details, it is hardly surprising that medical extermination of the so-called unfit proceeded so smoothly.

Before being dispatched to the euthanasia centers, the patients were first sent to what were called observation hospitals. The official reason given for the establishment of these intermediate institutions was to insure the granting of "dying aid" only to the most severely afflicted patients. At the Nuremberg Doctors' Trial, defendant Viktor Brack contended that the patients were carefully observed for a one to three-month period. After this, the physician in charge allegedly had the authority to overrule the decision for euthanasia made by top experts.[6] If he really had this authority, it is doubtful it was ever exercised for the true benefit of the victims; once they reached the observation hospital it was already beyond the point of no return.

A far more plausible reason for the existence of observation hospitals is indicated by author Gitta Sereny: "for camouflage purposes when the public first began to be suspicious about the destination of the blacked-out buses which fetched patients from mental hospitals."[7] This constituted window dressing to reassure the public that the patients were being scrupulously cared for in reputable institutions. It reinforced the desired overall image projected of euthanasia as a legitimate medical enterprise. The victims continued to feel reassured; a program with so much time and energy devoted to such thorough examinations could not help but be strictly for the benefit of the patient. In actuality, the observation hospitals were simply way stations to destruction.

Upon arrival at the euthanasia hospitals, the patients were led to an area where they were helped to undress. They thought they were going to take a shower. The next room they entered looked like a bath house but was really a gas chamber.

After the gas chambers had been moved to the concentration camps, the destruction still continued but in an altered form. What happened at the Hadamar Hospital illustrates how the euthanasia institutions adapted their facilities to accommodate the influx of Russian and Polish inmates allegedly afflicted with incurable tuberculosis. They were processed in an orderly and impeccably medical manner: registration, an examination of medical records, a promise of treatment to alleviate and cure their ailments, the preparation of rooms for rest, the presence of nurses and attendants to help the victims undress and get into bed. The staff members were very solicitous. The administrator of Hadamar, Alfons Klein, even took the trouble to go up to the wards in the evening and see first hand how severely the patients suffered. The real purpose of his visit was to justify Hadamar Hospital's unique way of dealing with such patients. "I myself believe," said Klein, "it is cruel if one would let them live longer." [8]

The particular method of "dying aid" granted to the patients was primarily the injection of lethal doses of morphine and scopolamine or the oral administration of poisonous pills. Sometimes the doctor in charge carried out the destructive procedure, but this task more commonly fell to members of the nursing staff. The tranquil atmosphere continued to prevail right up until the deadly injections were made. The nurse "talked very nicely to them and told them that they would receive a vaccination against infectious diseases." [9]

After death claimed the victims, the medical sham persisted as death certificates were filled out to make it appear as if they died from the trumped-up illnesses. Most patients were killed within several hours after arrival. The falsified dates gave the impression that the victims came "almost at death's doorstep... and that they lingered and suffered there for a few days, in some instances for a few weeks, and finally met their death from the ravages of the disease." [10] At the Hadamar Trial the prosecution asked Dr. Adolf Wahlmann, Hadamar's head physician, why he filed false death certificates even though he felt the destructive activities were legal. His response reflects the great sensitivity toward public relations possessed by many of the perpetrators: "I did not want to scare the population by not filling in a diagnosis. I could not put down on the death certificate, 'We killed them.'" [11]

The final reassurance was usually communicated in a form letter sent to surviving relations:

We sincerely regret the need for advising you that your daughter, ... died here suddenly and unexpectedly on August 5, 1940, of a brain edema. Because of her grave mental illness life was a torment for the deceased. You must therefore look on her death as a release. Because danger of epidemic currently threatens in this Institution, the police authorities ordered the body to be cremated immediately. We request notification to which cemetery we are to advise the police authorities to ship the urn with the mortal remains of the deceased. [12]

The medically initiated and operated process of extermination in the euthanasia hospitals was meant not only to pacify the victims, their relatives, and the public in general, but also to facilitate the continuation of active involvement by medical participants. The fact that the killing was being implemented in a hospital setting with proper medical equipment according to standard medical procedures proved to be very consoling. Also of inestimable value was the purported painlessness of the procedure and the humane intentions underlying its application: a merciful release from a painful incurable condition. Other devices such as banquets, celebrations, and noble-sounding speeches had the effect of bolstering morale and reducing the possibility of emotional disturbance resulting from involvement in the destruction process. In 1941, for instance, a special ceremony was held at Hadamar Hospital in commemoration of the cremation of the ten-thousandth patient. "Psychiatrists, nurses, attendants, and secretaries all participated. Everybody received a bottle of beer for the occasion." [13]

Two further points regarding the euthanasia program should be highlighted. One concerns the establishment of hospitals entirely or partially dedicated to the extermination of human life. The other has to do with the ease of transferability of personnel from curing to killing.

The removal of the mentally ill, incurables, and others away from the rest of the hospital population into separate institutions was considered a major innovation. On the one hand, the victims were placed a safe distance away from those patients receiving legitimate medical care. It was deemed too risky for the perpetrators, especially in a psychological sense, to combine both killing and healing under the same roof. On the other hand, the appearance of respectable medical care was retained under the guise of specialized hospitals devoted to treating patients with certain illnesses.

Specialization reached its height when entire institutions were taken over for the exclusive purpose of putting to death idiot, malformed, retarded, and mentally ill children. The killers, however, grew bolder and did not even bother to remove the doomed children from some of the legitimate hospitals. They set up, instead, special "pediatric wards" within these hospitals for killing purposes. One of the reasons for this was strictly utilitarian: the transfer of the victims to other locales of destruction was considered a waste of time, personnel, and gasoline. [14] Another reason was to more effectively conceal the killing; it was inconceivable to believe that hospitals that continued to provide genuine medical care would also exterminate helpless children.

The other component of the euthanasia killings, the

transformation of health-care personnel into killers or killer accomplices, is probably the most extraordinary part of the whole destruction process; all the more remarkable because of how easily many participants made the shift. And the change did not occur only among incompetent or mediocre professionals with sadistic inclinations. Some of the most active participants had records of long and devoted service to caring for severely afflicted individuals. A typical example of this is reflected in the answer nurse Margaret Borkowski gave when asked why she continued to work at Hadamar even though she believed that what was going on was wrong: "I belonged to the Institution of Hadamar for over 20 years. . . . I did not have any reason to go away from Hadamar." [15]

Contemporary Hospitals

Many physician-abortionists, whether specialists in hospital or abortion-clinic killing, receive their training and develop their destructive skills in the hospital setting. It is in the hospital that the modern techniques of assembly-line killing of the unborn are often first planned, tested, and gradually perfected. A number of hospitals today, like the euthanasia hospitals of Nazi Germany, serve as training grounds or schools for learning the most advanced ways of exterminating human lives.

The techniques of killing unborn children have already become an integral part of the obstetrics-gynecology residency program in many hospitals. In some programs obstetrical residents opposed to abortion must take their training in hospitals where abortions are performed. Some obstetrics professors believe that "pregnancy termination should most definitely be a required part of a residency program" even for those residents "who from personal conviction will not do abortions." [16] A survey conducted in 1976 of US hospitals with residency programs in obstetrics and gynecology revealed that 26 percent already *require* residents to perform first-trimester abortions and 23 percent require the performance of second-trimester abortions.[17] Unfortunately, many residents agree with the incorporation of unborn baby killing as a legitimate professional function. Too few of those who disagree, however, are willing to express their disapproval by resigning. They generally stay on and conform to the requirement, or at least do nothing to actively challenge it.

Too many present-day hospitals have been converted into super-sophisticated death factories for the unborn. For a massive destruction process to become so fully assimilated by those institutions whose very purpose is to save and preserve human life itself is a perversion of the highest magnitude. How readily hospital operating rooms have been used for child-destruction as well as childbirth! How much easier it is to disguise destruction in the antiseptic and clinically proper surroundings of modern hospital settings!

To destroy an unborn child in a hospital generally necessitates a stay of several days. This is not true for early abortions performed in the first three months of pregnancy, because these can usually be completed within half a day or less on an outpatient basis. Although many hospitals still do early abortions, non-hospital abortion clinics have taken over a lion's share of killing younger unborn babies. Hospitals still retain exclusive domain over the destruction of older unborn victims. The reason for this particular division of labor is strictly technological. To kill older, larger, and better developed children in the second and third trimester of pregnancy requires a great deal of technical expertise, advanced killing methods, sophisticated· equipment, close cooperation and intense psychological support among participants, and back-up life support system equipment in case the killing procedure employed endangers the aborting woman. Only in a well-stocked, efficiently functioning hospital can all the essential elements for disposing of these bigger babies be effectively integrated and operationalized.

The analysis of the destruction process in the modern hospital setting that follows will therefore focus on those later abortions performed by such techniques as saline induction, prostaglandins, and hysterotomy. Here we have a division of destructive labor somewhat akin to what happened in Nazi

Germany. Euthanasia institutions specialized in doing away with one category of victims, both young and old defective Germans. Contemporary hospitals have become quite proficient in getting rid of another category of victims, older unborn children and defective newborns.

When women enter hospitals to have their unborn children killed, they are given the same kind of service as that received by any other surgical patient. Abortion patients are systematically and scrupulously dispatched through a series of preparatory steps before the actual killing takes place. Much of this involves the usual medical preliminaries, including blood pressure, urinalysis, medical history, and other tests. These preliminary assessments indicate whether the woman is physically capable of having the child aborted out of her womb without undue complications. Psychologically, her encounter with a variety of technical specialists, frequently clad in white uniforms expertly manipulating impressive looking medical instruments, serves to convey the image of a valid medical enterprise rather than baby killing.

The passage through the hospital destruction process is meant to be more than simply a non-traumatic journey. In some hospitals the goal is even more ambitious: abortion is organized as a unique opportunity for personal growth. This stance is helped along by the presence of kind, empathetic, and technically competent staff members who literally hover over the abortee's every need and whim. The whole experience amounts to an intense ego trip, an orgy of introspection and self-centeredness unmatched by the most fanatic identity seekers.

There is a method to this madness besides the bolstering of the abortee's ego. By becoming preoccupied with her own body and welfare, she becomes less able to concentrate on the needs of her unborn child. The more tender loving care showered upon her, the more readily can she erase the image of the child from her awareness and conscience. The perpetrators are so busy caring for the aborting woman and she is so taken up with being the recipient of this care that there is no time or energy left over to consider the about-to-be-destroyed child.

The actual death of the child in the uterus after administration of saline solutions or prostaglandins commonly takes
anywhere from one to several hours. These compounds, however, do not ordinarily induce strong enough contractions to
expel the dead child until some twelve to thirty-six hours
later. The labor process itself may last from six to twelve
hours.[18] Although it takes longer to kill an unborn child in
today's modern hospital than a German defective in a euthanasia hospital, both victims, nevertheless, have been assured
a technological death at the hands of a medical executioner.

The ploy of false death certificates is not usually required
when the victims are killed early in gestation. This helps the
perpetrators maintain the stance that abortion does not involve the killing of a human being because if someone were
killed, a death certificate would surely be required. In the case
of later abortions performed in hospitals, a fetal death certificate is necessary. In New York, for example, a fetal death
certificate is supposed to be filed with the Department of
Health for every abortion performed.[19] Just what is put as the
cause of death on such documents? Again, a fraud parallel
to the falsified death certificates filled out by physicians in the
euthanasia hospitals is currently being repeated by physicians
responsible for certifying hospital abortion deaths. The cause
of death, similarly, is never truthfully recorded as physician-
induced destruction but something attributed to such accidental forces as prematurity or stillbirth. The reassuring quality
of these bogus certificates for the perpetrators and the public
is evident.

The labor that saline and prostaglandin abortees undergo
closely parallels the labor experience of a woman about to
give birth. It is not surprising, then, that some hospitals
manage the abortion patient very much like a maternity patient. Obstetricians and obstetrical nurses assume the responsibility for abortions in hospital maternity wings. One student
nurse explained how she was able to reconcile moving directly
from a maternity to an abortion unit.[20] Technicians specializing
in natural childbirth methods have even used their skills to
help women through abortion labor. A nurse specialist with
extensive experience in helping women prepare for childbirth

through the Lamaze technique of breathing and relaxation seemed to be just as much at home applying these same methods to women undergoing abortions. The results of her efforts with 416 saline abortees is set forth in the pages of a nursing journal.[21]

This illustrates another disturbing aspect of the whole destruction process, one which also characterized hospital killing in Nazi Germany: the interchangeability of technology and personnel. Apparently, the same techniques and people can be employed to support either life or destruction with equal proficiency. This has to be the ultimate in schizophrenic adaptability!

Other hospitals have found that placing abortion patients in or near the maternity section is not the most diplomatic way of running a flawless destructive operation. From the standpoint of using an already existing and well-established service, it seems to be a logical choice. Technology, however, also covers psychological factors as well as those related to efficiency. Abortion candidates as a rule do not wish to be reminded of how closely mid-trimester abortions resemble procedures associated with childbirth. At this point in their lives they are not particularly child oriented and any procedural set-up that evokes images or thoughts of babies could prove quite unnerving. To be placed in an area of the hospital "within hearing distance of the wails of the newborn" [22] is too great a confrontation with conscience. The abortee's prime psychological defense — denial that abortion is the intentional destruction of another human life — would be placed in danger of imminent collapse.

Women undergoing hospital abortions are not the only ones adversely affected when abortion and childbirth are so closely intertwined both in a technological and geographical sense. After passage of the 1967 liberalized abortion law in Colorado, staff members in the obstetrics unit at a Colorado general hospital became very upset by their involvement in saline abortions because "delivery of a dead fetus was directly opposed to the goals and values of the staff." They started to raise questions about their participation in "killing rather than delivering babies." [23] A similar reaction was expressed by nurses in Hawaiian hospitals after repeal of the state's abortion law took effect in March 1970. It was difficult for them to reconcile the incompatible demands made: "They had entered obstetrical nursing in order to save life, not prevent or take it." [24] From the Hawaiian experience, Drs. John F. McDermott and Walter F. Char draw a conclusion that they contend is based on the practices of some less-developed cultures: "That maternity experiences must not exist in general medical settings, that life and death cannot exist geographically or psychologically together." [25]

A typical resolution of this dilemma is for hospitals to separate abortions from obstetrical services. This involves setting up a department in the hospital exclusively devoted to performing abortions. This may not be such a costly or impractical step, since some hospitals already kill more babies than they deliver alive; abortion, the public is continually told, is the most common surgical procedure in America next to tonsillectomy.[26] Another variation is the incorporation of abortions into the surgical instead of the obstetrics unit. A rationale for this particular practice is offered by one nurse writing in the *American Journal of Nursing* of July 1971: "The logical placement would be the surgical unit; not only would the patient be likely to encounter a less emotionally involved nurse, but it seems healthier — and more accurate — to regard abortion as surgical intervention rather than as a failure of pregnancy." [27]

The assignment of unborn baby killing tasks to a separate department of the hospital is done for the same reason that defective children were destroyed in the special pediatric wards of Nazi hospitals: to mask the killing within the confines of a reputable medical setting.

Concentration Camps

It is in the concentration camps that the killing reached unprecedented heights in Nazi Germany. It is in these death factories that the process of destruction as a rational, bureaucratic, assembly-line enterprise came of age. Although killing by lethal injections in the euthanasia institutions and by shooting brigades in the eastern territories consumed many lives, nothing could match the camps for sheer killing power. The system of destruction developed destroyed millions, did it more quickly and efficiently, and left fewer traces than anything ever before devised. Raul Hilberg indicates how quickly and efficiently the killing centers functioned: "A man would step off a train in the morning, and in the evening his corpse was burned and his clothes packed away for shipment to Germany." [28] What the technicians of Auschwitz, Dachau, Buchenwald, Treblinka, and other camps did was build upon, improve, perfect, and extend a destruction process that had begun when physicians started exterminating German patients in psychiatric hospitals.

Part of the reason for the phenomenal success of the death camps was the ability of the designers to erect installations that appeared to be resettlement camps rather than locales for mass destruction. This is quite an achievement when one considers the fact that the camp architects did not have the luxury of ready-made medical settings with which to fool the inmates. Most camps were huge compounds consisting of many barracks-type structures, all surrounded by high barbed wire fences. Sand, stone, and wood dominated the environment while grass, trees, and vegetation were almost nonexistent.

Even in the midst of such desolate surroundings, the camp planners possessed the energy and ingenuity to create an atmosphere that would alleviate anxiety and hide destruction. At the Treblinka death camp a false railway station surrounded by flower beds gave the whole area "a neat and cheery look," related survivor Jean-Francois Steiner. "The flowers, which were real, made the whole scene resemble a pretty station in a little provincial town." [29]

A number of other environmental innovations were instituted at various camps to help smooth the path of the condemned. When the victims disembarked onto the platforms, they were greeted by the reassuring sight of ambulances, doctors, and medical orderlies. The elderly, the sick, and children were ushered into the waiting vehicles and ostensibly taken to the camp hospital for medical treatment. As the internees passed into the camp compound they looked up and saw another hopeful sign: a large inscription over the gate read "Arbeit Macht Frei" (Labor Gives Freedom).[30] Many thought this meant they would soon be allowed to become productive workers once more. Just before entering the gas chamber area they saw another pleasant scene: a lovely well-kept lawn in which mushroom-shaped concrete objects stood at regular intervals.[31] Little did the passers-by realize that these were shafts through which the gas crystals were dropped onto the victims in the chambers below.

All this was merely a tune-up for the biggest masquerade of all. The entire layout, beginning with the journey through the long underground viaduct and ending up inside the gas chamber, was a gigantic, perverse hoax. The brightly lit ante-rooms adjoining the gas chambers were made to look like dressing rooms. The perpetrators even thought of including clothes hangers with plaques underneath declaring in every European language, "If you want your effects when you go out, please make note of the number of your hanger." A "bath director" dressed in white was also on hand to pass out towels and soap. It was inside the gas chambers that the decor reached the height of unadulterated deception. The interiors actually resembled huge bath houses. The placement of shower faucets overhead played a significant role in reinforcing this impression. Morale and hope had to be maintained up to the very end.[32]

Among concentration camps, Dachau had one of the most pleasant appearances; its medical front was especially impressive:

> At first glance Dachau would appear to be a model camp. The visitor (assuming that his entry were possible) would be impressed by the football ground, the clothing stores full of garments, the fine showerbaths with their modern heating installation, the spotless kitchens, and the charming lay-out of the buildings with flower-beds and an avenue of poplars. The *Revier* (sick-bay) would seem amazingly clean and tidy.

It included rooms for eye and E.N.T. clinics, a physiotherapy room with the most modern apparatus (even an electrocardiograph), a big dressing-station, two magnificent operating theatres with a sterilization room, an x-ray department, a dental clinic, a well-fitted laboratory, a well-stocked dispensary, and beautiful parquet floors to the wards.[33]

The truth of the matter was a far cry from what appeared on the surface. "The Nazis—including the Nazi physicians—pursued but one aim: *extermination*. The whole medical apparatus was nothing but a *décor*, nothing but a lie intended to disguise the massacre." [34]

The careful planning that went into the design of the death settings paid off handsomely. Few victims actively rebelled; most were deceived or consoled by the subterfuges employed. The entrance to Treblinka had a definitely positive effect on survivor Richard Glazar: "We all crowded to look out of the windows. I saw a green fence, barracks, and I heard what sounded like a farm tractor. I was delighted." [35] Dr. Miklos Nyiszli recalled how the "Baths and Disinfecting Room" sign allayed the misgivings of even the most suspicious inmates: "They went down the stairs almost gaily." [36]

The victims were not the only ones consoled by all the window dressing; the perpetrators also needed soothing. Franz Stangl, commandant of Treblinka, blotted out the harsh realities of the daily liquidations by concentrating on creating an idyllic atmosphere: "gardens, new barracks, new kitchens, new everything; barbers, tailors, shoemakers, carpenters. There were hundreds of ways to take one's mind off it; I used them all." [37]

Auschwitz was the largest and most productive of all the killing centers. Although Auschwitz was also a huge complex that supplied slave labor for the German war effort, it best functioned as an extermination plant. Such a success story was due largely to dedicated technicians, careful planning, advanced equipment and resources, and the most up-to-date killing methods. A brief description of the destruction process at Auschwitz and other concentration camps provides further insight into how the various phases operated to bring about a near perfect outcome.

The victims usually got off trains with their luggage and immediately descended onto large unloading platforms. Awaiting their arrival was a good-sized contingent from the camp, including the camp commandant, camp physicians, guards, and prisoner work groups. Sometimes an orchestra composed of inmates led by a well-known Jewish violinist greeted the newcomers. As the doctors proceeded to select who would live and who would die, the orchestra played a medley of tangos, jazz numbers, and popular ballads.[38]

The throngs were divided into two basic groups: on the left were the aged, the ill, and women with children under fourteen; on the right were able-bodied men. The reason given to the victims for this particular division was that the aged and women would care for the sick and the children while the men would have to work. In actuality, those sent to the left were quickly dispatched to their deaths in the gas chambers, and those on the right temporarily survived as slave laborers for camp maintenance or to serve the German industrial war effort.

The victims usually had to walk to the area of the camp where the extermination machinery awaited them. The strains of music could be heard as the marchers made their way through the carefully-drawn route. The music emitted a soothing, almost hypnotic quality, which facilitated the flow of victims in an incident-free manner. It was a scene truly reminiscent of the Pied Piper's irresistible spell over the children of Hamlin. Still, there was the ominous presence of huge chimneys spewing forth great smoke and sickeningly sweetish odors to mar the journey. An explanation served to dispel the victims' anxiety: they were told the buildings housing these chimneys were bakeries.[39]

The processions moved relentlessly onward through the remaining phases preceding the ultimate destination. At each step along the way, SS troops barked out directions and escorted the hordes through the process. They were often polite and took the time to offer reassurances to the victims.

The next stop was inside a large underground hallway or

anteroom adjacent to what resembled a bathhouse. The bathhouse was really a huge gas chamber that could accommodate two thousand people. The inmates had to take off their clothes and place their valuables on a large table.

It was in such a trusting frame of mind that millions allowed themselves to be herded into what was in effect an underground crypt. Once inside, the deceptions built into the entire destruction process began to evaporate rapidly: no water was forthcoming from the showers; the lights were turned off; the heat given off from the overcrowded conditions resulted in death by suffocation. When the temperature had increased sufficiently, cylinders of highly poisonous gas were dropped into the chamber from a square opening in the ceiling. The effects of the gassing were devastating. Within just three minutes, two thousand individuals could be annihilated in one spot.[40]

The process did not end with gassing. Much still remained to be accomplished, including the disposing of corpses and the salvaging of valuable body by-products such as human hair, gold teeth, and specimens for anatomical and experimental studies. The final episode consisted of transporting the remains to the crematoriums for incineration in huge ovens. Sometimes the crematoriums were supplemented by burning in open pits on specially constructed funeral pyres.

Destruction at most extermination camps followed a similar pattern with some variations. At Treblinka, for instance, an assembly-line procedure was initiated as soon as the deportees disembarked at the railway station. The men and women were separated. The women had their hair cut off. The men were stripped of their clothes via an elaborate production line and then directed to the right hand barracks; there they waited until the women had been sent to the gas chambers. Those who threatened to slow down the process because of illness or age were taken to fake hospitals where the treatment administered was a bullet in the back of the head.[41]

The naked victims, in rows of five, were made to run the final hundred-meter path leading to the gas chamber. This particular innovation was prompted by a desire to speed up destruction, the underlying theory being a simple one: "A winded victim dies faster. Hence, a saving of time. The best way to wind a man is to make him run — another saving of time." That the system worked remarkably well can be attested to by the fact that it took only three-quarters of an hour "from the moment the doors of the cattle cars were unbolted to the moment the great trap doors of the gas chambers were opened to take out the bodies." [42] This represented a decided improvement over the previous system, where the destruction process took as long as two hours.

Besides bringing about a quick death for many, concentration camps also had an associated goal: to reduce the victims to a severe state of subhumanity long before they actually perished. For some this point was reached early; they died in the incredibly crowded cattle cars on the way to the killing centers. Those given a temporary reprieve because of robust health gradually succumbed to the back-breaking labor and living conditions in the camps. Disease, hunger, malnutrition, and dysentery soon overcame even the hardiest physical specimens. They took on the appearance of the living dead: walking skeletons; empty shells of humanity; hideous caricatures of what had once been an attractive and vibrant people.

Other indignities built into the destruction process helped to dehumanize the victims and therefore facilitate the work of destruction. Completely shearing hair from the victims' heads had the effect of reducing them to an indiscriminate mass. Camp survivor Dr. Gisella Pearl gives an account of the devastating impact on female inmates:

> Its purpose was to deprive its unwilling clients of even their last remnants of beauty, freshness, and human appearance. . . . we felt the heavy, blunt shears in our hair, and when we looked up again, we hardly knew one another any longer. . . . our heads had acquired a nightmarish appearance . . . so horrible to look at that we did not know whether to laugh or to cry. [43]

The intolerable living conditions in the camps created an atmosphere in which the law of the jungle prevailed. Inmates argued, fought, and even killed one another in vying for scarce resources. As reported by Pearl, it was particularly amusing for the captors "to watch our gradual deterioration and see how long it took for the most cultured twentieth-century intellectuals to reach the moral standards of a hyena." [44]

It is little wonder that the consciences of the perpetrators remained intact. They were not killing human beings, but simply removing a low-grade species from the face of the earth. The victims did not look human, nor did they act human. The previous steps of the destruction process had made sure of that. By the time they were herded into the gas chambers, many had become pitiful creatures with few resemblances to human beings left. Their deaths, therefore, came to be viewed as a humane deliverance rather than an atrocity. What better way for the technicians to justify their involvement and at the same time soothe their consciences!

Abortion Clinics

Modern hospitals exact a heavy toll of unborn lives in a highly efficient and technologically sophisticated manner. Such a record, though impressive, cannot match that established by the many free-standing abortion clinics that have cropped up almost overnight to constitute what has become one of the fastest growing industries in America. Within the chambers of today's abortion clinics, destruction has been elevated to a process of unbelievable perfection. A woman can get off an airplane, out of a taxi or car in the morning, and by early afternoon all the remnants of her unborn baby's corpse and intrauterine life-support membranes are completely disintegrated by an assembly-line system that would make the most avid Nazi technician gasp in awe. The speed of the destruction process at two abortion clinics in midtown Manhattan is described in the following manner:

> The two clinics each occupying an entire floor worked incessantly around the clock. . . . The entire

process from beginning to end — laboratory work, history-taking, counseling, operation, recovery, and discharge — was accomplished in three hours. After this, the building's special limousine transported the girls back to the airport for the speedy return trip home.[45]

Another candid account of the factory-like processing of individuals through legal abortion chambers came to public awareness in 1978. Investigators from the Better Government Association and reporters from the *Chicago Sun-Times* exposed the fraudulent and horrendous practices of what they called "abortion mills" located in the midst of Chicago's posh Magnificent Mile. The choice of headlines used to inaugurate a series of *Sun-Times* articles on the clinics is extremely revealing. One of the front-page headings blared: "Making a Killing in Michigan Av. Clinics." A caption spread across two pages declared: "Life on the abortion assembly line: Grim, grisly and greedy." [46]

These headlines were intended to disclose how blatantly doctors and others abuse and exploit women in the relentless pursuit of amassing enormous fortunes. How much more appropriately do they unveil the massive killing of unborn children on an assembly line of destruction operated by medical executioners and their dedicated accomplices!

Like the concentration camps, today's abortion clinics are killing centers solely directed toward one overriding goal: the extermination of human life. Their proficiency is also due to building and improving upon the prior experiences of those skilled physician-executioners who so perseveringly pioneered the science of unborn baby killing in the hospital setting. Again, a totally committed staff, careful planning, and the most modern equipment, resources, and killing techniques make up the major ingredients of a formula for destruction that will prove difficult if not impossible to surpass. An indication of how well an abortion clinic operates is supplied by Ardis Hyland Danon, nurse supervisor at Parkmed, a large abortion clinic in New York City: "On a busy day, I'm always amazed at how smoothly and efficiently the service is running." [47]

Abortion clinics do not give the appearance of being ultramodern death factories, but legitimate and respectable medical establishments where superior patient care is the only prime concern. The amazing thing is that this medical charade is pulled off so well that neither the pregnant woman nor some of the clinic perpetrators are aware of the real underlying purpose of their superbly-functioning enterprise. In fact, the essence of the whole destruction process consists of the many built-in reassurances that what the aborting woman and staff members are doing is not only legal and moral, but even meritorious. Reassurance dominates every facet of the clinic set-up, ranging all the way from the comfortable furnishings and impressive medical equipment to the kind and empathetic faces of the staff. This serves to allay individual consciences and conceal harsh and disturbing realities.

Abortion clinic designers have been more successful than concentration camp architects in insuring that the unpleasant aspects of killing be hidden behind, or at least minimized by, an attractive and functional setting. Most abortion clinics resemble, as one close observer so aptly pointed out, professionally decorated beauty salons.[48] Their plush interiors and furnishings are not unlike those funeral establishments, brilliantly satirized in Evelyn Waugh's *The Loved One*, so completely dedicated to the art of denying and cosmetizing death.[49]

The lengths to which abortion clinic designers have gone in their efforts to cover up destruction and alleviate tensions associated with participation in scientific killing of the unborn is nowhere more analytically and comprehensively covered than in architect Herbert McLaughlin's report on the design features of an ultra-modern abortion clinic located in New York City. Regarding the total atmosphere of the clinic, "it was generally agreed that the feeling should be soft and yet, crisp and clear." This was achieved mainly through the "widespread use of incandescent lighting, comfortable but contemporary furnishings, and the use of curving walls." The design team did not want to overdo the curves; they were concerned that too many curves might be "misinterpreted as a kind of ovarian architecture."[50]

The rest of the clinic layout was planned with comparable taste and delicacy. The purpose of constructing the patient waiting room as a "large, high-ceilinged, open space with wood bookshelves, plants and contemporary furniture of bright, bold colors and solid fabrics" was to create "a cheerful and anxiety-free environment." The hallways leading to the counseling rooms were decorated with "bold graphics" and "carpeted," while the counseling rooms were "extremely understated to create a very direct, nondistracting focus on the interaction and education process." The anterooms just outside the procedure rooms were decorated with "brightly printed wallpaper and curtains to provide a domestic and specifically reassuring tone." A different kind of reassurance was built into the procedure room: "a medical environment of manifest cleanliness and surgical correctness." And finally, in the recovery room there was a conscious attempt to establish "a college dormitory atmosphere, using simple wood bed frames with plaid bedspreads." [51]

The painstaking attention to the psychological aspects of clinic design highlights the ambitious aspirations entertained for this and many other abortion facilities: "That an abortion be a learning process and not merely a medical procedure." [52]

While the decor of abortion clinics varies, as one experienced observer expressed it, "from small Middle West cozy to huge Alphaville labyrinthine," all clinics are "clean, tastefully decorated, and staffed by kind people." [53] At the Parkmed clinic, nurse administrator Danon expressed pride in being given the responsibility for such tasks as choosing furniture, color schemes, and interior designs. Her final selections for the waiting room consisted of "soft, recessed lighting, light oak-paneled walls, light-green rug, and multicolored, vinyl-cushioned chrome chairs." [54]

The opening of many abortion clinics has been greeted with a great deal of fanfare and hoopla. The major appeal generally made is that abortions would be performed in an attractive, antiseptic, safe, and well-equipped setting. It is this kind of thrust that dominated a picture story on abortion written by Paul Berg in the May 20, 1973 issue of the *St. Louis Post-Dispatch*. [55] Some of the pictures selected to embellish this story are particularly revealing. In the inside pages the reader is treated to scenes glorifying the virtues of an abortion clinic's roomy and lovely interiors. One shows two women busily decorating a clinic room, another provides a glimpse of an immaculate and well-equipped procedure room, and still another shows smiling staff members seated in a beautifully furnished reception room. In addition, there is also a picture of the various contraceptives used in the clinic's counseling program. This is intended to give credibility to the contention that the abortion clinic is not exclusively in business to kill babies but to stop them from being conceived.

The overriding view that emerges from these pictures is a highly slanted one to say the least. Abortion is portrayed in a very positive manner, with special emphasis on the desirable and beautiful setting in which it occurs. The victims of abortion are rarely given an afterthought; they are pictured so nebulously that the viewer can hardly be motivated to identify or side with them as actual human beings. The horrors of dead human victims are conveniently expunged from these and most abortion related pictures released by the media for public consumption.

It is revealing to note that this same Paul Berg of the *Post-Dispatch* pictures staff is also the author of a picture story written several months later on the Nazi holocaust.[56] In this article he displayed little reticence about publishing horrifying pictures of concentration camp victims. One is a large detailed picture of starved Jewish corpses with agonized expressions and clenched fists crammed into a freight car. Also included are pictures of charred bodies found in the furnaces of the Buchenwald camp, and a "living dead" blind survivor with a horribly battered face.

One wonders what would have happened had Berg chosen to present the holocaust in the same way as he handled the topic of abortion. What if he chose to glorify the holocaust with pictures of smiling doctors and nurses stationed in the euthanasia hospitals and concentration camps? What if he chose to show photos of the nicely furnished quarters of the body disposal squads? What if he chose to include pictures of the most technically advanced equipment for exterminating

human lives? If his decision were to do just this and refuse
to publish any pictures of destroyed victims out of fear of
being offensive to readers' sensibilities, there would likely be
an immediate outcry from the American Jewish Congress,
B'nai B'rith, the American Civil Liberties Union, and many
other Jewish and non-Jewish organizations and groups.

Why such a reaction? The answer is simple: the awful
truth of the concentration-camp holocaust is the unwarranted
destruction of unwanted human lives; to depict it otherwise
is more than misleading — it is grossly untruthful. The terrible truth of the abortion-chamber holocaust is likewise the
unwarranted destruction of unwanted human lives; to portray
it otherwise, as many media people have done, is also being
equally misleading and grossly untruthful.

Apparently, killing is far more acceptable and even easily
denied when it is clothed in the finery of pleasant, antiseptic
surroundings. The abortion clinic environment always comes
out ahead when contrasted with the dirty back rooms in which
illegal abortions have occurred. Abortion clinic promoters
rarely fail to make this point in the course of extolling their
brand of sanitized destruction.

The effectiveness of the abortion clinic atmosphere in relieving anxiety is one of the most frequently heard themes
coming from women who have had abortions. One abortee
mentioned that her fears began to fade the moment she was
ushered into a "small, modernized one story white concrete
building on the outskirts of the city." [57] Another expressed de-
lightful surprise with the setting: "I didn't expect a place as
nice as this. I expected a dingy room and all kinds of people
like you see at a bus stop. . . . I thought it was going to be all
hush-hush and hurry up. But nobody in the waiting room seems
very upset — they're all sitting there socializing." [58] The
physical decor is also seen by some aborting women as helping
them to feel "nice" about themselves. [59] Even an emotionally-
detached, wise-cracking, sophisticated coed from a major
Eastern university was able to acknowledge her gratitude for
being given the opportunity to have her abortion "in a sanitary
hospital environment rather than the dusty back rooms that
housed death beds for many victims." [60]

The setting, the milieu, the environment, then, seems to make all the difference in the world. It is not killing per se that is so intolerable, but killing conducted in septic, non-medical surroundings. Never have so many lives been extinguished in such utterly benign atmospheres!

This is similar to the overall impression conveyed by the concentration camps: not that of a massive destruction facility but simply a place where people would be cared for. If they were ill they would be taken to the camp hospital in Red Cross trucks; if able bodied, their alleged treatment was a shower and then rest and resettlement. All this was a monumental facade, and its purpose — to facilitate destruction.

Typically, the trip through the abortion clinic begins with a warm greeting from a receptionist in an attractive waiting area. From there the women are ushered through a sequence of information gathering, counseling, and lab tests. A common explanation given for these tests is to establish whether the clinic clients are medically able to undergo what is persistently communicated as a very minor, non-hazardous medical procedure. An unstated purpose of the test results is to help the doctor determine if the child in the womb can be destroyed without causing his or her mother undue physical and psychological complications.

An overwhelming majority pass these preliminaries with flying colors and are quickly escorted to the abortion clinic procedure rooms, where their offspring are vacuumed into extinction. Once a woman embarks on her trek through an abortion clinic, rarely does she ever change her mind about having an abortion. Few unborn children ever leave the inside of an abortion clinic alive; the only ones who escape are those whose mothers cannot pass the clinic's prelims. One of the main reasons for disqualification is that the child is too large and developed for the vacuum aspirator to have any appreciable destructive effect. It is only a temporary reprieve; referral is soon made to a hospital where killing can be readily accomplished by saline or prostaglandin abortion.

As the women are led toward the very heart of the abortion clinic, the procedure room, they are never isolated or lonely. Someone is always present to make the journey a pleasant and relaxing one. The fact that other intelligent, attractive, and like-situated women are simultaneously making this same trip proves to be very consoling. After all, it is concluded, it would be unthinkable for so many nice people to be gathered together for anything but the most honorable intentions, and surely never for anything even remotely associated with a massive destruction process.

Their movement through the maze of clinic corridors, rooms, and waiting areas is far more leisurely but just as purposive as that which took place in the concentration camps. Although there is no live orchestra to greet and accompany the unborn children to their demise, the world's most beautiful and soothing music, piped in at every crucial spot, is a standard feature of many abortion clinics. Information about the simplicity and safety of the procedure is steadily fed to the participants all along the way. At the Margaret Sanger Center in New York City and other abortion clinics, transparent plastic models of the woman's reproductive system are frequently employed to give a more concrete explanation of what the abortion procedure involves.[61] Despite this, none of the information conveyed actually touches upon the truth. None of it indicates precisely what happens to the unborn child during an abortion. The abortion candidates are never told what the vacuum aspirator really does — literally tear apart the tiny body of the growing and developing child in the womb. What they are commonly told is that some nondescript tissue or contents are gently evacuated.

In a similar vein, concentration camp inmates were not told they were going to be killed either, but that they were simply going to the bathhouse for a group shower. Truth-in-telling was not an ingredient of the Nazi destruction process, nor is it found in today's killing centers.

Just before entering the procedure room, the woman takes off her street clothes and puts on a hospital gown in one of the adjoining dressing rooms. Like the phony bathhouses in the concentration camps, the interior of the procedure room comes across as a place for caring and not killing. Everything about the procedure room, including its design, equipment, and technically trained and clad inhabitants reinforces the deception of a legitimate enterprise before, during, and after the lethal instruments are applied. The following description of the Preterm abortion center procedure room is typical: "The woman is brought to a procedure room which is painted in a restful color and is as free of extraneous and anxiety-producing equipment as is possible." [62]

It is inside such a reassuring environment that millions of women have allowed highly skilled doctors and their assistants to scrape or suck the dismembered limbs and organs of their unborn progeny to oblivion. Although the procedure room is much smaller than the gas chamber and can accommodate only one victim at a time, there are many more procedure rooms in operation today than there were gas chambers in Nazi Germany. In terms of their destructive capabilities, procedure rooms are just as awesome. The consoling atmosphere and built-in deceptions help to make this possible. While the pretenses became evident once the destructive techniques began to operate in the gas chambers, this is not so in the procedure rooms. The vacuum aspirators function so swiftly and decisively on such small victims that the guise of a respectable medical procedure is rarely shattered, and the consciences of the perpetrators remain undisturbed. From the standpoint of the unborn child the aspirator is a devastating death machine; from the perpetrators' perspective it is merely an efficiently running medical device designed to remove some inconvenient tissue. In the abortion clinic there is no recognition given to the existence, let alone the viewpoint, of the unborn child.

Very little clinic effort is expended in trying to salvage the victims' remains. The vacuum aspirator so effectively tears apart the child's tiny body that there is nothing left to be exploited either commercially or scientifically. Periodically, small bits of arms, legs, hair, rib cages, and heads are identifiable as they zip through the aspirator's transparent tube. But by the time the aspirator is turned off, little remains except an indistinguishable mass of blood and tissue. In some clinics the victims' remains, if there are any to speak of, are subjected to pathological examination, the purpose of which is to make sure that all pieces of the baby's body have been scraped or sucked out of the woman's uterus. Their final destination is

often similar to what happened to the much larger gas chamber corpses: disintegration through incineration.

A typical aftermath to the destruction process is the recovery period. This is a time, usually several hours in duration,
when the no-longer-pregnant woman rests and has her body
and vital signs carefully checked. Concomitantly, propaganda
and reassurance continue to flow from the lips of counselors
and other clinic personnel, the main purpose being to alleviate
any residue of guilt not yet eradicated. This recuperation period is not only helpful to the aborted woman but also serves
to console the clinic perpetrators that they are performing
a valuable, medically valid, and humane service. It is also
in the recovery room that the counselors and staff members
join the woman in munching goodies and sipping juice, soup,
tea, or coffee. In the Margaret Sanger Center recovery room,
for example, she is treated to "a dazzling array of lovely cin-
namon toast, four kinds of lovely soup, and lovely tea or
coffee" and other choice morsels.[63] Thus, the grand finale of
the destruction process takes on an almost festive atmosphere
in which the participants celebrate with food and drink. This
resembles those celebrations that followed destruction at the
hands of euthanasia institution perpetrators, except that they
required stronger beverages to still their consciences.

The above description of the main ingredients making up
the destruction process points toward a fairly standardized
format for killing found to a greater or lesser extent in most
abortion clinics. The rationalization and routinization of killing are the major reasons for its astounding success. This is
not meant to minimize the diversity of destruction patterns
pioneered by modern-day abortion clinics. Where the differences exist among clinics, they are generally due to the degree
of ingenuity and creativity possessed by technological planners
and executors, in addition to the amount of financial and
other resources available.

At this juncture, a closer look should be taken at what goes
on in several different abortion clinics, in order to gain a
fuller appreciation of the destructive innovations developed
and the rationale for their development.

In most abortion clinics, the problem of pain is commonly

handled by administering a local anesthetic to that part of the woman's body involved in the abortion procedure. She stays awake throughout the entire operation, therefore reinforcing the contention that abortion is a very safe, simple, and painless matter. At Parkmed, though, general anesthesia is the overwhelming favorite among patients and perpetrators; so popular that each procedure room is equipped with an anesthesia machine plus a nurse anesthetist. If abortion is such a painless and simple procedure, why, then, do so many prefer to be asleep when it is performed? The reason given is a technological one: general anesthesia results in fewer cases of retained tissue ("incomplete emptying of uterine contents") because the physician can operate in a more leisurely manner without having to worry about hurting the patient.[64] The perpetrators often fail to mention that the act of technological destruction is easier to conceal from the woman when she is placed in a state of unconsciousness.

Another innovation concerns the question of how clinics deal with children already born. The last place one would expect to find young, postnatal children is in an abortion clinic. Few things could be more bizarre than seeing small children inside an establishment whose main preoccupation is the systematic destruction of prenatal infants. Most women getting abortions do not want to be reminded that what they are carrying is a growing, living child. Neither do they desire to be informed about what abortion does so flawlessly to this child. The presence of healthy, active children scampering around the clinic waiting rooms is hardly conducive to helping abortion aspirants deny reality. Besides, the sight of little ones on the scene might present a serious challenge to the many elaborate facades that form the very foundation of the clinic destruction process.

Despite the fact that abortion clinics are heavily committed to the business of unborn baby killing, some of them are actually broadminded enough to even allow women to bring their infants, toddlers, or preschoolers to the clinic. Rather than being threatened by the presence of young children, some abortion clinics appear happy to have them on the premises. One veteran twenty-two-year-old coed abortee tells of seeing children playing in the spacious "pulsating with activity" waiting room of a Pittsburgh abortion clinic.[65] Not to be out-done, the Margaret Sanger Center features the inclusion of a small playroom equipped with toys and blackboard next to the waiting room.[66] Their commitment to already-born children does have some limits. They do not, for example, provide a play person to watch the children while the mother aborts; she must bring along her own baby sitter. This ranks as one of the slickest psychological coups ever pulled off. It has the effect of strengthening and not weakening abortion clinic claims to credibility as a legitimate medical establish-ment. After all, so the reasoning goes, how could an organi-zation so accommodating to young children possibly be in-volved in baby killing?

Abortion clinics, like the Nazi camps, have also developed some unique ways of reducing their victims to a state of sub-humanity. One approach used is to shower such exquisite care on the aborting woman that there is no time to give a thought to the possibility of the existence of a victim. One close obser-ver of abortion clinic operations concluded that a major pur-pose for the scrupulous care given to the woman before, during, and after abortion is to direct attention away from the fetus: "Psychologically, the stage is set: she is there for something that involves *her* emotional and bodily health, not for a crime against a fetus." [67] The abortion clinic is one up even on the concentration camp: its victims are reduced to a level lower than that of subhumanity — the level of non-existence. The more elaborate the attention devoted to the women the better the clinic is able to get away with this par-ticular ploy.

Furthermore, the age and size of the victim plus the type of killing method employed help to solidify the subhuman or nonexistent status. Since free-standing abortion clinics spe-cialize in destroying individuals during the first three months of pregnancy, many abortion victims, particularly those in the early weeks after conception, have not developed enough to clearly possess all identifiable human features. This is quite consoling for the perpetrators, because, to their way of thinking, if the products of their technology do not look human, they surely cannot be human.

An overwhelming amount of scientific data indicates that the child in the uterus has a decidedly human form and appearance as early as six to seven weeks past conception.[68] The clinic perpetrators do not want to be bothered with such facts. They do not see, nor do they care to see, the small but obviously human two or three-month-old unborn child swimming inside the amniotic sac. Technology comes to the rescue and insures that they will never see what the intact child looks like before destruction. All they become aware of is the inconsequential aftermath of destruction. Thus, the most common term used to describe first-trimester victims, the products of conception — a veritable designation of subhumanity — is closely aligned with what the perpetrators actually see — a non-identifiable mass of blood and tissue at the bottom of a glass container.

The patterns of technological killing serve to reinforce further the distorted images of subhumanity imposed on unwanted victims by today's medical executioners.

Annihilation assembly-line style is not the creation of impulsive psychopaths seeking revenge against hated enemies. It is the product, rather, of emotionless, analytical minds obsessed with perfecting the technical details of killing. Despite the diversity of destruction processes developed at the various killing sites, the common focus on careful planning, coordination, and specialization of tasks has been responsible for consuming huge numbers of victims in both Nazi Germany and contemporary America. The heavy investment of doctors in every phase of destruction has endowed the killing with an incomparable imprint of power, prestige, scientific knowledge, and technical skill. Their leadership role in the killing has been a major factor in helping to enlist the services of other professions and technicians in the monumental task of destroying human beings.

CHAPTER 6

Killing Methods

Some of the methods of destruction employed in Nazi Germany are very dissimilar from those used in contemporary America. A majority of today's victims are not shot in the back kneeling in front of huge ditches or dispatched to gas chambers. Instead, most have met their end by being cut or sucked out of the womb. There are, nevertheless, some remarkable parallels between past and present killing techniques. Destruction by injection of lethal substances was a favorite means of German physicians for disposing of unwanted defectives and mentally ill individuals in the euthanasia hospitals. Deadly injections are likewise preferred by contemporary doctors as a means of getting rid of unwanted, unborn children during the second trimester of pregnancy. The only significant difference has to do with the substances injected: morphine, scopolamine, and phenol in Nazi Germany, and saline and prostaglandins in today's society. Moreover, the withholding of treatment from defective children, followed by enforced starvation, was a common practice in the pediatric divisions and euthanasia institutions of the Third Reich, and this practice has also continued up to the present — today's targets being newborn mongoloids with intestinal obstructions and other seriously afflicted infants.

Whatever the differences or similarities in destructive technology, each method has had to live up to a very ambitious objective: the killing of millions. Those methods finally chosen did not develop overnight but were the products of

careful planning and testing. Killing effectiveness was determined according to how well each method measured up to
certain criteria. Techniques that killed rationally, quickly,
safely, and cleanly while successfully concealing the destructive act were given the highest ratings.

The last criterion in particular is of the utmost importance.
With reference to this, psychoanalyst Erich Fromm made an
astute observation about the massive destruction wrought by
bomber crews in World War II and the mass exterminations
in the gas chambers. While on the surface both methods of
killing appear quite different, they actually have a lot in common. Their most important similarity is the proficiency with
which each hid the destructive acts from the eyes of the perpetrators. Intellectually, the bomber crew teams understood
the purpose of their mission, but because they could not see
human beings getting killed, maimed, or burned, they failed
to be emotionally affected. They remained preoccupied with
carrying out their technological tasks. The same goes for
those who had responsibility for manning the gas chambers.
Although closer geographically to the victims than the aircraft members, the gas chamber experts likewise remained
emotionally impervious to human suffering, because destruction also took place out of sight, hidden inside the chamber
walls.[1]

This same type of comparison can be readily extended
to the application of abortion technology. In most abortion
procedures the child is killed inside the womb, where the
physician cannot see the tiny victim being torn apart, burned,
or poisoned. This helps the doctor to perceive the act of abortion as a strictly rational, cerebral task devoid of any emotional
significance.

It is in situations like these that Fromm's insights are
especially pertinent: "The technicalization of destruction,
and with it the removal of the full affective recognition of
what one is doing." The implications of this are far-reaching
and absolutely horrendous. Again, according to Fromm, the
die is cast, and "once this process has been fully established
there is no limit to destructiveness because nobody *destroys*;

one only serves the machine for programmed — hence, apparently rational — purposes." [2]

In Nazi Germany, many millions perished because of this supreme triumph of methodology over emotionality. The holocaust, tragically, was not the ending but just the beginning — if one is willing to grant any credibility to the figure of 40-55 million abortions per year on a worldwide basis.[3] This is truly one of the most extreme cases of unlimited destruction in history. And it can be largely attributed to the development of techniques that effectively conceal both the victim and the act of killing, thereby blunting any emotional awareness toward what is actually being done.

The remainder of this section will examine some Nazi and modern killing procedures. Special attention will be given to the question of how well each meets the criteria for successful destruction.

Shooting

The shooting of victims by specially trained units called *Einsatzgruppen* reached its peak during the German attack against Russia, begun on June 22, 1941. A great majority of *Einsatzgruppen* officers were not sadists, hoodlums, or criminals, but intellectuals who "brought to their new task all the skills and training which, as men of thought, they were capable of contributing." [4] Following on the heels of the German army, they led their men in a systematic hunting down of Jews, Gypsies, communist party functionaries, and the insane. The vast area of destruction included the Baltic states, White Russia, the Ukraine, and the Crimea-Caucasus.[5]

The killing procedures became standardized whatever the area of implementation or the particular unit carrying them out. The condemned were summoned, escorted, or forced to gather at designated collecting points in various towns or cities. From there they were taken to remote wooded areas and lined up in front of enormous pits. Some had been originally constructed as antitank ditches, while others were specially dug as depositories for the newly destroyed. A shooting platoon, armed with rifles and sometimes submachine guns, carefully aimed and fired at the backs of the victims' necks; they promptly toppled over into the massive graves. One batch after another were quickly lined up in the same manner and the shooting continued until the capacity of the holes was consumed with layers of corpses.

The system worked very well, with little resistance coming from the victims. It efficiently combined the processes of killing and body disposal in one site. Shooting by these kinds of firing squads was considered a traditional method of execution having time-honored roots in many countries and civilizations. Because the victims had been defined as dangerous and subversive partisans, systematic shooting was viewed as an appropriate and legitimate way of dealing with them. The executioners saw themselves as professionals carrying out an unpleasant but necessary order.

Shooting as a technique of destruction rated highly according to most of the criteria for effective destruction, but was deficient in one aspect: concealment of the victim. Unlike the abortionist, bomber crew member, or gas chamber technician, the one who pulls the trigger does not have the luxury of denying the commission of a lethal act on a living human being. What is even more significant, he sees the direct consequences of his actions. The killer could not even close his eyes to the reality of what was taking place; he had to be alert and attentive; he had to make sure the bullet struck the right part of the victim's anatomy.

Realizing the shortcomings of shooting technology, the perpetrators devised a number of operational procedures to depersonalize the process and make it more psychologically palatable for the firing squad members. The humanity of the victims was reduced by having them kneel and face the open ditch with their backs toward the perpetrators. This way the killers did not have to look at the agonizing and pleading expressions of doomed human faces; it was far easier to shoot at their expressionless backsides. While there was considerable agreement on this aspect of destruction, spirited controversies arose over which particular type of shooting strategy best removed the emotional element from the procedure. On October 4, 1941, General Bohme, the plenipoten-tiary commanding general of Serbia, issued a set of detailed instructions for shooting 2,100 inmates at the Sabac and Belgrade camps: officer-led detachments, shooting at a distance of eight to ten yards with rifles, and placement of the candidates at the edge of the graves in order to "avoid un-necessary touching of corpses."[6] Other commanders in the field felt that shooting victims in the back of the neck was too personalized a technique and opted instead for "massed firing from a considerable distance."[7]

Another approach, designed to combine efficiency with impersonality, was called the "sardine method": "The first batch had to lie down on the bottom of the grave. They were killed by crossfire from above. The next batch had to lie down on top of the corpses, heads facing the feet of the dead. After five or six layers, the grave was closed."[8]

Commander Otto Ohlendorf devised a plan to minimize the horrors of the executions by making them less interesting:

> Undressing was not permitted. The taking of any personal possessions was not permitted. Publicity was not permitted, and at the very moment when it was noted that a man had experienced joy in carrying out these executions, it was ordered that this man should never participate in any more executions. The men could not report voluntarily, they were ordered.[9]

Furthermore, there were so many victims to get rid of that the perpetrators could not concentrate on anything ex-cept carrying out the tasks of aiming and pulling the trigger. There was no time to dwell on the humanity of the victims — as soon as one batch disappeared into the massive holes another one was lined up. It didn't take long for the entire destructive operation to become a routine, emotionally-de-tached endeavor where speed, efficiency, and technological perfection were the only things that mattered.

Even with all the elaborate mechanisms devised to reduce personal guilt and responsibility for destruction, shooting still had serious drawbacks. Participants continued to be dis-

turbed by their involvement. One of the most dramatic examples of this occurred in August 1941, when Heinrich
Himmler viewed an execution of one hundred inmates of the
Minsk prison. Not only were the firing squad members
adversely affected, but Himmler himself was visibly shaken.[10]
As a result of this experience he ordered the perpetrators to
find a less conspicuous method of execution.

Gassing

1. Vans

The search for a perfect killing technique had been going
on for a number of years before Himmler's confrontation with
the harsh realities of firing-squad technology. Physicians,
scientists, and technicians had been active in developing an
approach that promised to fit the bill: execution by gassing.
As previously indicated, gas chambers had been tested out
on patients in mental hospitals in the late 1930s. Getting rid
of Jews and other unwanted individuals in the battle zones,
however, required a more mobile method than gassing in permanent, stationary chambers.

The answer to this dilemma seemed to be resolved by the
construction of gas vans, which retained the mobility of shooting while eliminating its more gruesome features. They were
designed especially for women and children. The procedure
involved herding the victims into the enclosed cabin section
of the vehicle and driving toward the outskirts of town. On
the way they died from the exhaust fumes piped into the
interior of the cabin. By the time these deathmobiles reached
their final destination deep in the forest, all the passengers
inside were dead. They were then removed and dropped into
the gaping holes of the waiting pits.

One technician provided some details regarding the operation of this gassing procedure and his own ideas about improving its effectiveness:

The application of gas is usually not undertaken

correctly. In order to come to an end as fast as possible, the driver presses the accelerator to the fullest extent. Thus the persons executed die by suffocation and not by dozing off as planned. My directions have proved that by correct adjustment of the levers death comes faster and the prisoners fall asleep peacefully. Distorted faces and excretions, such as could be seen before, are no longer noticed.[11]

This type of destruction had several meritorious features. First of all, it was a quiet and inconspicuous way to go about exterminating individuals. Gone were the piercing sounds of gunfire and the screams of the doomed. The gas spread smoothly, gradually easing the victims into a state of eternal sleep. At other times, the gas worked its deadly effect so swiftly that the victims had no chance to raise even a cry of agony. And even if they did, the mobile death chambers were sealed tight enough to keep the sounds from reaching the ears of the killers.

Secondly — and this was of particular importance — the victims and the act of destruction were hidden from sight. Along with this the feelings of revulsion generally associated with horrible atrocities were also conveniently wiped out. Although the pressure of the driver's foot on the accelerator actuated the release of the lethal gas, he did not see the victims being killed; he was simply driving the van. The technicians responsible for designing the gassing apparatus did not see the horrifying results of their technology; it wasn't their feet that released the gas. Those who removed the corpses did not see anyone being killed; they were merely carrying out the job of the disposal of corpses.

Furthermore, gas-induced destruction did not leave nearly the same mess as shooting did. Firing on victims was a very bloody affair and frequently produced corpses with contorted and agonized expressions. The products of gassing were far more likely to have fewer overt signs of destruction; they were cleaner, less bloody, and more intact. Their removal was therefore viewed as a less nasty job than getting rid of screaming, bleeding, and bullet-ridden victims.

From many standpoints, then, the gas vans approached the ideal in the development of destructive technology. Nevertheless, a few flaws still existed, the main one being an inadequate capacity to cope with the large numbers of victims that had to be disposed of in a short period of time. Not that many gas vans were available and just so many individuals could be crammed into the limited space within the cabin. It was also considered a time-consuming task to transport them from the collecting points to the disposal sites. In addition, the gassing mechanism did not always operate effectively and sometimes left a mess comparable to the shooting massacres. These deficiencies could be tolerated, but only temporarily. The quest for a more effective method equal to the challenge of massive extermination continued to consume the energies of physicians, scientists, and other technicians.

2. Chambers

The ultimate step in the advancement of destructive technology was reached with the installation of large gas chambers in the concentration camps.

Before this particular method of killing was implemented on a large scale in the death camps, it was first tested out in euthanasia hospitals by physicians. Prominent Nazi hunter Simon Wiesenthal provides a chilling account of the total preoccupation of medical scientists at the Hartheim euthanasia center with the precise details of gassing as an effective method of scientific extermination:

> Various mixtures of gases were tried out to find the most effective one. Doctors with stopwatches would observe the dying patients through the peephole in the cellar door of Castle Hartheim, and the length of the death struggle was clocked down to one tenth of a second. Slow-motion pictures were made and studied by the experts. Victims' brains were photographed to see exactly when death had occurred. Nothing was left to chance.[12]

Among the first recipients of permanent gas chambers were four camps devoted to the exclusive task of extermination — Chelmno, Belzec, Sobibor, and Treblinka. Each was located within a two-hundred-mile radius of Warsaw. The transport of victims from the large population centers of Poland to the death camps was easily facilitated through a vast railway system. The main instrument of destruction at each camp consisted of pumping carbon monoxide gas from diesel engine exhausts into large, permanent chambers. As many as several hundred victims could be accommodated in each chamber at one time. Some of the victims succumbed immediately to the deadly fumes, while it took others several hours to become fully asphixiated. The gassing mechanism did not always work and at times the death selectees had to wait inside the chamber for hours before the system became operational.

One graphic account of what went on in these chambers was provided by Kurt Gerstein, one of the leading gas technicians of the Third Reich. The date was August 19, 1942, and the place the Belzec concentration camp:

Heckenholt tried to set the Diesel engine going, but it would not start.... The people waited in their gas chambers — in vain. One could hear them cry. "Just as in a synagogue," says SS Sturmbannfuehrer, Professor Dr. Pfannenstiel, Professor for Public Health at the University of Marburg/Lahn, holding his ear close to the wooden door.... After 2 hours and 49 minutes — as registered by my stop watch — the Diesel engine started. Up to that moment the people in the four chambers already filled were still alive — 4 times 750 persons in 4 times 45 cubic meters! Another 25 minutes went by. Many of the people, it is true, were dead by that time. One could see that through the little window as the electric lamp revealed for a moment the inside of the chamber. After 28 minutes only a few were alive. After 32 minutes all were dead! From the other side, Jewish workers opened the wooden doors.... The dead were still standing like stone statues, there having been no room for them to fall or bend over. Though dead, the families could still be recognized, their hands still clasped. It was difficult to separate them in order to clear the chamber for the next load. The bodies were thrown out blue, wet with sweat and urine, the legs covered with excrement and menstrual blood.[13]

Once this system of destruction got off the ground the gas fumes worked quickly; it took only one-half hour to kill everyone inside the chamber. Despite periodic delays due to technological breakdowns, over a half-million were exterminated at Belzec alone in a nine-month period.[14]

Like the gas van operators, those who manned the gas chambers neither saw nor heard the destruction process actually consuming its victims. That would have been too psychologically disturbing, to say the least. But not so for Professor Pfannenstiel. Listening to the mortal struggles of the victims provided a unique opportunity for him to display his perverted sense of humor. For Gerstein it was strictly a matter of scientific interest. He was hired to methodically evaluate carbon monoxide gas as an effective method of destruction. His precise observations helped to improve its killing capability.

As the potential pool of death candidates increased into the millions, the carbon monoxide chambers could not handle the immense work load. They were too small, broke down too often, took too long to kill, and left too great a mess.

The death technicians did not give up, and their persistence finally paid off. The ideal method and equipment for massive unlimited killing was put together at Auschwitz. The gas that did the most damage went by two common names, Zyklon B or hydrogen cyanide. Originally, Zyklon B had been used for a number of purposes including fumigating buildings, disinfecting clothes, delousing human beings, and exterminating insects. The perpetrators thought it only logical to extend its use to encompass the extermination of Jews and others considered on the same level as insects. Huge chambers able to accommodate two thousand at a time were considered the worthy arenas for the use of the extraordinarily powerful Zyklon.

A comprehensive picture of the ultra-efficient Zyklon destruction was supplied by Auschwitz survivor Dr. Miklos Nyiszli:

> Everyone was inside. A hoarse command rang out: "SS and Sonderkommando leave the room." They obeyed and counted off. The doors swung shut and from without the lights were switched off.
>
> At that very instant the sound of a car was heard: a deluxe model, furnished by the International Red Cross. An SS officer and a SDG (*Santätsdienstgefreiter:* Deputy Health Service Officer) stepped out of the car. The Deputy Health Service Officer held four green sheet-iron canisters. He advanced across the grass, where, every thirty yards, short concrete pipes jutted up from the ground. Having donned his gas mask, he lifted the lid of the pipe, which was also made of concrete. He opened one of the cans and poured the contents — a mauve granulated material— into the opening. The granulated substance fell in a lump to the bottom. The gas it produced escaped through the perforations, and within a few seconds filled the room in which the deportees were stacked. Within five minutes everybody was dead. . . .
>
> In order to be certain of their business the two gas-butchers waited another five minutes. Then they lighted cigarettes and drove off in their car. They had just killed 3,000 innocents.[15]

The process of destruction perfected at Auschwitz represented the culmination of years of research and testing, and exactly how the advances introduced softened the harshness of killing for the perpetrators should be carefully noted.

For one thing, Zyklon killed the gas chamber inhabitants very quickly. Rudolph Höss, commandant of Auschwitz, estimated that the killing took anywhere from three to fifteen minutes, depending upon the weather and how many individuals were locked in the chamber.[16] Because of the speed of the destruction process, the agony of dying was likewise abbreviated. This was a far cry from the prolonged suffering that frequently accompanied carbon monoxide asphixiation. Furthermore, when the chamber doors were opened the Auschwitz body disposal squads did not have to contend with the unnerving spectacle of still living, moving, gasping, and twitching bodies, as was so often the case in camps where carbon monoxide was used. Zyklon did a far better job of producing bodies without any life signs.

Like other gassing techniques, the Zyklon procedure kept the act of destruction hidden from the eyes and therefore the consciences of the perpetrators. The health officer who dropped the gas canisters into the chamber did not see the deadly result of his action. The same can be said for those who led the hordes into the chambers and those who removed the dead bodies afterwards. No one saw anyone being killed through the thick, impenetrable walls of the gas chamber.

Another major improvement pioneered at Auschwitz was the inclusion of both killing and body disposal under the same roof. The compactness of the killing process featured the anteroom, gas chamber, and crematory ovens working together in close harmony to insure a near flawless performance. The technicians were totally engrossed in the task of operating and maintaining the destruction machinery. There was no time to personalize those slated for extinction. The whole process was structured as a strictly rational, technical endeavor, devoid of any emotionality.

Destruction by the Zyklon method was also found to be safe and secure for the perpetrators. Although there were periodic episodes of inmate resistance to destruction, few death technicians found themselves targets of attack by the condemned. One of the truly phenomenal things about the killing procedure at Auschwitz is that such a small number of perpetrators were responsible for dispatching millions to their deaths. This is surely a tribute to the technological ingenuity and psychological acumen built into the gassing process! The naked victims had been thoroughly demoralized before entering the chamber doors; there was little will or resistance left.

All the perpetrators had to do was direct traffic and once in a while push a recalcitrant inmate through the chamber entrance. Never has participation in a massive destruction process been so free of personal danger! This also carried over into the psychological realm. Although there are a number of reports indicating adverse psychological complications from involvement in firing squads, few such accounts can be found among Zyklon B participants.

The success of Zyklon killing can be attributed to the efforts of men like Rudolph Höss. He took great pride in his particular technological innovations and expressed contempt toward those who promoted the carbon monoxide method.[17] Höss set out to demonstrate the superiority of Zyklon, something he accomplished quite conclusively. Moreover, the intense controversy between advocates of Zyklon B and carbon monoxide illustrates the highly competitive atmosphere in which destructive techniques developed, grew, and flourished. Individuals were literally vying with one another to see who could come up with the safest, quickest, and most effective method of killing. This unwavering commitment of such participants at each step of the way eventually spelled doom for millions.

Cutting

1. Dilatation and Curettage

Before vacuum aspirators came on the scene, the most frequently used method of destroying unborn children in the first three months of pregnancy was through dilatation and curettage (hereafter referred to as D & C). This technique is initiated with a local anesthetic being applied to either side of the cervix (mouth of the womb) and the uterus. A general anesthetic, which puts the woman to sleep, is also commonly employed. The doctor then begins the dilatation process by sliding metal instruments of varying diameters called dilators into the cervical opening with the purpose of dilating or stretching this opening. The cervix is a firm muscle; it does not ordinarily dilate until the end of pregnancy, when the woman goes into labor. It must therefore be forcibly stretched and opened wide enough before the doctor can get at the tiny victim inside.

The physician then proceeds with the curettage phase of the killing process. What he does is insert a rod-shaped instrument called a curette through the dilated opening into the uterus. At the end of the curette is a spoon-shaped knife with sharp serrated edges. This instrument is used to methodically cut the child's body into shreds and scoop out the fragments. Sometimes the child's head is too large and solid for the curette to obliterate entirely, and a ring forceps is generally employed to crush the head. Its pieces are then small enough to extract. The curette and forceps are used together to cut up and scrape out not only the baby's body but also the intrauterine life-support systems, including the umbilical cord and placenta.

An ex-abortionist, Dr. Richard Ough, provides some revealing details about what is involved in a D & C abortion:

> Only when I performed an abortion myself did I finally realize the essence of the procedure, with euphemisms and semantics brushed aside. It was a D and C termination, the method used in early pregnancy.
>
> Under the direction from a senior colleague, I dismembered the living fetus, and with my instruments extracted the tiny arms, legs, torso and finally the head, which came out reluctantly, as its firm roundness tended to slip from the forceps' grasp. The patient had scarcely missed her second period, yet the tiny feet and hands were almost perfectly formed. I laid the parts on the green surgical sheet to ensure that none had been left behind. Had it not been for my violent intervention, this "Tom Thumb" would have remained in his secure environment, his heart still beating, his brain still functioning.[18]

Some nurses in Hawaiian hospitals have described what goes on as the slicing and chopping up of babies.[19]

D & Cs are typically promoted as quick, simple, and safe procedures; it takes only a matter of from five to fifteen minutes to completely destroy the baby and those associated structures that sustain intrauterine existence. Nevertheless, the physician-abortionist is still faced with a formidable challenge: he must forcibly invade the sanctuary of the womb and literally attack, in most instances, a perfectly healthy, developing child with a lethal weapon without damaging the abortee's internal organs and tissues. From the standpoints of the ecology of pregnancy and the often delicate hormonal and other balances in the intrauterine environment, one can hardly imagine a more severe disruption of natural processes than that induced by a D & C abortion.

Moreover, according to obstetrician-gynecologist Dr. William J. Sweeney, the D & C is a blind procedure, inasmuch as the physician cannot see or feel what he is doing: "A pregnant uterus on which you perform an abortion is soft. You can't feel the top of it. It's like curetting a cloud. You can perforate that uterus without ever knowing it and then have to go back and operate abdominally to repair the damage you might have done." Despite such technological limitations, Dr. Sweeney concludes with the old practice-makes-perfect adage. "Well, we've gotten pretty good at this since the law went into effect," he explained. "We're doing quadruple the number of abortions we did at first." [20]

The D & C qualifies as a near perfect type of killing technique on several counts. Besides being quick and efficient, its most prominent virtue is that the victim remains hidden from the executioner before, during, and after he proceeds with his acts of scientific butchery. Concealment of a bona fide victim is abetted by three factors — the victim's non-visibility, his tiny size, and the technological skill of the killer. The perpetrators never see, nor do they wish to see, the intact, growing child who is conveniently hidden from sight under layers of skin, tissue, and abdominal muscles. The blindness of the D & C procedure also helps the physician to remain blind to what he is actually doing. Because the individual in the womb is so small, especially during the first six to seven weeks after conception, it is a fairly easy task for the curette to destroy all vestiges of humanity with a few short strokes before scooping and scraping it out of the womb. All the doctor and nurse attendants usually see are indistinguishable fragments of tissue and blood.

Between the eighth and the twelfth week of pregnancy, however, the unborn child, although still quite small, has attained a distinctly human form, is very active, and grows dramatically in size and smoothness of functioning. During this time it takes more surgical skill to slice up the victim thoroughly enough so that the perpetrators will not have to directly observe the reality of what is in essence a wholesale slaughter of a defenseless human life. Many doctors, nonetheless, have become quite adept at so dismembering the victim's arms, legs, organs, rib cage, and head inside the womb that when they are scraped out nothing recognizably human can be detected. This goes a long way toward sustaining the perpetrators in the fiction that all they are doing is simply removing tissue, contents, or protoplasm from the uterine cavity. Even when some dismembered body parts are identifiable, they are usually so small and fragmented that they have little impact on the killers. The perpetrators do, though, have a stake in being able to identify any intact parts; it is important to make sure that the uterus is entirely emptied of all body components and other related tissues. Neglect of this post-destruction examination could lead to inadvertently leaving remnants inside the woman and thereby causing bleeding, infection, and other possibly harmful complications.

Although D & Cs are highly successful on most counts, they do not quite make the grade as a perfect method of destruction. Much of this is due to the technological limitations inherent in a procedure where sharp instruments are applied blindly. Enough instances of uterine perforation, retained fetal and placental parts, infection, and excessive blood loss have occurred to make physicians cautious about employing D & C procedures for abortion.

Furthermore, the act of dismembering the small human bodies sometimes proves to be anguishing because some of the parts cut and pried out of the uterus are recognizably human. According to one experienced physician-abortionist:

> When you do a D & C most of the tissue is removed by the Olden forceps or ring clamp and you actually get gross parts of the fetus out. So you can see a miniature person so to speak, and so even now I occasionally feel a little peculiar about it, because as a physician I'm trained to conserve life and here I am destroying life.[21]

2. Dilation and Extraction

Another method of destroying unborn humans with sharp instruments is called dilation and extraction (D & E). This is similar to the D & C except it is employed beyond the twelfth week of pregnancy and therefore involves killing, dismembering, and extracting larger and more fully developed individuals. It is being promoted as superior to the more common method of destroying human lives in the womb during the second trimester, the intraamniotic injection (IAI), on several counts: it is cheaper, safer, quicker, and less traumatic for the woman. With a D & E, there is also no possibility that the victim could ever be aborted alive, as sometimes happens when an IAI is employed.

While D & E may qualify as an excellent, relatively flawless method of eliminating midtrimester humans as far as the aborting woman is concerned, it still contains some unnerving features for the physician-executioner to contend with. A study conducted at the University of California in San Francisco (UCF) found that "D & E is apt to bruise doctors' psyches . . . even give them nightmares." The reason for such reactions, according to a report in *Medical Tribune* of January 25, 1978, has to do with the nature of the procedure:

> Dilation and extraction (D & E) is being shunned by physicians, who would rather not stare at a bloody

and butchered reminder that they have actually destroyed a fetus. . . .

Wielding forceps with no-slip transverse edges, a doctor extracts the fetus piece by piece. "The gynecologist is aware of being the active agent in the D & E procedure" because he "is the one who is crushing and dismembering the fetus," Dr. Sadja Goldsmith, a gynecologist on the UCF team, told MEDICAL TRIBUNE.[22]

At a meeting of the Association of Planned Parenthood Physicians in October 1978, Dr. Warren M. Hern likewise reported on the psychological anguish experienced by some physicians who employed the D & E method of destruction. "Some part of our cultural and perhaps even biological heritage," he explained, "recoils at a destructive operation on a form that is similar to our own." The main reason for this, admits Dr. Hern, is that "there is no possibility of denial of an act of destruction by the operator. It is before one's eyes. The sensations of dismemberment flow through the forceps like an electric current." [23]

Here is unadorned violence staring the doctor in the face. In this procedure it is difficult to deny the existence of a human victim and what the physician is doing to the victim. Things are too stark and overt; causality is crystal clear. This type of killing fails to meet the most crucial criteria of successful methods of destruction because the victims' body parts are too large and visible, the killing procedure is too conspicuous and messy, and the fact that the physician is the actual agent of destruction is undeniable.

Despite such serious technical and psychological drawbacks, D & E is still being touted as a better method of destroying individuals in the second trimester of gestation than IAI. If physicians are to meet the needs of abortion patients and spare them the physical and psychological complications of the riskier IAI abortions, then, according to Dr. Mildred Hanson, they must learn to put up with the negative facets of D & Es. "There's no reason," she stated, "we should avoid this unpleasant aspect and expect the patient to bear a deeper burden of guilt." [24] According to Dr. Goldsmith and colleagues, "doctors have found that these negative reactions decrease as they get used to the procedure." [25]

It is frightening when one realizes how totally brutalized some members of the medical profession can become. Apparently, given enough time and experience, even this most obvious act of scientific barbarism can be taken in stride, can become routine and devoid of any emotional significance. Whatever vestiges of conscience some doctors start out with are soon destined to be obliterated by the frequent and skillful application of scientific instrumentation for destructive purposes. This must certainly rate as the ultimate in desensitization to destruction.

3. Hysterotomy

Hysterotomy is another method of killing the unborn that involves cutting. After administering a general anesthetic, the doctor makes a long incision on the lower part of the woman's abdomen. He then places his fingers through the opening, reaches into the uterus, and carefully tears the placenta and the child inside the amniotic sac away from the wall of the uterus. This in effect is the crucial destructive act: it separates the child and his intrauterine life-support system, his life-sustaining sources of oxygen and nutrients. This is more than enough to bring about rapid suffocation. The doctor then removes the dead child, umbilical cord, and placenta from the uterus.

Although hysterotomies are performed less frequently than other methods of killing children in the mid point of pregnancy and beyond, they are employed often enough in situations where other techniques are inadvisable or fail to work. Coincidentally, hysterotomy abortion is quite similar to a cesarean section birth, but while the procedures are almost identical their outcomes are miles apart. When the c-section child is taken out of the uterus he is immediately placed on such necessary extrauterine life-support aid as special incubators, intravenous nourishment, or resuscitory equipment. Not so for the victim of hysterotomy abortion. Instead, nourishment, oxygen, and other life-sustaining treatments are withheld in a manner reminiscent of what is done with unwanted, defective newborns.

Obviously, hysterotomy is not an ideal technique of destruction; there are too many serious drawbacks. The one given the most prominence has to do with the risks involved in undergoing major surgery of this nature. For one thing, general anesthesia always presents greater dangers than local anesthesia. For another, the probability of complications and maternal mortality from an act that cuts into the abdomen and tears the child out is far greater than from any other type of abortion procedure. A study of 402,000 legal abortions performed in New York City from mid-1970 to mid-1972 revealed a maternal mortality rate of 208.3 per 100,000 abortions when hysterotomy was the technique used. This far exceeded the maternal death rates from other abortion methods: saline, 18.8; D & C, 2.4; suction, 1.1[26]

Psychologically speaking, hysterotomy is a formidable technique to contend with. Unlike other abortion methods, the procedure is not done blindly; it conceals neither the victim nor the act of destruction. As the doctor invades the sanctuary of the womb he can see a well-formed human being moving inside the transparent amniotic sac. After shearing away the child's life line from the uterine wall, the doctor can also observe him waging a hopeless battle against this devastating physician-induced action. Under such circumstances it is difficult, if not impossible, for the doctor to deny his role as the major technical perpetrator. It is not hard to understand why most physicians try to avoid performing hysterotomies.

In light of the psychological adversities associated with hysterotomy technology, it is a wonder that any are being performed at all. Nonetheless, there seem to be enough doctors around to do quite a few of them. In an interview conducted by Gloria Steinem for *Ms* magazine, Dr. Kenneth Edelin estimated that 2 percent of the legal abortions performed in the United States are hysterotomies. On the basis of 900,000 abortions reported in 1975, this means at least

18,000 hysterotomies were performed. From this, Dr. Edelin had to admit, "that's a lot of hysterotomies." [27] Those who engage in this type of killing may very well constitute one of the fastest growing breeds of medical executioners, a group that has become so desensitized toward violence that when it stares them in the face they continue to remain detached and unperturbed.

One other technical and psychological problem connected with doing hysterotomies is the greater chance of producing victims who are still alive or at least contain visible life signs such as movement or a beating heart after being aborted and removed from the uterus. Although the doctor performing the procedure may not be bothered personally by the sight of such a disquieting event, he cannot be sure that those assisting him possess an equivalent degree of emotional immunity. In order to shield others from the shock of confronting a still-living human victim, some doctors have tacked on a supplemental procedure to the hysterotomy technique. What they do is keep the child in the uterus for three to five minutes after detachment from the wall of the uterus. During this period the child's oxygen supply is conclusively cut off by pressure on the umbilical cord. By the time the victim is removed from the the uterus into the view of others in the operating room, all visible signs of life have been completely extinguished. This, by the way, is the very thing that Dr. Edelin was convicted of before being exonerated on appeal.

Some research-minded physicians even prefer the removal of aborted babies with life signs. Hysterotomy "products" are considered excellent research material because of their intact condition and still-functioning life processes. Such specimens are particularly valuable for experiments aimed at testing and developing equipment designed to salvage wanted premature infants.

Vacuuming

In the meantime, technicians have been far from idle. Their pursuit of a better way to exterminate first-trimester

humans is unrelenting. They have come up with what many
believe is a final solution to the problem of unwanted pregnancies: vacuum aspiration abortion. This technique involves
tearing to smithereens living, growing unborn human beings
and sucking their remains out of the womb through cannulas
and tubes hooked up to a vacuum pump.

Like most destruction methods developed by medical
scientists, vacuum aspiration abortion did not appear on the
scene suddenly but has had a long history of scrupulous testing
and experimentation before its widespread adoption. One of
the first uses of negative pressure for inducing abortion was
carried out by Dr. S. G. Bykov as far back as 1927. His contribution to destructive technology featured a syringe with
enough suction force to destroy and reduce the body within to
an indiscriminate blob of protoplasm. It was not until 1958
that Chinese physicians reported on a more extensive development and utilization of this same method.[28] Suction abortion
has since become the most common method of killing unborn
babies throughout Japan and Eastern Europe. More recently,
this has also been the case for western countries, including the
United States, where vacuum aspirators have largely replaced
D & Cs in popularity among physicians. The extent to which
vacuum aspirators dominate the weaponry employed in the
physicians' war against the unborn is strikingly evident in
statistics compiled by the US Center for Disease Control: of
the 1,966,067 legal abortions performed in the United States
from 1972 to 1974, 1,436,120 involved the use of a suction
machine.[29]

The mechanics of vacuum aspiration destruction are similar
to what happens in D & Cs in several respects: the abortion
area is anesthetized with either a local or general anesthetic
and the cervix must be forcibly dilated beforehand. The aspirator also tears apart the child's body inside the womb. The
damage is not done by cutting with a sharp instrument but
by the sucking force of a suction curette attached to a vacuum
pump. This type of curette is a slender hollow tube about
six inches long with different-sized openings at its rounded
tip, depending upon the duration of pregnancy. Its other end
is attached to a long pressure tubing made of rubber or poly-

ethylene, which is in turn connected to an electrical pump. After placement of the curette through the dilated cervix into the uterus, the motor pump is turned on. It sounds like a vacuum cleaner, but the suction pressure is twenty-nine times more powerful.[30]

Destruction takes place rapidly. The child's small body is immediately reduced to a nondescript fluid mass of tissue, blood, and cartilage. The force of the pressure sucks the obliterated remains out of the uterus through the holes in the curette, through the tubing, and finally into a collecting bottle. It usually takes no more than several minutes for the suction apparatus to complete the destruction-disintegration process. It is not surprising, then, that nurses in one Hawaiian hospital referred to the aspirator as "the murder machine." [31]

Vacuum aspiration is one of the most effective killing procedures ever devised. It is frequently promoted as the neatest, quickest, and least painful technique of all. And much medical literature appears to be directed toward proving these claims.

Neatness is an important ingredient, and makes aspiration a particularly attractive method of destruction. It is not as messy as a D & C; sucking rather than cutting out the baby is a cleaner and less bloody process. This is particularly the case in early pregnancy, when the suction device can rapidly demolish and remove the miniscule victim with little blood loss. The flow of blood is also reduced because the soft, flexible curette often used for aspiration in pregnancies of up to eight weeks gestation is less likely to perforate the uterus than the sharp-edged steel or metal curettes used in D & C abortions. The establishment of vacuum aspiration abortion as a cleaner method of destruction than D & Cs brings to mind the similar advantage that Zyklon B had over carbon monoxide gassing in the concentration camps of the Third Reich: it left less of a mess.

The speed with which the aspirator destroys and gets rid of the victim is one of its most distinctive characteristics. *Medical World News* was sufficiently impressed with the quickness of this procedure to pose the question, "Two-Minute Abortion is Here — Are We Ready?" [32] In a review of the

literature on the use of the uterine aspirator in Japan and
Eastern Europe, Drs. Dorothea Kerslake and Donn Casey of
the department of obstetrics and gynecology at Newcastle-
upon-Tyne, England, found that aspiration of the parts usually
took even less than two minutes.[33] Psychologist Dr. Harvey
Karman, one of the most prolific innovators in the field of
first-trimester abortion technology, has a unique way of expressing how fast his own version of suction abortion actually
works. His typical answer to the abortee's question, "When
are you going to start?" is "We're already finished; you can
go home."[34] Dr. Ming K. Hah, reputed to be the fastest
abortionist in Chicago, vacuums the unwanted unborn to
smithereens at a breakneck pace: eight abortions per hour,
forty per day. At times, he is quick enough to perform two
abortions simultaneously.[35]

The painlessness of vacuum aspiration is another endearing
quality of this method given much hoopla in the literature.
A number of aspiration specialists have stated that the me-
chanical stretching of the cervix is apt to hurt more than the
abortion itself. Anesthetics help to alleviate the pain of the
dilating of the cervix, which is particularly unyielding early
in pregnancy, especially among women who have never been
pregnant before.

A certain amount of technical energy has also been devoted to doing abortions without having to dilate at all. The
ubiquitous Dr. Harvey Karman is once again found in the
forefront. He claims to have come up with what he calls an
"a-traumatic abortion" procedure. The atraumatic nature of
the technique is due primarily to Karman's unique technological creation: a soft, narrow, flexible, blunt-edged cannula
(like a suction curette except it is flexible and narrower),
which is introduced into the cervical canal without the necessity of either dilation or anesthesia. His cannula is reputed to
be slender enough to slip into an undilated cervix and still
complete the job of sucking out the child's remains without
anesthetics as late as possibly twelve weeks after the woman's
last menstrual period.

Another component designed to enhance the atraumatic
character of his procedure is the use of a hand-operated plas-

tic syringe — similar in appearance to a hypodermic syringe — to supply the necessary pressure. Apparently, a silent-operating portable syringe is far less psychologically painful than a noisy vacuum pump. A picture of Karman with his two-piece minisuction kit, consisting of cannula and plastic syringe, next to the forty-three instruments generally recommended for D & C abortions is intended to highlight the simplicity and superiority of his method.[36] Karman has so much confidence in his product that he is even willing to allow its implementation to fall into the hands of paramedics.[37] For this he has become a veritable patron saint to some women's liberation groups, who see his methodology as making it possible for them to realize their fondest dream: the maintenance of control over their bodies through painless, self-administered technology.

With regard to removing all traces of the victim, suction abortion does a better job than even a D & C. Much of this can be attributed to the speed and thoroughness with which the pressure destroys, obliterates, and evacuates, thereby resulting in "no need for continuous manipulation and searching for small parts of tissue as happens in curettage."[38] Again, as in D & Cs, the physician-executioner and medical accomplices do not see the victim before or during the time of destruction; what they do see are the insignificant, indistinguishable results. This kind of killing is limitless because nobody kills; nobody kills because there is no perceptible victim; the only thing, as was so poetically expressed by obstetrician-gynecologist resident Dr. T. Keith Edwards of the Bluefield Sanitarium in Bluefield, West Virginia, is "the budding promise of a new individual crumpled into a red, pink and white mass in a bottle."[39] Because aspiration technology is so effective in hiding the remnants of a destroyed human being, it is easy for the perpetrators to view themselves simply as experts in the removal of tissue and contents.

Although most abortion participants are reluctant to acknowledge concealment of the evidence of destruction as a major reason for employing such early abortion methods as vacuum aspiration, some periodically do so. "It isn't so bad when the embryo has been taken away before the form is

214 MEDICAL HOLOCAUSTS I

recognizable as a human being," declared a nurse in Hawaii. She expressed reservations about involvement in abortions performed already in the third month of pregnancy because "there it is, a recognizable boy or girl, and you know that you have been part of the operation that caused its life to be terminated." [40]

An equally astounding revelation comes from obstetrician-gynecologist Dr. William Sweeney:

> Before twelve weeks, I'll abort someone if that's what she wants. Then the fetus is just an amorphous mass as far as I'm concerned. But when it gets to where I can recognize it as a human baby, or if it's twenty weeks old it may even have a fetal heart, then I won't perform an abortion except under unusual circumstances. [41]

What an incredible statement for a medical doctor who prides himself on the many children he has brought into the world, often heroically, under severe circumstances! Dr. Sweeney, like many of his illustrious colleagues, does not want the facts of prenatal life to get in the way of his own personal biases. What makes it possible for him and others to sustain the fantasy of the three-month-old-and-under unborn child as nothing more than an amorphous mass? The almost unerring capability of the vacuum aspirator to reduce the tiny victims to just that. The message is quite clear: kill the child before he or she becomes recognizably human. If this is not done, the scientific killers might become too upset by having to confront the reality of what they are doing.

Dr. Sweeney does have one criticism to level against vacuum aspirators: "they're not very nice aesthetically." More specifically, he is bothered by the *"sworrpp"* and "splash" of the "fetus or baby that just got sucked out" into a bottle. He is also upset by the practice of not changing the bottle between abortions. "Can you imagine," he asks, "walking into a room where there was a bottle full of other people's abortions?" [42]

The deplorable thing here is that his objections are based on technical rather than moral considerations. Just as in Nazi

Germany, there is no room for raising questions about the morality of killing. In the world of exterminative medicine, technology is everything and morality is nonexistent.

The efforts of modern medical technicians to develop, test, and promote their destructive wares is a common phenomenon in the intensely competitive world of abortion technology. In a manner akin to the activity of the German gas experts, today's physicians are embroiled in a deadly game of scientific one-upmanship, the purpose of which is to see who can come up with the most effective and unobtrusive method of exterminating unborn children. The medical literature is loaded with endless success stories about the comparative virtues of vacuum aspirators as opposed to D & Cs and other destructive techniques. Professors at the most prestigious medical schools are grinding out numerous research articles on this very topic. The publish-or-perish rat race predominates. Only this time, the professional survival of some in the upper rungs of academic medicine is coming to depend on how many unborn victims can be salvaged for purposes of research and scholarly output before, during, or after they are killed. Rarely has making a living for so few been so closely tied in with the destruction of so many!

Lethal Injections

1. Morphine, Scopolamine, and Phenol

Patients in the euthanasia institutions of Nazi Germany were commonly killed by injecting morphine, scopolamine, phenol or other poisonous substances into various parts of the body with hypodermic syringes. The fact that this particular method was carefully administered and supervised by doctors and nurses in a medical setting under the guise of inoculations against disease facilitated its successful implementation. The victims remained calm and manageable, while the perpetrators experienced little difficulty sustaining the myth of a legitimate medical endeavor. Most of this can be attributed to the killing method employed. Some of those on trial for participation in the euthanasia killings, for example, kept persistently referring to the injections as treating or putting the victims to sleep rather than killing them.[43]

Moreover, the doctor or nurse who administered the injection was not always present when the victim actually died. Sometimes it took several hours for the poison to cause death. The killers therefore did not have to directly confront the ultimate consequences of their scrupulously applied medical procedure. The most they saw was an immediate falling into a seemingly deep and peaceful sleep. If they happened to be present to pronounce the victims dead, so many were killed that it was difficult to distinguish between those they killed and those killed by other staff members. The doctors, nurses and attendants who had to deal with the dead victims several hours after the injection had its deadly effect were often not part of the team that had responsibility for its administration. They could console themselves that their participation was strictly limited to caring for the deceased; they had no control over what went on beforehand. This convenient division of labor went a long way toward diffusing personal responsibility for destruction.

The medical killers became quite taken up with the scientific details of the destruction technique employed. A great deal of curiosity and discussion ensued regarding a number of questions: How long did it take for the poisonous injections to have a lethal effect? What was there about the solutions that caused death? How were various organs affected? What particular mixture of morphine and scopolamine was necessary to kill the victims? These are questions relating to a field of study that Dr. Leo Alexander dubbed ktenology, the science of killing.[44] The answers to these and other questions required testing the various dosage levels employed and close scientific observation of their differential effectiveness in bringing about the desired outcome, which in this case was the victim's demise.

The complete absorption of the perpetrators in the scientific aspects of destruction technology is nowhere better illustrated than in Hadamar defendant replies to questioning by the prosecutor about the fatal dosage levels. Nurse Heinrich

Ruoff answered carefully, "That depended. You have to judge that from the person. The smallest dose was 2½ to 3 c.c. for children, up to 8 to 10 c.c. for adults." [45] Dr. Adolf Wahlmann's response to the same question was likewise expressed with scientific precision. When the prosecutor first asked him what was the lethal dose of morphine or scopolamine, he replied, "There is no lethal dose. There is a maximum dose which can be given without death coming, and in morphine it is .03 til .1." The prosecutor followed this up with a question about the maximum dosage likely to bring about death. Dr. Wahlmann experienced no further problem with the question worded in this more concise manner: "That is very different. If I have a very strong person, then I have to use more. If I have a person who is used to morphine, then I have to use very much. If I have a very weak person, then I need very little." [46]

Another facet of destruction given considerable attention is the time interval between the injections and the actual death of the victims. The speed with which killing could be accomplished was a crucial factor because the perpetrators had the task of getting rid of many individuals over short periods of time. In the euthanasia institutions the traffic at times got quite heavy. Several transports of victims arrived within a twenty-four-hour period; one group had to be exterminated and removed from view before the next batch arrived. This required setting up shifts of workers, smooth handling of the doomed patients, and, above all, killing techniques that worked quickly enough to prevent undue overlapping between the various groups of human expendables.

At the Hadamar Trial, Nurse Ruoff furnished some details regarding the length of survival after the injections were administered: "Half an hour — an hour — sometimes even two hours. It depended. Sometimes it was only a quarter of an hour." Interest also focused on whether poison administered through injections or tablet form produced death faster; the answer — both were equally swift. [47]

Killing by injection was not confined to the euthanasia hospitals; it also became a popular method of exterminating "unworthy patients" in the concentration camps. Care for

sick patients in the Auschwitz camp infirmary consisted of
phenol injections through the heart. Since many could be done
in an hour, this was considered an efficient method of treating
typhus epidemics among inmates.[48]

Auschwitz survivor Dr. Vilem Jurkovic provided grim
details about destruction by phenol injections and the amount
of time it generally took to bring about the victims' deaths:

> In a little room at the end of the corridor, opposite
> the bathroom, an SS hospital orderly administered an
> injection of phenol straight to the heart. The prisoner
> died in a few seconds, or a minute at the most. It was
> a quick death, administered without any great effort
> or financial outlay. A little farther on, two prisoner
> orderlies had to stack the bodies in the bathroom, like
> so many logs of wood.[49]

Injections of petrol took a longer period of time to kill
than phenol. "Whilst at Auschwitz I saw S.S. male nurses
Heine and Stribitz inject petrol into women prisoners," related survivor Dr. Ada Bimko. "All five of these died within
three to ten minutes." [50]

Dr. Waldemar Hoven, chief physician at Buchenwald,
specialized in doing away with aged inmates in poor health
by injecting undiluted raw phenol into their arms. According
to the testimony of Dr. Erwin Schuler-Ding, presented at the
Doctors' Trial, as the victims sat quietly in a chair a nurse
had the task of blocking a vein in the arm while Dr. Hoven
administered the injection:

> I talked to the doctor about the composition of
> the phenol injection and, as far as I can remember, it
> consisted of undiluted raw phenol, which was to be
> administered in doses of 20 cc.
>
> One by one, four or five prisoners were led in.
> The upper part of the body was naked. . . .
>
> They sat down quietly on a chair, that is without
> any sign of excitement, near a light. A male nurse
> blocked the vein in the arm and Dr. Hoven quickly

injected the phenol. They died in an immediate total convulsion during the actual injection without any sign of other pain. The time between the beginning of the injection and death I estimate at about ½ second. The rest of the dose was injected as a precautionary measure, although part of the injection would have been enough for the fatal result (I estimate 5 cc.).[51]

In terms of sheer speed, this method received the highest rating because the injection caused almost instantaneous death. With the use of quick-acting phenol, however, the perpetrators could not easily conceal the act of destruction from their awareness, since they directly and immediately saw the destructive impact of the injections. In such circumstances it was hard to view their involvement as anything other than an intentional act of medical-induced killing.

How, then, could they continue their active participation in the midst of so much undisguised destruction? Part of the answer is revealed in a description of the effects of phenol poisoning on the victims: "They died in an immediate total convulsion during the actual injection without any sign of other pain." Apparently, the perpetrators were able to function in a situation where destruction took place before their very eyes as long as it was over quickly and its observable consequences disappeared with equal rapidity. They had no time to reflect on the harsh reality of what they were doing. Their task continued to be viewed in its technological and scientific aspect, while disturbing philosophical and moral considerations were kept under cover. Moreover, the quickness of the destructive act was interpreted as a very humane way of disposing of the victims; they were mercifully put out of their misery with no prolonged suffering. It is almost as if the perpetrators were doing the victims a favor. The only thing that mars this portrayal is the existence of what is described as an "immediate total convulsion." Because no "sign of other pain" was detected, this was considered a minor irritant in the implementation of an otherwise swift, reliable, and flawless technique of killing.

The amount of phenol necessary to bring about such a rapid death constituted one other prominent facet of killing efficiency. The dosage usually administered was 20 cc's. But it was estimated that 5 cc's of phenol were sufficient to produce a fatal outcome. What accounts for the remaining 15 cc's also being injected? The efficiency-minded medical killers were surely not about to squander anything so valuable as destructive resources, especially during wartime. On the other hand, they were also very concerned about effectiveness. They wanted to avoid the situation where 5 cc's might not be enough to kill some individuals. It would be upsetting as well as embarrassing if any of the victims happened to survive, even temporarily, an insufficient dose of phenol. The balance between efficiency and effectiveness swung in favor of effectiveness. This meant administering the entire dosage of 20 cc's "as a precautionary measure" to increase the certainty of death.

Phenol injections, even in the hands of skilled medical personnel, had one major shortcoming — they left a telltale odor with the corpse. This was too conspicuous a method for executing prominent prisoners or high-ranking Nazi party members, where secrecy was of the utmost importance. The search went on for a method of execution that would result in autopsy findings that gave the appearance of death from natural causes. After extensive testing was conducted, often on children, Professor Dr. Heissmeyer, a physician associated with the Hohenlychen Hospital, came up with the ideal method — intravenous injections of a suspension of live tubercle bacilli.[52] Medical science again demonstrated its incomparable ingenuity in the field of killing methodology.

2. Saline, Prostaglandins, and Stabbing

The most common method of killing unborn children after the third month of pregnancy is through the injection of a saline solution (a mixture of salt and water) or sodium chloride into their amniotic sacs. The procedure generally involves, first of all, injecting a local anesthetic into the woman's abdomen. This type of anesthetic is preferred over putting her to sleep (a general anesthetic) because it is safer; it is necessary for the woman to be awake in order to tell the physician in case the saline is accidently infused into her uterus or bloodstream instead of the amniotic sac. The next step consists of inserting a $3\frac{1}{2}$ inch 18-gauge spinal needle through the anesthetized area into the sac enclosing the baby. Anywhere from 100 to 250 ml of amniotic fluid surrounding the baby is slowly withdrawn and replaced with an equivalent amount of 20 percent sodium chloride injected into the amniotic sac. It takes from one to seven hours before the concentrated salt solution works its deadly effect on the child. Approximately sixteen to twenty-four hours later or longer the woman goes through a labor of from six to twelve hours [53] and delivers a dead, intact baby. Intravenous injections of oxytocin are often started after saline instillation in order to shorten the injection-abortion time interval.

Even though saline injections have extinguished hundreds of thousands of unborn lives, no medical perpetrators have ever seen the saline solution actually killing the victims. This is truly a tribute to the fantastic capability of saline technology, keeping the unpleasant horrors of destruction concealed from the eyes of the medical executioners. Saline abortion, like other abortion methods, has a decided advantage over many other killing techniques insofar as neither the physician administering the lethal substance nor the medical attendants present ever see a victim being killed. Without an observable victim, the technical killers can content themselves with participating in what gives the appearance of being a valid medical operation. The only thing they see and help to facilitate is the careful application of medical instrumentation on behalf of the woman having the abortion; all medical skill is directed toward keeping her comfortable and making sure she receives the best of care.

What are the real facts of destruction that saline abortion technology so effectively hides? One is unlikely to find an honest portrayal in the medical literature of what happens to the saline victim. Most medical journal articles on saline abortion are preoccupied with assessing the efficacy of saline

as a safe (for the aborting woman) method of inducing second-trimester abortions. Rarely is the fact of fetal death ever
acknowledged, and when it is, it is given scant attention.

An exception to this are the findings from autopsies conducted at the Columbia University College of Physicians and
Surgeons on 143 victims destroyed by saline solutions. The
purpose of this scientific butchery was "to assess the mor-
phologic effects of hypertonic saline solutions on the fetus in
the hope of gaining an insight into the actual mechanism of
death." [54] Any lingering doubts about saline abortion being a
method of destruction by poisoning are laid to rest in the
researchers' explanation of the lethal effects of the saline
solution employed:

> That severe fetal dehydration is the direct result
> to be expected from such an extensive exchange is
> supported by our findings of generalized visceral con-
> gestion, striking perivascular hemorrhages, edema, and
> shrinkage of renal convoluted tubules. These findings
> are comparable to those described in acute salt poison-
> ing of infants.... The fatal dose of sodium chloride
> in human subjects has been calculated at about 0.8
> Gm. per kilogram of body weight by the oral route.
> The amounts of sodium chloride administered during
> most saline abortions far exceed the lethal dosage as
> far as the fetus is concerned. [55]

Further nuances regarding the dynamics of destruction
from saline poisoning are also provided:

> The rapidity with which the fetus dies very likely
> influences the pattern and/or degree of tissue damage.
> The time interval between saline instillation and fetal
> death has varied from as early as 1 hour to as late
> as 7 hours, with a mean of 4 hours. The rapidity of
> fetal death has suggested that hypertonic saline might
> cause spasm of the cord vessels with cessation of cord
> blood flow as the primary cause of death....
> Finally, the possibility must be considered that

fetal shock may actually constitute the most important intermediary mechanism of fetal death during saline abortion, as well as in other instances of acute salt poisoning. The widespread sludging and engorgement of blood vessels occurring in these conditions may effectively reduce the circulating blood volume and thus initiate and/or perpetuate a state of shock. . . .

In conclusion, the evidence from this study and other studies strongly suggests that the infusion of hypertonic saline solutions into the amniotic cavity directly results in acute salt poisoning of the fetus. Development of fetal hypertonicity (hypernatremia) leads to widespread vasodilatation, edema, congestion, hemorrhage, shock, and death.[56]

Another unusually frank and detailed description of how saline kills the child in the womb was furnished by abortionist Dr. William B. Waddill at a preliminary hearing before the Municipal Court of the West Orange Judicial District of California on April 18, 1977. The purpose of this hearing was to determine if there was sufficient evidence to bring Dr. Waddill to trial for the strangulation death of a newborn baby girl who survived a saline abortion attempt. Dr. Waddill tried to impress upon the court that it was the saline that killed the baby and not him. In the process of doing this, he freely elaborated the following theories about how saline brings about the baby's death:

20 percent hypertonic saline is an extremely caustic solution. The mechanism of death of the fetus is not absolutely known. There are a number of different theories on it. . . . The baby has respiration or active respiration at at least 16 weeks gestation. It also has active sucking and swallowing at 16 weeks gestation. The hypertonic saline goes into the amniotic fluid. This goes into the fetus. It goes in also through the skin. The hypertonic saline causes a tremendous change in the electrolyte balance inside the uterine cavity. There's a tremendous influx of fluid

from the maternal circulation into the cavity. The uterine cavity increases its size. Probably some of the increase in size has to do with the precipitation of labor. The hypertonic saline destroys the placenta for all intents and purposes as far as its endocrine or hormonal production is concerned. Probably one of the main ways it affects the fetus is through the umbilical cord. The umbilical cord is probably about 99 percent water. The hypertonic saline causes a tremendous amount of dehydration by withdrawing fluid.

Hypertonic saline causes tremendous basal dilatation of the blood vessels. In other words, the vessels just dilate and just stay dilated and with the extreme dehydration that occurs throughout the baby through the lungs, the gastrointestinal tract, the kidneys, through the vasculature, the cardiovascular system inside the baby, and the blood vessels of the baby, the brain is, I'm sure, destroyed from lack of blood supply, but then I know — no one, I guess, could probably give you an absolute time estimate on this thing, but it is such a caustic and tremendously bad and hostile environment for the baby that it just creates an enormous destructive process.[57]

The purpose of Dr. Waddill's candor was not to shed light on the harsh realities of intrauterine destruction but to save his own skin. His frankness is unlikely to set a precedent of truth telling among other medical executioners of the unborn. Most abortionists would neither admit that what is in the womb is a baby, nor would they dare state saline kills this baby. Why is one form of killing (lethal injection) permissible while the other (manual strangulation) is not? Could it be because one is far less noticeable and easier to conceal than the other?

The following less technical but comparably rhetoric-free account provides additional insight into the destructive impact of saline on the baby within:

A concentrated salt solution is injected into the

amniotic fluid. The baby breathes and swallows it, is poisoned, struggles, and sometimes convulses. It takes over an hour to kill the baby. . . .

The corrosive effect of the concentrated salt, often burns and strips away the entire outer layer of the baby's skin. This exposes the raw, red, glazed looking subcutaneous layer. The baby's head sometimes looks like a "candy apple."

Some have also likened this method to the effect of napalm on innocent war victims. It is probably every bit as painful.[58]

Like their Nazi predecessors, modern medical men also pay close attention to the time interval between injection and destruction. Because technology is not yet developed enough to directly visualize the moment of death in the womb, more indirect methods are used, such as electronic devices for recording the fetal heart rate. At the University Medical School of Szeged in Hungary, intrauterine fetal death was indicated when fetal heart actions could no longer be picked up by the Doptone fetal pulse detector applied every other hour.[59] The time lapse from injection to death for saline abortion victims killed at the University of Cincinnati College of Medicine varied from thirty minutes to two hours. Fetal death in this instance was measured by monitoring fetal heart sounds with an ultrasonic detector.[60] A more elaborate technique of determining fetal death was developed at Mount Sinai Hospital in New York City: in case the fetal heart beat could not be detected by auscultation or a Doppler device, radiological or ultrasonic equipment was used for purposes of further validation.[61]

Why all this concern about pinpointing the time of fetal death? One must keep in mind that those who specialize in destroying unborn children are not just ordinary executioners but, even more important, scientific executioners. As such their approach to killing is to combine the elements of both curiosity and efficiency. Being scientifically trained, they have a built-in desire to know the precise mechanism of fetal death even though it cannot be viewed directly; efficiency dictates that killing proceed as quickly and smoothly as possible. A more specific knowledge of how long it takes the saline to kill the child is viewed as a valuable step toward improving the efficiency of destruction.

Besides, having documented evidence that the child in the womb no longer has a heart beat gives the doctor the reassurance that he has prevented the physician-abortionist's most dreadful fear, the delivery of a live baby, from becoming a reality. If heart action is still detected even hours after the saline has been administered, the doctor can then apply what is defined as preventive medicine: another shot of saline to make sure the child is dead before the time of actual delivery. To the medical executioner, fetal death is a strictly technological task to be accomplished with the utmost dispatch. It is not a personalized event vested with feelings but simply a cerebral, intellectual occurrence; an abstraction to be given concrete form through time intervals. The fact that the victim's death cannot be seen reinforces this emotionally-detached orientation.

Contemporary doctors, like their Nazi counterparts, also display considerable interest in what dosage levels are most apt to bring about the victim's demise. Today's medical journals are literally saturated with articles containing detailed information about the destructive effectiveness of various amounts of saline. The three crucial factors commonly identified are the amount of amniotic fluid removed preceding saline infusion, the concentration of saline used, and the volume of saline injected.

While a 20 percent solution of concentrated saline is considered deadly enough to kill most midtrimester humans with few if any hitches, Dr. Paul C. Jenks of Waterloo, New York switched to a stronger 23.4 percent concentration in order to "secure the abortion" and avoid making a second injection. Dr. Jenks is no armchair theorist. His personal contribution to today's physician-run death industry is substantial. As of May 1973 he claimed credit for performing 530 saline abortions with only minor complications for the aborted women.[62] On the other hand, one must not make saline concentrations too strong, because although they might more conclusively destroy the child in the womb they could also have severe or even disastrous effects on the aborting woman. A number of maternal deaths in the past have been attributed to supersaturated 35 percent concentrations of saline.[63] The scientific killers must maintain an often delicate balance between killing the unborn as quickly and efficiently as possible while at the same time insuring the safety and well-being of the abortee.

Dr. David H. Sherman's experience with nine thousand saline-induced deaths performed in a special hospital saline unit provides an impressive base from which to draw conclusions about fatal dosage levels. Regarding the amount of amniotic fluid withdrawn according to the stage of pregnancy, Dr. Sherman found the following most effective: 75 ml up to seventeen weeks of gestation; 100 to 125 ml from seventeen to twenty weeks; 200 to 225 ml above twenty weeks. With respect to the volume of saline it took to bring about destruction and expulsion, he has these rules of thumb to offer: small volumes of saline solution, as little as 50 to 75 ml, have induced abortion but not always with predictable success; up to 250 ml are required for pregnancies of twenty-one to twenty-four weeks duration.[64]

After a review of the literature and a detailed study of 143 unborn babies destroyed by saline, Dr. Robert S. Galen and several colleagues made a revealing observation regarding fatal dosage levels: "The amounts of sodium chloride administered during most saline abortions far exceed the lethal dosage as far as the fetus is concerned."[65] This constitutes a precautionary measure: an overdose enhances the certainty of death before expulsion into the extrauterine environment. It is this same kind of preoccupation with technological proficiency that prompted Nazi doctors to inject their victims with an overabundance of phenol.

Further information on the dynamics of fetal death is starting to receive greater attention from today's medical scientists. Their interest is not motivated by concern for the victim. They have little or no desire to comprehend how saline death is experienced by the child in the womb; the fact that it is often a prolonged and agonizing process does not seem to penetrate the perpetrators' awareness. Since technology spares them from the ordeal of actually seeing the child's hopeless battle against the deadly assault of saline poisoning, they can calmly discuss and describe with a fair degree of scientific detail something they have never emotionally or ethically grasped.

The closest the technical killers come to the brutal reality of saline destruction is in the autopsy room, where the small corpses are carefully examined for objective evidence of the destructive aftermath. Here the impact cannot be denied — the scorched and dehydrated outer layer of skin, the subcutaneous hemorrhages, the engorged blood vessels, the striking pools of blood in the lungs and other organs — findings which, according to Dr. Galen and others, are closely akin to "acute salt poisoning of infants." [66] Still, dissecting and analyzing already-deceased bodies is miles away from and far less disturbing than having to watch living, moving human beings slowly succumb to the corrosive effects of a poisoned environment. The emotional impact on the perpetrators is considerably muted; it is an entirely technical, after-the-fact matter. The pathologist who conducts the autopsy is not usually a participant in the abortion procedure. He therefore finds it possible to go about the business of assessing the destructive damage with a clear conscience.

It should be kept in mind that the reason underlying most legitimate autopsies is to shed greater light on the cause of death in order to better medically counteract or prevent that which brought about the death. This stands in sharp contrast to the major purpose for performing autopsies on saline abortion victims: to perfect the technology that killed the child. Only in a world dominated by technological destruction could such a perversion attain respectability! Physicians in the Third Reich also excelled in doing autopsies for improving destructive technology instead of fighting disease. Contemporary American doctors appear to have no qualms about continuing this tradition.

Another facet of the saline procedure that helps the medical participants continue their involvement despite the advanced age and size of the victims is the extended period of time between instillation of the poisonous salt and expulsion of the dead baby in abortion labor. The doctor who administers the lethal substance can conveniently avoid confronting the unpleasant outcome of his meticulously applied technique by not being present when the child is delivered dead.

It is a common practice in many hospitals for nurses to handle abortion labor and delivery. Resident physicians at the North Carolina Memorial Hospital found saline procedures less stressful than D & Cs because they did not have to be in attendance when the dead baby was actually aborted; this part of the procedure was taken care of by the nursing staff.[67] Doctors in Hawaiian and New York hospitals were also likely to be absent when the deceased victims were finally expelled. Again, it was a nursing task to care for the aborted woman and remove the dead child.[68]

Although discarding a dead "product" is not a particularly attractive job, nurses can console themselves that they have nothing to do with a destructive activity that has already taken place hours and sometimes days before. Nurses at some hospitals become so absorbed in coaching the aborting woman in the use of natural childbirth breathing techniques that they have little time available to focus on the aborted victim. Their main purpose is not only to keep occupied with a "professional" task during a period of potential anxiety, but also "to distract the woman and to help her relax." [69] Those who have a more difficult time dissociating their involvement in the death-delivery process from the act of destruction frequently opt to work in the much more convivial atmosphere of the recovery room, where, as one nurse put it, "We don't see the fetus being passed." [70] The division of labor in saline killing closely resembles the allocation of "professional" tasks in the Hadamar Hospital and other euthanasia institutions of Nazi Germany, where a time interval occurred between the injections of morphine and scopolamine and the actual deaths of the victims.

Injection of prostaglandins into the amniotic sac is another technique found especially suitable for destroying second-trimester unborn children. Prostaglandins are a family of chemical compounds that stimulate uterine contractions strong enough to kill the baby and produce the delivery of a dead victim. The administration of prostaglandins is similar to the saline procedure, except that the removal of amniotic fluid is not a necessary preliminary step. The most sucessful approach is to inject a single intraamniotic instillation of prostaglandins or several doses at different time periods. A total of 40 to 50 mg is considered sufficient to kill the child and bring about abortion expulsion. It has been demonstrated that prostaglandin-induced fetal death is a more prolonged process than death precipitated by saline induction. A study done at the University Medical School in Szeged, Hungary backs this up: "Fifty per cent of the fetuses in the saline group died at the early period of the abortion process ... whereas 50 per cent of the fetuses in the PGF_2a [prostaglandin] group died much later." [71]

The prolonged suffering that prostaglandin victims often go through before succumbing is rarely if ever admitted. To the medical abortion mentality it is simply an abstract passage of time to be meticulously measured and recorded rather than a horrendous, personalized tragedy to be denounced. In 1976, however, Dr. Richard Selzer, a surgeon affiliated with Yale University, departed from the medical herd and supplied an unusual rhetoric-free glimpse into what prostaglandin abortion is really like. The abortion was performed in a university hospital on a twenty-four-week-old unborn victim. Dr. Selzer was there as an observer to learn the truth. Apparently he got more than he bargained for. He expected to see a flawless, incident-free procedure, but what he actually saw shook his perception and conscience to their very foundations and left a profound and indelible imprint. In a dramatic and candid fashion, Dr. Selzer likens the unborn child's agonizing battle for life against the intrusion of a lethal needle methodically thrust far into the heart of his intrauterine environment to the death struggle of a sunfish hooked by a fishing line. [72]

While it takes prostaglandins longer to kill the child than is the case with saline, they seem to be more effective in reducing the time interval between injection and actual abortion. A comparison of prostaglandin and saline abortions performed at the New York Hospital-Cornell Medical Center revealed a mean injection-abortion time span of 20.34 hours for saline and 15.16 hours for prostaglandins.[73] A similar conclusion was reached by Dr. Charles H. Hendricks of Chapel Hill, North Carolina in his discussion of a paper on the efficacy of prostaglandins authored by Dr. Thomas F. Dillon and associates in New York: 90 percent of women aborted by prostaglandins did so within thirty-two hours, while 90 percent of those aborted by saline had not done so until fifty-five hours after injection.[74]

Prostaglandins incorporate many of the same features that make saline such an effective method of killing: advanced scientific equipment and instruments, hidden destruction perpetrated on a concealed victim, and a long enough instillation-abortion time period to allow for dispersion of responsibility among different individuals. Like the euthanasia experts of Nazi Germany and the contemporary saline technicians, prostaglandin specialists have also become obsessed with the technological details of destruction. The medical literature on prostaglandins is dominated ad nauseam by such issues as the type of prostaglandin used (F2a, E1, or E2), the route of administration (intravenous, intravaginal, intrauterine, intrauterine-extraovular, intrauterine-extraamniotic, intraamniotic, or oral), and the appropriate dosages and regimen schedules. If one were not aware of the true purpose underlying all this painstaking attention to technical precision, it would be easy to be seduced into accepting it as another illustration of the marvels of medical science in operation.

A unique quality that helps to make prostaglandin abortions more palatable for the perpetrators has to do with its impact on the doomed child. Besides taking longer to kill, its destructive effect is not nearly as prominent as that of saline. In prostaglandin destruction the child is delivered dead, but in a far more intact and less deteriorated condition. The prostaglandin victim resembles in outward appearance a spontaneous abortion, stillbirth or prematurely born deceased infant. Death can therefore be more easily attributed to accidental rather than contrived forces. Prostaglandin-induction outcome is also comparable to the appearance of death from natural causes left by Nazi physician-administered inoculations of tubercle bacilli. Not only do the perpetrators remain at an emotional distance from the act of destruction, but they are also spared the unpleasant aftermath often accompanying saline destruction: the sight of the raw red undersurface where the outer layer of the child's skin has been stripped away by the corrosive effects of hypertonic saline.

Furthermore, the intact condition of prostaglandin corpses makes them ideal specimens for research-oriented physicians. Drs. I. James Park, Ann Wentz, and Howard Jones of the department of obstetrics and gynecology at the Johns Hopkins University School of Medicine indicated that fetal skin and tissue obtained from "prostaglandin abortuses" continued to grow after being implanted in a culture medium. The lack of growth exhibited by similar tissue samples excised from "saline abortuses" demonstrated their unsuitability for biological, chemical, and cytogenetic studies.[75] Thus, contributions to experimental medicine serve as an irresistible bonus derived from prostaglandin-induced abortions. This in turn confers even greater credibility upon this particular technique of killing.

Although today's medical abortionists do not inject phenol directly into the hearts of their victims like the Nazi doctors did, they have come up with a destructive technique that bears a disquieting resemblance to that method. Dr. Anders Aberg, director of the mother-care unit at Lund University Hospital in Sweden, killed an unborn twin by sticking a needle through the heart. Eleven weeks later the dead twin was removed by labor and the living sister by cesarean section. This destructive procedure was set in motion after a biochemical examination by Dr. Michael Cantz of amniotic fluid from fraternal twins in utero revealed that one of them had Hurler's syndrome, a malady that is usually fatal by the age of ten.

The horrendous details of what is touted as a bold, unprecedented, and scientifically-precise procedure appear in *Medical World News* of May 15, 1978:

Using real-time ultrasonic scanning as a guide, Dr. Aberg pierced the heart of the Hurler's fetus with an amniocentesis needle during the 24th week of gestation. Ultrasound enabled him to tell precisely when the needle hit the heart and it stopped. The physicians had kept track of the fetuses' positions by ultrasound after the original amniocentesis, and their relative positions did not change in the five weeks.

A second sample of fluid was taken from the amniotic sac of the abnormal fetus just before the needle pierced its heart, and Dr. Cantz made a second diagnosis of Hurler's — several weeks afterward.[76]

American medical reaction to what is actually the stabbing death of an afflicted human being before birth is almost as horrendous as what was done to this individual. "Amazing," commented fetologist Neil K. Kochenour of the University of Louisville School of Medicine. "I think it sounds like a very good solution, and obviously it worked." Case Western Reserve anatomy professor Dr. M. Neil Macintyre was so awestruck that the most telling remark he could muster was, "I'll be damned." Dr. Michael Kaback, director of the prenatal diagnosis and genetic counseling center at UCLA Harbor General Hospital, referred to the operation as an "extraordinary approach." He did express some vague qualms about "ethical aspects," but was quick to add, "I'm not criticizing; I don't think they did anything wrong." The thing that bothered Dr. Henry L. Nadler, professor of pediatrics at Northwestern University, was not the destructive procedure itself, but the difficulty involved in trying to explain to a parent about sticking a needle into the heart of a twin. Otherwise, he thought that the approach used was not unreasonable.[77]

The above responses provide a glimpse into the appalling mindset spawned by exterminative medicine. No questions are raised about the morality of perverting medical technology for destructive ends. The only issue that matters is the efficiency and effectiveness with which the technology accomplishes its goal. It is another example of a Nazi-style medical ethic in operation: the treatment of afflictions by eliminating the afflicted.

Imposed Starvation

Death by starvation engulfed the victims of Nazi Germany at every phase of the destruction process. Its first effects were felt in the cattle cars on the way to the death camps. The intolerably crowded living conditions without food or water during trips lasting as long as eight days is movingly told by an Auschwitz survivor, Dr. Gisella Pearl: "The small children cried with hunger and cold, the old people moaned for help, some went insane, others gave life to their babies there on the dirty floor, some died and their bodies travelled on with us." [78]

If they happened to survive this ordeal and then escaped selection for the gas chambers, their fate was often slow starvation within the confines of the camp compound. A combination of back-breaking labor and a deplorably meager diet reduced many inmates to a state of "Musulmans," a term commonly used to describe the walking skeletons of Auschwitz.[79] Water was in such short supply that the prisoners gladly exchanged their rations for just a half-pint of it. Many even drank the putrid water from rusted washroom pipes in a final desperate attempt to relieve their parched throats. Dysentery, disease, and death frequently resulted from such actions.

Enforced starvation was also one of the prime methods of destruction employed in the euthanasia program after the gas chambers were dismantled and moved out of the psychiatric institutions. This approach was considered appropriate for defective and disturbed children languishing in the special children's divisions of various hospitals throughout Nazi Germany. One rare inside view of how this was accomplished was revealed to psychology student Ludwig Lehner on a tour he had taken of the Eglfing-Haar mental hospital in the autumn of 1939:

In about fifteen to twenty cribs lay the same number of children, aged one to five. In this ward Pfann-
müller went to particular length to set forth his views.

"These creatures" (he meant the children in
question) "represent to me as a National Socialist
merely a drain on our body politic. We kill" (or he
may have said "We do the thing") "not by poison,
injection, or such methods — that would be merely
furnishing new propaganda material to the foreign
press. . . . No, our method is much more natural and
simple, as you see." With these words he drew one
of the children from its crib, aided by a nurse evidently on regular duty in the ward. He showed around
the child like a dead rabbit and with a knowing expression and a cynical grin said words to this effect:
"This one, for example, may take another two or
three days." I can never forget the sight of this fat,
grinning man, a whimpering bundle of skin and bones
in his fleshy hands, surrounded by the other starving
children. The murderer explained further that food
was not withdrawn from the children all at once
but by gradual reduction of the rations.[80]

To the Nazi mentality of individuals like Dr. Pfann-
müller, death by gradual starvation was viewed as a most
natural and fitting way to dispose of those so frequently referred to as "useless eaters."

Unfortunately, enforced starvation did not end with the
fall of the Third Reich. It is now employed as a method of
dealing with defective and retarded children in the prestigious
medical centers of contemporary America. This was first
brought to the public's attention in 1971 when the Joseph
P. Kennedy, Jr. Foundation produced a twenty-five-minute
film entitled "Who Should Survive?"[81] The film portrayed
an actual case in which a mongoloid infant (also commonly
known as a Down's syndrome baby) born with an intestinal
obstruction (duodenal artresia) was permitted to starve to
death because the parents refused permission for simple cor-
rective surgery to be performed. This did not take place at

the Eglfing-Haar euthanasia hospital in 1939, but at the Johns
Hopkins University Hospital of Baltimore, Maryland in 1963.
At the beginning of the film, Johns Hopkins is described by
Eunice Kennedy Shriver as one of the world's great medical
centers.

The doctor-narrator of the film described some of the
agonizing details involved in the case of no treatment and
involuntary starvation. The explanation for doing this offered
to the nurses was that the parents did not want the operative
procedure done on the child and it was therefore decided
to "respect their decision." The order was given to cease any
artificial means for prolonging the baby's life. A sign, "Nothing by Mouth," was then placed on the bassinet and the
child was wheeled to an isolated room at the end of the
corridor. The doctor-narrator continued to share his feelings
about the prolonged death watch: "I tried to avoid going in
and seeing the baby. If I did look I tried excruciatingly hard
not to touch him. It was difficult to handle or even examine
him." Considerable concern was expressed over the impact
on the nursing staff: "Their initial reaction was one of horror and disbelief that we were made to do this. We were
going to take a baby, a really healthy baby, healthier than
many patients they were caring for, going to a bassinet in a
dark corner and starve to death." The physician-narrator
concluded with an observation on the prolonged nature of
the dying process: "It took 15 days for the baby to become
severely dehydrated enough that he finally died and that was
an awful long time."

The similarities between this case and what happened to
defective and unwanted children in Nazi Germany are disturbingly close. In both instances doctors and nurses acquiesced to the decision to let the children die; in both instances doctors and nurses failed to treat the children's afflictions in addition to withholding food and nourishment;
in both instances the process of starvation and dehydration
was prolonged; in both instances the children were checked
daily to determine their condition and how much longer it
would take them to die.

The procedure of imposed starvation death used at Johns

Hopkins is significant from several technological and psychological vantage points. First, by placing the child in a remote spot the reality of death is hidden. Most hospital personnel are therefore spared the unnerving experience of having to watch the child deteriorate. Then they are not likely to be personally bothered; the whole matter remains distant and abstract. Second, those who had the responsibility of looking after the child and keeping track of his degeneration could soften their moral scruples by viewing the child's dying as if it were a natural occurrence. The order, "Nothing by Mouth," had already been given. Their job was to minister to the child as was ordinarily done with any other dying patient — in a caring manner. This helped them maintain a sense of decency to the very end. Such a stance is similar to that of those nurses who acted compassionately and talked nicely to the victims as they succumbed in the euthanasia hospitals of Nazi Germany. Third, it is important to note why prolonged death by starvation was preferred over quick death from lethal injections. Basically, it was a matter of legality — hastening the child's death through medication was viewed as "clearly illegal" by the Johns Hopkins medical and nursing staff, while not operating and then allowing "nature to take its course" was considered a much more legally acceptable course of action.[82]

Another and perhaps even more fundamental reason for not using death-dealing medication was expressed by one doctor: "No one would ever do that. No one would ever think about it, because they feel uncomfortable about it. . . . A lot of the way we handle these things has to do with our own anxieties about death and our own desires to be separated from the decisions that we're making." [83] The direct administration of lethal drugs is too overt an act. The withholding of treatment and the failure to provide sustenance are acts that are more passive and less obviously related to destruction. Although doing nothing kills as conclusively as doing something, the extended time lapse between the withdrawal of treatment and actual death helps the participants to obscure this connection.

What happened to the mongoloid child at the Johns

Hopkins University Hospital is not, however, just a once-in-a-lifetime aberration. Three previous cases of infants at Johns Hopkins Hospital being allowed to die of starvation and dehydration were also acknowledged in 1971.[84] Just how often this method for dealing with unwanted defective children has been used by other hospitals and medical centers will never be known. But it is far more often than realized if the practice at Johns Hopkins is an example of what is going on elsewhere.

Deplorably, allowing retarded children to die by withholding treatment and nourishment did not cease with the Johns Hopkins revelations. If anything, such a practice in all probability has increased rather than subsided. One indication of this is the boldness with which some physicians have admitted employing this brand of infanticide for mongoloids and seriously afflicted newborns.

Dr. Anthony Shaw of the pediatric division of the University of Virginia Medical Center in Charlottesville, writing in the *New England Journal of Medicine* of October 25, 1973, reported on a situation very similar to the Johns Hopkins case:

> Baby B was referred at the age of 36 hours with duodenal obstruction and signs of Down's syndrome. His young parents had a 10 year old daughter, and he was the son they had been trying to have for 10 years; yet, when they were approached with the operative consent, they hesitated. They wanted to know beyond any doubt whether the baby had Down's syndrome. If so, they wanted time to consider whether or not to permit the surgery to be done. Within 8 hours a geneticist was able to identify cells containing 47 chromosomes in a bone-marrow sample. Over the next 3 days the infant's gastrointestinal tract was decompressed with a nasogastric tube, and he was supported with intravenous fluids while the parents consulted with their ministers, with family physicians in their home community and with our geneticists. At the end of that time the B's decided not to permit

surgery. The infant died 3 days later after withdrawal
of supportive therapy.[85]

The main difference here is that this child was not as hardy
as the Johns Hopkins baby; it took him only three days to die.

In the same issue of the *New England Journal of Medicine*, Drs. Raymond S. Duff and A. G. M. Campbell disclosed that forty-three defective infants were allowed to die
in the Yale University special-care nursery between January 1,
1970 and June 30, 1972. At least one of these victims had
Down's syndrome and intestinal artresia. Treatment was not
given because "his parents thought that surgery was wrong
for their baby and themselves. He died seven days after
birth." [86]

In the technologically-charged, fiercely competitive world
of exterminative medicine, the controversy is not over killing
per se; this is a given, an acceptable and noncontroversial
part of professional life. What is debated is the method of
killing. The destructive procedures that finally win out in
the mad, relentless race to destroy more and more human
expendables are those that kill rationally, swiftly, efficiently,
effectively, and inconspicuously. The preeminence of methodology in the hands of prestigious medical executioners has
pushed the scope of antiseptic destruction far beyond the
boundaries of any reasonable restraints. This model of exclusive dedication to perfecting the techniques of killing is an
alarming commentary on the abominable state of medical
ethics. Prospects for the survival of future generations,
whether they be declared unfit, imperfect, unwanted, or inconvenient, are exceedingly dim, as the growing insensitivity
to unmitigated violence spawned by destructive medical technology threatens to engulf all of civilized society.

CHAPTER 7

Body Disposal

The perpetrators are not only intent on killing the victims but also on getting rid of their remains as quickly as possible. The presence of undiscarded corpses poses too great a threat for a destruction process whose very credibility depends on concealing the true nature of its activities from public view. The Nazi body-disposal squads had a challenging job because most of the bodies they dealt with were large and intact. Burying in mass graves and burning in huge ovens and open pits came to be the most common technological means of total annihilation. Although contemporary body disposers specialize in removing much smaller and less intact corpses, they still have the arduous task of making sure that all the victims' body parts are scraped, sucked, ejected, or cut out of the womb. Their destination after this is often mass burial or incineration in hospital furnaces along with the trash. The medical executioners of both Nazi Germany and today's America have consistently seized upon the destruction-disposal process as an opportunity to exploit their human guinea pigs for commercial and scientific purposes before erasing the evidence of mass extermination entirely. The insidious cycle of selection, destruction, exploitation, and disintegration becomes irrevocably entrenched and along with it comes the extreme brutalization of medical science.

Burying and Burning

1. Nazi Techniques

Although the Nazi destruction of millions was a monumental challenge requiring considerable technological expertise and commitment, this constituted but one part of the destruction process. Getting rid of the corpses proved to be an even more formidable undertaking. The problem of body disposal was acknowledged by Auschwitz commandant Rudolph Höss, in an interview with psychologist Dr. G. M. Gilbert during the Nuremberg trials: "The killing itself took the least time. You could dispose of 2,000 head in a half hour, but it was the burning that took all the time." [1] The other methods of body disposal — burying, commercial utilization, and scientific exploitation — were also time consuming. The technique used in removing the corpses varied according to where the killings took place, the methods employed, and the number of victims killed.

In the euthanasia institutions, a common pattern was killing the patients in gas chambers and then burning their remains in furnaces. As early as December 1939, the Court of Appeals at Frankfurt-on-Main reported on stories circulating among the populace about the destruction-disposal procedure at the Hadamar Hospital:

> The arrivals are immediately stripped to the skin, dressed in paper shirts, and forthwith taken to a gas chamber, where they are liquidated. . . . The bodies are reported to be moved into a combustion chamber by means of a conveyor belt, six bodies to a furnace. The resulting ashes are then distributed into six urns which are shipped to the families. The heavy smoke from the crematory building is said to be visible over Hadamar every day. [2]

That this practice continued into 1941 can be gleaned from a protest issued by the Bishop of Limburg in August 1941:

After the arrival of the busses the people of Hadamar observe smoke rising from the chimney and are shaken by the constant thought of the poor victims, especially when the wind carries the noxious odors in their direction. One effect of the program here being put into effect is that children in chiding each other say: "You're not quite bright, they'll put you in the oven at Hadamar!" [3]

Additional public outcries resulted in the cessation of incineration as a means of disposal at Hadamar and other euthanasia institutions. The belching smoke stacks were too ominous. Later, lethal injections replaced gassing and mass burials supplanted burning. From August 1942 on at Hadamar the process involved carrying the bodies in special stretchers from the wards into the basement. There they were stacked until early in the morning, when the actual burial took place. The bodies were carried to the institution's cemetery in coffins, two bodies to a coffin. Sometimes as many as thirty to thirty-four bodies were dumped into a common grave. The body disposal operation periodically got bogged down, due primarily to the large numbers killed at one time. While the burial squad tried to catch up, the backlog of cadavers filled, according to body-disposal expert Philipp Blum, much of the storage space in the various cellars of the basement. [4]

When the mobile killing units expanded their destructive activities, the practice of doing away with the victims through mass burial in huge pits concomitantly spread throughout the occupied territories of Russia and other countries. This was considered a highly efficient operation; both destruction and disposal took place at the same time in the same site. When the concentration camps first got into the business of large-scale killing, burial in huge ditches continued to persist as a common method of eliminating the evidence of destruction.

Mass burials, however, contained problems that became evident only when the pace of the killing increased. Covering the bodies proved to be a far more complicated task than anticipated. The earth tended to collapse and odors were emitted over a large area. Field commanders found it necessary to issue special orders about doing a better job of covering the graves.[5] Even when adequately covered, the huge masses of destroyed humanity did not always stay submerged. The practice of placing large numbers of bodies in the pits had calamitous consequences at the Belsec concentration camp. "They had put too many corpses in it and putrefaction had progressed too fast, so that the liquid underneath had pushed the bodies on top up and over and the corpses had rolled down the hill."[6]

A more serious deficiency associated with mass burials was that they left tell-tale signs of destruction. As greater numbers of bodies occupied larger tracts of space underground, the perpetrators began to get worried. Discussions focused on finding more conclusive methods of obliterating all traces of the killings. Dr. Herbert Linden, sterilization expert in the Ministry of the Interior, did not hesitate to express his opinion on this matter to SS Police Leader Odilo Globocnik: "But would it not be better to burn the bodies instead of burying them? A future generation might think differently of these matters!" Globocnik, on the other hand, continued to favor burial on idealistic grounds: "But, gentlemen, if after us such a cowardly and rotten generation should arise that it does not understand our work which is so good and so necessary, then, gentlemen, all National Socialism will have been for nothing. On the contrary, bronze plaques should be put up with the inscription that it was we, we who had the courage to achieve this gigantic task."[7]

In the end, reality won out over idealism and the order was given to destroy the mass graves. This necessitated exhuming the bodies and then disintegrating the remains. The intricacies of body-disposal technology associated with making the transition from mass burial to mass burning is well illustrated by what went on at the Treblinka concentration camp. After a number of unsuccessful attempts at incinerating the huge number of bodies to be disposed of, cremation expert Herbert Floss was called in:

According to his investigations ... the old bodies burned better than the new ones, the fat ones better than the thin ones, the women better than the men, and the children not as well as the women but better than the men. It was evident that the ideal body was the old body of a fat woman. Floss had these put aside. Then he had the men and children sorted too. When a thousand bodies had been dug up and sorted in this way, he proceeded to the loading, with the good fuel underneath and the bad above. He refused gasoline and sent for wood. ...

As a first innovation, the excavators would extract the bodies and set them in a pile outside the ditch, where the prisoners would find and transport them to the fires at a ratio of two prisoners per body ... New problem: below a certain level the bodies extracted were dismembered and the prisoners transported them in pieces, a leg under one arm and a torso under the other. As a result they transported many less. Herbert re-enlisted the litters that had been used to carry the bodies from the gas chambers to the ditches: progress.

The output was now two thousand bodies per day. One evening at roll call Floss made a speech.

"Today we burned two thousand bodies. This is good, but we must not stop here. We will set ourselves an objective and devote all our efforts to reaching it. Tomorrow we will do three thousand, the day after tomorrow four thousand, then five thousand, then six thousand, and so on until ten thousand." [8]

Before the construction of permanent gas chambers and crematoriums, the destruction-disposal process at Auschwitz consisted of killing the victims in two thatched cottages made over into primitive gas chambers, and burying them in deep pits. This method of getting rid of the corpses proved unsatisfactory and had to be abandoned in favor of burning:

After a few months, although the corpses were

covered with chlorine, lime and earth, an intolerable stench began to hang around the entire neighborhood. Deadly bacteria were found in springs and wells, and there was a severe danger of epidemics.

To meet this problem, the Sonderkommando was increased in size. Day and night, working in two shifts, the prisoners in the squad dug up decaying corpses, took them away on narrow-gauge trucks and burnt them in heaps in the immediate vicinity. The work of exhuming and burning 50,000 corpses lasted almost til December, 1942. After this experience the Nazis stopped burying their victims and cremated them instead.[9]

After the installation of more modern facilities for extermination, the bodies were cremated in huge ovens and open pits. Auschwitz survivor Dr. Miklos Nyiszli provided an account of how this particular phase of body removal and incineration actually worked:

The Sonderkommando squad, outfitted with large rubber boots, lined up around the hill of bodies and flooded it with powerful jets of water. This was necessary because the final act of those who die by drowning or by gas is an involuntary defecation. Each body was befouled, and had to be washed. Once the "bathing" of the dead was finished . . . the separation of the welter of bodies began. It was a difficult job. They knotted thongs around the wrists, which were clenched in a viselike grip, and with these thongs they dragged the slippery bodies to the elevators in the next room. Four good-sized elevators were functioning. They loaded twenty to twenty-five corpses to an elevator. . . . The elevator stopped at the crematorium's incineration room, where large sliding doors opened automatically. . . . Again straps were fixed to the wrists of the dead, and they were dragged onto specially constructed chutes which unloaded them in front of the furnaces.

There they were laid by threes on a kind of push-cart made of sheet metal. The heavy doors of the ovens opened automatically; the pushcart moved into a furnace heated into incandescence.

The bodies were cremated in twenty minutes. Each crematorium worked with fifteen ovens, and there were four crematoriums. This meant that several thousand people could be cremated in a single day. . . . Nothing but a pile of ashes remained in the crematory ovens. Trucks took the ashes to the Vistula, a mile away, and dumped them into the raging waters of the river.[10]

Another Auschwitz survivor, Dr. Olga Lengyel, furnished several other body-disposal details not mentioned by Dr. Nyiszli. Because it was often impossible to separate the compressed and entangled corpses, the body-removal squads "invented special hook-tipped poles which were thrust deep into the flesh of corpses to pull them out." Just before the corpses were shoved into the furnaces they were carefully sorted: "the babies went in first, as kindling, then came the bodies of the emaciated, and finally the larger bodies."[11]

Getting rid of the victims' remains reached a high level of scientific proficiency at Auschwitz. At first much of this success was due to the construction of large enclosed crematoriums for incineration. Further information on the fantastic capacity of the four Auschwitz crematory units is again supplied by Dr. Lengyel:

Above each rose a high chimney, which was usually fed by nine fires. The four ovens of Birkenau were heated by a total of thirty fires. Each oven had large openings. That is, there were 120 openings, into each of which three corpses could be placed at one time. That meant they could dispose of 360 corpses per operation. That was only the beginning of the Nazi "Production Schedule."

Three hundred and sixty corpses every half hour, which was all the time it took to reduce human flesh to ashes, made 720 per hour, or 17,280 corpses per twenty-four hour shift. And the ovens, with murderous efficiency, functioned day and night.[12]

It was not until the summer of 1944 that their true capabilities for total annihilation were put to the ultimate test. But even they could not handle the enormous job of burning the bodies of 400,000 Hungarian Jews within a forty-six-day period. The versatility of destructive technology, however, proved triumphant. The ovens, augmented by the addition of eight open pits, each about sixty yards long and four yards wide, accomplished this incredible task in good order.[13] The human fat that accumulated on the bottom of the ditches was collected and poured back into the fire in order to speed up the disintegration process. Any remnants of body parts were periodically consumed by flame throwers.[14]

Burning alive in furnaces or pits came to be a favorite method of eliminating the children of Auschwitz at the peak of the killing season. An exchange between witness S. Szmaglewska, a Polish writer, and Soviet prosecuting attorney Smirnov before the International Military Tribunal at Nuremberg in 1946 brought to light the horrifying details:

> *Witness:* When the extermination of the Jews in the gas chambers was at its height, orders were issued that children were to be thrown straight into the crematorium furnaces, or into a pit near the crematorium, without being gassed first.
> *Smirnov:* How am I to understand this? Did they throw them into the fire alive, or did they kill them first?
> *Witness:* They threw them in alive. Their screams could be heard at the camp. It is difficult to say how many children were destroyed in this way.
> *Smirnov:* Why did they do this?
> *Witness:* It's very difficult to say. We don't know whether they wanted to economize on gas, or if it was because there was not enough room in the gas chambers.[15]

Even the most intense and widespread inferno did not always obliterate all signs of destruction. The victims' bones or bone fragments sometimes survived the flames of the crematoriums or pits. Bone-crushing machines were developed to extinguish these final traces of mass extermination. A Soviet-Polish Extraordinary Commission established to investigate crimes committed in the concentration camps discovered that the body-disposal experts resorted to "grinding small bones in a special 'mill.'" At one camp they found "over 1,350 cubic meters of compost consisting of manure, ashes of burned bodies and small human bones." [16]

Survivor Motek Strigler revealed that a bone mill was used to pulverize any remaining vestiges of destruction after the corpses had been exhumed and cremated at the Skarzisko Kamienno extermination center:

> In our own plant the detail, during its sojourn, had to dig up the thousands of bodies that had been buried on the rifle range and cremate them. The site of the mass graves was filled in, graded and planted with grass, but we were still able to find tell-tale traces — fragments of bone, fingers cut off for their rings, melted down gold. The exhumed bones were not burned but loaded into a truck containing a bone mill. [17]

2. Contemporary Techniques

Getting rid of the remains of millions of unborn children after destruction in the womb is not nearly such an overwhelming problem as that confronted by the Nazi body disposers. The main reason for this, obviously, is due to the small size of contemporary victims. Nevertheless, the body-disposal process today is plagued with some vexing difficulties. As was the case in Nazi Germany, it is still far easier to kill the victims than to dispose of all of their remnants. By and large in most abortions the victim is killed inside the womb. The real technological challenge is to remove all of his or her body parts plus the umbilical cord and placenta from the uterine cavity, and then dispose of them.

The body-disposal techniques used today, like those of Nazi Germany, depend upon the killing methods employed. In early abortions, the tiny bodies are rapidly reduced to a gelatinous mass of tissue, fluid, and blood, which literally flows out into a collecting bottle. It is a relatively simple task to get rid of this liquidy substance. According to a Lincoln, Nebraska physician who performs early abortions in his office, the "material" removed in a procedure he referred to as "endometrial aspirations" amounts to approximately two tablespoonsful of blood and is disposed of in the sewer system.[18]

Since abortion is a blind procedure, however, the doctor is not always sure he has drained all the body parts out. The curette or aspirator might miss a limb, part of a head, or rib cage. Therefore, a common practice, even in early abortions, is to carefully examine what are frequently labeled the "products of conception" and send them to the pathology lab for microscopic analysis. This is done as a precautionary measure to insure that everything is completely removed. The retention of fetal parts inside the womb is a known cause of infection, bleeding, fever, and other complications.

Planned Parenthood's Margaret Sanger Center in New York has the tissue "sent to a laboratory for analysis, as is all tissue removed during any surgical procedure."[19] An operational, planning, and staffing model for abortions in New York City specifies that pathological exams be routinely performed on "all tissue removed from the uterus."[20] Other places are not as thorough in the perusal of aborted tissue and body parts. At the Hillcrest Clinic and Counseling Service in Atlanta, Georgia "the fetal matter is examined by the doctor performing the abortion and then destroyed."[21]

With more advanced pregnancies — beyond the eighth week — the process of removing all the body parts by vacuum aspiration becomes more and more problematical, as the child is larger and more solid. Although the aspirator still kills very effectively, the suction force is not always powerful enough to suck out all of the baby's body and rip the placenta away from the uterine wall. "Occasionally, the cannula became blocked (most frequently by the umbilical cord of a large fetus) and had to be withdrawn completely," related Dr. M. Vojta of the Institute of Care for Mother and Child in Czechoslovakia. "The passage of the placenta through the cannula was readily recognized due to the organ's granular appearance. It was followed by parts of the fetal skeleton which were mixed with blood." [22] Dr. A. Peretz and associates in Haifa, Israel reported on four cases of late, incomplete abortions where parts of the child's body got stuck in the uterus because "limbs were suctioned into the tube, making it impossible to complete the evacuation." [23]

Dr. Dorothea Kerslake and Donn Casey of the department of obstetrics and gynecology at the Newcastle General Hospital in England have worked out a procedure for removing body parts that get clogged in the suction curette: the withdrawal of the curette "until its mouth appears outside the cervix where the normal pressure will clear it." If this does not work, "the blockage is cleared with forceps, or by increasing the suction." The degree of suction is controlled by putting one's thumb over an air hole at the base of the curette or by regulating a device on the pump.[24]

The piecemeal removal of body parts by cutting or negative pressure is usually not feasible after the twelfth week of pregnancy, because by then the child inside the womb is too large and hard. This may soon change, nevertheless, as more medical abortionists begin to rely on D & E (dilatation and extraction) as the preferred method for destroying babies in the second trimester of pregnancy. In fact, D & E procedures are increasingly touted as being safer than saline instillations (the most common method for late-term abortions) as well as having other advantages, such as taking less time and being less expensive, painful, and emotionally traumatic for the abortion patient.[25]

Still, the technique of removing the large, fully developed remains of the victims with sharp instruments continues to be potentially traumatic surgically and psychologically for the doctor. The problems associated with the extraction of these body parts are acknowledged by nurse-midwife and epidemiologist Judith Bourne Rooks and Dr. Willard Cates, both staff members of the Center for Disease Control headquartered in Atlanta, Georgia:

> Ossified parts, such as the skull, must often be crushed. The bone fragments must be extracted carefully to avoid tearing the cervix. Reconstruction of the fetal sections after removal from the uterus is necessary to ensure completeness of the abortion procedure. Cleary, D & E transfers much of the possible psychological trauma of the abortion from the patient to the professional.[26]

Dr. A. Alberto Hodari and colleagues are acutely aware of the technical problems involved in "evacuating a uterus past the eighteenth menstrual week." They have even specified that "it was harder to remove the more ossified fetal parts" and "the cervical os was more likely to be lacerated when a large head was removed." [27] Despite such drawbacks, this group of abortionists seemed to experience little difficulty in tearing apart and extracting the bodies of 2,500 unborn human beings of fifteen to eighteen weeks gestation destroyed by D & Cs at the Detroit Memorial Hospital from the middle of March 1974 through the end of March 1976. Such lethal weapons as ring forceps and sharp curettes in the hands of skilled executioners overcame the usual obstacles connected with this form of late-term body mutilation, removal, and disposal.

The more typical later abortion methods such as hypertonic saline and prostaglandins not only kill the child but also usually eject the corpse from the uterus in an intact condition. Getting the body out sometimes proves to be a very demanding technological feat. While saline generally kills the victim within an hour or two, it may take days or even longer before the woman goes into labor and expels a deceased child. After four years of experience in destroying unborn human lives with saline, Drs. Charles and Francis Ballard of the University of Southern California Medical

Center revealed that the time from infusion of saline to abortion ranged anywhere from 7 to 333 hours.[28]

Physicians administering deadly solutions into the amniotic sac are very concerned about getting the dead victim out of the uterus as soon as possible. The longer the child's corpse remains inside the woman the more likely it is that she will become susceptible to infections and other complications. Maternal death is also a possible outcome. Bleeding and sepsis were among the most significant factors leading to ten maternal deaths from saline abortions performed in New York City from July 1, 1970 through June 30, 1972. In one of these cases the woman was found "in extremis in the bathroom of her home, hemorrhaging and with partial extrusion of the fetus. The patient was dead on arrival at a nearby hospital." [29]

In addition to the physical hazards associated with extended instillation-abortion time intervals, it is extremely discomforting psychologically to walk around carrying a dead body within for any prolonged length of time; it might stir up guilt and awareness of what abortion really is. The quicker the abortion is over and the evidence of destruction done away with, the better for the woman's psyche. The last thing she wants to be burdened with are any reminders of pregnancy or pregnancy destruction.

A number of procedures have been devised to deal with expelling the corpses of late abortions resistant to being dislodged from the uterus. If labor had not begun forty-eight hours after injection of saline, Drs. Charles and Francis Ballard employed intravenous infusion of oxytocin over a period of twenty-four hours. If after another twenty-four hours the child still had not been expelled, they administered another dose of hypertonic saline.[30] This approach, however, is not entirely hazard free. The use of such substances as oxytocin to shorten the time it takes to get the deceased child out of the uterus is fraught with some additional complications, including water intoxication and ruptured uteri.[31]

Intervention with cutting instruments, forceps, and vacuum machines may also be used when other methods fail to dislodge the victim. When the administration of saline or prostaglandins over a three-year period (January 1973 through December 1975) to 2,045 women resulted in a failure to eject fifty-eight unborn victims from the womb, doctors at the Fertility Control Center associated with Johns Hopkins Hospital and School of Medicine employed "vaginal uterine evacuation" to get the bodies out. The first step was to make sure they were dead before proceeding. A doppler examination verified the "absence of fetal heart tones." Then, using a combination of ring forceps, sharp-edged curettes, and vacuum aspirators, the doctors set about the task of pulling, cutting, and sucking parts of stubborn bodies out of the uterus until all segments were entirely disposed of. These acts of scientific mutilation were simply called "removing" the "products of conception." [32]

Hysterotomy and hysterectomy may even be resorted to. In one instance of saline failure, Ballard and Ballard employed hysterectomy as the method of body removal, and "the uterus was found to contain twins." [33]

Such surgical procedures, nonetheless, are still considered formidable and subject to serious complications. Dr. Harold Schulman of the Albert Einstein College of Medicine and the Bronx Municipal Hospital does not perform any surgical operations when saline fails to bring on labor. He cuts the victim's body out with a curette, but only after the uterus has shrunk to a small size. This may take as long as three months. "Suction curettage is not useful for this procedure," explained Dr. Schulman, "because the tissue is too firm to be aspirated." [34] If the dead child's body is only partially expelled during abortion labor, the doctor then pulls it all the way out with either his hands or ovum forceps. This is the technique employed by Dr. Thomas F. Dillon and fellow abortionists at the Roosevelt Hospital and the Columbia University College of Physicians and Surgeons to extract prostaglandin corpses lodged in the vagina or external cervical os. [35]

Once the aborted bodies and body parts are outside the woman's body, the main goal is to get rid of them quickly and efficiently. This is a simple matter when all that has to be disposed of are the tiny fragments resulting from early abortions. A far greater challenge is the growing number of large, intact bodies to be dispensed with. The variety of methods evolved by modern body-disposal experts are comparable to those developed by the disposal squads of the Third Reich.

During the early phases of legalized killing in the state of New York, some hospitals asked women aborting at home to deliver the bodies of their babies to the hospital, where they could be discarded in a scientific manner. At a symposium on legal abortion held during the annual meeting of the American College of Obstetricians and Gynecologists in the Bahamas in the fall of 1970, Dr. Harold Schulman discussed his experiences with implementing such a practice:

> Originally, when we started the program, we instructed all patients to bring the fetuses back. As I indicated in my presentation, 70 per cent of the patients undergoing saline instillation were released following the procedure, and delivered at home. We'd then receive telephone calls confirming the abortion, some typically as follows:
>
> > Patient: "Well I passed everything. It's just like you described."
> > Hospital: "Well, then everything is O.K.?"
> > Patient: "Yes."
> > Hospital: "Well, then: Why don't you bring it in to us in the morning?"
> > Patient: "Do I have to?"
>
> We thought about this. Certainly, if the patient felt alright and really didn't want to bring the fetus in, I really couldn't think of a good reason to force this issue. Currently, we do not force her to bring it in; she may dispose of it any way she wants.[36]

It is distasteful enough to be saddled with the responsibility for aborting large, intact babies without the presence of high status professionals to soften the trauma, but to ask these women to prolong their contact with such stark evidence of destruction was, apparently, expecting too much. Currently, midtrimester abortions are no longer performed on an outpatient basis but in the hospital setting, where both the destruction and disposal phases can be carried out by members of the medical staff. Since doctors are not generally on hand when the victims of saline or prostaglandin assaults are ejected from the womb, it is the nurses who are frequently charged with the dirty work of handling and discarding the corpses. All too typical of what happens is the procedure followed in one prestigious American university medical center, where "the products of conception are placed in a basin, covered and are removed immediately from the bedside" by the nursing staff.[37]

A New York nurse furnished a detailed description of what it is like to assist at a saline abortion and then discard the baby's body:

> I kept the now damp sheets over her knees, looking beneath occasionally and telling her everything was going fine, she was doing well. I felt like a natural childbirth coach, and I had to remind myself that this wasn't a birth.
>
> I was afraid I would look down and see a chubby pink baby boy popping up; then I would uncontrollably congratulate Irene for a fine job and a healthy offspring.
>
> When I looked again, a blue-black lump had appeared. With the next contraction, a beautifully formed blue-veined head passed smoothly out. The bedpan was tipped upward with the weight of the new "mother," and the head, once out, fell downward, towards the back of the shiny metal container, where it sank into the primordial fluids that preceded it.
>
> A dull thud sounded. We both knew it was out.
>
> Strange ones have I emptied in the flush and grind of a bedpan hopper. But never had I carried such an unwieldy pan. The "utility" room is crowded with equipment and stuffy beyond odor. I sat the pan

down on the shining stainless steel table and looked for a specimen cup. I found a large plastic container lined with a transparent plastic bag. The "specimen" had to sit inside the sac inside its white plastic womb.

A bedpan has only one real side you can pour from, but pouring was the only way I could get it into the container. With plastic gloves, I had just accidently touched the well-formed but soft head and the immature body, and I knew I couldn't touch it again.

I noticed that the head and neck collapsed when it touched the sides of the pan. It curled up automatically, just like a doodle bug that, out of fear and instinct, becomes an instantly rolling ball when its hind quarters are brushed.

Lifting the heavy pan, I quickly poured its contents into the container. The fluid ran in fine, but the large, thick fetus was caught on the rim of the pan, its tiny, transparent blue legs and buttocks facing me. The glistening placenta pressed against its mute companion, and when I finally managed, with shaking hands, one last push of the pan, both plopped noisily into the container.

The index finger of the left hand, I noticed, was out of line. He held a tight fist, except for this jutting, poking, pointing finger, which was obviously emphasizing some astute *in utero* point about the situation. Reluctantly, I poured formaldehyde over and around its delicate features.[38]

Abortion counselor Joan McTigue provides another glimpse into the distasteful task of placing dead bodies into containers: "It's exhausting, draining. We need space, time to deal with what it means to be dropping five fetuses a day into formaldehyde jars. Nobody wants to confront that." [39]

The next step is the pathology lab, where the remains are carefully scrutinized. Sometimes the backlog of bodies awaiting pathological analysis becomes inordinate. This is likely to happen on weekends when the labs are not usually open. As reported by one nurse in a New York hospital, "You could populate a whole village with the fetuses in cartons lined up on the table on Monday morning." [40] After the pathology exam is completed, the bodies are ordinarily burned in the hospital incinerator.

Little has been published regarding the grisly details of incinerating aborted babies, but some information is beginning to surface. One of the first revelations came to public attention in the case of a male child aborted by hysterotomy on January 20, 1969 at Stobhill General Hospital in Glasgow, Scotland. At this particular hospital it was learned that a baby of from twenty-six to thirty-two weeks gestation was aborted in the gynecological operating theater in the presence of a consultant, two assistant doctors, an anesthetist, a theater sister, and a theater attendant. After the aborted body was observed for a brief period by the theater sister, it was placed in a bag and taken by the theater attendant to the hospital incineration room, where it was up to an incinerator attendant to toss it into the furnace. [41] In testimony presented before the House Judiciary Committee on November 25, 1974, Dr. Ada B. Ryan of Flushing, New York disclosed another variation on the cremation theme at one large city hospital: "Babies were being thrown into the incinerator while they were still whimpering." [42] One cannot help but recall that many children were also burned alive in the ditches and crematoriums of Nazi death camps.

In her study of an abortion hospital in New York, psychologist Magda Denes supplies an unusually frank account of her reactions to observing and handling the bodies of saline abortion victims slated for the hospital incinerator. She is particularly fascinated by the paper buckets in which they are kept before being disposed of. Attached to the lid of each bucket, she relates, "there is a white cardboard label bearing — printed in ink — the mother's name, the doctor's name, the time of delivery, the sex of the item, the time of gestation." Denes continues:

> I look inside the bucket in front of me. There is
> a small naked person in there floating in a bloody

liquid. . . . the body is purple with bruises and the face has the agonized tautness of one forced to die too soon. . . . A death factory is the same anywhere, and the agony of early death is the same anywhere. . . .

Finally, I lift a very large fetus. . . . I look at the label. Mother's name: Catherine Atkins; doctor's name Saul Marcus; sex of item: male; time of gestation: twenty-four weeks. . . . This is Master Atkins — to be burned tomorrow — who died like a hero to save his mother's life. Might he have become someday the only one to truly love her? The only one to mourn her death? [43]

The next day the aborted bodies, bunched together in a plastic bag, are packed in a cardboard box. Then a technician takes them by taxi to a hospital with a furnace large enough to complete the process of disintegration. While initially upset at seeing the victims' remains being burned, the task of disposal soon became a fairly routine matter to this particular body-disposal messenger. The only bothersome element remaining — the smell discharged from the corpses — got so bad at times that it was hard to get a taxi.[44]

What is considered a more personalized approach toward the incineration of aborted babies is taken at University Hospital in Omaha, Nebraska, First of all, the bodies are dispatched to the hospital laboratory for observation and analysis. Two weeks later they are burned in a crematorium on the hospital grounds. Then the ashes are dropped into a special container and buried at a local cemetery. A brief ceremony featuring a eulogy by a clergyman is conducted at the burial site. Dr. Joe Scott, chairman of University Hospital's obstetrics and gynecology department, characterized it as "a thoughtful procedure . . . done out of respect for the people involved." [45]

A similar type of thoughtfulness prompted Nazi doctors to dump the ashes of those exterminated in the euthanasia hospitals into urns and then to ship them off to relatives.

Humane Society incinerators have even served as receptacles for removing all traces of mass destruction of the unborn. Under the guise of removing "human tissue specimens" or "surgical tissue," Columbus Pathology Incorporated was able to succeed in burning the bodies of abortion victims in the facilities of the Capital Area Humane Society of Columbus, Ohio. This went on for a ten-month period before the true nature of the affair was uncovered in May 1979. Particularly repugnant to the society administrator Elaine Black was the deception employed by Columbus Pathology and the behavior of those who delivered the bodies to be burned. On one occasion, the delivery men left boxes full of aborted bodies outside in the sun because they objected to the presence of "carcasses of dead dogs waiting to be incinerated." On another occasion, "the young woman who brought the material opened some of the boxes and made a big show of throwing the fetuses around." [46]

The number of aborted bodies erased through incineration sometimes becomes so great as to arouse community concern. A London gynecologist told reporters Michael Litchfield and Susan Kentish that the smell of burning flesh seems to be the most distasteful aspect:

> Local residents in the vicinity of my clinic have been complaining about the smell of burning flesh. The smell comes from the incinerator. It does make a stink. They say it smells like a Nazi extermination camp during the last War. . . . So I am always looking for ways of disposing of the foetuses, other than burning them. [47]

Although burning continues to be one of the most popular methods of destroying the remains, contemporary technologists have tried almost every conceivable alternative. Aborted bodies have been buried, stuffed in garage cans, left at dumps, dropped near the seashore, and obliterated in garbage disposers.

On August 6, 1975, a plastic bag containing six aborted babies, test tubes, petri dishes, and human tissue from the Elmhurst City Hospital in New York City fell off the back of a sanitation department truck. It took an hour before the broken bottles and test tubes were cleared away and the scattered bodies taken to the Queens morgue by ambulance technicians. Marvin Durell, associate director of the Elmhurst City Hospital, elaborated on the hospital's policy for discarding aborted human beings: those "weighing less than 500 grams — slightly more than a pound — are incinerated. Those which weigh more than 500 grams are buried at a city cemetery." [48] In this situation, apparently, something went awry and the bodies got mixed up with the hospital trash.

An article in the *Los Angeles Times* brought to light more information on the sordid practices of the body-disposal business. It was disclosed that bodies from area hospitals and abortion clinics were being sent to the Medical Analytical Labs, Inc. in Santa Monica, California for pathological analysis. From there they were transported to a warehouse before being disposed of. The exact method of disposal, however, was not indicated. The only thing mentioned by the *Times* was that the bodies were then taken care of in "a prescribed manner." Knowledge of this became public when it was learned that unsealed boxes stacked up near the Santa Monica Medical Building's pharmacy and elevators contained more than one hundred fetal bodies, "each in its own numbered, transparent plastic container, ranged in age from one or two months, to as much as six months. Most showed advanced development, with tiny hands and feet perfectly formed." [49]

In New York, small hospitals and abortion clinics without incinerators handled the problem of body disposal by leaving small bodies and body parts in bags strewn along the Long Island shoreline. Needless to say, this attracted birds in addition to incurring the wrath of nearby residents. The public conscience was offended, albeit only temporarily. The evidence of destruction was too visible to be denied or ignored. The health department would not give permission to have the bodies buried through local undertakers. What Dr. Ada Ryan aptly referred to as "the final solution for disposal of the dead babies" came to pass when the health department suggested that some arrangements be made with the larger hospitals to use their incinerators. [50]

The bone-crushing machines pioneered in the Nazi death

camps to eradicate all traces of mass annihilation are not entirely extinct. Today's counterparts are garbage-disposal units installed in the scrub sinks of abortion clinics. Such a revelation accidentally came to public attention on May 31, 1978, when plumber Rick Gray found some body parts in a garbage disposer he had removed from the "Ladies Center," an abortion chamber located in Omaha, Nebraska. "I saw what looked like a miniature arm. There was a miniature hand. It was very distinctive," he reported. "I saw something that looked like a rib cage. You could see miniature finger-nails on the hands." [51]

Attending physician Dr. John Epp told police investigators that only recently had the clinic used the garbage-disposal method. Previously, the "fetuses" were transported to a pathology lab, where they were examined and disposed of. The switch to the disposer was made, he explained, because sending fetal remains through the mail required too much handling. [52]

A medical aide at one of Chicago's legal abortion mills divulged another approach to eliminating aborted body parts: "I just throw it in the garbage." The supervisor disapproved of this method "because it starts to smell if you leave it in the garbage in the sterilization room." She had a different solution to the problem of getting rid of the mutilated mass of humanity. "Throw it down the toilet," she said. "Bickham says we pay $10,000 a month rent here so the toilets should be able to handle it. If they get clogged, the building should take care of it." [53]

Commercial Utilization

1. Nazi Profiteering

Before the obliteration of all traces of destruction, the possessions and bodies of the condemned underwent the most thorough exploitation ever initiated. Ironically, although the victims were viewed as little more than subhuman, their clothes, the gold in their mouths, the hair on their heads, their bodies, and even their ashes were considered valuable products with potential payoff for industry. A vast salvage operation grew up in the concentration camps, which is best illustrated by Auschwitz-Birkenau, where a huge building referred to as Canada was set aside for the exclusive purpose of sorting clothes, shoes, food, and other valuables taken from the victims. Upon the liberation of Auschwitz in January 1945, part of this incredible inventory was uncovered: 348,820 men's suits, 836,255 women's outfits, 5,525 pairs of women's shoes, and hundreds of thousands of additional items of apparel.[54]

The technicians also became quite adept at salvaging various parts of the destroyed bodies. The teeth-pulling brigade stationed in front of the ovens stood as a prime example of the thoroughness with which this aspect of body exploitation was carried out.

> Consisting of eight men, this kommando equipped its members with two tools. . . . In one hand a lever, and in the other, a pair of pliers for extracting the teeth. The dead lay on their backs; the kommando pried open the contracted jaw with his lever; then, with his pliers, he extracted, or broke off, all gold teeth, as well as any gold bridgework and fillings. All members of the kommando were fine stomatologists and dental surgeons.
>
> The gold teeth were collected in buckets filled with an acid which burned off all pieces of bone and flesh. . . . Gold is a heavy metal, and I would judge that from 18 to 20 pounds of it were collected daily in each crematorium.[55]

In addition to teeth, other body parts turned out to be valuable products. Hair was found to be appropriate material for detonating action bombs as well as filling mattresses and cushions.[56] Although not fully authenticated, enough reports and stories circulated to indicate that some of the fat from the corpses was used for manufacturing soap. Testimony presented to a session of the National Council of Danzig

in Danzig, Poland on May 5, 1945 by Mayor Kotus-Jankow-
ski revealed the existence of a factory producing soap derived
from human remains at the Danzig Institute of Hygiene:
"We found a cauldron with the remains of boiled human
flesh, a box of prepared human bones, and baskets of hands
and feet and human skin, with the fat removed." [57]

Human skin was a popular commodity at the Dachau
death camp. Testimony presented at Nuremberg by Czech
physician Dr. Franz Blaha recounted the wide variety of
commercial products derived from the skin of the victims:

> It was common practice to remove the skin from
> dead prisoners.... Dr. Rascher and Dr. Wolter in
> particular asked for this human skin from human
> backs and chests. It was chemically treated and placed
> in the sun to dry. After that it was cut into shapes
> for use as saddles, riding breeches, gloves, house
> slippers and ladies' handbags. Tattooed skin was espe-
> cially valued by SS men.... This skin had to be from
> healthy prisoners and free from defects. Sometimes we
> did not have enough bodies with good skin and
> Rascher would say, "All right, you will get the bodies."
> The next day we would receive 20 or 30 bodies of
> young people. They would have been shot in the neck
> or struck on the head so that the skin would be un-
> injured. [58]

Another use found for human skin was in the manufacture of lampshades. Frau Ilse Koch, wife of the commandant
of Buchenwald, had a special affinity for lampshades fashioned out of tattooed skin. Former Buchenwald inmate
Andreas Pfaffenberger related to the Nuremberg tribunal
the ghastly details of how her desires were fulfilled:

> All prisoners with tattooing on them were ordered
> to report to the dispensary.... After the tattooed pris-
> oners had been examined, the ones with the best and
> most artistic specimens were kept in the dispensary,
> and then killed by injections.... The corpses were

then turned over to the pathological department, where the desired pieces of tattooed skin were detached from the bodies and treated. The finished products were turned over to SS Standartenfuehrer Koch's wife, who had them fashioned into lampshades and other ornamental household articles.[59]

A German embalmer who assisted Dr. August Hirt in dissecting the corpses of victims exterminated in the gas chambers testified that Hirt used human heads for something besides trying to prove the inferiority of the Jewish race through skull measurements. "One day I had prepared a head for him," the embalmer said. "Well, do you know what the professor did with it? He gave it to the commander of the Natzweiler camp, who used it as a paperweight." [60]

And finally, even the ashes of the corpses had utility. Auschwitz survivor Dr. Olga Lengyel revealed that they served as fertilizer for farms and gardens.[61] Besides being employed as fertilizer, the cremated remains at the Natzweiler camp were placed in urns and sold to families of the destroyed:

> Cremation of one corpse required fifteen minutes. The ashes were used to fertilize flowers and vegetables in the gardens of the commanding officer. In a storehouse, shelf after shelf was filled with cinerary urns, priced at 60 and 120 marks apiece.[62]

The amount of perverse ingenuity and imagination poured into body exploitation for financial gain was virtually unlimited.

2. Contemporary Profiteering

Increasing numbers of contemporary physicians can be found who are interested in not simply getting rid of but also exploiting aborted bodies for commercial purposes. Although today's victims do not have any gold teeth to pull or much hair to cut, there is evidence that their bodies are being subjected to the same type of abuse as went on in Nazi Germany.

Commercially speaking, the bodies of aborted children have been used for various profit-making ventures. The manufacture of soap and other ingredients from human fat did not cease with the fall of the Third Reich. That there are modern purveyors of this pernicious form of exploitation was revealed to British reporters Litchfield and Kentish. They were told of a gynecologist who "sells the foetuses to a factory... a chemical factory... they make soap and cosmetics... and they... pay very well, indeed, for babies because animal fat is very precious, gold dust in their line." [63] This story was corroborated later when Litchfield and Kentish arranged a meeting with him under the guise of working out a business deal. In what is surely one of the most disturbing admissions to date, this doctor elaborated upon his role in selling aborted bodies to soap and cosmetic firms:

> You see, there isn't much money in flogging them for research. It's all a question of what is worth my while... and how they can be taken away without my breaking the law....
>
> You see, I get some very big babies. It's such a shame to toss them in the incinerator, when they could be put to so much better use. We do a lot of late terminations.
>
> Now, many of the babies I get are fully-formed and are living for quite a time before they are disposed of. One morning, I had four of them lined up crying their heads off. I hadn't the time to kill them there and then because we were so busy. I was so loathe to drop them in the incinerator because there was so much animal fat that could have been used commercially. [64]

In a story published on February 29, 1976, the *Washington Post* disclosed that between 1972 and the middle of 1974 D.C. General Hospital's obstetrics and gynecology department sold the bodies and organs of babies aborted by hysterotomy to Flow Labs of Rockville, Maryland. Flow used them to produce cell cultures, which were sold to medical pharmacological researchers and firms. It was also revealed that $75 was paid to D.C. General for each body supplied; this reached a total of $3,532 for a 2½ year period. The money was expended for such things as departmental equipment, a TV set, attendance at educational meetings, and cokes and cookies for visiting professors. The hospital's pathology department had also been trafficking in the preparation and sale of aborted human bodies and organs to commercial firms for the past ten years. For this activity it received over $68,000.[65]

An interesting sidelight to this whole reprehensible business is the leadership displayed by Dr. Frank Bepko, head of D.C. General's obstetrics and gynecology department. Although Dr. Bepko is described as being personally opposed to abortion, it is he who made the arrangements with Flow Labs in the first place. He refuses to kill unborn babies but is not adverse to having their destroyed bodies dismembered for monetary benefit!

The greater number of bodies available for disposal due to legalization of abortion was acknowledged by Dr. Bepko:

> They ordered me to personally process patients for abortions. . . . so what we did was set the (abortion) program up. What happened then was just like Humpty Dumpty: All the king's horses and all the king's men couldn't put Humpty together again. We has to dispose of them (the fetuses).[66]

An investigation of Dr. Bepko's department by the D.C. division of municipal audits put an end to this particular form of monetary exploitation. Since midterm unborn babies continued to be destroyed at D.C. General, Dr. Bepko and his staff were confronted with the task of finding more suitable methods of body disposal. "What I am going to have to do now is have the patients sign for a funeral, or disposal by incineration," declared Dr. Bepko. "We're going to have to sit down and decide how to handle the problem." [67]

The intricacies of erasing the evidence of destruction seem to be as problematic for modern body-disposal experts as they were for those who performed these same duties during the time of the Third Reich.

In 1976 it was learned that a Chicago biological supply firm offered for sale human embryos and other organs encased in a "paperweight" type of plastic block to customers throughout the United States. The costs advertised in its catalogue were $90 for a human brain, $60 for intestines, and $70 for lungs. A human foot encased in plastic was priced at $70, and "embedments of human embryos" were listed for $97.80.

Those interested in purchasing the small corpses were provided with the following details:

> These embryos range from 3 to 4 months in age. They have been bisected along the median, cleared, and mounted naturally. Specify age or ages desired. ... Occasionally ages other than those listed can be furnished. Please write us for current information. [68]

This flagrant monetary exploitation of the huge supply of aborted babies is distressingly similar to the mentality that existed in Nazi Germany. There, it was fashionable to find on display in the homes of Nazi officials decorative lampshades and paperweights made from the remains of concentration camp victims. Is it possible that some individuals in contemporary American culture derive comparable esthetic pleasure out of supplementing their collection of knickknacks with a human foot, brain, or embryo embedded in plastic?

Another perversity in the growing abuse of aborted bodies came to light on August 12, 1977, when police confiscated the corpses of thirteen unborn babies found floating in jars of formaldehyde. They were discovered in Gibsonton, Florida in the backyard of a carnival man who had used them in the World Fair Freak Show. Just two weeks earlier he had been barred in Illinois from displaying the corpses of twenty babies and fetuses as part of a carnival sideshow.[69]

Experimental Exploitation

Massive killing, whether in Nazi Germany or today's society, is characterized by an amazing degree of efficiency. Both past and present physician perpetrators of destruction are not content with simply killing human beings. Nor are they satisfied with their role in pioneering some of the most technically advanced methods of killing the world has ever known. They have also devised further ways to exploit the products of their destructive technology. Various tissues, organs, and body parts have been systematically observed, measured, weighed, analyzed, manipulated, cut up, and preserved in the relentless process of squeezing every possible ounce of data out of the subjects.

Experimentation is in essence a by-product of destruction; it did not get off the ground until widespread destruction became an established practice. Then an incomparable pool of potential research subjects suddenly became available. In Nazi Germany the experimental population was primarily composed of concentration camp inmates destined for extermination. In contemporary society a growing number of experimental subjects are being supplied from the ranks of babies slated for abortion destruction. In fact, the condemned unborn are now the principal targets of experimental procedures formerly directed against captive expendables in orphanages, prisons, and institutions for the mentally retarded.

1. Nazi Manipulation and Mutilation

A report authored by Dr. Sigmund Rascher provided what was considered valuable information on how various organs of Dachau inmates were affected by exposure to high altitudes without oxygen. The following observations were made as

a result of dissections performed on one subject who failed
to survive these high-altitude experiments:

> When the cavity of the chest was opened the
> pericardium was filled tightly (heart tamponade).
> Upon opening of the pericardium 80 cc. of clear
> yellowish liquid gushed forth. The moment the tam-
> ponade had stopped, the right auricle began to beat
> heavily, at first at the rate of 60 actions per minute,
> then progressively slower. Twenty minutes after the
> pericardium had been opened, the right auricle was
> opened by puncturing it. For about 15 minutes, a thin
> stream of blood spurted forth. Thereafter clogging of
> the puncture wound in the auricle by coagulation of
> the blood and renewed acceleration of the action of
> the right auricle occurred.
>
> One hour after breathing had stopped, the spinal
> marrow was completely severed and the brain re-
> moved. Thereupon the action of the auricle stopped
> for 40 seconds. It then renewed its action, coming to
> a complete standstill 8 minutes later. A heavy sub-
> arachnoid oedema was found in the brain. In the veins
> and arteries of the brain a considerable quantity of
> air was discovered. Furthermore, the blood vessels in
> the heart and liver were enormously obstructed by
> embolism.
>
> The last-mentioned case is to my knowledge the
> first one of this type ever observed on man. The above-
> described heart actions will gain particular scientific
> interest, since they were written down with an electro-
> cardiogram to the very end.[70]

Autopsies also constituted a standard procedure for fatalities occurring among the subjects immersed in the freezing
waters of the human experimental laboratories of Dachau:

> The experimental subjects (VP) were placed in
> the water, dressed in complete flying uniform.... In
> one experimental series, the occiput (brain stem) pro-

truded above the water, while in another series of experiments the occiput (brain stem) and back of the head were submerged in water.

Fatalities occurred only when the brain stem and the back of the head were also chilled. Autopsies of such fatal cases always revealed large amounts of free blood, up to one-half liter, in the cranial cavity. The heart invariably showed extreme dilation of the right chamber. As soon as the temperature in these experiments reached 28°, the experimental subjects died invariably, despite all attempts at resuscitation.

Other important findings, common in all experiments, should be mentioned, marked increase of the viscosity of the blood, marked increase of hemoglobin, an approximate five-fold increase of the leukocytes, invariable rise of blood sugar to twice its normal value. Auricular fibrillation made its appearance regularly at 30°.[71]

At Auschwitz a pathology laboratory was set up under Dr. Josef Mengele. Dr. Mengele, like many other Nazi physicians, was preoccupied with proving the inferiority of Jews and other condemned individuals. He therefore exhibited a special fascination for inmates with abnormalities. Rather than have their corpses burned outright, they were dispatched to Auschwitz's pathology lab. There the brains, hearts, and other organs were dissected, preserved in alcohol, specially packed, and shipped to the Institute of Biological, Racial, and Evolutionary Research at Berlin-Dahlem. On one occasion, a fifty-year-old hunchback and his sixteen-year-old son with a deformed foot were singled out for special experimental treatment because Dr. Mengele believed "he had discovered, in the person of the hunchback father and his lame son, a sovereign example to demonstrate his theory of the Jewish race's degeneracy."[72] After destruction their skeletons were prepared for the Anthropological Museum in Berlin.

By February 1942, some German medical scientists became alarmed that the Jews were destined for total extermi-

nation. Their concern, however, was not motivated by humanitarian considerations; they were actually worried about the
dearth of Jewish skulls available for research purposes.
Among the concerned medical researchers was Dr. August
Hirt, professor of anatomy at the University of Strasbourg.
Like many of his colleagues, Dr. Hirt was infected with the
elitist, super-race ideology and believed that Jews and other
victims were of an inferior stock. Not only did he believe
this in theory — he also wanted to provide scientific support
through the collection of photographs, measurements, and
other data from the skulls and heads of the victims.

The documented details of this research project are contained in a report written by Dr. Hirt and submitted to
Heinrich Himmler, from whom it received final approval.
Hirt gave precise instructions on the tasks of data collection
and procurement of the experimental specimens:

> This special deputy, commissioned with the col-
> lection of the material ... is to take a prescribed se-
> ries of photographs and anthropological measure-
> ments, and is to ascertain, insofar as is possible, the
> origin, date of birth, and other personal data of the
> prisoner. Following the subsequently induced death
> of the Jew, whose head must not be damaged, he will
> separate the head from the torso and will forward it
> to its point of destination in a preserving fluid in a
> well-sealed tin container especially made for this pur-
> pose. On the basis of the photos, the measurements
> and other data on the head and, finally, the skull it-
> self, comparative anatomical research, research on
> racial classification, pathological features of the skull
> formation, form and size of the brain, and many other
> things can begin.[73]

In August 1942, at least three separate shipments of
bodies were sent from the Natzweiler concentration camp to
Dr. Hirt's Anatomical Institute at the University of Strasbourg for the purpose of anthropological research. They
were preserved in the cellars of the institute in tanks. In the

fall of 1944, Hirt ordered his two assistants to cut up and cremate the eighty-six corpses remaining before they could be discovered by the allied armies. The job of body disintegration proved too formidable a task to complete on time.[74] The evidence of Dr. Hirt's experiments in scientific body exploitation was made known to the world through pictures taken by the French occupational forces.[75]

Dr. Julius Hallervorden, a prominent German neuropathologist, also initiated an extensive program of research on the human brain. Over five hundred specimens were shipped to him in order to facilitate his scientific pursuits. Just where did these heads come from and how were they obtained? Again, they were severed from the bodies of exterminated victims. In this instance, however, German mental patients rather than Jews comprised the pool of experimental material. Their deaths provided Dr. Hallervorden with an irresistible opportunity to gratify his scientific passion for skull research. His unbounded enthusiasm for this project is reflected in remarks made at the time of the Nuremberg trials:

> I heard that they were going to do that, and so I went up to them and told them, "Look here now, boys (*Menschenskinder*), if you are going to kill all these people, at least take the brains out so that the material could be utilised." They asked me: "How many can you examine?" and so I told them "An unlimited number — the more the better." I gave them the fixatives, jars and boxes, and instructions for removing and fixing the brains, and then they came bringing them in like the delivery van from the furniture company. The Charitable Transport Company for the Sick brought the brains in batches of 150-250 at a time. . . . There was wonderful material among those brains, beautiful mental defectives, malformations and early infantile diseases.[76]

The medical experimental laboratory at Buchenwald

featured the preservation of human organs, especially heads, in bottles:

> In one laboratory where captured scientists were forced to work on fellow prisoners, shelves were filled with bottles containing human organs. One bottle held a human head, cut lengthwise to show a section of the inside. A dozen death masks, skulls and shrunken heads were in another room. Their inscriptions read: "Polish Jew, age 38" and "Aryan from Breslau, married to Jewess, age 52." [77]

Babies aborted in an intact condition were also preserved and sent to scientific institutes in Berlin. In fact, it was an eight-week-old fetus brought out "in one piece" that saved the life of Dr. Gisella Pearl at Auschwitz just as Dr. Mengele was on the threshhold of sending her to the gas chamber. When she showed him "the jar containing the fetus" and explained "only rarely is it possible to bring it out in one piece," Dr. Mengele calmed down, forgot his anger and replied, "Good... beautiful... Take it to Crematory No. II tomorrow. We are sending it to Berlin." [78]

Even though the experimental products of destruction were lowered to the level of beasts, subjected to cruel and painful indignities, and killed before, during, or after the process of experimentation, the German researchers came to view their charges as valuable human research material. This was especially the case for experiments conducted to benefit the German armed forces. Dr. Pearl disclosed how "the undernourished emaciated bodies" were robbed of their last remaining drops of blood for the aid of German soldiers:

> The German army needed blood plasma! The guinea pigs of Auschwitz were just the people to furnish that plasma. *Rassenschande* or contamination with "inferior Jewish blood" was forgotten. We were too "inferior" to live, but not too inferior to keep the German army alive with our blood. [79]

2. Contemporary Manipulation and Mutilation

The attitude of Nazi physicians toward subjects procured from euthanasia institutions and concentration camps for scientific utilization, unfortunately, has not disappeared. The mentality of today's medical scientists toward the bodies of babies aborted in hospitals and clinics is alarmingly similar. This is particularly so for the larger bodies because they offer a greater range of possibilities for medical manipulation and mutilation. Every imaginable indignity is being inflicted on the victims, including testing for any remaining reflexes and cutting apart and preserving the bodies and body parts for further investigation and experimentation.

Physicians affiliated with the Columbia University College of Physicians and Surgeons performed autopsies on the bodies of 143 children aborted by hypertonic saline. Sections of their hearts, lungs, livers, kidneys, spleens, and other body parts were cut out and preserved for microscopic analysis. The purpose of this scientific butchery was to assess the effects of the saline solution on the fetal organs.[80]

The same kind of curiosity prompted medical researchers at Saint Luke's Hospital Center in New York City, also affiliated with Columbia University, to slice portions of skin, thigh muscle, liver, heart, brain, stomach, and intestine from the bodies of twenty-three saline abortion victims. In addition to placing these dissected parts in flasks, the remaining portions of the bodies were dropped into a blender and reduced to a gelatinous mass. These contents were then poured into a flask for the purpose of chemical analysis.[81]

The following excerpt provides some more specifics on what was actually done to these human guinea pigs:

As soon as the delivery occurred, the abortus was transferred to the laboratory in a sealed plastic bag. To avoid any loss of water, the investigational weighing procedures were undertaken immediately.

After removal from the plastic container, the fetal surface was blotted gently with sponges to remove amniotic fluid, and weighed on a scale. . . . immediately

after body volume measurement, the fetus was transferred onto an operating table and covered with ab-
sorbent pads. The fetus was then reblotted to remove
any water on the body surface. Three 100 mg. samples
were taken from the skin, thigh muscle (above the
knee), liver, heart, brain, stomach, and intestine of
the fetus. The dissected samples were transferred into
tared 50 ml. flasks and weighed rapidly.... The remainder of the fetal body was reweighed and homogenized for 20 minutes in a blender with 50 to 100 ml.
distilled water. The homogenized sample was then
transferred into a tared 2 L. flask. The blender was
washed with distilled water, and analysis was made
of total body chemical composition. Each sample was
then dehydrated at 105°C until constant weight was
reached; overnight incubation sufficed for small samples, and 72 hours was required for the total body
sample.[82]

A noteworthy feature of this description is the utter care
with which the newly destroyed bodies were handled just
before being cut up, homogenized, dehydrated, and analyzed.
If only such dedicated care were channeled toward saving
and preserving rather than destroying and mutilating human
lives!

An experiment conducted in Hungary and reported on
in an American medical journal illustrates another research
utilization of aborted fetal bodies. The scope of this study
is more narrowly circumscribed because its exclusive focus
is on the functioning of the human heart, the organ most
closely and fundamentally associated with life itself. The
procedure employed involved removing unborn children from
the womb, cutting out their beating hearts, and placing them
in a nutrient solution in order to observe and record their
contraction rates. In the words of the researchers:

We studied the spontaneous contraction rate of
hearts obtained from apparently healthy human fetuses
at legal termination of pregnancy. The estimated

gestational (menstrual) age of the fetuses ranged
from 5 to 15 weeks. The hearts were dissected from the
fetuses and were mounted in a thermostatically controlled bath.... Under these circumstances the hearts
survived for many hours without any significant
change in their spontaneous contraction rate.[83]

Contemporary medical researchers have not abandoned
the kind of interest in human skulls that consumed the scientific energies of the German doctors Hirt and Hallervorden. Professor Paul Ramsey reported on a discussion he
had with the representative of a pharmacological firm located
in New Jersey. This individual told Ramsey about a research
project emanating from Japan that involved keeping some
"previable" fetuses alive up to three days after being aborted.
During this period minerals were injected into their umbilical
cords and then their heads were systematically cut off. The
purpose of this research was to study how quickly the mineral
substances reached the fetal jawbone.[84]

Another modern version of skull research is reflected in
the work of Dr. Peter A. J. Adam, a professor of pediatrics
at Case Western Reserve Medical School in Cleveland, Ohio.
Dr. Adam has displayed an intense preoccupation with the
metabolism of human fetal brains. He and a team of colleagues from the Children's Hospital in Helsinki, Finland
learned that glucose and D-B-Oh-Butyrate serve equally well
as energy sources for fetal brain metabolism. While there
is nothing wrong in studying brain functioning per se, the
means and procedures utilized to accomplish such a laudable
goal is where Dr. Adam's research comes so close to what
the German doctors did to get their information. The main
procedure employed is identical to the one used by German
physicians: the heads of the subjects were severed from the
rest of the bodies.

A detailed account of this experiment appeared in a 1975
issue of *Acta Paediatrica Scandinavica*. Under the "Methods
and Materials" section of the study a description of the subjects is provided:

Human fetuses were obtained by abdominal hysterotomy from 12 pregnant women undergoing legal
therapeutic abortion between 12 and 21 weeks of
gestation. Fetal crown-rump length ranged from 8.5
to 18.0 centimeters. None of the fetuses had a physical
abnormality discernible during dissection.[85]

The authors also include a schematic drawing of the
"closed" recirculating system through which the brains were
perfused after being cut away from the victims' bodies. The
procedure followed was carefully recorded:

In fetuses weighing more than 100 g (6 of 12),
a polyethylene catheter was introduced into each internal carotid artery by threading from the root of the
aorta, and the catheters were joined with a Y-connec-
tor. The catheters were secured in place with surgical
tape encircling the internal carotid artery. In fetuses
weighing less than 100 g (6 of 12) a single catheter
was introduced into the aortic arch, and the ... vessels occluded with either surgical tape or ligature. ...
The head was then isolated surgically from the other
organs. Venous return was obtained by incising the
sagittal sinus, which permitted the perfusate to flow
through the organ chamber and to recirculate.[86]

In a footnote to this study, it is emphasized that the experiment was not begun until "after the fetal heart beat
had ceased." How thoughtful and humane of the researchers
to wait for the child to die first! This is the same sentiment
that motivated Drs. Hirt and Hallervorden of Nazi Germany
to issue instructions that experiments on human skulls were
not to commence until after the subjects had expired in the
gas chambers. Apparently, medical scientists feel justified in
initiating any type of experimental procedure, including
chopping off subjects' heads, as long as they are killed or
die beforehand. Never have such acts of sheer butchery been
so closely bound up with such an array of respectable professionals and impressive scientific paraphernalia!

Auschwitz survivor Dr. Gisella Pearl's observation that concentration camp guinea pigs were considered too inferior to live but not too inferior to make vital blood donations to the German army closely mirrors present-day realities. Unborn children, particularly the previable brand, are not deemed significant enough to merit the right to life, but their value jumps dramatically when it comes to draining from them every possible ounce of information, blood, and tissue for the benefit of the wanted born and unborn.

This type of scientific debasement is not just confined to the beginnings of the human life continuum. Psychiatrist Dr. Willard Gaylin, writing in the pages of *Harper's Magazine*, indicated that declaring those with total or even partial brain damage as legally dead might well usher in a new era of research involving the newly dead or, as he prefers to call them, "neomorts." Respiration and circulation of these "living cadavers" could possibly be maintained indefinitely while researchers harvest a vast assortment of scientific, educational, and humanitarian benefits, including training medical students, performing operations, testing drugs, intentionally damaging parts of the heart to determine if new diagnostic tools are capable of detecting the damage, and testing antidotes after deliberately inducing various diseases and maladies.[87]

Dr. Gaylin also envisions warehouses of the living dead as a steady source for periodic blood donations and as a storage bank for transplanting major organs. The possibilities appear to be extensive. The Nazi medical-research mentality of unlimited exploitation lives once again! Those lingering on in the wards of hospitals for the chronically ill are considered burdensome or even worthless when alive; it is only through redefining them as legally dead that they begin to possess any value.

A great tragedy associated with these experiments, besides the destruction, is that of the researchers' perspectives. What they have done is lost the big picture — the human being as an irreducible entity whose dignity requires the utmost respect and loving care. Instead, humanity is shorn away and relegated to its most gross level, that of sheer anatomy;

the subjects are perceived as purely experimental material, as disparate congeries of tissues, organs, and biochemical elements. Components of the human being become of prime importance while the human being as an indivisible whole is rendered totally dispensable.

Where has the dignity and respect for the most vulnerable of human lives gone? Is there no limit to what can be done in the name of science? How long will public apathy allow these kinds of medical atrocities to continue unabated? The tyranny of destructive technology run amok is as much with us today as it was in the darkest days of the Third Reich. Its inexorable movement is steamrolling to oblivion many of the values that once differentiated human beings from the beasts!

Another tragedy, absolutely frightening in terms of future ramifications, is how utterly impervious to death and destruction the body-removal experts remain while being totally absorbed in perpetrating their own unique brand of medical violence on and rank exploitation of defenseless human discards. This is so whether their specialty involved dragging bodies out of gas chambers with hook-tipped poles, cutting and sucking body parts out of the womb with sharp curettes and vacuum pumps, burying the victims in the mass graves of Treblinka, stuffing the remains of aborted babies in plastic garbage bags and dropping them along the shoreline, burning the victims in open pits, crematoriums or hospital incinerators, manufacturing soap, lampshades and saddles from the hides of camp inmates, displaying embryonic bodies on coffee tables and at freak shows, or beheading, slicing, extracting, and homogenizing organs, and initiating other experimental atrocities. These symptoms of extreme desensitization toward violence have become deeply embedded in a profession known for its healing and preservative tasks and have spread to the rest of society. Surrounded by such a grim state of affairs, the humanizing attributes of empathy and compassion for the most unwanted and defenseless lives stand on the edge of virtual extinction.

CHAPTER 8

The Management of Breakdowns in Destruction

Any technological enterprise, no matter how efficient and effective, has its imperfections. When the technology dispatches such huge numbers to oblivion it is bound to break down once in a while. Sometimes the problem involves a defect in the equipment or the technical procedure; other times the difficulty is with those manning the destructive machinery. The most vexing situation faced by the Nazi technicians was what to do when the firing squads and gas chambers failed to kill some of the victims. Today's medical executioners face a similar dilemma when they are confronted with babies who are still alive after being aborted. How such difficulties were managed in Nazi Germany and how they are dealt with in contemporary society demonstrates, like nothing else can, the triumph of technology over humanity.

The Aftermath of Technological Blunders

1. The Temporary Survivors of Nazi Technology

The large number of lives so quickly and efficiently destroyed in the euthanasia institutions and concentration camps of the Third Reich attests to how very successfully the technology actually worked. However, even the most perfect killing procedure occasionally broke down. Sometimes the particular method employed did not kill as swiftly as anticipated or did not kill at all. And the one thing the perpetrators wished to avoid was the sight of living victims whose survival was due to faulty equipment or inadequate knowledge of how to properly use it.

In the Hadamar Hospital, the injection of morphine and scopolamine usually killed most patients quickly. Once in a while, however, the dosage was insufficient to accomplish this goal. Even overdoses did not always kill all the victims. These drugs reduced their respiratory rates to such low levels that some individuals appeared to be dead but were actually alive.[1] The other method of killing at Hadamar, the administration of deadly pills, did not always attain its destructive end immediately either.[2]

In the summer of 1941, Dr. Eysele killed groups of tubercular patients at Buchenwald by injecting sodium-evipan into their veins or directly into their hearts. While most died, those with particularly strong hearts were still living after as many as two injections.[3]

Shooting in front of huge ditches also had its technical drawbacks, one of the major ones being that some individuals were only wounded by the gunfire. After a mass execution in Zhitomir an old man with a white beard and cane on his arm was seen lying among the corpses in an enormous grave. He had been shot seven times but was still breathing.[4] In other shooting massacres, some of the wounded worked themselves out of the graves.[5] When the perpetrators got drunk in the midst of the killing operations, many of the victims were "left for a whole night breathing and bleeding." Others had enough strength to drag themselves, naked and covered with blood, to the nearest town.[6]

Although the gas chambers claimed the greatest number of victims in the most efficient manner, they too did not always live up to their destructive capabilities. This was particularly the case when carbon monoxide gas was pumped into the chambers. More often than not, after the chamber doors were opened a number of victims were still breathing, moaning, or twitching. Removing corpses from the gas chambers was considered a nasty enough task without having to compound it with the additional burden of beholding individuals with some visible signs of life.

While killing at Auschwitz, where Zyklon B gas was employed, left fewer temporary survivors than at places where carbon monoxide was used, there were more technological failures than were acknowledged. Rudolph Höss, the staunch promoter of destruction by Zyklon B, claimed that "In all the years I knew of not a single case where any one came out of the chambers alive." [7] This was sheer overexaggeration on Höss' part. In actuality, many Zyklon victims were still alive when the body disposers began to remove the corpses. The technicians frequently economized too much on the amount of gas applied, and some victims had high resistances and did not succumb immediately to the noxious fumes. [8]

2. The Temporary Survivors of American Technology

Today's sophisticated methods of exterminating millions of unborn children have worked with a high degree of proficiency. Nevertheless, periodically something goes awry somewhere and they do not always succeed in killing the victims before expulsion outside the woman's body. Just how often technical malfunctions produce live babies will never be truly known. Such an embarrassing and disturbing state of affairs is not something physician perpetrators are prone to personally acknowledge, let alone bring to the public's attention. With the huge number of abortions being performed, it is not surprising that enough technological failures have occurred to mar the image of a flawless, trouble-free operation. Stories of babies temporarily surviving the assaults of destructive technology and waging a hopeless struggle for existence have always been the stuff of conjecture, rumor, and vivid imagination. Now they have begun to appear in the pages of books and prestigious medical journals, though in a far more muted form.

In December 1970, Dr. Jean Pakter, director of the New

York City Health Department's Maternity and Newborn Services, revealed that "26 fetuses had remained alive after legal abortions." Nothing more was said about these babies except that one survived and was put up for adoption while the others died after living for a few minutes.[9] A study published in 1976 in the *American Journal of Obstetrics and Gynecology* provided information on thirty-eight babies born alive following abortions induced in upstate New York between July 1970 and December 1972. A large majority (twenty-six) resulted from saline abortion attempts. In addition, seven live births from abortion failures were reported in 1973 and fifteen in 1974.[10] The final fate of these survivors was summarized as follows:

> Seven (18 per cent) died within one hour after birth, 19 (50 per cent) died between one and four hours after birth; and 10 (26 per cent) died between four and 24 hours after delivery. Two infants (5 per cent) survived longer than 24 hours. Of the latter, one died 27 hours and 5 minutes after birth, and the other survived and was eventually discharged into the mother's care.[11]

The article also contains an extensive discussion of why the saline abortion procedure failed to accomplish its goal (destruction before expulsion from the uterus). The large size of the victims plus the inadequate doses of saline injected were factors considered significant in contributing to the delivery of living rather than dead babies.

Dr. Helen I. Glueck and medical scientists at the University of Cincinnati College of Medicine at one time successfully aborted eight dead babies following injections of hypertonic saline. Then something went wrong with either the procedure or the amount of saline injected, because a ninth victim was aborted alive.[12] Dr. Niels H. Lauersen and associates at the New York Hospital-Cornell Medical Center found themselves faced with a prostaglandin victim aborted "with the heartbeat still present. . . . the heartbeat subsided within 3 minutes after delivery."[13] Drs. Charles and Francis Ballard of the University of Southern California Medical Center also mentioned the delivery of two "live fetuses" of about twenty-two to twenty-four weeks gestation. It seems someone had miscalculated and thought they were younger than they actually turned out to be. Their survival, however, was only temporary, and they suffered a fate similar to that of most individuals aborted alive — "they subsequently died." [14]

Another source of information regarding breakdowns in abortion technology are those few doctors and nurses willing to testify in court as to the destructive practices employed by colleagues in handling the still-living victims of induced abortion. The fear of losing their jobs or other reprisals are obstacles that prevent many medical personnel from initiating similar challenges. What has been brought to public attention so far can be considered, therefore, only the tip of the entire reprehensible iceberg.

In October 1973, nurses at the University of Minnesota Hospitals became distraught when two infants were still alive after being aborted by the experimental drug rivanol. They died about one to two hours after being aborted. A nurse indicated that one of the aborted babies cried while being picked up. Another nurse signed a statement to the effect that she had been asked to change the hospital records after she had noted the operation produced "the delivery of a living fetus." Further protests from the nursing staff resulted in a suspension of rivanol abortions. [15]

A coroner's inquest regarding a late-term abortion performed by Dr. Leonard E. Laufe at the West Penn Hospital in Pittsburgh on March 19, 1974 provided information on the final responses of a three-pound-one-ounce victim of thirty weeks gestation. Anesthesia director Nancy Goskey saw "a gasping respiration," which she believed was evidence of life being present. Nurse Monica Bright remembered observing the baby in the pathology lab fifteen minutes after abortion, still gasping and with a visible pulse in the upper chest and neck. Some of the nurses indicated that the child might have survived if appropriate resuscitation efforts had been attempted. Furthermore, an obstetrics technician said she saw

Dr. Laufe alter the medical records to give the impression that the baby was smaller than was actually the case after a controversy erupted over her large size and the presence of life signs.[16]

A preliminary examination held at the West Orange County Municipal Court of California from April 11, 1977 through April 25, 1977 resulted in Dr. William B. Waddill being bound over to a California superior court to stand trial for killing an infant who survived a botched saline abortion. The testimony presented at this hearing contains stark details of how a small victim reacted after a breakdown in destructive technology. Nurse Patricia A. Olvera testified that the baby whined weakly, moved, and gasped for air. She also checked for a heart beat and detected a regular rate of eighty-eight beats per minute.[17] Nurse Patricia Ann Hanes indicated she saw movements of the mouth and breathing attempts.[18] Dr. Ronald J. Cornelsen indicated that the baby's heart was beating, she was breathing fairly rhythmically, and her arms had moved up and down. In addition, she was heard to utter a cry or an expiratory grunting sound.[19]

The Perpetrators' Responses

Active involvement in destroying human lives even under technically perfect conditions can prove to be unnerving for the participants. All the more so when periodic hitches develop in the killing procedures. Malfunctions in destructive technology bring to the killers' awareness unpleasant realities usually concealed when the killing operations function flawlessly. The perpetrators' responses to the technological failure to kill run the gamut all the way from intense anxiety to emotional indifference. Tragically, not that many participants appear to suffer severely enough psychologically to cause any appreciable reduction in the killing. A far greater number seem to be able to maintain a stance of personal aloofness while perpetrating acts of unspeakable violence. Even direct confrontation with the horrendous consequences of breakdowns in the killing machinery is not strong enough to shatter or even penetrate their firmly entrenched preoccupation with the strictly procedural and technical aspects of destruction.

1. Anxiety

The sight of dead, not-yet-dead, and dismembered bodies is very upsetting to some perpetrators — so much so that they find it impossible to participate in the killing any longer. The harsh realities reach into the deepest recesses of consciences that have been all but totally obliterated by the omnipresence of flawless technlogy. Others, equally disturbed, continue their involvement in destructive activities, but only with the aid of such supports as morale-building speeches, medical intervention, consumption of alcoholic beverages, or counseling sessions.

A particularly excruciating experience for the Nazi perpetrators was to behold the not-quite-dead victims making a last-ditch but hopeless effort to live. Even Himmler was disturbed by an incident in August 1941, when he saw a firing squad fail to kill outright two out of one hundred victims. General von dem Bach-Zelewski explained to Himmler how adversely affected the shooting squad members were by this incident: "Look at the eyes of the men in this *Kommando*, how deeply shaken they are! These men are finished for the rest of their lives. What kind of followers are we training here? Either neurotics or savages!" [20]

Himmler thereupon made a speech in which he attempted to console the perpetrators and provide legal and ideological justification for participation in what was admittedly a "repulsive duty" and a "bloody business." He emphasized that their consciences need not be bothered since they were carrying out necessary, noble, and legally authorized orders against subhumans.[21] From this point on, commanders in the field kept careful track of how their charges were holding up under the strain. The number of speeches and discussions intended to boost morale continued to increase as the killings expanded. Doctors were called in to treat those perpetrators who broke down or showed signs of cracking under the pressure of direct involvement in the killings. Dr. Ernst Grawitz attributed General von dem Bach-Zelewski's stomach and intestinal ailments to "hallucinations in which he relived his experiences in the East, particularly the shooting of Jews." [22]

Overindulgence in alcohol also constituted a typical means of the perpetrators for dealing with the task of handling the dead and nearly dead victims of extermination. Personnel in the euthanasia institutions spent alot of their off-duty hours frequenting bars and drinking heavily.[23] Use of alcohol was also noted at the numerous celebrations held to honor the successes at various killing centers such as the one that took place at Hadamar in 1941, marking the cremation of the ten-thousandth mental patient.[24] The same held true in the cases of those who shot victims in the East or herded them into or removed them from the gas chambers. At some of the shooting sites drunkenness became so prevalent that the victims were left breathing and bleeding for an entire night.[25]

Alcoholic consumption was especially prevalent among physicians who participated in the killing. The doctors of Auschwitz sometimes found their destructive tasks "too much for them" and therefore "needed the solace of drink to deaden their senses." [26] Dr. Koenig became so disturbed by his involvement in the death-selection process that "he had to drink a lot of alcohol to stick it out." [27]

Just how successful these efforts were in counteracting the psychological strains of managing malfunctions in the technology of destruction is uncertain. The perpetrators' accounts give the impression that speeches, discussions, medical help, and alcohol were enough to sustain the killers. It seems that the reception of the right type of psychological consolation at the appropriate time was enough to aid them in carrying out their destructive duties.

Although too few in number to make any appreciable impact on the mainstreams of medical thought, some of those involved in today's massive scientific assaults against human life before birth have become distressed enough to actually question the acceptance of abortion as a legitimate medical procedure. If such a response ever became widespread, the entire credibility of abortion and its proponents would be placed in serious jeopardy. The leaders of abortion technology are fully aware of this and are ever alert to the winds of potential revolt among medical and nursing personnel. In a manner paralleling the Nazis, today's medical perpetrators are primed to intervene the moment abortion participants experience any difficulty carrying out their tasks. A look at several cases of technological and subsequent psychological breakdown provides insight into how some doctors and nurses have been affected by their abortion work and how such problems were handled.

The first individual confronted with the sight of an intact, living aborted infant is invariably the woman undergoing a saline or prostaglandin abortion. It is not that unusual for her to be left unattended when the baby is expelled. Having been fed a heavy diet of semantic hypocrisy featuring the unborn as a nondescript lump of cells, it is not surprising that she is unprepared for the shock of beholding a small, perfectly formed baby, sometimes gasping to survive.

Some women get so agitated by the experience of viewing the "products" of saline abortion that they have to be hospitalized for psychiatric problems. In one such case, a young woman was admitted to an inpatient psychiatric unit fifteen months after an abortion. Her condition, diagnosed as an obsessive-compulsive neurosis, was directly linked to seeing "the baby's fingers and toes." Because she "had expected to see a lump or something," she was "surprised that it was so developed." Her reaction to this startling revelation was one of overwhelming guilt. She became so consumed with thoughts of feeling dirty that she washed her hands thirty to forty times a day.[28]

A psychiatric answer meant to prevent the recurrence of such an unnerving situation is "to shield the expelled fetus from the patient's view because of the potential for precipitation of a significant psychologic illness." [29]

The details of implementing this kind of proposal were

revealed to abortion researcher Linda Bird Francke by a nurse with some experience in second-trimester abortions:

> We tried to avoid the women seeing them. They always wanted to know the sex, but we lied and said it was too early to tell. It was better for the women to think of the fetus as an "it." Then we'd scoop up the fetuses and put them in a bucket of formaldehyde, just like Kentucky Fried Chicken. I couldn't take it any longer, and I quit.[30]

But who is to shield the nurses from exposure to the horrifying aftermath of destructive technology? They are frequently the ones saddled with the dirty work of handling and getting rid of the dead and nearly dead bodies. This is not that far removed from the tasks performed by the body-disposal experts of the Third Reich. Many nurses have become extremely distraught by their participation in this phase of the destruction process.

Only six weeks after permissive abortion became legal in Hawaii on March 11, 1970, nurses began to show severe psychological reactions to their abortion involvement. Urgent requests for psychiatric consultation issued forth from several Hawaiian hospitals. It is important to note that a large majority of the nurses had favored repealing the anti-abortion law, but once they became intimately and personally involved in abortion procedures their attitudes changed dramatically. Common responses included symptoms of depression and anxiety, bad dreams, unhappiness, anger, fatigue, crying too easily, confusion, uncertainty, and difficulty in assimilating two irreconcilable functions into their nursing roles: "they were trained to save life and now they were asked to assist in the termination of life." [31]

Many of the nurses' disturbed responses were due to the failure of the abortion procedure to conceal evidence of destruction, plus the disquieting experience of having to discard still-living victims. They became particularly alarmed when they "saw fetal parts sucked or scraped out in the operating room, or saw in the bed dead fetuses or pieces of limbs, fingernails and hair." [32] Another unnerving part of the abortion process was revealed in a nurse's reaction to handling a living aborted baby:

> She showed how she rocked a fetus in her arms, an aborted fetus which she said had been warm and breathing, one which she would formerly ordinarily put in an incubator, but now was supposed to go into formaldehyde. Crying in desperation, she carried the fetus and searched for a doctor to help her with her dilemma, but she could not find one as the physicians were not always available when the fetus delivered on the unit. [33]

Two psychiatrists, Drs. John F. McDermott and Walter F. Char, moved in adroitly to quell the disturbance. A series of group-therapy sessions were set up with the nurses in which they were encouraged to ventilate their feelings, communicate their conflicts, identify with the psychiatrists and the woman undergoing abortion rather than with the fetus, and redefine their professional roles to incorporate abortion as a legitimate medical procedure in light of the "changing ways of looking at birth, life, death, sex, morality and medical care." In a manner reminiscent of Heinrich Himmler's speech to the emotionally shaken members of a firing squad in August 1941, Char and McDermott see the fruits of their counseling efforts as resulting in abortion being viewed not as "an inherent good in itself," but "a last resort and as the lesser of two evil types of solution" when compared with the alternative of unwanted children. [34]

A similar request for psychiatric help was made of Dr. Howard D. Kibel by a general hospital in New York early in July 1970, just after New York's permissive abortion law went into effect. The delivery room staff threatened to quit due to a breakdown in destruction technology: a twenty-week-old saline victim moved after expulsion from the womb. The nurses "found it intolerable to deliver a 'live' infant, only to dispose of it." [35] The same kinds of emotional reactions found among nurses in Hawaiian hospitals were also evident here. In addition, Dr. Kibel acknowledged that the nurses unconsciously experienced the act of abortion as an act of murder. This was equally true of those strongly committed intellectually to the new law. Their feelings of guilt and shame were reflected in the dream of one nurse involving an antique vase:

> In the dream she was stuffing a baby into the mouth of the vase. The baby was looking at her with a pleading expression. Around the vase was a white ring. She interpreted this as representing the other nurses looking upon her act with condemnation.[36]

Psychiatric intervention in this situation consisted of five group sessions, each one lasting from 1 to 1½ hours. Kibel places great store in the power of mutual group ventilation of feelings to relieve guilt and shame. "Channeling feelings into words" is also seen as a feasible approach toward helping the nurses overcome their anger, confusion, and conflicts. He suggested trying out a variety of ways to handle crises stemming from abortion participation — such as separate groups for doctors, delivery room nurses, maternity floor nurses, aides, and others.[37]

Disturbed emotional reactions were also experienced by both doctors and nurses involved in abortions at the North Carolina Memorial Hospital in Chapel Hill. Staff and resident physicians were beset with periodic bouts of depression, anxiety, and obsessive reflection on their abortion participation. The stress became so unbearable for one doctor that he withdrew from the abortion unit for several months. One comment typified the feelings of most doctors: "I'm seldom aware of my operative schedule except when it is my turn to do abortions. I find myself thinking about it weeks in advance with feelings of dread!" Failure of the saline procedure to kill the victims precipitated a crisis among nurses who had the distasteful job of getting rid of the breathing, moving bodies. One nurse handled the situation by crying until the movement stopped, while another one was horrified when she observed an aborted infant with movement left to expire in a basin in the operating room.[38]

Dr. Francis J. Kane of DePaul Hospital in New Orleans and colleagues from the University of North Carolina School of Medicine offered some recommendations for dealing with doctors and nurses bothered by various aspects of scientific baby killing. Again, high on the list of guidelines is the importance of group discussions led by physicians, preferably psychiatrists, as a means of aiding abortion participants to continue their duties without further psychological complications. Priority is also given to the development of training programs to better prepare medical and nursing personnel for coping with the emotional problems associated with performing abortions.[39]

As far back as 1967, experiences with staff at the Denver General Hospital indicated how "philosophically disturbing" the whole idea of abortion was, particularly for obstetricians and obstetrical nurses who "have traditionally been trained to preserve rather than destroy life." There was also awareness of the magnitude of the task at hand: "In a short period of time to break down the traditions, beliefs, and mores of society and suddenly change the whole attitude in regard to unborn human life." Despite the enormity of the job, Dr. Horace Thompson and others at Denver General agree it can be accomplished. A combination of time plus "a considerable amount of in-service training and re-education" are viewed as the essential ingredients for success.[40]

Another startling example of what involvement in the destruction of unborn children does to the medical killers was divulged by Dr. Bernard N. Nathanson. He spoke of doctors and nurses being troubled by deep depression and recurring nightmares dominated by images of blood. In the words of Dr. Nathanson to two *Good Housekeeping* writers, "I was seeing personality structures dissolve in front of me on a scale I had never seen before in a medical setting.... Very few members of the staff seemed to remain fully intact through their experiences."[41]

One member of the nursing staff at a New York hospital related how disturbed she felt about working in a hospital where abortions were performed. Simultaneous involvement with abortion and non-abortion patients as well as the expulsion of a baby aborted alive were particularly traumatic:

> I used to have nightmares. I would open a door and there would be a giant fetus in it. It just didn't make sense. At one point I had a patient in one room who was going through her fifth miscarriage even though the doctors had sewed her cervix shut to try to retain it, while in the room across the hall I was taking care of four women having salines. It freaked me out. We had one saline born alive.[42]

Some physician-abortionists, like the medical executioners of the Third Reich, are resorting to excessive use of alcohol as a means of blotting out any bothersome residues of guilt. Heavy drinking is mentioned as one of the ways in which medical staff at the North Carolina Memorial Hospital coped with the more repugnant parts of their abortion work.[43] Dr. Nathanson also recalled how alcohol came in handy when physicians started "losing their nerve in the operating room." He clearly "remembered one sweating profusely, shaking badly, nipping drinks between procedures." [44]

Writer Norma Rosen's interviews with abortion doctors revealed a pattern of guilt, despair, heavy drinking, and nightmares among some of them.[45] Dr. William Rashbaum of the Albert Einstein College of Medicine admitted to being troubled by what was referred to as "a fantasy in the midst of every abortion: He imagined that the fetus was resisting its own aborting, hanging onto the walls of the uterus with its tiny fingernails, fighting to stay inside." And how did he manage to deal with it? In the words of Dr. Rashbaum, "Learned to live with it. Like people in concentration camps." [46]

The medical literature is just beginning to own up to the psychological problems of doctors and nurses resulting from participation in the process of killing and discarding the dead and not-yet-dead aborted victims. The sparse material published on this topic conveys the impression that the emotional distress associated with killing in the womb is only a temporary aberration and can be easily remedied by the presence of understanding authority figures (psychiatrists) and a resocialization process characterized by ventilation and peer support within the medium of group-therapy sessions. Just how fanciful or valid these claims are is difficult to assess. If, as the physician-abortionists contend, killing unborn children can be so readily incorporated as a valid part of medical practice among those who must deal with the undeniable and distasteful evidence of deceased and not entirely deceased human victims, it indicates the alarming lengths to which involvement in destruction can be tolerated, embraced, and routinized.

2. Emotional Detachment

One of the most horrifying accomplishments of past or present holocausts, in addition to the huge numbers efficiently dispatched to extinction, is the ability of those carrying out the killing operations to remain psychologically distant from the daily task of removing corpses, body parts, and dying victims who may move, moan, and even plead for their lives. This is surely an indication of how tenaciously the technical orientation of the perpetrators is maintained even under the most adverse circumstances. The unwavering dedication to emotionless and depersonalized destruction, regrettably, is sufficiently powerful to override any challenge, whether psychological or technological.

The Nazi planners did not expect an entirely trouble-free technical performance every time; they did assume, nevertheless, that the perpetrators would not be bothered seriously even when the methods failed to kill all the victims right away. True to expectations, many technicians did not seem to be disturbed by the hideous aftermath of mass extermination. The sight of dead bodies and individuals uttering their last agonizing gasps of breath was taken in stride. The cleanup crews were there to perform a strictly technological task — the removal and disposal of dead or dying sub-humans.

This extreme lack of feeling was pronounced among those doctors who performed the horrendous death-dealing experiments on concentration camp inmates. They had no trouble compiling meticulous scientific records while observing the death agonies of their experimental expendables. A typical illustration is the immense satisfaction felt by Dr. Sigmund Rascher because the heart actions of a high-altitude research victim "were written down with an electrocardiogram to the very end." [47]

Another destructive experiment conducted by Dr. Rascher was made known to the Nuremberg tribunal in 1946. It featured the employment of scientific terminology to depict the killing of prisoners for the purpose of experimenting with the hemostatic preparation "Polygal 10":

> The Russian was shot in the right shoulder from above.... The bullet emerged near the spleen. It was described how the Russian twitched convulsively, then sat down on a chair and died after 20 minutes. In the dissection protocol the rupture of the pulmonary vessels and the aorta was described. It was further described that the ruptures were tamponed by hard blood clots. That could have been the only explanation for the comparatively long span of life after the shot. [48]

Many death technicians likewise remained emotionally dissociated from their destructive taks. "I had no feelings in carrying out these things," one gassing technician told the Nuremberg court. "That, by the way, was the way I was trained." [49]

Dr. Hans Hermann Kremer maintained the same air of emotional indifference as he watched and participated in mass atrocities. The diary he kept of his experiences while at Auschwitz is a ghastly document, characterized by the ease with which Dr. Kremer was able to move back and forth between participating in killing and leading a normal life of enjoying food, drink, and recreational activities. Sample

entries from his diary reflect "a peculiar mixture of detachment and of the eager excitement of a child attending a
party."

6 September 1942 —
Today, Sunday, excellent lunch: tomato soup, half a
hen with potatoes and red cabbage (20 g. fat), sweets
and marvellous vanilla ice.... in the evening at
8:00 hours outside for a *Sonderaktion* [special action;
this phrase was commonly employed to describe any
action in which a killing took place].

8 November 1942 —
Took part in two *Sonderaktionen* last night in rainy
weather (12th and 13th).... In the afternoon another *Sonderaktion* which was the 14th I took part in.
In the evening we had a nice time in the leaders' club.
...We had Bulgarian red wine and Croatian plum-
schnapps.[50]

Most contemporary medical killers of the unborn likewise appear to be emotionally unaffected by the sight of dead
bodies or body parts being cut, sucked, ripped, yanked, or
ejected out of the womb. They also remain impervious to the
heartbeats and gasps of still-living aborted babies. While
some medical perpetrators become upset when they first see
the "products" of mass extermination move or whimper, it
is astonishing how quickly such an experience ceases to bother
them. Killing and its alarming aftermath become old hat.

A common attitude upon confronting a not-yet-dead
"product" of abortion destruction is expressed by Dr. Richard
W. Stander of the obstetrics and gynecology department at
the University of Cincinnati College of Medicine. He described the experience as "the single unhappy case in which
a living fetus was delivered after intra-amniotic injection of
hypertonic saline."[51] A similar mentality was expressed by
Dr. Arthur L. Hoskins of Baltimore, Maryland, who views
the "production of a surviving fetus" as one of the complications associated with saline abortion.[52] This has gone far

beyond the level of pure sentiment: the notation "two living aborted fetuses" is part of a table listing "complications occurring in 47 of 401 patients undergoing saline instillation" in a study of abortions at Bellevue Hospital in New York City by Drs. J. Joshua Kopelman and Gordon W. Douglas.[53] *Medical World News* of November 14, 1977 incorporated identical sentiments in an article entitled, "Avoiding Tough Abortion Complication: A Live Baby." [54] Only in a distorted world dominated by mass assembly-line destruction is it possible to define babies aborted alive as unhappy cases or complications! To the killers this is simply the consequence of technological fallibility, a rare phenomenon entirely devoid of any emotional significance.

One of the problems encountered in the saline destruction procedure is a bloody tap: the removal of bloody fluid from the amniotic sac instead of the usual yellow colored liquid. This sometimes happens because the needle thrust into the sac hits the baby rather than the fluid surrounding the baby. As long as the blood is not coming from the maternal circulatory system the physician abortionist is unperturbed. As one doctor put it, "The needle stuck something it shouldn't have. I hope it's the fetus. That's the least problematic possibility." [55]

Other doctors are not quite so callous; the periodic realization of what the needle does to the baby causes them to experience some uneasiness. As explained by an expert in saline killing:

> On a number of occasions with the needle, I have harpooned the fetus. I can feel the fetus move at the end of the needle just like you have a fish hooked on a line. This gives me an unpleasant, unhappy feeling because I know that the fetus is alive and responding to the needle stab. When you put in the needle, theoretically you go in the sac and take out fluid and put in salt water. But there are times when you hit the fetus and you can feel the fetus wiggling at the end of that needle and moving around which is an unpleasant thing. No one has ever mentioned this, but

I've noticed it a number of times. You know there is something alive in there that you're killing. . . .

In my own case I never had any psychological adverse reaction. Except an occasional feeling that one was destroying life.[56]

For this medical killer, like many of his contemporary colleagues, the placement of the needle in the wrong spot is only a minor, unpleasant, and awkward feature of an otherwise flawless killing procedure. It induces a fleeting moment of discomfort that never reaches the feelings or conscience of the perpetrator. Neither does it last long enough to put an end to the killing.

Today's physician-abortionists and fetal experimenters are living the same kind of schizophrenic existence so clearly illustrated in the diary kept by German physician Dr. Hans Hermann Kremer. They can inflict the most violent acts imaginable on the human being in the womb with the utmost skill and watch with intense rationality and scientific curiosity as the last sparks of life flicker out. They can live an otherwise exemplary professional, civic, and family life while remaining personally untouched by the death and destruction perpetrated in the name of medical science. This is indeed a tragedy of the highest magnitude!

Debugging the Machinery of Destruction

In killing actions where millions are exterminated, one cannot always depend on the perpetrators remaining emotionally dissociated from their victims. Nor can speeches, counseling, or alcohol always succeed in keeping their anxiety at a low enough level for them to keep on killing. In such massive destructive operations so completely dominated by technology what could be more fitting than a strictly technological resolution! This means ironing out the kinks in the machinery of destruction in order to shield the killers from the potentially unnerving situation of having to handle victims with some life signs still intact. It also means working out a standardized procedure for disposing of those who happen to temporarily survive the most technically advanced and superbly operating methods of killing.

1. Nazi Repairs and Modifications

The first series of experiments conducted at Buchenwald involved testing out various poisons on human guinea pigs. Dr. Erwin Ding placed poison in the food of inmates without their knowledge. When it failed to kill them, they were strangled in a crematorium and autopsies were performed on their remains.[57]

The preoccupation of German physicians with the dosage levels of poison necessary to kill the victims was motivated by a desire to prevent the possibility of survivors after the lethal substances were injected. This is what prompted Buchenwald chief physician Dr. Waldemar Hoven to inject 20 cc's of undiluted raw phenol into the arms of aged inmates in poor health. Although only 5 cc's would ordinarily bring about death, the 20 cc's actually injected were viewed as a "precautionary measure" to insure a fatal outcome.[58]

In some instances, however, the medical perpetrators underestimated the amount of poison required to kill the victims. If this happened, the usual procedure was to inject them with additional doses of lethal drugs. When a few tubercular patients at Buchenwald did not die after as many as two injections of sodium-evipan, Dr. Eysele administered a third injection.[59] This was sufficient to finally finish them off.

A similar procedure was followed at the Hadamar Hospital. If after the initial injection of morphine and scopolamine the patients were not dead, "they were given another shot." [60] At the Hadamar Trial, Nurse Minna Zachow told what happened when the other method of killing used at Hadamar, deadly pills, did not accomplish its goal: "They received tablets, and the next morning everyone of them who was not dead received an injection." [61]

Identical principles were applied to the killings at the shooting sites. The usual way of handling the wounded was to shoot them again. To make it a more psychologically palatable procedure for the shooting brigades, a doctor was sometimes on hand to give the order for the so-called "mercy shots." [62] At a shooting massacre in Zhitomir, an old man was not yet dead after being shot seven times. Rather than shooting him "for good," it was decided to let him "perish by himself." [63]

The technological answer to the failure of carbon monoxide gas to kill everyone in the gas chamber was the use of a more lethal gas, Zyklon B, which killed more people in a shorter period of time. [64]

Even the ultraefficient hydrogen cyanide did not always kill all of its victims. The perpetrators also handled this problem in the typical technological manner, with the application of a more conclusive method of killing. An example of this is the case of a teenage girl who temporarily survived the horrendous ordeal of gassing at Auschwitz. Inmate-physician Dr. Miklos Nyiszli revived her and pleaded for her life. The response of the perpetrators was to carry the young girl into a room where another method of killing was employed: "a bullet in the back of the head." [65]

The same fate awaited the child of a dead mother found in the gas chamber, who was "so firmly pressed against her breast that it was still alive." Other technology was again called into action: "They shot it forthwith and threw it among the other corpses." [66]

Whatever the type of gas used, the perpetrators had to contend with the distasteful chore of removing from the chambers individuals who were still alive. The questioning of one of the defendants at the Nuremberg War Crimes Trials revealed his way of dealing with survivors of the gassing process:

Q. In case the inmates would not have been killed following the introduction of the gas done by you, would you have killed them with a bullet?
A. I would have tried once again to suffocate them with gas, by throwing another dose of gas into the chamber. [67]

In most instances, however, it was considered neither economical nor efficient to handle the situation by closing the chamber door again and then dropping more canisters of gas into the chambers. Time rather than the further application of destructive technology finished off many of the remaining half-dead survivors; they expired on the journey from the gas chambers to the incinerators. The hardiest chamber survivors were burned alive with the already deceased. As one camp survivor phrased it, "Still breathing, the dying victims were taken to the crematory and shoved into the ovens." [68]

One of the most chilling and detailed accounts of how secondary methods of killing took up the slack when the primary ones broke down was supplied by convicted killer Dr. MO (pseudonym) during a prison interview conducted in 1969 by Professor Henry V. Dicks of the Columbus Centre, a research institute located at the University of Sussex in Great Britain. At the time of the interview Dr. MO, a former public health physician in the Nazi regime, was serving simultaneous life sentences for putting twenty-six patients to death at a small hospital for the mentally deficient in 1945. Excerpts from the exchange between Dicks and Dr. MO reveal a disturbingly persistent commitment to getting the job done by overcoming the methodological limitations inherent in destructive technology:

> So MO in his official capacity goes to the little hospital's pharmacy. "But of course the pharmacist had evacuated it already." All the lethal poisons — the opiates, etc.— had gone. But MO found a white powder lying around: "I don't any longer remember what it was," he interposes, "I hoped it would work if taken in sufficiently large doses." (*Between us we could not deduce the likely chemicals, as from what follows.*) "Well it didn't go right at all" — none died on the first dosage by mouth, and even on the second day when he doubled the dose these poor people were just nauseated or vomited. With this result on the third morning, MO had found some ampoules of what he believed was called "Novalgin" (on which

I commented it sounded like a compound for pain alleviation); he hoped that intravenous injections of this would do the trick. . . . Two or three of the patients died soon after his injections — but even MO could not be sure whether it was from the effects of the injection or from long malnutrition and stress. "So then we shot," he said laconically. "I had to certify death and indicate those still alive who should receive the mercy shot. . . . That's all." [69]

2. Contemporary Repairs and Modifications

Contemporary doctors have become quite concerned about technological breakdowns that result in the abortion of living rather than dead babies. Dr. Rafael A. Del Valle of Concord, California was sufficiently worried to seek advice from fellow obstetricians and gynecologists about how to deal with the case of "a 300 gram fetus who still had an active fetal heart and showed muscle movements" after a prostaglandin abortion.[70] Today's physician-abortionists, like the Nazi technicians before them, experienced little difficulty in coming up with a variety of suggestions for getting rid of the wounded and dying survivors of destructive technology.

In some hospitals the emphasis is on prevention. What the perpetrators do is modify the technology or apply it earlier in order to increase the probability of the child dying before expulsion outside the woman's body. Dr. Nils Wiqvist of the Karolinska Hospital in Stockholm, Sweden concluded that since muscle movements and even gasps are more likely to occur beyond the twentieth week of gestation, it is the policy at his hospital to refrain from performing prostaglandin abortions after that period of time.[71] At the University of Southern California Medical Center in Los Angeles County it was likewise decided to restrict abortions to less than twenty weeks gestation after two babies from twenty-two to twenty-four weeks were aborted alive.[72] However, even babies aborted below or close to the twenty-week limit may show signs of struggling for breath and life. This is exactly what Dr. Thomas D. Kerenyi and fellow abortionists found in their saline induction unit at Park East Hospital in New York City: babies of seventeen and twenty weeks gestation respectively unexpectedly survived the onslaughts of saline and then died three hours later. The doctors lost no time in working out a way to prevent the recurrence of such a potentially upsetting experience. From then on, the procedure was altered by making routine ultrasonic checks for intrauterine fetal heartbeats at two-hour intervals after infusion of saline. If after six hours the fetal heartbeat was still present, another injection of saline was administered.[73]

At the annual meeting of the Planned Parenthood Federation of America in late 1977, Dr. Wing K. Lee, director of fetal medicine at Mount Sinai Hospital in Hartford, Connecticut, discussed problems relating to infants surviving midtrimester abortion attempts. He reported that 45 out of 607 midtrimester abortions performed at Mount Sinai between April 1974 and October 1976 resulted in live births, including a set of twins.[74]

Doctors in attendance did not lack for suggestions on how to avoid the medical executioner's most bothersome irritant: the delivery of a living baby. The most common proposal made was to substitute one method of killing for another when the original one failed to bring about the desired result. A 1975 live-birth controversy prompted physicians at the Nassau County Medical Center in East Meadow, New York to once again employ hypertonic saline injections beyond twenty weeks of pregnancy. Dr. Joel Robins, associate professor of obstetrics and gynecology at the State University of New York Stony Brook Health Sciences Center, and a team of doctors expressed support for switching from the prostaglandin to the saline method. Based on a comparison of 700 prostaglandin and 170 saline abortions, they found that the number of live births dropped from seven with prostaglandin to none with saline.[75]

Despite the precautionary measures taken and the sophistication of contemporary destructive technology, living victims are still being expelled and removed from the uterus.

A number of strategies have been developed to deal with such a situation.

According to one of the approaches used, the physician refuses to provide treatment for the child aborted alive. What he does instead is either declare the survivor to be already deceased or define the victim as a form of subhumanity that does not merit life-sustaining help. When a nurse in a New York hospital pointed out to the doctor on duty the existence of an aborted infant with a visibly strong heartbeat, he simply replied, "For all intents and purposes it's dead. Leave it there." [76] Another nurse, also employed in New York, related a similar type of experience with a baby who temporarily survived a saline abortion. "I raced to the nursery with it and put it in an incubator," she recounted. "I called the pediatrician to come right down, and he refused. He said, 'That's not a baby. That's an abortion.' " [77]

Like their Nazi predecessors, today's medical executioners also rely upon time as a crucial factor in extinguishing the embarrassing presence of life signs. At one Planned Parenthood clinic located in Brooklyn, New York, for example, "the doctors would remove the fetus while performing hysterotomies and lay it on the table, where it would squirm until it died." [78]

Dr. Ronald J. Bolognese of Philadelphia, an avid proponent of the "time will take care of things" school of thought, explains how this works out in practical application:

> With Prostaglandin, fetal demise usually occurs during the process of labor and delivery. At the time of delivery, it has been our policy to wrap the fetus in a towel. The fetus is then moved to another room while our attention is turned to the care of the gravida. She is examined to determine whether complete placental expulsion has occurred and the extent of vaginal bleeding. Once we are sure that her condition is stable, the fetus is evaluated. Almost invariably all signs of life have ceased. [79]

Similar types of delaying tactics are suggested by Dr. William E. Brenner from the University of North Carolina at Chapel Hill:

> Since viewing the abortus may be traumatic to the patient, the abortus should be separated from the patient and removed from her room, keeping it out of her view as soon as possible. If respirations or other movements continue for a few minutes, and are not just reflex movements, the patient's physician, if he is not in attendance, should probably be contacted and informed of the situation. The pediatrician on call should probably be appraised of the situation if signs of life continue. The physician may institute those measures he believes are appropriate based on his estimate of the probability of the fetus surviving from the weight, gestational age, and condition of the fetus.[80]

By the time the doctor goes through all these motions and rituals, the living victims most certainly would have expired.

Legal actions brought against physicians for negligence, manslaughter, or homicide in cases where babies temporarily survive abortion attempts illustrate what destructive procedures were resorted to when the initial ones failed to kill the victims. In 1973, doctors at the University of Minnesota Hospitals were accused of not treating two infants aborted alive after the experimental drug rivanol failed to kill them inside the womb.[81] At a coroner's inquest held in 1974, Dr. Leonard E. Laufe of the West Penn Hospital in Pittsburgh was charged with homicide for leaving unattended to die a 3½ pound baby girl of thirty weeks gestation who survived a hysterotomy abortion. A medical student in attendance during the abortion had suggested another method for doing away with the baby: a dose of morphine.[82] On October 3, 1973, after three unsuccessful attempts had been made to kill a black male child of advanced gestation by saline induction, Dr. Kenneth C. Edelin switched to the hysterotomy method. At Edelin's trial, Dr. Enrique Gimenez-Jimeno testified that when the baby was found to be still breathing after his placenta was peeled off the uterine wall, Dr. Edelin held him inside the uterus for three minutes to make sure he died before being removed.[83]

Physician-attorney Dr. Cyril H. Wecht concluded his analysis of the Laufe and Edelin cases with some guidelines for getting doctors off the legal hook in situations where babies are born alive after botched abortions. One of the guidelines includes a recommendation for using another method of killing. It would be applied, of course, before there is any possibility that the child would be declared a legal person. In the words of Dr. Wecht:

> If medically feasible, the physician could seek to avoid criminal liability by administering a toxic substance to the fetus before the "critical point." This recommendation, while understandably morally and theologically reprehensible to many physicians, nevertheless would appear to be prophylactically sound from a legal standpoint, based upon the Laufe and Edelin cases.[84]

Testimony presented at a preliminary hearing on April 11, 1977 by Dr. Ronald J. Cornelsen was the key factor responsible for bringing Dr. William B. Waddill to trial for the strangulation death of an hour-old infant following a saline abortion attempt. Dr. Cornelsen's testimony is absolutely unique. Not only does it provide unprecedented information on the method used to kill the child — manual strangulation — but also stark details on a range of other destructive methods considered. The following excerpts are taken from a transcript of the responses of Dr. Cornelsen to questions asked by Deputy District Attorney Robert D. Chatterton regarding what happened to the aborted baby on the evening of March 2, 1977, in the nursery of Westminster Community Hospital, Westminster, California:

Q. When he [Dr. Waddill] turned to look at you, did you have a conversation?
A. He told me that he was sorry to get me into this

mess. . . . Then he said, "We have a baby here that
came out alive from the saline abortion". . . .

Q.   And then what happened?

A.   He put his hand into the isolette, into one of the
portholes. . . . I saw him put his hand about the baby's
neck. . . . I saw him pushing down with his hand and
with his hand around the neck pushing down on
the neck.

Q.   In your experience as a pediatrician, what you
saw him doing with the baby's neck, was that medical
procedure?

A.   None that I'm familiar with. . . .

Q.   Was he saying anything as he was pressing down
on the neck of the baby?

A.   He said that he couldn't find the GD trachea.

Q.   What do you mean by GD?

A.   God damned trachea. . . .

Q.   Would you tell the court what the trachea is.

A.   The trachea is the main windpipe that carries
air down into the bronchus or into the lungs from the
mouth or nose. . . .

Q.   What is the next thing that happened?

A.   And then he took his hand out and said, "Ron,
why don't you listen to the baby's heart?". . . . I heard
the baby's heart beat; and I heard respiratory movement, air going in and out of the lung. . . . I told him
that the heart was still beating.

Q.   Now, after having examined and determined a
heart rate and after having heard the breathing and
having informed Dr. Waddill of your observations,
what next occurred?

A.   He put his hand back into the isolette. . . . He
began pushing down on the baby's neck again. . . .
I could see the baby's head bend up forward and the
chest kind of make a V position with the head and
the chest on the baby. . . .

Q.   What is the next thing that occurred after you
observed him doing that?

A.   I mentioned . . . why not let the baby alone, that

probably it would die on its own anyway. . . . He then turned . . . and asked for some potassium chloride.

Q. Did you say anything when he asked for potassium chloride?

A. I asked what that was for? . . . Well, he just said he could use it to inject into the baby, and it would stop the heart right away. . . . and I said that this probably would be detected on autopsy. And then I said, "Or is autopsy done?"

Q. And what did he say to that?

A. Well, he said he didn't know if autopsies were normally done on saline abortions.

Q. What next occurred?

A. Then he asked for the potassium chloride again. . . . I said, "We don't keep that stuff in here in the nursery."

Q. Then what was said or done?

A. Dr. Waddill suggested that we could get some potassium chloride from the floor. . . . Then he said, "Better not do that or that would be missed on the drug count."

Q. Okay. Then what?

A. Then he asked Nurse Kennedy if she could get a bucket or a pail of water. . . . He said we could hold the baby's head under the water, and that would stop it then. . . . She said, "I don't believe we have a bucket or a pail here in the nursery."

Q. Did he say anything to Nurse Kennedy then?

A. He told her to get back out. . . .

Q. And after she had left the nursery, what was it that you next saw or heard?

A. Dr. Waddill put his hand back into the isolette and pushed on the baby's neck again. . . . just between the head and the shoulders, pressing down and then just pushing a little higher down. . . .

Q. Okay. Before we discuss what you did when you got out of that area . . . did you see any movements by the baby?

A. When the use of potassium chloride was being

discussed and at the time the water was asked for, I noticed that the baby was breathing fairly rhythmically on its own.... The arms had moved up and down. And I thought I heard either a cry or an expiratory grunting sound of the baby.

Q. All right. So then you had an occasion to leave the nursery. And at the time you left it, what was Dr. Waddill doing?

A. He had his hand in the isolette up in the porthole pushing on the baby's neck.

Q. So what did you do?

A. I went ... to make a phone call. ...

Q. When you completed that phone call what occurred?

A. Dr. Waddill was standing there by me in the work area.... He said, "Ron, the baby won't quit breathing. Can you think of something else?".... Then I said, "Why not leave the baby alone. It looks pretty gone now. And it probably will die on its own." ....

Q. What was the next thing either said or done between the two of you?

A. He said that he could run — put the water in the sink and hold the baby's head under the water.... I said it would be crazy because an autopsy would find water in the trachea which could be different than just amniotic fluid that might be in the trachea....

Q. What did he do? ...

A. And then he went back to the isolette.... He just put his hand about the baby's neck again.

Q. Did you spend any time watching him on this occasion?

A. No.... I turned and found the baby that I was to examine and undressed the baby to examine it....

Q. What's the next thing that you either saw or observed about Dr. Waddill?

A. Well, he came into the nursery where I was examining; and he said, "Ron, I think the baby is dead. Would you listen to the baby's heart?" ....

Q. Having examined the baby, hearing no heartbeat, hearing no breathing, observing its condition, what did you tell Dr. Waddill?

A. I told him that the baby was dead. . . .

Q. Can you give us an estimation of its size when you saw it?

A. When I first saw the baby and listened to the heart for the first time, I'd guess it was probably about a three-pound baby. . . . it would have to be somewhere around seven—seven to eight months.[85]

Never before has the hitherto hidden world of destructive technology aimed at the smallest and most vulnerable members of the human community been so fully undraped. Not since Dr. MO of Nazi Germany employed a succession of killing techniques on victims in a home for the mentally defective has anyone displayed such a total dedication to getting the job accomplished despite the obstacles. If Dr. Cornelsen's testimony is accurate, it shows the fanatic persistence with which Dr. Waddill sought and found an alternate killing method when the primary one failed. This is an alarming commentary on how firmly the goal of destruction has become embedded in the fabric of medical practice. Given the overriding premise underlying the ethic of destruction — to kill — what Dr. Waddill is charged with doing is perfectly logical. When the zealous commitment to technological destruction is added to this, killing is easily reduced to a matter of sheer technique: if one method of killing does not work, another one will be quickly found that does.

What about those sturdy individuals aborted alive who are not choked, drowned, or poisoned? As was the fate of the gas chamber survivors of the concentration camps, if the lapse of time does not take its toll, the flames of an incinerator surely will. One need only recall Dr. Ada Ryan's testimony before the House Judiciary Committee to realize that aborted babies have been tossed into the furnaces of American hospitals while still whimpering.[86] According to information uncovered by reporters Litchfield and Kentish in

England, a similar fate awaited those crying aborted victims not scheduled for scientific or commercial exploitation.[87] If the incinerator attendant at the Stobhill General Hospital in Glasgow, Scotland, had not "heard a whimper from the bag" with a newly aborted baby in it, this child would have ended up being burned alive in the hospital incinerator.[88] How many children aborted alive out of the womb have been burned to death because their feeble cries of agony have gone unheeded or undetected?

The sight of individuals breathing, gasping, and struggling to survive momentary lapses in destructive technology is still not enough to deter most perpetrators from continuing to kill. Some retain sufficient residues of conscience to be so shaken by such an encounter that they can no longer participate in the destruction. Others, while bothered initially, become immune to the harsh consequences of their technical ministrations. With the passage of time and psychological support from fellow perpetrators, killing and its disturbing aftermath become routine. Not even the disarming presence of temporary survivors phases the perpetrators any more. Their typical response is to either let the victims die or employ a more conclusive method of destruction, one that will finish them off for good. When this point is reached, it is an undeniable sign that the process of desensitization has set in permanently. This point was reached by those physicians and technicians who operated the machinery of destruction in the euthanasia hospitals, concentration camps, and gas chambers of the Third Reich. The same thing is happening among the doctors and technicians who man the killing equipment in the hospital abortion units and abortion clinic chambers of contemporary society.

CHAPTER 9

Death Statistics

The effectiveness of destructive technology is nowhere more tellingly revealed than in the statistics compiled on those exterminated. The number of lives destroyed in the Nazi holocaust ran into the millions; the number of unborn lives destroyed in today's holocaust likewise runs into the millions. As the figures mount, so does the propensity to depersonalize the victims. Adolf Eichmann expressed this mentality perfectly in 1944: "One hundred dead is a catastrophe. Five million dead is a statistic." [1] This is precisely how modern statisticians view today's victims: as strictly a matter of numbers and not human beings.

Nazi Body Counts

The picture that emerged from the Nazi holocaust is one of virtually unlimited destruction. This was one of the few instances in history when such terms as unlimited, massive, and enormous can be taken literally. The inclusion of physicians, scientists, and technicians in every facet of the death-inducing production lines could not help but lead to an extraordinarily successful outcome.

Nazi thoroughness extended to evaluating the effectiveness of the destructive activities through body counts. The perpetrators wanted to make sure that all the planning, equipment, and personnel that went into the holocaust was worth the effort. They tried to keep track of how many died from the various methods applied — shooting, gassing, injections, imposed starvation, and others. It was no easy job; the victims often succumbed faster than the perpetrators could count. Sometimes the numbers exterminated were exact counts; other times they were estimates.

No one will ever really know how many lives were actually extinguished. Whatever the figure, the executioners took great pride in the rapidly mounting numbers. How they enjoyed demonstrating the numerical superiority of one method of killing as opposed to another! The prize for sheer delight in the huge numbers exterminated must surely go to Adolf Eichmann. He was so elated by his role in the destruction of five million Jews that he said he would jump laughingly into his grave.[2]

To gain a better appreciation of how well the extermination machinery worked one only has to look at some of the statistics gathered at the various killing centers. Estimates of the numbers killed in the euthanasia program vary from 50,000 up to 300,000. Viktor Brack, one of the euthanasia leaders, testified before the Nuremberg tribunal that 50,000 to 60,000 were killed in euthanasia institutions from the autumn of 1939 to the summer of 1941.[3] This figure is based on the erroneous assumption that euthanasia ended in 1941. The killing of mental patients and other defectives actually continued until the time of the allied occupation of Germany. On July 2, 1945, for example, an American occupational force found a state hospital in the town of Kaufbeuren still in operation. The doctor in charge related that "the last child patient had been killed on May 29th, 33 days after the occupation of the nearby village. The last adult had died twelve hours before."[4]

A report of the Czechoslovak War Crimes Commission, which puts the number of mental patients and aged killed at 275,000, appears much closer to the truth of what happened.[5] Psychiatrist Dr. Fredric Wertham's analysis results in an almost identical figure: about 275,000. This is based on the existence of from 300,000 to 320,000 patients in psychiatric hospitals in 1939 and only 40,000 in 1946.[6]

Numerical accounts of the destructive activities perpetrated by the mobile killing units in Russia and Eastern Europe were also kept. The reports consisted of daily situation bulletins and monthly resumés until the end of March 1942, and after that a series of weekly communiqués. A Dr. Knobloch then compiled and edited them for distribution to Hitler, Himmler, Heydrich, and other Reich leaders. If the totals seemed too low, Knobloch had the prerogative of juggling the figures to make them appear more impressive. How proud the Nazis were of flaunting their statistics! An example of what they included is contained in a report drafted in the winter of 1941/42. The number of Jews killed were listed as follows: Estonia, 2,000; Latvia, 70,000; Lithuania, 136,421; White Russia, 41,000.[7]

A long report sent to Heydrich by a chief executioner, Franz Stahlecker, included not only a figure of 229,052 Jews executed in the eastern territories, but also a new twist, "a map, tastefully marked with coffins at appropriate points."[8]

Although the mobile killing operations were responsible for a mind-boggling 1.4 million lives,[9] this was simply a prelude to the more massive destructive activities of the concentration camps. Among them Auschwitz was the biggest and most productive death factory. Data on the rates of destruction at Auschwitz vary according to who compiled them, but they all demonstrate the incredible speed and efficiency with which human lives were extinguished.

The highest estimate for the daily rate of destruction was furnished by the Central Commission for Investigation of German Crimes in Poland: "When operations were in full swing in August 1944, the number of corpses burnt daily rose to 24,000."[10] Information from Auschwitz survivor Dr. Olga Lengyel provides a stark account of extermination efficiency:

The four ovens of Birkenau were heated by a total of thirty fires. Each oven had large openings. That is, there were 120 openings, into each of which three corpses could be placed at one time. That meant they could dispose of 360 corpses per operation. That was only the beginning of the Nazi "Production Schedule."

Three hundred and sixty corpses every half hour, which was all the time it took to reduce human flesh to ashes, made 720 per hour, or 17,280 corpses per twenty-four hour shift. And the ovens, with murderous efficiency, functioned day and night.

However, one must also reckon the death pits, which could destroy another 8,000 cadavers a day. In round numbers, about 24,000 corpses were handled each day. An admirable production record — one that speaks well for German industry.[11]

Another statistical picture was furnished by Rudolph Höss, commandant of Auschwitz. His estimates are lower, but staggering nevertheless. Based on the crematories' capacity of eight thousand bodies per day plus the virtually unlimited capacity of burning in open pits, Höss concluded that "it was therefore possible to exterminate and get rid of as many as 10,000 people in twenty-four hours." [12]

Daily statistics secretly kept by a French Sonderkommando physician, Dr. Pasche, were smuggled to Dr. Lengyel. They reveal the period of May through July of 1944 to be the record season of death factory operations at Auschwitz:

May, 1944	360,000
June, 1944	512,000
From the 1st to the 26th of July, 1944	442,000
	1,314,000 [13]

In less than a quarter of a year the Nazis "liquidated" more than 1.3 million persons at Auschwitz-Birkenau! The Hungarian Jews bore the biggest brunt of this unprecedented destruction: 400,000 gassed in the summer of 1944.[14]

Furthermore, during the period of Höss' tenure at Auschwitz (May 1940-December 1943), 2.5 million perished in the gas chambers and another half million died of illness and starvation. When prison psychologist Dr. G. M. Gilbert asked Höss how it was technically possible to exterminate 2.5 million people, he replied in "a quiet, apathetic matter-of-fact tone of voice":

> That wasn't so hard — it would not have been hard to exterminate even greater numbers.... The killing was easy; you didn't even need guards to drive them into the chambers; they just went in expecting to take showers and, instead of water, we turned on poison gas. The whole thing went very quickly.[15]

Although not as efficient or productive as Auschwitz, other concentration camps contributed their share of victims to the death statistics. Based on the number of trains that arrived at Treblinka from July 23, 1942 until it closed down on November 23, 1943, "the number of victims murdered at Treblinka amounts to at least 731,600."[16] Even those transferred to the so-called privileged camp of Theresienstadt — a supposed refuge for the old, the enfeebled, and decorated war veterans — did not fare any better. Of the 139,654 Jews sent there, only 17,320 still remained in May 1945.[17]

The total number of Jewish lives extinguished in the holocaust is unknown, but several figures give some idea regarding the huge scope of destruction. Six million is one of the most common figures cited. This is said to have come from Adolf Eichmann in a report to Heinrich Himmler. Eichmann estimated that four million were killed in the concentration camps and another two million were shot by the mobile killing units in the East. Himmler was not happy with Eichmann's report; he thought it was an underestimate. He therefore sent a statistical expert to check up on the authenticity of the estimates. Eichmann later toned down his figure to five million.[18]

The figure of 5.7 million Jewish victims was furnished by the World Jewish Congress during the Nuremberg trials. English historian Gerald Reitlinger believes this to be an overestimate compiled at a time when reliable data was unavailable. He claims that a more careful scrutiny of what information exists would place the number killed between 4,204,400 and 4,575,400.[19] His estimates are based in large part on a balance sheet compiled from the resettlement lists of Himmler's final-solution statistics expert Dr. Korherr. Reitlinger, nevertheless, admits his own figures must be regarded as conjectural. Whatever the exact figures, he provides a necessary perspective to the whole issue of numbers: "Whether six million died, or five million, or less, it was still the most systematic extermination of a race in human history." [20]

It must be remembered that Jews were not the only victims annihilated. Many Germans, Poles, Russians, and others were also killed. When these are added to the number of Jews annihilated, the grand total reaches upwards to ten million or more. The numbers are absolutely staggering.

American Body Counts

If the Nazi assault against human life can be legitimately depicted in such terms as massive, enormous, and gigantic, so too can these same words be used to characterize the contemporary medical onslaught against human life in the womb. Nazi physicians would be hard put to match the number of lives snuffed out by modern medicine. Not only do contemporary doctors kill more human beings than their Nazi counterparts — they also keep better records of their destructive activities. Death statistics today are carefully tabulated, coordinated, and communicated by physicians, researchers, and scientists with the aid of high-speed, sophisticated computers and advanced reporting systems.

Even with such an impressive array of record-gathering technology, some lack of clarity still exists as to the number of unborn children actually being exterminated. There is consensus, however, on two aspects of destruction: the number of victims killed is prodigious and the medical executioners delight in dazzling the public with a torrent of formidable statistics on the virtues of safely and cleanly discarding the remains of induced abortions. To the death statisticians, the huge numbers involved do not reflect a horrendous tragedy, but simply a medical service designed to root out subhuman elements perceived as inconvenient, bothersome, and even dangerous to personal and public health.

Recent studies provide more precise insights into how well contemporary killing centers are functioning. Acquaintance with the production rates of some of them as well as with the broader national and worldwide figures will close out the statistical picture.

Before and after the 1973 Supreme Court decision on abortion, hospitals have served as a major locale for unborn baby killing. Some of the most prestigious hospitals have also been among the most productive of all the death factories. Only recently have figures become available that give a more comprehensive picture of how much destruction is being perpetrated in contemporary hospitals. A survey of American hospitals, clinics, and private physicians conducted by the Planned Parenthood Federation's Alan Guttmacher Institute revealed that in 1973 hospitals performed 394,300 abortions while non-hospital abortion clinics were responsible for 337,800. Since 1974, however, non-hospital clinic abortions have surpassed the number done in hospitals.[21]

When compared with the number of lives exterminated in the euthanasia institutions of Germany from 1939 until 1945 (aproximately 275,000), the number of unborn lives killed in American hospitals in 1973 alone (394,300) is an absolutely staggering figure indeed.

Among abortion clinics, Preterm is one of the oldest and most productive. Established in the District of Columbia in March 1971 as a "total family planning" agency, it has accumulated an imposing set of statistics: "An average schedule of 60 vacuum aspirations/day, six days a week" with 24,000 abortions performed during the first twenty-three months of operation.[22] Two freestanding abortion clinics located in the same building in midtown Manhattan were responsible for a grand total of forty-thousand abortions in one year's time. Dr. Abner I. Weisman characterized these facilities as examples of abortion production-line style, with waiting rooms jam-packed like the salon of a local beauty parlor.[23]

Probably the most active of all the abortion clinics was the now-defunct Center for Reproductive and Sexual Health of New York City. During the time it was in operation it held the distinction of being the largest abortion clinic in the western world. Its record of massive destruction is hard to top. Former director Dr. Bernard N. Nathanson reported the clinic had performed sixty thousand abortions in just 1½ years. In one of the most candid revelations to date, Dr. Nathanson admitted this meant he "had in fact presided over 60,000 deaths." [24]

In the final months of his tenure as director, Nathanson at last began to feel that "the clinic was a mill and we were grinding people through it, even though we did one-to-one counseling." [25] An earlier report on the clinic's productivity gave a statistical indication of how valid Nathanson's feeling was. During its first thirteen months of operation — July 1, 1970 through August 1, 1971 — 26,000 unborn lives were exterminated. This total was made possible by a sixteen-hours-a-day, seven-days-a-week schedule. The only time this death factory shut down was on legal holidays. The average monthly rate of abortions reached 2,300.[26]

This, though, was just a warm-up. The rate of destruction began to climb higher:

> From eight in the morning until midnight, seven days a week, doctors working in ten operating rooms performed vacuum aspirations on an endless parade of pregnant wombs. In peak months more than 3,000 patients paying $150 a piece passed through.... Doctors regularly worked 12-hour shifts.[27]

Nathanson remembered one particularly ambitious doctor who "commuted weekly from Kentucky, flying up for a long weekend during which he manned the vacuum aspirator almost around-the-clock, and returned Monday to his regular practice." [28] With this kind of untiring dedication it is little wonder that the death statistics mounted so astonishingly!

No one abortion clinic or facility, of course, can compete with the 2.5 million or so exterminated at Auschwitz. Nevertheless, there are many more killing centers for the unborn than there were destruction sites during the time of the Third Reich. The number of hospitals and clinics that either specialize in killing the unborn or provide this service as an avocation run into the thousands. According to an Alan Guttmacher Institute survey, in the United States alone "abortions were reported in 1975 by a total of 2,398 clinics, hospitals and physicians in their private offices." [29] These destructive establishments exist not only in just about every geographical section of the United States, but also in almost every country of the world. The statistics pouring forth from killing centers for the unborn all over the world are truly staggering; they dwarf anything churned out by the Nazis. There are more lives extinguished by physician-abortionists in *one year* than all the lives destroyed by physicians and non-physicians during the entire *twelve years* of the Nazi regime!

Analysis of the national and international situation indicates the vast magnitude of death and destruction currently taking place.

If sixty thousand abortions at one clinic within the span of 1½ years seems like an unbelievable figure, statistics on the number of unborn children legally killed in one year in the United States as a whole are even more incredible. According to the previously cited study conducted by the Alan Guttmacher Institute, 745,000 legal abortions were performed in 1973 and 892,200 in 1974. [30] Because not everyone who was surveyed responded, these totals may well represent underestimates of from 5 to 10 percent. Therefore, the figures for 1973 and 1974 are probably closer to 800,000 and 900,000 respectively. A more recent survey indicates that the number of legal abortions reported increased to 1,034,200 in 1975 and 1,115,000 in 1976. [31]

A way of gaining further perspective on the number of legal abortions performed annually is to compare them with the most common of other surgical procedures performed in America, tonsillectomy. In 1974 abortion ran a close second, 900,000 abortions to 917,000 tonsillectomies. [32] Based on a projection that "the utilization of legal abortion services has not yet reached a plateau, and that the number of legal abortions will continue to increase," there was a good chance that physician-induced intrauterine baby killing would replace tonsillectomy as the most frequently performed "surgical procedure." The official fulfillment of this forecast was announced in the May/June 1977 issue of *Family Planning Perspectives*. "Legal abortion," acknowledged body counters Sullivan, Tietze, and Dryfoos, "now appears to be the most frequently performed surgical procedure in this country." [33]

Another indicator of how massive legal abortions have become is to compare the number of abortions performed with the number of live births. As of 1973 in the Middle Atlantic states, for example, there were 537 abortions for every thousand live births. New York led the way with 921 abortions for every thousand live births. In the District of Columbia an even more astounding statistical portrait was unveiled: far more babies were aborted than born (4,208 abortions per thousand births). [34] At this rate it is not inconceivable that some day abortions may exceed births on a national rather than just a local level.

The principal investigator of this study is none other than Dr. Christopher Tietze of the Population Council. Dr. Tietze has made a career out of keeping meticulous records on the number of unborn children destroyed through induced abortion. He is far and away the leading collector, compiler, and interpreter of death statistics in America. In this sense, he holds a position paralleling that of Nazi statisticians Drs. Knobloch and Korherr. Dr. Tietze is a consummate professional. His reports on the results of medical destruction are models of scientific analysis, always embellished with an impressive series of graphs, statistical tables, charts, and succinct conclusions.

One would think that one million or so abortions is a huge number of human beings for any civilized society to execute in one year, even if the executioners are licensed physicians. Apparently, however, Dr. Tietze and others like him are dissatisfied with the statistical results; they actually believe the numbers should be higher! There are several things that keep the number of legal abortions down to what Dr. Tietze considers the too-low figure of 800,000 in 1973: not enough public hospitals were performing abortions, non-hospital abortion clinics were beginning to perform the bulk of abortions, often on a profit-making basis, and not enough states were assuming their fair share of abortions. Dr. Tietze was especially perturbed with eleven states for their lack of abortion output in 1973: "Not a single public hospital reported performance of a single abortion for any purpose whatsoever." [35]

Statistically speaking, then, how many abortions does Dr. Tietze think should have been performed in 1973 instead of the 800,000 reported? In answer to this question, he comes up with an interesting numerical response: "Between approximately one-half and one million women who needed abortions were not able to obtain them in 1973." [36] If what Tietze refers to as the unmet need for legal abortion services is added to the number of abortions reportedly done, then a figure of from 1.3 to 1.8 million abortions is what he has in mind as an appropriate figure for 1973.

Dr. Tietze is clearly unhappy with the present state of abortion consumption in the United States. He places much of the failure to perform more abortions on the shoulders of uncooperative hospitals: "The shocking fact is that the Supreme Court decision of 1973 has had little effect on hospitals. Most of the unmet abortion needs end up in the cradle." [37] Obviously, Dr. Tietze would much prefer that they end up in the grave. If individuals like him continue to get their way, this is precisely what will happen. At the rate things are now moving, an annual American legal extermination output of two million unborn lives is well within the realm of possibility. Perhaps it is already upon us. Future statistical reports promise to keep the public fully apprised of the situation.

While a million abortions per year has become a commonplace phenomenon in some countries, the number of unborn children extinguished on the international scene cannot help but impress even the most blasé among the pro-death statisticians. A United Nations study, authored by

Lester R. Brown and Kathleen Newland of the Worldwatch Institute, estimated that 40 to 55 million abortions are now performed each year on a worldwide basis. Furthermore, two-thirds of the world's population live in countries with liberal abortion laws already in effect.[38]

The figure of 40 to 55 million promises to soar higher as the abortion law liberalization-repeal movement continues to make inroads into the remaining one-third of the world's population located in countries with restrictive abortion laws. Is it far-fetched to assume that in the not-too-distant future the annual international destruction of the unborn could reach 100 million? In retrospect, the Nazi record of six to ten million victims in a twelve-year period is a mere drop in the bucket compared with the current global slaughter of defenseless unborn lives.

Rather than being appalled by the massive destruction borne out in the statistics, today's corpse counters welcome each numerical increase as a "humane and practical step" toward legally ending unwanted pregnancies. Brown and Newland depict the numbers aborted as representing a positive, sweeping, and irreversible social change. They find it odd that abortion has not been resorted to more frequently as a means of bringing down birth rates in an overpopulated world.[39] They are unbothered by the fact that each abortion constitutes the intentional destruction of another unique human life. As researchers, they can remain aloof, totally absorbed in the abstract world of numbers, estimates, formulas, and numerical projections.

Conclusion

Responsibility for today's massive destruction of human lives, even more so than during the Nazi era, must be placed squarely on the shoulders of the medical profession. It was upstanding doctors, and not the so-called backalley butchers, who committed most of the mayhem against the unborn even when abortion was illegal. Physicians were behind many of the propaganda campaigns aimed at getting the anti-abortion laws abolished. The fall and decline of American medicine is most starkly epitomized in the statistic that destruction of the unborn is now the most frequently performed surgical procedure in America, surpassing even tonsillectomy. Physicians are also in the forefront of the current movement to legalize euthanasia. Under the cloak of the law and technology, medical doctors continue to violate the ethics of humanity and their professional *raison d'etre* by killing human beings before birth at a staggering rate. The number of postnatal discards snuffed out under the aegis of medical science is expanding far more rapidly than most people are aware of. If physicians would take a united stand against abusing their medical skills for destructive purposes, there would be very few abortions and acts of euthanasia performed, either legal or illegal. Too many doctors, however, lack the fortitude to oppose a reprehensible trend that reduces the physician to the unconscionable role of technical executioner.

An uphill battle confronts anyone who dares to challenge this appalling state of affairs. Armed with an awesome arsenal of scientific weapons, fortified with an endless stock of technical terms, and supported by prestigious medical organizations and vast economic resources, physicians are formi-

dable adversaries indeed. The domination of American medicine by elitist, amoral technocrats who possess no qualms
about perverting their skills to destroy the unwanted shows
no signs of abating. In fact, it may become even worse in the
future. The fiercely competitive atmosphere in which thousands of candidates vie for the sparse number of medical
school openings is hardly conducive to developing doctors
geared toward placing restraints on destructive technology.
Those who survive the cutthroat competition are likely to
become part of an increasingly arrogant breed of physicians,
convinced of their infallibility and intolerant of criticism from
God and mortals alike.

Although things appear bleak and time is running out
for the survival of a humane social order where all human
lives are considered of inestimable value, an opportunity still
exists to alter the monstrous course of events. Grassroots
resistance to the medical destruction of millions has grown
tremendously. Right-to-life organizations from almost every
geographical area of America now constitute a potent voice
for those who cannot defend themselves from the assaults
of medical perpetrators. Another encouraging sign is the
growing number of doctors who not only refuse to participate
in the killing, but even take the almost unprecedented step
of openly criticizing colleagues who do.

The task of educating the medical profession and public
regarding the beauty, dignity, and worth of human life at
all stages of development and the harsh realities of what
abortion, euthanasia, and other medical atrocities do to this
life remains enormous. Despite the flurry of activities in opposition to medical violence, the killing continues at an alarming pace. Nothing less than a revolution in attitudes, perceptions, and values is called for.

To those who are trying to sow the seeds of religious
warfare by calling the right to life a uniquely Catholic issue,
a Mormon issue, or one of Orthodox Jewry, several points
should be made abundantly clear. It was the American Medical Association that led the way in getting statutes protective
of life before birth enacted during the mid to late 1800s.
Organized medicine's role was so significant that historian

James C. Mohr, in his book *Abortion in America*, referred to it as "The Physicians' Crusade Against Abortion, 1857-1880." The Association's opposition to abortion was not based on the tenets of any one religious body but on the fact that abortion constituted what the AMA in 1859 called the "slaughter of countless children" and the "unwarrantable destruction of human life," and in 1871 the "wholesale destruction of unborn infants." Such statements, significantly, did not emanate from the Catholic Church, speaking through its bishops. They represented, rather, the voice of American medicine being expressed through its most influential body, the American Medical Association. Furthermore, the many state legislatures that followed the lead of the physicians by passing laws designed to protect human life in the womb were overwhelmingly Protestant, and not Catholic, in composition.

In the current drive to establish a nonviolent community, a basic principle needs to be continually emphasized: the right to life is not a narrow sectarian matter but a broad universal one that transcends the boundaries of race, religion, and creed. It is the bottom line from which all other rights proceed. Unless the right to life is restored as self-evident and inalienable for everyone, all other rights are meaningless.

It should be kept uppermost in mind that annihilation assembly-line style is not the creation of impulsive psychopaths venting aggression against hated enemies, but the handiwork of highly trained technicians preoccupied with developing and perfecting the machinery of destruction. Although the inhumanity of respectable professionals is a difficult reality to grasp, there is a far greater likelihood of mass extermination being perpetrated at the hands of dispassionate scientists than enraged maniacs. The unwanted of today and the future have much more to fear from credentialed medical executioners than they ever will from mobs in the streets.

The application of scientific know-how to the development of destructive techniques not only keeps brutal acts against helpless victims hidden from view, but also results in the brutalization of the medical profession and public alike. The pervasive insensitivity toward the plight of the most vulnerable and least visible members of humanity has been facilitated considerably by the creation of killing procedures that dispatch millions to oblivion in a swift, proficient, and unobtrusive manner. Technology has the insidious effect of robbing killing of its most repugnant features and reducing it to the trivial level of a technical procedure.

The exercise of raw medical power against weak, immature, or defenseless human beings must be stopped. Persistent appeals and challenges must be addressed to members of organized medicine to cease their war on the unborn and increasingly on the born; to lay down their weapons and put aside their curettes, forceps, and other lethal instruments; to pull out the plugs on their suction machines and remove the deadly solutions from their syringes. Now, more than ever, doctors need to become acquainted with the ancient roots of their profession and dedicate themselves to the sanctity-of-life ethic embodied in the Hippocratic Oath, a document that condemns both abortion and euthanasia, and is the very cornerstone of civilized medicine.

Today, some thirty-four years after the defeat of Nazism, we are just awakening to the realization of how fully implicated physicians were in Germany's holocaust. Hopefully, it will not take another thirty-four years to become conscious of the extent to which contemporary medical involvement in abortion on demand, hospital infanticide of defective infants, and euthanasia of underpar aged constitutes a repetition of history's most grievous errors. Such parallels stand little chance of exposure, let alone examination, unless the medical profession and public alike are willing to confront the harsh realities of massive destruction so thoroughly obscured under the guise of lovely decors, sophisticated equipment, antiseptic methods, and prestigious technicians. The whole area of past and present medical barbarities, heavily shrouded by a mushrooming barrage of clinical procedures and devices, must be opened up for public awareness, scrutiny, and action. A thorough acquaintance with the medical horrors of the Third Reich and their kinship with those of contemporary society represents an essential step toward the kind of consciousness raising so urgently needed to end the monstrous bloodbath currently being implemented by respectable medical executioners.

Appendix

THE AMERICAN MEDICAL ASSOCIATION ON ABORTION: AN ANATOMY OF CONTRASTING POLICY STATEMENTS

What Is Abortion?

1859 — "The slaughter of countless children; no mere misdemeanor, no attempt upon the life of the mother, but the wanton and murderous destruction of her child; such unwarrantable destruction of human life."

1871 — "The work of destruction; the wholesale destruction of unborn infants."

1967 — "The interruption of an unwanted pregnancy."

1970 — "A medical procedure."

Who Should Perform Abortions?

1871 — "It will be unlawful and unprofessional for any physician to induce abortion or premature labor ... and then always with a view to the safety of the child — if that be possible."

1970 — "Abortion should be performed only by a duly licensed physician and surgeon in an accredited hospital."

Who Are Physician-Abortionists?

1871 — "Men who cling to a noble profession only to dishonor it; false brethren; educated assassins; these modern Herods; these men, who, with corrupt hearts and blood-stained hands, destroy what they cannot reinstate, corrupt souls, and destroy the fairest fabric that God has ever created ... under the cloak of that medical profession; monsters of iniquity."

1967 — "Conscientious practitioners performing therapeutic abortions for reasons other than those posing a threat to the life of the mother; equally conscientious physicians who believe that all women should be masters of their own reproductive destinies and that the interruption of an unwanted pregnancy, no matter what the circumstances, should be solely an individual matter between the patient and her doctor."

What Should Be Done To Physician-Abortionists?

1871 — "The members of the profession should shrink with horror from all intercourse with them, professionally or otherwise; these men should be marked as Cain was marked; they should be made the outcasts of society; it becomes the duty of every physician in the United States ... to resort to every honorable and legal means in his power to crush out from among us this pest of society."

1970 — They should be allowed to perform abortions as long as they are done "in an accredited hospital acting only after consultation with two other physicians."

What Should The Ethics of Abortion Be?

1871 — "Thou shalt not kill; this commandment is given to all and applies to all without exception; it matters not at what stage of development his victim may have arrived — it matters not how small or how apparently insignificant it may be — it is a murder, a foul, unprovoked murder, and its blood, like the blood of Abel, will cry from earth to Heaven for vengeance."

1967 — "The Committee does not intend to raise the question of the rightness or wrongness of therapeutic abortion; this is a personal and moral consideration which in all cases must be faced according to the dictates of the conscience of the patient and her physician."

Notes

Citations listed in the notes beginning with one or several letters followed by a series of numbers are the actual initials and page numbers of court transcripts circulated during the war crimes trials held at Nuremberg. Among the abbreviations used, "EC" refers to the "Economic Case," a group of documents processed by the Economic Section of the Office of the United States Chief Counsel (OCC) at Frankfurt. The letter "L" stands for documents processed by the London office of the OCC. "PS," short for "Paris-Storey," indicates material processed by OCC offices in Paris and Nuremberg. Documents translated by Lt. Walter Rothschild are designated by the letter "R" while those processed by the British prosecuting staff are covered by the letter "D." The initials "NO" refer to Nazi organizational documents and "NG" to documents issued by agencies and ministries of the German government.

Complete photostats of the original court testimony are available at major depository libraries such as the Library of Congress and the Columbia Law Library. Where printed collections of Nuremberg documents are available, they are employed as text sources. Some of the major collections can be found in the following publications: International Military Tribunal, *Trial of the Major War Criminals* (Nuremberg, 1947-1949), 42 vols.; Office of United States Counsel for Prosecution of Axis Criminality, *Nazi Conspiracy and Aggression* (Washington, D.C.: U.S. Government Printing Office, 1946-1948), 11 vols; Nuernberg Military Tribunals, *Trials of War Criminals* (Washington, D.C.: U.S. Government Printing Office, 1947-1949), 15 vols.

PREFACE

[1] Bernard N. Nathanson, "Deeper Into Abortion," *New England Journal of Medicine* 291 (November 28, 1974): 1189.

Chapter 1

PHYSICIANS AS HEALERS

[1] Ralph H. Major, *A History of Medicine*, 2 vols. (Springfield, Ill.: Charles C .Thomas, 1954), 2: 787-808.

[2] Ibid., p. 876.

[3] Thomas H. Huxley, Address on "Liberal Education," cited by Abraham Flexner, *Medical Education: A Comparative Study* (New York: Macmillan Company, 1925), p. 38.

[4] Richard H. Shryock, *Medicine in America: Historical Essays* (Baltimore, Maryland: Johns Hopkins Press, 1966), p. 29.

[5] Flexner, *Medical Education*, p. 38.

[6] Fredric Wertham, *A Sign for Cain: An Exploration of Human Violence* (New York: The Macmillan Company; London: Collier-Macmillan Limited, 1966), p. 174.

[7] Esther Fischer-Hamberger, "Germany and Austria," in *World History of Psychiatry*, ed. John G. Howells (New York: Brunner/Mazel, Inc., 1975), p. 273.

[8] Shryock, *Medicine in America*, pp. 1-45.

[9] Ibid., p. 36.

[10] Horatio R. Storer et al., "Report on Criminal Abortion," *Transactions of the American Medical Association* 12 (1859): 75-78.

[11] Eugene Quay, "Justifiable Abortion — Medical and Legal Foundations," *Georgetown Law Journal* 49 (Spring 1961): 437.

[12] Storer et al., "Report on Criminal Abortion," pp. 75-76.

[13] In 1847 the distinguished histologist Dr. Albert von Kolliker "first demonstrated the true development of the spermatozoa, showing that they are not extraneous bodies, but originate in the testicular cells and fertilize the ovum." Fielding H. Garrison, *An Introduction to the History of Medicine*, 4th ed., reprint. (Philadelphia and London: W. B. Saunders Company, 1929), p. 461.

[14] Storer et al., "Report on Criminal Abortion," p. 77.

[15] Ibid., pp. 77-78.

[16] D. A. O'Donnell and W. L. Atlee, "Report on Criminal Abortion," *Transactions of the American Medical Association* 22 (1871): 250.

[17] Ibid., pp. 240-257.

[18] Ibid., p. 257.

[19] Ibid., p. 258.

[20] Ibid., pp. 257-258.

[21] James C. Mohr, *Abortion in America: The Origins and Evolution of National Policy, 1800-1900* (New York: Oxford University Press, 1978), pp. 324-325.

[22] Ibid., p. 200.

Chapter 2

THE ILLEGAL KILLERS

[1] Leo Alexander, "The Molding of Personality Under Dictatorship: The Importance of the Destructive Drives in the Social-Psychological Structure of Nazism," *Journal of Criminal Law and Criminology* 40 (May-June, 1949): 14.

[2] Leo Alexander, "Destructive and Self-Destructive Trends in Criminalized Society: A Study of Totalitarianism," *Journal of Criminal Law and Criminology* 39 (January-February, 1949): 558.

[3] Leo Alexander, "War Crimes: Their Social-Psychological Aspects," *American Journal of Psychiatry* 105 (September 1948): 174.

[4] Alexander, "Molding of Personality Under Dictatorship," p. 21.

[5] Gisella Pearl, *I Was A Doctor In Auschwitz* (New York: International Universities Press, 1948), p. 80.

[6] Ibid., p. 28.

[7] Affidavit of Fritz Friedrich Karl Rascher, M.D., 31 December 1946, Concerning the Life and Activities of Dr. Sigmund Rascher, *Trials of War Criminals before the Nuernberg Military Tribunals, The Medical Case,* 2 vols. (Washington D.C.: U.S. Government Printing Office, 1947-1949), 1: 676-678. (Hereafter cited as *The Medical Case.*)

[8] Diary of the Division for Typhus and Virus Research at the Institute of Hygiene of the Waffen SS, 1941 to 1945 (Ding Diary), *The Medical Case,* 1: 557-572.

[9] Ravensbrueck Experiments Concerning Sulfanilamide and Other Drugs; Bone, Muscle, and Nerve Regeneration and Bone Transplantation, *The Medical Case,* 1:45.

[10] Olga Lengyel, *Five Chimneys: The Story of Auschwitz* (Chicago and New York: Ziff-Davis Publishing Company, 1947), p. 177.

[11] Ibid., p. 173.

[12] Pearl, *Doctor In Auschwitz*, p. 129.

[13] Lengyel, *Five Chimneys*, p. 146.

[14] Pearl, *Doctor In Auschwitz*, pp. 110-111.

[15] Lengyel, *Five Chimneys*, p. 147.

[16] Pearl, *Doctor In Auschwitz*, p. 84.

[17] Abraham J. Rongy, *Abortion: Legal or Illegal?* (New York: Vanguard Press, 1933), p. 89.

[18] Frederick J. Taussig, *Abortion Spontaneous and Induced: Medical and Social Aspects* (St. Louis: The C. V. Mosby Company, 1936), p. 422.

[19] Jerome E. Bates and Edward S. Zawadzki, *Criminal Abortion: A Study in Medical Sociology* (Springfield, Ill.: Charles C. Thomas, 1964), p. 3.

[20] Marie E. Kopp, *Birth Control in Practice: Analysis of Ten Thousand Case Histories of the Birth Control Clinical Research Bureau* (New York: Robert M. McBride & Co., 1934).

[21] Lawrence Lader, *Abortion* (Indianapolis: The Bobbs-Merrill Company, Inc., 1966), pp. 8, 64-65.

[22] Bates and Zawadzki, *Criminal Abortion*, pp. 173-174.

[23] Ibid., p. 95.

[24] Ibid., pp. 37, 95.

[25] Ibid., pp. 175-186.

[26] Raul Hilberg, *The Destruction of the European Jews* (Chicago: Quadrangle Books, Inc., 1967), p. 649.

[27] Stanley Milgram, *Obedience to Authority: An Experimental View* (New York: Harper & Row, 1974), pp. 5-6.

[28] Hannah Arendt, *Eichmann in Jerusalem: A Report on the Banality of Evil* (New York: The Viking Press, 1963), pp. 22-23.

[29] Opening Statement of the Prosecution by Brigadier General Telford Taylor, 9 December 1946, *The Medical Case*, 1:27, 28, 68-74.

[30] Ibid., 1: 67.

[31] Fredric Wertham, *A Sign for Cain: An Exploration of Human Violence* (New York: The Macmillan Company; London: Collier-Macmillan Limited, 1966), pp. 154-155, 168-169.

[32] Ibid., pp. 171-176.

[33] Gitta Sereny, *Into That Darkness: From Mercy Killing to Mass Murder* (London: Andre Deutsch Limited, 1974).

[34] Direct Examination of Alfons Klein, *Trial of Alfons Klein et al. (The Hadamar Trial)*, ed. Earl W. Kinter (London: William Hodge and Company, 1949), p. 89. (Hereafter cited as *The Hadamar Trial*.)

[35] Letter from Hitler to Karl Brandt and Bouhler, 1 September 1939, Charging Them With the Execution of Euthanasia, *The Medical Case*, 1: 848.

[36] Wertham, *A Sign for Cain*, p. 166.

[37] Ibid., pp. 164-165.

[38] Rongy, *Abortion: Legal or Illegal?*, p. 97.

[39] Ibid., p. 130.

[40] Taussig, *Abortion Spontaneous and Induced*, p. 449.

[41] Proceedings of a Conference of the National Committee on Maternal Health, *The Abortion Problem* (Baltimore: Williams and Wilkins Company, 1944), p. viii.

[42] Paul H. Gebhard et al., *Pregnancy, Birth and Abortion* (New York: Hoeber-Harper, 1958), pp. 197-199.

[43] Mary S. Calderone, "Illegal Abortion as a Public Health Problem," *American Journal of Public Health* 50 (July 1960): 949.

[44] William B. Walker and J. F. Hulka, "Attitudes and Practices of North Carolina Obstetricians: The Impact of the North Carolina Abortion Act of 1967," *Southern Medical Journal* 64 (April 1971): 441-445.

[45] Jerome M. Kummer, "Abortion: The Rearguard in Birth Control," *Journal of Reproductive Medicine* 5 (October 1970): 71.

[46] Alan F. Guttmacher, "Therapeutic Abortion in a Large General Hospital," *Surgical Clinics of North America* 37 (April 1957): 468.

[47] Alan F. Guttmacher, "The Law That Doctors Often Break," *Redbook Magazine*, August 1959, p. 96.

[48] Sanford R. Wolf, Tom T. Sasaki, and Irving M. Cushner, "Assumption of Attitudes Toward Abortion During Physician Education," *Obstetrics and Gynecology* 37 (January 1971): 143.

[49] "Therapeutic Abortion," *Proceedings of the American Medical Association House of Delegates* (June 1967), pp. 42-43.

[50] Mary S. Calderone, ed., *Abortion in the United States* (New York: Hoeber-Harper, 1958), p. 59.

[51] Horatio R. Storer et al., "Report on Criminal Abortion," *Transactions of the American Medical Association* 12 (1859): 75-78; D. A. O'Donnell

and W. L. Atlee, "Report on Criminal Abortion," *Transactions of the American Medical Association* 22 (1871): 239-258.

[52] Calderone, ed., *Abortion in the United States*, p. 59.

[53] Lader, *Abortion*, p. 47.

[54] Calderone, ed., *Abortion in the United States*, p. 62.

[55] Ibid., p. 60.

[56] Wertham, *A Sign for Cain*, p. 164.

[57] "King of the Abortionists," *Newsweek*, February 17, 1969, p. 92.

[58] Ibid.

[59] Lader, *Abortion*, pp. 44-45.

[60] Ibid., p. 45.

[61] O'Donnell and Atlee, "Report on Criminal Abortion," pp. 240-257.

[62] Guttmacher, "Law That Doctors Often Break," p. 96.

[63] Somers H. Sturgis, "Alan Guttmacher, M.D.— A Life Fulfilled," *New England Journal of Medicine* 290 (May 9, 1974): 1085.

[64] John F. McDermott et al., "The Concept of Child Advocacy," *American Journal of Psychiatry* 130 (November 1973): 1203-1206.

[65] Walter F. Char and John F. McDermott, "Abortions and Acute Identity Crisis in Nurses," *American Journal of Psychiatry* 128 (February 1972): 952-957.

[66] Dennis J. Horan et al., "The Legal Case for the Unborn Child," in *Abortion and Social Justice*, ed. Thomas W. Hilgers and Dennis J. Horan (New York: Sheed & Ward, 1972), pp. 133-134.

Chapter 3

MEDICAL AGITATION FOR LEGAL DESTRUCTION

[1] Extract from the Final Plea for Defendant Beiglboeck, *The Medical Case*, 2: 77.

[2] Nicholson J. Eastman, "Induced Abortion and Contraception: A Consideration of Ethical Philosophy in Obstetrics," *Obstetrical and Gynecological Survey* 22 (February 1967): 11.

[3] Robert B. Benjamin, "Abortion or Compulsory Pregnancy?," *Minnesota Medicine* 52 (March 1969): 457.

[4] Daniel Gasman, *The Scientific Origins of National Socialism: Social Darwinism in Ernst Haeckel and The German Monist League* (New York: American Elsevier Publishing Company, Inc., 1971), p. 40.

[5] Ernst Haeckel, *The History of Creation: Or The Development of the Earth and Its Inhabitants by the Action of Natural Causes*, trans. E. Ray Lankester, vol. 1, 4th ed. (New York: D. Appleton & Co., 1892), pp. 175-176.

[6] Ernst Haeckel, *The Wonders of Life: A Popular Study of Biological Philosophy*, trans. Joseph McCabe (London: Watts & Co., 1904), p. 22.

[7] Ibid., pp. 121-123.

[8] Ibid., pp. 114, 119.

[9] Haeckel, *History of Creation*, p. 178.

[10] Gasman, *Scientific Origins of National Socialism*, pp. 90-91.

[11] Ibid., p. 93.

[12] Ibid., p. 95.

[13] Ernst Haeckel, *The Riddle of the Universe: At The Close of the Nineteenth Century*, trans. Joseph McCabe (New York and London: Harper & Brothers, 1900), pp. 324-325.

[14] Gasman, *Scientific Origins of National Socialism*, p. 14.

[15] Karl Binding and Alfred Hoche, *The Release of the Destruction of Life Devoid of Value* (Leipzig, Germany: Felix Meiner, 1920), comp. Robert L. Sassone (Santa Ana, Calif.: A Life Quality Paperback, 1975).

[16] Ibid., p. 16.

[17] Ibid., pp. 17-18.

[18] Ibid., pp. 37-38.

[19] Ibid., pp. 36-37.

[20] Ibid., pp. 38-40.

[21] Extracts from the Closing Brief Against Defendant Brack; Extracts from the Closing Brief Against Defendant Karl Brandt, *The Medical Case*, 1: 810, 827.

[22] Hans Löhr, "The Physician Must Come To Terms With the Irrational," in *Nazi Culture: Intellectual, Cultural and Social Life in the Third Reich*, ed. George L. Mosse, trans. Salvator Attanasio et al. (New York: Grosset & Dunlap, Universal Library, 1968), p. 233.

[23] "Abortion and Race Hygiene," *Journal of the American Medical Association* 105 (July 20, 1935): 213.

[24] Ibid.

[25] Opening Statement of the Prosecution by Brigadier General Telford Taylor, 9 December 1946, *The Medical Case*, 1: 58.

[26] Leo Alexander, "Medical Science Under Dictatorship," *New England Journal of Medicine* 241 (July 14, 1949): 39.

[27] "Statement by Dr. Leo Alexander," in *Doctors of Infamy: The Story of the Nazi Medical Crimes*, by Alexander Mitscherlich and Fred Mielke, trans. Heinz Norden (New York: Henry Schuman, 1949), p. xxxi.

[28] Helmut Ehrhardt, *Euthanasia and Destruction of Life Devoid of Value* (Stuttgart, Germany: Ferdinand Enke Publishers, 1965), p. 26.

[29] Alexander, "Medical Science Under Dictatorship," p. 39.

[30] Alice Platen-Hallermund, *The Killing of Mental Patients in Germany* (Frankfurt am Main: Verlag Der Frankfurter Hefte, 1948), pp. 12-13.

[31] Abraham J. Rongy, *Abortion: Legal or Illegal?* (New York: Vanguard Press, 1933), p. 10.

[32] Ibid., pp. 29-30.

[33] Ibid., pp. 51-53.

[34] Ibid., p. 54.

[35] Ibid., p. 130.

[36] Ibid., p. 212.

[37] Frederick J. Taussig, *Abortion Spontaneous and Induced: Medical and Social Aspects* (St. Louis: The C. V. Mosby Company, 1936).

[38] Ibid., pp. 29-30.

[39] Ibid., pp. 29, 396, 404, 449.

[40] Ibid., p. 422.

[41] Jerome M. Kummer, "Criminal Abortion: A Consideration of Ways to Reduce Incidence," *California Medicine* 95 (September 1961): 173.

[42] Jerome M. Kummer, "New Trends in Therapeutic Abortion in California: Complete Legalization is Imminent," *Obstetrics and Gynecology* 34 (December 1969): 886.

[43] Jerome M. Kummer, "Abortion: The Rearguard in Birth Control," *Journal of Reproductive Medicine* 5 (October 1970): 71-74.

[44] Harold Rosen, "Psychiatric Implications of Abortion: A Case Study in Social Hypocrisy," *Western Reserve Law Review* 17 (1965): 464.

[45] Robert E. Hall, "Abortion: Physician and Hospital Attitudes," *American Journal of Public Health* 61 (March 1971): 519.

[46] Natalie Shainess, "Abortion: Social, Psychiatric, and Psychoanalytic Perspectives," *New York State Journal of Medicine* 68 (December 1, 1968): 3070-3073.

[47] Natalie Shainess, "Abortion Is No Man's Business," *Psychology Today,* May 1970, pp. 18, 76.

[48] Natalie Shainess, "Abortion: Inalienable Right," *New York State Journal of Medicine* 72 (July 1, 1972): 1772-1773.

[49] "The Playboy Foundation Annual Report," *Playboy,* January 1974, p. 59.

[50] Shainess, "Abortion: Inalienable Right," pp. 1773-1774.

[51] Ibid., p. 1772.

[52] Ibid., p. 1773.

[53] Group for the Advancement of Psychiatry, *The Right to Abortion: A Psychiatric View* (New York: Charles Scribner's Sons, 1970), pp. 20, 26.

[54] Ibid., p. 49.

[55] Zigmond M. Lebensohn, "Abortion, Psychiatry, and the Quality of Life," *American Journal of Psychiatry* 128 (February 1972): 950.

[56] Zigmond M. Lebensohn, "Legal Abortion as a Positive Mental Health Measure in Family Planning," *Comprehensive Psychiatry* 14 (March/April 1973): 97-98.

[57] "A Statement on Abortion by One Hundred Professors of Obstetrics," *American Journal of Obstetrics and Gynecology* 112 (April 1, 1972): 992-998.

[58] Ibid., p. 992.

[59] Ibid.

[60] Herbert Ratner, "Editor's Comments," *Child and Family* 12, No. 3 (1973): 286.

[61] "A Statement on Abortion," p. 992.

[62] Ibid.

[63] James D. Watson, "Children From The Laboratory," *Prism,* May 1973, p. 13.

[64] Ibid.

[65] James M. Gustafson, "Mongolism, Parental Desires, and the Right to Life," *Perspectives in Biology and Medicine* 16 (Summer 1973): 529-557.

[66] Raymond S. Duff and A. G. M. Campbell, "Moral and Ethical Dilemmas in the Special-Care Nursery," *New England Journal of Medicine* 289 (October 25, 1973): 890.

[67] Ibid., p. 894.

[68] Marya Mannes, *Last Rights: A Case For The Good Death* (New York: William Morrow and Company, Inc., 1973), pp. 1-7.

[69] Gila Berkowitz, "Desperate Measures," *Medical Dimensions,* October 1975, p. 9.

[70] Walter W. Sackett, "I've Let Hundreds of Patients Die. Shouldn't You?," *Medical Economics* 50 (April 2, 1973): 92-97.

[71] "British Doctor Tells of Mercy Killings," *St. Louis Post-Dispatch,* November 8, 1974, p. 14A.

[72] "The Session of the League of German Medical Societies," *Journal of the American Medical Association* 85 (October 17, 1925): 1237.

[73] "Interruption of Pregnancy from Eugenic Indications," *Journal of the American Medical Association* 86 (February 27, 1926): 639.

[74] "Birth Control," *Journal of the American Medical Association* 92 (January 26, 1929): 330.

[75] "Indications for Abortion and the Law," *Journal of the American Medical Association* 96 (May 23, 1931): 1810.

[76] "Session of League of German Medical Societies," p. 1237.

[77] Taussig, *Abortion Spontaneous and Induced*, p. 394.

[78] "Changes in the Penal Code," *Journal of the American Medical Association* 101 (September 23, 1933): 1011.

[79] "Protection to Posterity in Relation to Social Politics," *Journal of the American Medical Association* 78 (February 11, 1922): 447-448.

[80] "Hereditary Transmission and Natural Selection," *Journal of the American Medical Association* 76 (May 21, 1921): 1415-1416.

[81] "Meeting of the Prussian Council on Health," *Journal of the American Medical Association* 99 (August 20, 1932): 666.

[82] "Sterilization to Improve the Race," *Journal of the American Medical Association* 101 (September 9, 1933): 866.

[83] "The Congress of Gynecology," *Journal of the American Medical Association* 102 (January 6, 1934): 57.

[84] "New Decisions on Sterilization and Castration," *Journal of the American Medical Association* 104 (June 8, 1935): 2109.

[85] "Congress of the European Society of Mental Hygiene," *Journal of the American Medical Association* 111 (December 24, 1938): 2404.

[86] Alexander, "Medical Science Under Dictatorship," p. 39.

[87] Platen-Hallermund, *Killing of Mental Patients in Germany*, p. 34.

[88] "Eugenics in Germany," *Journal of the American Medical Association* 101 (July 22, 1933): 295.

[89] Extract from the Affidavit of Dr. Ludwig Sprauer, 23 April 1946, Concerning the Organization of the Euthanasia Program, *The Medical Case*, 1: 853.

[90] Wertham, *A Sign for Cain*, pp. 168-169.

[91] Joseph C. Harsch, *Pattern of Conquest* (Garden City, New York: Doubleday, Doran and Co., Inc., 1941), p. 257.

[92] Bernhard Schreiber, *The Men Behind Hitler: A German Warning To The World*, trans. H. R. Martindale (Les Mureau, France: La Haye-Mureaux, n.d.), p. 41.

[93] Proceedings of a Conference of the National Committee on Maternal Health, *The Abortion Problem* (Baltimore: Williams and Wilkins Company, 1944), p. vii.

[94] Ibid., p. 144.

[95] Ibid., p. 104.

[96] Ibid., pp. 51-52.

[97] Ibid., p. 178.

[98] Mary S. Calderone, ed., *Abortion in the United States* (New York: Hoeber-Harper, 1958), pp. 9-13.

[99] M. F. Ashley Montagu, Foreword to *Abortion in the United States*, ed. Mary S. Calderone, p. 4.

[100] Calderone, ed., *Abortion in the United States*, p. 115.

[101] Ibid., pp. 162-167.

[102] Ibid., p. 168.

[103] D. A. O'Donnell and W. L. Atlee, "Report on Criminal Abortion," *Transactions of the American Medical Association* 22 (1871): 239-258.

[104] Calderone, ed., *Abortion in the United States*, p. 164.

[105] Ibid., p. 170.

[106] Ibid., pp. 103-104.

[107] Ibid., pp. 183-184.

[108] Robert E. Hall, ed., *Abortion in a Changing World*, 2 vols. (New York and London: Columbia University Press, 1970), 1: 363-370.

[109] Betty Sarvis and Hyman Rodman, *The Abortion Controversy* (New York and London: Columbia University Press, 1973), p. 14.

[110] Hall, ed., *Abortion in a Changing World*, 1: v.

[111] Hall, ed., *Abortion in a Changing World*, 2: 60.

[112] Ibid., p. 64.

[113] Ibid., p. 43.

[114] Ibid., pp. 86-87.

[115] Ibid., p. 203.

[116] Ibid., p. 205.

[117] Ibid., pp. 185-186.

[118] Ibid., p. 137.

[119] Ibid., pp. 158-160.

[120] "AMA Policy on Therapeutic Abortion," *Journal of the American Medical Association* 201 (August 14, 1967): 544.

[121] Ibid.

[122] "Therapeutic Abortion," *Proceedings of the American Medical Association House of Delegates* (June 1967), pp. 46-48.

[123] "Therapeutic Abortion," *Proceedings of the American Medical Association House of Delegates* (June 1970), p. 221.

[124] "Mercy Death Law Ready for Albany," *New York Times*, February 14, 1939, p. 2.

[125] Norman Podhoretz, "Beyond ZPG," *Commentary*, May 1972, pp. 6-8.

[126] Joann Rodgers, "Is There a Right to Death?" *Sunday Herald Advertiser*, October 28, 1973.

[127] "Panelists' Views on Killing Child Not Recommendation," *Pediatric News*, April 1977, p. 32.

[128] "Attack on the Law Concerning Abortion," *Journal of the American Medical Association* 96 (February 14, 1931): 541.

[129] "The Attitude of Women Physicians Toward the Abortion Question," *Journal of the American Medical Association* 98 (April 30, 1932): 1580.

[130] Ralph M. Crowley and Robert W. Laidlaw, "Psychiatric Opinion Regarding Abortion: Preliminary Report of a Survey," *American Journal of Psychiatry* 124 (October 1967): 559-562.

[131] "Abortion: The Doctor's Dilemma," *Modern Medicine* 35 (April 24, 1967): 12-13.

[132] "Modern Medicine Poll on Sociomedical Issues: Abortion-Homosexual Practices-Marihuana," *Modern Medicine* 37 (November 3, 1969): 19.

[133] Hall, ed., *Abortion in a Changing World*, 1: 90.

[134] "Abortion: The Doctor's Dilemma," p. 13.

[135] "Modern Medicine Poll on Sociomedical Issues," p. 19.

[136] Raymond C. Lerner, Charles B. Arnold, and Sylvia Wassertheil, "New York's Obstetricians Surveyed on Abortion," *Family Planning Perspectives* 3 (January 1971): 56.

[137] Sylvia Wassertheil-Smoller, et al., "New York State Physicians and the Social Context of Abortion," *American Journal of Public Health* 63 (February 1973): 145.

[138] Sanford R. Wolf, Tom T. Sasaki, and Irving M. Cushner, "Assumption of Attitudes Toward Abortion During Physician Education," *Obstetrics and Gynecology* 37 (January 1971): 141-144.

[139] Paul R. Mascovich et al., "Attitudes of Obstetric and Gynecologic Residents Toward Abortion," *California Medicine* 119 (August 1973): 30.

[140] Arthur Peck, "Therapeutic Abortion: Patients, Doctors, and Society," *American Journal of Psychiatry* 125 (December 1968): 802-803.

[141] Robert H. Williams, "Our Role in the Generation, Modification, and Termination of Life," *Archives of Internal Medicine* 124 (August 1969): 229-233.

[142] Norman K. Brown et al., "The Preservation of Life," *Journal of the American Medical Association* 211 (Janurary 5, 1970): 76-79.

[143] E. Harold Laws et al., "Views on Euthanasia," *Journal of Medical Education* 46 (June 1971): 540-542.

[144] Brown et al., "Preservation of Life," p. 542.

[145] "Statement by Dr. Andrew C. Ivy," in *Doctors of Infamy*, p. xi.

[146] Roe v. Wade, 410 U.S. 149 (1973).

Chapter 4

DEATH SELECTION

[1] "Criteria for the Interruption of Pregnancy," *Journal of the American Medical Association* 88 (February 19, 1927): 582.

[2] "Criteria for the Interruption of Pregnancy," *Journal of the American Medical Association* 102 (January 13, 1934): 144.

[3] "Problems of Heredity," *Journal of the American Medical Association* 105 (September 28, 1935): 1052.

[4] Circular, 5 April 1943, Containing the Decree of Reich Health Leader Dr. Conti, Concerning the Interruption of Pregnancy of Female Eastern Workers, *Trials of War Criminals before the Nuernberg Military Tribunals: "The RuSHA Case,"* vol. 4 (Washington D.C.: U.S. Government Printing Office, 1951-1952), pp. 1094-1095.

[5] Abortions on Eastern Workers, *The RuSHA Case*, 5: 109-112.

[6] Extract from the Affidavit of Defendant Brack, 14 October 1946, Describing Administrative Details and Procedure of the Euthanasia Program, *The Medical Case*, 1: 843.

[7] Leo Alexander, "Medical Science Under Dictatorship," *New England Journal of Medicine*, 241 (July 14, 1949): 40.

[8] Extracts from the Closing Brief Against the Defendant Karl Brandt, *The Medical Case*, 1: 796.

[9] Ibid., p. 801.

[10] Affidavit of Julius Muthig, April 17, 1945, NO-2799.

[11] Extract from Letter from Dr. Fritz Mennecke to His Wife, 25 November 1941, Concerning His Activities as Physician Selecting Inmates of Concentration Camp Buchenwald for Euthanasia, *The Medical Case*, 1: 861-862.

[12] The International Military Tribunal, *Trial of the Major War Criminals*, vol. 11 (Nuremberg, Germany, 1947), p. 417.

[13] Statement of S.S. Obersturmfuhrer Franz Hoessler, *Trial of Josef Kramer Defendant and Forty-Four Others (The Belsen Trial)*, ed. Raymond Phillips (London: William Hodge and Company, 1949), pp. 714-715.

[14] Evidence for the Prosecution, *The Belsen Trial*, pp. 66-67.

[15] Evidence for the Defendant Klein, *The Belsen Trial*, p. 184.

[16] Statement of Obersturmfuhrer Dr. Fritz Klein, *The Belsen Trial*, p. 717.

[17] Olga Lengyel, *Five Chimneys: The Story of Auschwitz* (Chicago and New York: Ziff-Davis Publishing Company, 1947), p. 145.

[18] Miklos Nyiszli, *Auschwitz: A Doctor's Eyewitness Account*, trans. Tibere Kremer and Richard Seaver (New York: Frederick Fell, Inc., 1960), p. 90.

[19] Howard Hammond, "Therapeutic Abortion: Ten Years' Experience with Hospital Committee Control," *American Journal of Obstetrics and Gynecology* 89 (June 1, 1964): 353.

[20] Ibid., p. 349.

[21] Ibid., pp. 352-353.

[22] B. J. Lindberg, "What Does the Abortion-Seeking Woman Do When the Psychiatrist Refuses It?" *Svenska Lak-Tidn* 45 (1948): 1381.

[23] Myre Sim, "Abortion and the Psychiatrist," *British Medical Journal* 2 (July 20, 1963): 147.

[24] Mary S. Calderone, ed., *Abortion in the United States* (New York: Hoeber-Harper, 1958), p. 140.

[25] Ibid., p. 141.

[26] Group for the Advancement of Psychiatry, *The Right to Abortion: A Psychiatric View* (New York: Charles Scribner's Sons, 1969), p. 11.

[27] Magda Denes, *In Necessity and Sorrow: Life and Death in an Abortion Hospital* (New York: Basic Books, Inc., 1976), p. 226.

[28] Edward Wilson, "The Organization and Function of Therapeutic Abortion Committees," *Canadian Hospital*, December 1971, p. 39.

[29] Roe v. Wade, 410 U.S. 166.

[30] Letter from Hitler to Karl Brandt and Bouhler, 1 September 1939, Charging them with the Execution of Euthanasia, *The Medical Case*, 1: 848.

[31] Doe v. Bolton, 410 U.S. 208.

[32] Bernard N. Nathanson, "Deeper Into Abortion," *New England Journal of Medicine* 291 (November 28, 1974): 1189-1190.

[33] James F. Gustafson, "Mongolism, Parental Desires, and the Right to Life," *Perspectives in Biology and Medicine* 16 (Summer 1973): 529-557.

[34] Eric L. Zoeckler, "Life or Death Up to Parents in Some Births," *St. Louis Post-Dispatch*, October 19, 1971, p. 1.

[35] Raymond S. Duff and A. G. M. Campbell, "Moral and Ethical Dilemmas in the Special-Care Nursery," *New England Journal of Medicine* 289 (October 25, 1973): 891.

[36] Ibid., p. 894.

[37] Elizabeth Hall with Paul Cameron, "Our Failing Reverence For Life," *Psychology Today*, April 1976, p. 104.

[38] O. Ruth Russell, *Freedom to Die: Moral and Legal Aspects of Euthanasia* (New York: Human Sciences Press, 1975), p. 161.

Chapter 5

ASSEMBLY-LINE PROCESSING AT THE KILLING SITES

[1] Extract from the Affidavit of Defendant Brack, 14 October 1946, Describing Administrative Details and Procedure of the Euthanasia Program, *The Medical Case*, 1: 844; Alexander Mitscherlich and Fred Mielke, *Doctors of Infamy: The Story of the Nazi Medical Crimes*, trans. Heinz Norden (New York: Henry Schuman, 1949), p. 115.

[2] Joseph Wechsberg, ed., *The Murderers Among Us: The Wiesenthal Memoirs* (New York: McGraw-Hill Book Company, 1967), p. 315.

[3] Ibid., pp. 315-316.

[4] Extracts from the Testimony of Defendant Brack, *The Medical Case*, 1: 877.

[5] Mitscherlich and Mielke, *Doctors of Infamy*, p. 102.

[6] Extract from Affidavit of Brack, *The Medical Case*, 1: 843.

[7] Gitta Sereny, *Into that Darkness: From Mercy Killing to Mass Murder* (London: Andre Deutsch Limited, 1974), p. 83.

[8] Recross-Examination of Alfons Klein, *The Hadamar Trial*, pp. 199-200.

[9] Direct Examination of Margaret Borkowski, *The Hadamar Trial*, p. 36.

[10] Opening Argument for the Prosecution, *The Hadamar Trial*, p. 216.

[11] Direct Examination of Adolf Wahlmann, *The Hadamar Trial*, p. 168.

[12] Mitscherlich and Mielke, *Doctors of Infamy*, p. 103.

[13] Fredric Wertham, *A Sign for Cain: An Exploration of Human Violence* (New York: The Macmillan Company; London: Collier-Macmillan Limited, 1966), p. 157.

[14] Ibid., p. 169.

[15] Cross-Examination of Margaret Borkowski, *The Hadamar Trial*, p. 39.

[16] Martin L. Stone, Myron Gordon, and Joseph Rovinsky, "The Impact of a Liberalized Abortion Law on the Medical Schools," *American Journal of Obstetrics and Gynecology* 111 (November 1, 1971): 731.

[17] Barbara L. Lindheim and Maureen A. Cotterill, "Training in Induced Abortion by Obstetrics and Gynecology Residency Programs," *Family Planning Perspectives* 10 (January/February 1978): 25.

[18] Burritt W. Newton, "The Art of Abortion," *Postgraduate Medicine* 50 (September 1971): 215.

[19] Mark D. Mandel, "An Operational and Planning Staffing Model for First and Second Trimester Abortion Services," *American Journal of Public Health* 64 (August 1974): 755.

[20] Alice Goldmann, "Learning Abortion Care," *Nursing Outlook* 19 (May 1971): 350-352.

[21] Nancy Whitley, "Second Trimester Abortion: A Program of Counseling and Teaching," *Journal of Obstetric, Gynecologic and Neonatal Nursing* 2 (September/October 1973): 15-21.

[22] Helen Dudar, "Abortion for the Asking," *Saturday Review: The Society*, April 1973, p. 33.

[23] Rothlyn Zahourek, "Therapeutic Abortion and Cultural Shock," *Nursing Forum* 10 (1971): 13.

[24] John F. McDermott and Walter F. Char, "Abortion Repeal in Hawaii: An Unexpected Crisis in Patient Care," *American Journal of Orthopsychiatry* 41 (July 1971): 622.

[25] Ibid., p. 625.

[26] Edward Weinstock et al., "Legal Abortions in the United States Since the 1973 Supreme Court Decisions," *Family Planning Perspectives* 7 (January/February 1975): 23.

[27] "Letters," *American Journal of Nursing* 71 (July 1971): 1349.

[28] Raul Hilberg, *The Destruction of the European Jews* (Chicago: Quadrangle Books, Inc., 1967), p. 555.

[29] Jean-Francois Steiner, *Treblinka*, trans. Helen Weaver (New York: Simon and Schuster, 1967), pp. 208-209.

[30] Elie A. Cohen, *Human Behaviour in the Concentration Camp*, trans. M. H. Braaksma (London: Jonathan Cape, 1954), p. 25.

[31] Miklos Nyiszli, *Les Temps Modernes*, April 1951, p. 1665, cited by Gerald Rietlinger, *The Final Solution: The Attempt to Exterminate the Jews of Europe 1939-1945*, 2d and aug. ed. (South Brunswick, New York: Thomas Yoseloff, 1968), p. 160.

[32] Olga Lengyel, *Five Chimneys: The Story of Auschwitz* (Chicago and New York: Ziff-Davis Publishing Company, 1947), pp. 72-73.

[33] Henri Rosencher, "Medicine in Dachau," *British Medical Journal* 2 (December 21, 1946): 953.

[34] A. A. D. Lettich, Trente-quatre mois dans les camps de concentration. Tremoignage sur les crimes "scientifiques" commis par les medecins allemands. These Faculte de medicine de Paris, 1946, cited by Cohen, *Human Behaviour in the Concentration Camp*, p. 261.

[35] Sereny, *Into that Darkness*, p. 148.

[36] Miklos Nyiszli, *Auschwitz: A Doctor's Eyewitness Account*, trans. Tibere Kremer and Richard Seaver (New York: Frederick Fell Inc., 1960), p. 49.

[37] Sereny, *Into that Darkness*, p. 200.

[38] Lengyel, *Five Chimneys*, p. 71.

[39] Ibid., p. 22.

[40] David S. Wyman, "Why Auschwitz Was Never Bombed," *Commentary*, May 1978, p. 37.

[41] Steiner, *Treblinka*, p. 211.

[42] Ibid., p. 158.

[43] Gisella Pearl, *I Was A Doctor In Auschwitz* (New York: International Universities Press, 1948), pp. 42, 44.

[44] Ibid., p. 89.

[45] Abner I. Weisman, "Abortion Is Not The Answer," *Journal of the American Medical Association* 217 (September 13, 1971): 1554.

[46] Pamela Zekman and Pamela Warrick, "The Abortion Profiteers: Making a Killing in Michigan Av. Clinics," *Chicago Sun-Times*, November 12, 1978, pp. 1, 5, 6.

[47] Ardis Hyland Danon, "Organizing an Abortion Service," *Nursing Outlook* 21 (July 1973): 460.

[48] Barbara Grizzuti Harrison, "Now that Abortion is Legal," *McCall's*, November 1973, p. 64.

[49] Evelyn Waugh, *The Loved One* (Boston: Little, Brown and Company, 1948).

[50] Herbert McLaughlin, "Clinic Design Emphasizes Restraint to Minimize Patients' Tension," *Modern Hospital* (September 1973): 74-75.

[51] Ibid., p. 75.

[52] Ibid., p. 74.

[53] Dudar, "Abortion For The Asking," p. 31.

[54] Danon, "Organizing an Abortion Service," p. 462.

[55] Paul Berg, "Battle Lines In A Moral and Legal Dispute," *Sunday Pictures — St. Louis Post-Dispatch*, May 20, 1973, pp. 1-15.

[56] Paul Berg, "The Story of How the Jews Fought Back," *Sunday Pictures — St. Louis Post-Dispatch*, November 11, 1973, pp. 32-39.

[57] "Personal Experience at a Legal Abortion Center," *American Journal of Nursing* 72 (January 1972): 110.

[58] Dudar, "Abortion For The Asking," p. 31.

[59] Harrison, "Now That Abortion Is Legal," p. 70.

[60] Pamela Dillett, "Inside an Abortion Clinic," *The National Observer*, February 15, 1975, p. 18.

[61] Planned Parenthood of New York City, Inc., *Abortion: A Woman's Guide* (New York: Abelard-Schuman, 1973), p. 51.

[62] Michael S. Burnhill, "Humane Abortion Services: A Revolution in Human Rights and the Delivery of a Medical Service," *Mount Sinai Journal of Medicine* 42 (September-October 1975): 436.

[63] Planned Parenthood, *Abortion: A Woman's Guide*, p. 51.

[64] Danon, "Organizing an Abortion Service," p. 462.

[65] Dillett, "Inside an Abortion Clinic," p. 18.

[66] Planned Parenthood, *Abortion: A Woman's Guide*, p. 49.

[67] Harrison, "Now that Abortion Is Legal," p. 70.

[68] Lennart Nilsson, Axel Ingelman-Sundberg, and Claes Wirsen, *A Child Is Born: The Drama of Life Before Birth*, trans. Britt Wirsen, Claes Wirsen, and Annabelle MacMilan (New York: Dell Publishing Co., Inc., 1966), p. 71; Roberts Rugh, Landrum B. Shettles, with Richard N. Einhorn, *From Conception to Birth: The Drama of Life's Beginnings* (New York, Evanston, San Francisco, and London: Harper & Row, Publishers, 1971), p. 54.

Chapter 6

KILLING METHODS

[1] Erich Fromm, *The Anatomy of Human Destructiveness* (New York: Holt, Rinehart and Winston, 1973), pp. 346-347.

[2] Ibid., p. 348.

[3] Lester R. Brown and Kathleen Newland, "Abortion Liberalization: A Worldwide Trend," A Worldwatch Institute Paper, 1976, p. 1.

[4] Raul Hilberg, *The Destruction of the European Jews* (Chicago: Quadrangle Books, Inc., 1967), p. 189.

[5] Gerald Rietlinger, *The Final Solution: The Attempt to Exterminate the Jews of Europe 1939-1945*, 2d rev. and aug. ed. (South Brunswick, New York: Thomas Yoseloff, 1968), p. 198.

[6] Bohme to LXV Corps, 704th Division, 764th Division, October 25, 1941, NOKW-907.

[7] Affidavit by Blobel, June 6, 1947, NO-3824. Affidavit by Ohlendorf, November 5, 1945, PS-2620. Statement by Walter Haensch, July 21, 1947, NO-4567.

[8] Affidavit by Alfred Metzner, September 18, 1947, NO-5558.

[9] Extracts from the Testimony of Defendant Ohlendorf, *Trials of War Criminals before the Nuernberg Military Tribunals, The Einsatzgruppen Case*, 15 vols. (Washington D.C.: U.S. Government Printing Office, 1946-1949), 4: 249.

[10] Hilberg, *Destruction of Jews*, p. 218.

[11] *Dokumentry i Materialy*, Lodz, 1946, III, p. 279.

[12] Joseph Wechsberg, ed., *The Murderers Among Us: The Wiesenthal Memoirs* (New York: McGraw-Hill Book Company, 1967), p. 315.

[13] Extract from the Field Interrogation of Kurt Gerstein, 26 April 1945, Describing the Mass Gassing of Jews and Other "Undesirables," *The Medical Case*, 1: 868-869.

[14] Nora Levin, *The Holocaust: The Destruction of European Jewry 1933-1945* (New York: Schocken Books, 1973), p. 307.

[15] Miklos Nyiszli, *Auschwitz: A Doctor's Eyewitness Account*, trans. Tibere Kremer and Richard Seaver (New York: Frederick Fell Inc., 1960), pp. 50-52.

[16] G. M. Gilbert, *The Psychology of Dictatorship* (New York: The Ronald Press Company, 1950), p. 246.

[17] Rietlinger, *Final Solution*, p. 154.

[18] Richard Ough, *Church Times*, September 5, 1975, cited by *National Right to Life News*, April 1976, p. 19.

[19] John F. McDermott and Walter F. Char, "Abortion Repeal in Hawaii: An Unexpected Crisis in Patient Care," *American Journal of Orthopsychiatry* 41 (July 1971): 621.

[20] William J. Sweeney with Barbara Lang Stern, *Woman's Doctor: A Year in the Life of an Obstetrician-Gynecologist* (New York: William Morrow & Company, Inc., 1973), p. 205.

[21] Magda Denes, *In Necessity and Sorrow: Life and Death in an Abortion Hospital* (New York: Basic Books, Inc., 1976), p. 140.

[22] "MDs Shun 16th Week D & E as Reminder of Destroyed Fetus," *Medical Tribune*, January 25, 1978, p. 9.

[23] Warren M. Hern and Billie Corrigan, "What About Us? Staff Reactions to the D & E Procedure," Paper Presented at the Annual Meeting of the Association of Planned Parenthood Physicians, San Diego, California, October 26, 1978, p. 9.

[24] "MDs Shun 16th Week D & E," p. 9.

[25] Sadja Goldsmith, Nancy B. Kaltreider, and Alan J. Margolis, "Second Trimester Abortion by Dilation and Extraction (D & E): Surgical Techniques and Psychological Reactions," Paper Presented at the Annual Meeting of the Association of Planned Parenthood Physicians, Atlanta, Georgia, October 13-14, 1977, p. 6.

[26] Christopher Tietze, Jean Pakter, and Gary S. Berger, "Mortality With Legal Abortion in New York City, 1970-1972: A Preliminary Report," *Journal of the American Medical Association* 225 (July 30, 1973): 508.

[27] Gloria Steinem, "Questions No One Asked Dr. Kenneth Edelin On The Witness Stand," *Ms*, August 1975, p. 78.

[28] M. Vojta, "A Critical View of Vacuum Aspiration: A New Method for the Termination of Pregnancy," *Obstetrics and Gynecology* 30 (July 1967): 28, 33.

[29] Willard Cates et al., "Legal Abortion Mortality in the United States: Epidemiologic Surveillance, 1972-1974," *Journal of the American Medical Association* 237 (January 31, 1977): 453.

[30] Dr. & Mrs. J. C. Willke, *Handbook on Abortion*, rev. ed. (Cincinnati: Hayes Publishing Co., Inc., 1976), p. 29.

[31] McDermott and Char, "Abortion Repeal in Hawaii," p. 621.

[32] "Two-Minute Abortion Is Here — Are We Ready?" *Medical World News*, May 12, 1972, p. 15.

[33] Dorothea Kerslake and Donn Casey, "Abortion Induced by Means of the Uterine Aspirator," *Obstetrics and Gynecology* 30 (July 1967): 35.

[34] Lisa Cronin Wohl, "Would You Buy an Abortion From This Man?: The Harvey Karman Controversy," *Ms*, September 1975, p. 61.

[35] Pamela Zekman and Pamela Warrick, "Dr. Ming Kow Hah: Physician of Pain," *Chicago Sun-Times*, November 15, 1978, pp. 1, 4-5.

[36] "Two-Minute Abortion Is Here — Are We Ready?," p. 16.

[37] Harvey Karman, "The Paramedic Abortionist," *Clinical Obstetrics and Gynecology* 15 (June 1972): 379-387.

[38] A. Peretz et al., "Evacuation of the Gravid Uterus by Negative Pressure (Suction Evacuation)," *American Journal of Obstetrics and Gynecology* 98 (May 1, 1967): 21.

[39] T. Keith Edwards, "What It's Like To Do An Abortion," *West Virginia Medical Journal* 71 (May 1975): 123.

[40] Helen Branson, "Nurses Talk About Abortion," *American Journal of Nursing* 72 (January 1972): 106.

[41] Sweeney with Stern, *Woman's Doctor*, p. 207.

[42] Ibid., pp. 206-207.

[43] Direct Examination of Margaret Borkowski; Direct Examination of Heinrich Ruoff, *The Hadamar Trial*, pp. 36, 176.

[44] Leo Alexander, "Medical Science Under Dictatorship," *New England Journal of Medicine* 241 (July 14, 1949): 41.

[45] Direct Examination of Heinrich Ruoff, *The Hadamar Trial*, p. 177.

[46] Direct Examination of Adolf Wahlmann, *The Hadamar Trial*, p. 167.

[47] Direct Examination of Heinrich Ruoff, *The Hadamar Trial*, p. 177.

[48] Reitlinger, *Final Solution*, p. 122.

[49] Ota Kraus and Erich Kulka, *The Death Factory: Document on Auschwitz*, trans. Stephen Jolly (New York: Pergamon Press, 1966), p. 74.

[50] Deposition of Dr. Ada Bimko, *Trial of Josef Kramer Defendant and Forty-Four Others (The Belsen Trial)*, ed. Raymond Phillips (London: William Hodge and Company, 1949), p. 741.

[51] Extract From a Sworn Statement by Dr. Erwin Schuler (Ding), 20 July 1945, Concerning Euthanasia with Phenol Injection, *The Medical Case*, 1: 687.

[52] Leo Alexander, "War Crimes: Their Social-Psychological Aspects," *American Journal of Psychiatry* 105 (September 1948): 171.

[53] Burritt W. Newton, "The Art of Abortion," *Postgraduate Medicine* 50 (September 1971): 215.

[54] Robert S. Galen et al., "Fetal Pathology and Mechanism of Fetal Death in Saline-Induced Abortion: A Study of 143 Gestations and Critical Review of the Literature," *American Journal of Obstetrics and Gynecology* 120 (October 1, 1974): 347.

[55] Ibid., p. 352.

[56] Ibid., pp. 353-354.

[57] The People of the State of California vs. William Baxter Waddill, Jr., Transcript of Preliminary Examination, In the Municipal Court of the West

Orange County Judicial District, State of California, Case No. 77W2085, April 18, 1977, pp. 39-40.

[58] Willke, *Handbook on Abortion*, pp. 30-31.

[59] Janos Herczeg, Bela A. Resch, and Ferenc E. Szontagh, "On the Time of Fetal Survival of Abortuses Induced by Hypertonic Saline or Prostaglandin F_2a," *American Journal of Obstetrics and Gynecology* 118 (April 15, 1974): 1154.

[60] Helen I. Glueck et al., "Hypertonic Saline-Induced Abortion: Correlation of Fetal Death with Disseminated Intravascular Coagulation," *Journal of the American Medical Association* 225 (July 2, 1973): 28.

[61] David H. Sherman, "Salting Out: Experience in 9,000 Cases," *Journal of Reproductive Medicine* 14 (June 1975): 241.

[62] "Saline Proves Safe for Late Abortions," *Medical World News*, May 10, 1974, p. 22.

[63] Charles A. Ballard and Francis E. Ballard, "Four Years' Experience with Mid-Trimester Abortion by Amnioinfusion," *American Journal of Obstetrics and Gynecology* 114 (November 1, 1972): 579.

[64] Sherman, "Salting Out," p. 241.

[65] Galen et al., "Fetal Pathology and Fetal Death in Saline Abortion," p. 352.

[66] Ibid.

[67] Francis J. Kane et al., "Emotional Reactions in Abortion Services Personnel," *Archives of General Psychiatry* 28 (March 1973): 410.

[68] McDermott and Char, "Abortion Repeal in Hawaii," p. 622; Howard D. Kibel, "Staff Reactions to Abortion: A Psychiatrist's View," *Obstetrics and Gynecology* 39 (January 1972): 131.

[69] D. F. Kallop, "Preoperative Instruction for the Patient Undergoing Elective Abortion," *Clinical Obstetrics and Gynecology* 14 (March 1971): 65.

[70] Enid Nemy, "Even Now, Helping With Abortions Is Traumatic Shock for Some Nurses," *New York Times*, February 1, 1972, p. 32.

[71] Herczeg, Resch, and Szontagh, "On the Time of Fetal Survival," p. 1154.

[72] Richard Selzer, "What I Saw at the Abortion," *Esquire*, January 1976, pp. 66-67.

[73] Niels H. Lauersen et al., "Comparison of Prostaglandin F_2a and Hypertonic Saline for Induction of Midtrimester Abortion," *American Journal of Obstetrics and Gynecology* 120 (December 1, 1974): 875.

[74] Thomas F. Dillon et al., "The Efficacy of Prostaglandin F_2a in Second-Trimester Abortion," *American Journal of Obstetrics and Gynecology* 118 (March 1, 1974): 698.

[75] I. James Park, Anne C. Wentz, and Howard W. Jones, Jr., "The Viability of Fetal Skin of Abortuses Induced by Saline or Prostaglandin," *American Journal of Obstetrics and Gynecology* 115 (January 15, 1973): 274-275.

[76] "Aborted Hurler's Twin is Delivered with Normal One," *Medical World News*, May 15, 1978, p. 12.

[77] Ibid., p. 16.

[78] Gisella Pearl, *I Was A Doctor In Auschwitz* (New York: International Universities Press, 1948), p. 26.

[79] Ibid., p. 36.

[80] Alexander Mitscherlich and Fred Mielke, *Doctors of Infamy: The Story*

of the Nazi Medical Crimes, trans. Heinz Norden (New York: Henry Schuman, 1949), p. 101.

[81] "Who Should Survive?" A film produced by the Guggenheim and Joseph P. Kennedy Jr., Foundation, 1971.

[82] James M. Gustafson, "Mongolism, Parental Desires, and the Right to Life," *Perspectives in Biology and Medicine* 16 (Summer 1973): 531.

[83] Ibid.

[84] Eric L. Zoeckler, "Life Or Death Up To Parents In Some Births," *St. Louis Post-Dispatch*, October 19, 1971, p. 1.

[85] Anthony Shaw, "Dilemmas of 'Informed Consent' In Children," *New England Journal of Medicine* 289 (October 25, 1973): 886.

[86] Raymond S. Duff and A. G. M. Campbell, "Moral and Ethical Dilemmas in the Special-Care Nursery," *New England Journal of Medicine* 289 (October 25, 1973): 891.

Chapter 7

BODY DISPOSAL

[1] G. M. Gilbert, *Nuremberg Diary* (New York: Farrar, Straus and Company, 1947), p. 250.

[2] Alexander Mitscherlich and Fred Mielke, *Doctors of Infamy: The Story of the Nazi Medical Crimes*, trans. Heinz Norden (New York: Henry Schuman, 1949), p. 105.

[3] Ibid., p. 108.

[4] Cross-Examination of Philipp Blum, *The Hadamar Trial*, p. 147.

[5] Affidavit by Josef Guggenberger, September 9, 1947, NO-4959.

[6] Gitta Sereny, *Into that Darkness: From Mercy Killing to Mass Murder* (London: Andre Deutsch Limited, 1974), p. 112.

[7] Extract from the Field Interrogation of Kurt Gerstein, 26 April 1945, Describing the Mass Gassing of Jews and Other "Undesirables," *The Medical Case*, 1: 866-867.

[8] Jean-Francois Steiner, *Treblinka*, trans. Helen Weaver (New York: Simon and Schuster, Inc., 1967), pp. 350-356.

[9] Ota Kraus and Erich Kulka, *The Death Factory: Document on Auschwitz*, trans. Stephen Jolly (New York: Pergamon Press, 1966), p. 127.

[10] Miklos Nyiszli, *Auschwitz: A Doctor's Eyewitness Account*, trans. Tibere Kremer and Richard Seaver (New York: Frederick Fell Inc., 1960), pp. 52-55.

[11] Olga Lengyel, *Five Chimneys: The Story of Auschwitz* (Chicago and New York: Ziff-Davis Publishing Company, 1947), p. 75.

[12] Ibid., pp. 68-69.

[13] Ibid., p. 69.

[14] Affidavit by Höss, March 14, 1946, NO-1210.

[15] Kraus and Kulka, *Death Factory*, p. 114.

[16] The Jewish Black Book Committee, *The Black Book: The Nazi Crime Against the Jewish People* (New York: Duell, Sloan and Pearce, 1946), p. 389.

[17] Eugen Kogon, *The Theory and Practice of Hell: The German Concen-*

tration Camps and the System Behind Them, trans. Heinz Norden (New York: Farrar, Straus & Company, Inc., 1950), p. 172.

[18] Jane Miller, "Fetal Tissue Disposed of Here Just As Other Specimens Are," *Lincoln Journal-Star*, June 11, 1978.

[19] Planned Parenthood of New York City, Inc., *Abortion: A Woman's Guide* (New York: Abelard-Schuman, 1973), p. 52.

[20] Mark D. Mandel, "An Operational and Planning Staffing Model for First and Second Trimester Abortion Services," *American Journal of Public Health* 64 (August 1974): 755.

[21] Cathy Yarbrough, "Hospitals Near Atlanta Clinics Use Anesthesia and Have Ambulances on Call," *Atlanta Constitution*, July 18, 1973, p. 3-B.

[22] M. Vojta, "A Critical View of Vacuum Aspiration: A New Method for the Termination of Pregnancy," *Obstetrics and Gynecology* 30 (July 1967): 30.

[23] A. Peretz et al., "Evacuation of the Gravid Uterus by Negative Pressure (Suction Evacuation)," *American Journal of Obstetrics and Gynecology* 98 (May 1, 1967): 20.

[24] Dorothea Kerslake and Donn Casey, "Abortion Induced by Means of the Uterine Aspirator," *Obstetrics and Gynecology* 30 (July 1967): 37.

[25] Judith Bourne Rooks and Willard Cates, "Emotional Impact of D & E vs. Instillation," *Family Planning Perspectives* 9 (November/December 1977): 277.

[26] Ibid.

[27] A. Alberto Hodari et al., "Dilatation and Curettage for Second-Trimester Abortions," *American Journal of Obstetrics and Gynecology* 127 (April 15, 1977): 850-854.

[28] Charles A. Ballard and Francis E. Ballard, "Four Years' Experience with Mid-Trimester Abortion by Amnioinfusion," *American Journal of Obstetrics and Gynecology* 114 (November 1, 1972): 575.

[29] Morton A. Schiffer, Jean Pakter, and Jacob Clahr, "Mortality Associated with Hypertonic Saline Abortion," *Obstetrics and Gynecology* 42 (November 1973): 761.

[30] Ballard and Ballard, "Four Years' Experience with Mid-Trimester Abortion," p. 577.

[31] Schiffer, Pakter, and Clahr, "Mortality Associated with Saline Abortion," p. 763.

[32] Ronald T. Burkman et al., "The Management of Midtrimester Abortion Failures by Vaginal Evacuation," *Obstetrics and Gynecology* 49 (February 1977): 233-236.

[33] Ballard and Ballard, "Four Years' Experience with Mid-Trimester Abortion," p. 578.

[34] Harold Schulman and Georgia Randolph, "The Relationship of Amnio Fluid Sodium to the Latent Period of Saline Abortion," *Obstetrics and Gynecology* 39 (May 1972): 681-682.

[35] Thomas F. Dillon et al., "The Efficacy of Prostaglandin F_2a in Second-Trimester Abortion," *American Journal of Obstetrics and Gynecology* 118 (March 1, 1974): 690.

[36] George Schaeffer et al., "Symposium on Legal Abortion," *Clinical Obstetrics and Gynecology* 14 (March 1971): 306.

[37] Beverly Yaloff, Margot Wade and Mildred Burlingame, "Nursing Care in an Abortion Unit," *Clinical Obstetrics and Gynecology* 14 (March 1971): 79.

[38] Sally Kilby-Kelberg, "The Abortion," *Medical Dimensions*, May 1974, p. 36.

[39] Helen Dudar, "Abortion for the Asking," *Saturday Review: The Society*, April 1973, p. 32.

[40] "Nurses are Reacting Against Abortions," *St. Louis Review*, November 6, 1970, p. 2.

[41] "Death of a Baby: Inquiry in Glascow," *British Medical Journal* 2 (June 14, 1969): 704-705.

[42] Statement of Ada B. Ryan M.D. before the House Judiciary Committee with Reference to the Nomination of Nelson Rockefeller, November 25, 1974, p. 9.

[43] Magda Denes, *In Necessity and Sorrow: Life and Death in an Abortion Hospital* (New York: Basic Books, Inc., 1976), pp. 58-61.

[44] Ibid., pp. 85-87.

[45] "Use of Disposal Sparks Abortion Fireworks," *Omaha World-Herald*, June 11, 1978.

[46] John T. Kady, "Fetus Burning Is Halted," *Daily Standard* of Celina, Ohio, May 18, 1978, p. 3.

[47] Michael Litchfield and Susan Kentish, *Babies for Burning* (London: Serpentine Press Ltd., 1974), pp. 147-148.

[48] Thomas Collins, "Fetuses in Street: 'Horrible,' " New York *Daily News*, August 7, 1975.

[49] Grahame L. Jones, "Storage of Fetuses in Corridor Stirs Furor," *Los Angeles Times*, February 8, 1976.

[50] Statement of Dr. Ada B. Ryan before House Judiciary Committee, p. 8.

[51] "Disposal Sparks Abortion Fireworks."

[52] "Reports Abortion Fetuses Put in Disposer are Probed," *Omaha World-Herald*, June 12, 1978.

[53] Pamela Zekman and Pamela Warrick, "12 Dead After Abortions in State's Walk-In Clinics," *Chicago Sun-Times*, November 19, 1978, p. 10.

[54] Filip Friedman, *This Was Oswiecim: The Story of a Murder Camp*, trans. Joseph Leftwich (London: The United Jewish Relief Appeal, 1946), p. 63.

[55] Nyiszli, *Auschwitz*, p. 54.

[56] Ibid., p. 53; Lengyel, *Five Chimneys*, p. 20.

[57] Friedman, *This Was Oswiecim*, p. 64.

[58] Affidavit of Franz Blaha, November 25, 1945, *Nazi Conspiracy and Aggression*, 11 vols. (Washington, D.C.: U.S. Government Printing Office, 1946), 5: 952.

[59] PW Intelligence Bulletin No. 2/20, December 19, 1944, *Nazi Conspiracy and Aggression*, 6: 122-123.

[60] Jewish Black Book Committee, *The Black Book*, p. 285.

[61] Lengyel, *Five Chimneys*, p. 75.

[62] Jewish Black Book Committee, *The Black Book*, p. 281.

[63] Litchfield and Kentish, *Babies for Burning*, p. 146.

[64] Ibid., p. 148.

[65] B. D. Colen, "Hospital Got Cash for Fetuses," *Washington Post*, February 29, 1976, pp. B1, B11.

[66] Ibid., p. B11.

[67] Ibid.

[68] John Boland, "Chicago Firm Offers Embryos, Human Organ 'Paper Weights,' " *The Wanderer*, June 10, 1976, p. 1.

[69] "Display Fetuses Seized by Police," *St. Louis Globe-Democrat*, August 13-14, 1977, p. 9D.

[70] First Interim Report on Low-Pressure Chamber Experiments in the Concentration Camp of Dachau, *The Medical Case*, 1: 146-147.

[71] Intermediate Report, 10 September 1942, On Intense Chilling Experiments in Dachau Concentration Camp, *The Medical Case*, 1: 220.

[72] Nyiszli, *Auschwitz*, p. 175.

[73] Letter from Sievers to Rudolph Brandt, 9 February 1942, and Report by Hirt Concerning the Acquisition of Skulls of Jewish-Bolshevik Commissars, *The Medical Case*, 1: 749.

[74] Extract from the Closing Brief Against Defendant Sievers, *The Medical Case*, 1: 740-741.

[75] Selections of Photographic Evidence of the Prosecution, *The Medical Case*, 1: 905-908.

[76] Bernhard Schreiber, *The Men Behind Hitler: A German Warning to the World*, trans. H. R. Martindale (Les Mureaux, France: La Haye-Mureaux, n.d.), p. 56.

[77] Jewish Black Book Committee, *The Black Book*, p. 255.

[78] Gisella Pearl, *I Was A Doctor In Auschwitz* (New York: International Universities Press, 1948), p. 122.

[79] Ibid., p. 74.

[80] Robert S. Galen et al., "Fetal Pathology and Mechanism of Fetal Death in Saline-Induced Abortion: A Study of 143 Gestations and Critical Review of the Literature," *American Journal of Obstetrics and Gynecology* 120 (October 1, 1974): 347-355.

[81] Jack Wang et al., "Body Composition Studies in the Human Fetus After Intra-Amniotic Injection of Hypertonic Saline," *American Journal of Obstetric sand Gynecology* 117 (September 1, 1973): 57-63.

[82] Ibid., p. 57-58.

[83] Bela A. Resch et al., "Comparison of Spontaneous Contraction Rates of In Situ and Isolated Fetal Hearts in Early Pregnancy," *American Journal of Obstetrics and Gynecology* 118 (January 1, 1974): 73-74.

[84] Paul Ramsey, *The Ethics of Fetal Research* (New Haven and London: Yale University Press, 1975), p. 22.

[85] Peter A. J. Adam et al., "Oxidation of Glucose and D-B-Oh-Butyrate by the Early Human Fetal Brain," *Acta Paediatrica Scandinavica* 64 (January 1975): 18.

[86] Ibid.

[87] Willard Gaylin, "Harvesting the Dead: The Potential for Recycling Human Bodies," *Harper's Magazine*, September 1974, pp. 23-30.

Chapter 8

THE MANAGEMENT OF BREAKDOWNS IN DESTRUCTION

[1] Cross-Examination of Philipp Blum, *The Hadamar Trial*, pp. 147-148.

[2] Cross-Examination of Minna Zachow, *The Hadamar Trial*, p. 20.

[3] Eugen Kogon, *The Theory and Practice of Hell: The German Concentration Camps and the System Behind Them*, trans. Heinz Norden (New York: Farrar, Straus & Co., 1950), p. 203.

[4] Deputy Commander of *Wehrkreis* IX to Chief of Replacement Army, January 17, 1942, enclosing Rosler report, dated January 3, 1942, USSR-293 (1), cited by Raul Hilberg, *The Destruction of the European Jews* (Chicago: Quadrangle Books, Inc., 1967), pp. 212-213.

[5] Kube to Lohse, November 1, 1941, PS-1104.

[6] Affidavit by Metzner, September 18, 1947, NO-5558.

[7] G. M. Gilbert, *The Psychology of Dictatorship* (New York: The Ronald Press, 1950), p. 246.

[8] Olga Lengyel, *Five Chimneys: The Story of Auschwitz* (Chicago and New York: Ziff-Davis Publishing Company, 1947), p. 73.

[9] Martin L. Stone, Myron Gordon, and Joseph Rovinsky, "The Impact of a Liberalized Abortion Law on the Medical Schools," *American Journal of Obstetrics and Gynecology* 111 (November 1, 1971): 730.

[10] George Stroh and Alan R. Hinman, "Reported Live Births Following Induced Abortion: Two and One-Half Years' Experience in Upstate New York," *American Journal of Obstetrics and Gynecology* 126 (September 1, 1976): 83-90.

[11] Ibid., p. 84.

[12] Helen I. Glueck et al., "Hypertonic Saline-Induced Abortion: Correlation of Fetal Death With Disseminated Intravascular Coagulation," *Journal of the American Medical Association* 225 (July 2, 1973): 28.

[13] Niels H. Lauersen et al., "Comparison of Prostaglandin F_2a and Hypertonic Saline for Induction of Midtrimester Abortion," *American Journal of Obstetrics and Gynecology* 120 (December 1, 1974): 881.

[14] Charles A. Ballard and Francis E. Ballard, "Four Years' Experience with Mid-Trimester Abortion by Amnioinfusion," *American Journal of Obstetrics and Gynecology* 114 (November 1, 1972): 580.

[15] Don Effenberger, "Minnesota Investigates Case of Babies Allowed to Die," *St. Louis Review*, March 8, 1974, p. 4.

[16] William McClinton, "Witnesses Claim Aborted Fetus Could Have Been Saved," *St. Louis Review*, November 8, 1974, p. 8.

[17] Direct Examination of Patricia O. Olvera, The People of the State of California vs. William Baxter Waddill, Jr., Transcript of Preliminary Examination, In the Municipal Court of the West Orange County Judicial District, State of California, Case No. 77W2085, April 11, 1977, pp. 14-17.

[18] Direct Examination of Patricia Ann Hanes, California vs. Waddill, April 11, 1977, pp. 68-69.

[19] Direct Examination of Ronald J. Cornelsen, California vs. Waddill, April 11, 1977, p. 148.

[20] *Aufbau* (New York), August 23, 1946, pp. 1-2, cited by Hilberg, *Destruction of Jews*, p. 218-219.

[21] Ibid.

[22] Grawitz to Himmler, March 4, 1942, NO-600.

[23] Alexander Mitscherlich and Fred Mielke, *Doctors of Infamy: The Story of the Nazi Medical Crimes*, trans. Heinz Norden (New York: Henry Schuman, 1949), p. 105.

[24] Fredric Wertham, *A Sign for Cain: An Exploration of Human Violence* (New York: The Macmillan Company; London: Collier-Macmillan Limited, 1966), p. 157.

[25] Affidavit by Metzner, September 18, 1947, NO-5558.

[26] Ota Kraus and Erich Kulka, *The Death Factory: Document on Auschwitz*, trans. Stephen Jolly (New York: Pergamon Press, 1966), p. 133.

[27] Ella Lingens-Reiner, *Prisoners of Fear* (London: Victor Gollancz Ltd., 1948), p. 74.

[28] Steven Lipper and W. Morton Feigenbaum, "Obsessive-Compulsive Neurosis after Viewing the Fetus during Therapeutic Abortion," *American Journal of Psychotherapy* 30 (October 1976): 666-667.

[29] Ibid., p. 673.

[30] Linda Bird Francke, *The Ambivalence of Abortion* (New York: Random House, 1978), p. 34.

[31] Walter F. Char and John F. McDermott, "Abortions and Acute Identity Crisis in Nurses," *American Journal of Psychiatry* 128 (February 1972): 953-954.

[32] John F. McDermott and Walter F. Char, "Abortion Repeal in Hawaii: An Unexpected Crisis in Patient Care," *American Journal of Orthopsychiatry* 41 (July 1971): 623.

[33] Ibid., p. 622.

[34] Char and McDermott, "Abortions and Crisis in Nurses," p. 956.

[35] Howard D. Kibel, "Staff Reactions to Abortion: A Psychiatrist's View," *Obstetrics and Gynecology* 39 (January 1972): 131.

[36] Ibid., p. 132.

[37] Ibid., p. 133.

[38] Francis J. Kane et al., "Emotional Reactions in Abortion Services Personnel," *Archives of General Psychiatry* 28 (March 1973): 410.

[39] Ibid., p. 411.

[40] Horace Thompson, David L. Cowen and Betty Berris, "Therapeutic Abortion: A Two-Year Experience in One Hospital," *Journal of the American Medical Association* 213 (August 10, 1970): 991-995.

[41] Charles Remsberg and Bonnie Remsberg, "Second Thoughts on Abortion from the Doctor who Led the Crusade for It," *Good Housekeeping*, March 1976, p. 130.

[42] Francke, *Ambivalence of Abortion*, p. 33.

[43] Kane, "Emotional Reactions in Abortion Personnel," p. 411.

[44] Remsberg and Remsberg, "Second Thoughts on Abortion," p. 130.

[45] Norma Rosen, "Between Guilt and Gratification: Abortion Doctors Reveal Their Feelings," *New York Times Magazine*, April 17, 1977, p. 71.

[46] Ibid., pp. 73. 78.

[47] First Interim Report on the Low-Pressure Chamber Experiments in the Concentration Camp of Dachau, *The Medical Case*, 1:147.

[48] Affidavit of Fritz Friedrich Karl Rascher, M.D., 31 December 1946, Concerning the Life and Activities of Dr. Sigmund Rascher, *The Medical Case*, 1: 677.

[49] Mitscherlich and Mielke, *Doctors of Infamy*, p. 86.

[50] Leo Alexander, "The Molding of Personality Under Dictatorship: The Importance of the Destructive Drives in the Social-Psychological Structure of Nazism," *Journal of Criminal Law and Criminology* 40 (May-June 1949): 22, 25.

[51] Russell K. Laros et al., "Coagulation Changes in Saline-Induced Abortion," *American Journal of Obstetrics and Gynecology* 116 (May 15, 1973): 284.

[52] Fritz K. Beller et al., "Consumptive Coagulopathy Associated with Intra-Amniotic Infusion of Hypertonic Salt," *American Journal of Obstetrics and Gynecology* 112 (February 15, 1972): 541.

[53] J. Joshua Kopelman and Gordon W. Douglas, "Abortions by Resident

Physicians in a Municipal Hospital Center," *American Journal of Obstetrics and Gynecology* 111 (November 1, 1971): 670.

54 "Avoiding Tough Abortion Complication: A Live Baby," *Medical World News*, November 14, 1977, p. 83.

55 Magda Denes, *In Necessity and Sorrow: Life and Death in an Abortion Hospital* (New York: Basic Books, Inc., 1976), p. 103.

56 Ibid., p. 141.

57 Extract from the Closing Brief against Defendant Mrugowsky, *The Medical Case*, 1: 632.

58 Extract from a Sworn Statement by Dr. Erwin Schuler (Ding), 20 July 1945, Concerning Euthanasia with Phenol Injection, *The Medical Case* 1: 687.

59 Kogon, *Theory and Practice of Hell*, p. 204.

60 Examination of Frederich Dickmann, *The Hadamar Trial*, p. 56.

61 Cross-Examination of Minna Zachow, *The Hadamar Trial*, p. 20.

62 Bohme to LXV Corps, 704th Division, 764th Division, October 25, 1941, NOKW-907.

63 Deputy Commander of *Wehrkreis* IX to Chief of Replacement Army, cited by Hilberg, *Destruction of Jews*, pp. 212-213.

64 Gilbert, *Psychology of Dictatorship*, p. 246.

65 Miklos Nyiszli, *Auschwitz: A Doctor's Eyewitness Account*, trans. Tibere Kremer and Richard Seaver (New York: Frederick Fell, Inc., 1960), p. 120.

66 Kraus and Kulka, *The Death Factory*, p. 142.

67 Mitscherlich and Mielke, *Doctors of Infamy*, p. 86.

68 Lengyel, *Five Chimneys*, p. 73.

69 Henry V. Dicks, *Licensed Mass Murder: A Socio-Psychological Study of Some SS Killers* (New York: Basic Books Inc., 1972), pp. 147-148.

70 Rafael A. Del Valle, "Mid-Trimester Abortion Life in Fetus," *Ob-Gyn Collected Letters of the International Correspondence Society of Obstetricians and Gynecologists* 15 (November 1, 1974): 163.

71 Nils Wiqvist, "Mid-Trimester Abortion Life in Fetus," p. 164.

72 Ballard and Ballard, "Four Years' Experience with Mid-Trimester Abortion," p. 580.

73 Thomas D. Kerenyi, Nathan Mandelman, and David H. Sherman, "Five Thousand Consecutive Saline Inductions," *American Journal of Obstetrics and Gynecology* 116 (July 1, 1973): 598.

74 "Avoiding Tough Abortion Complication," p. 83.

75 Ibid.

76 "Nurses Are Reacting Against Abortions," *St. Louis Review*, November 6, 1970, p. 2.

77 Francke, *Ambivalence of Abortion*, pp. 33-34.

78 Ibid., p. 33.

79 Ronald J. Bolognese, "Mid-Trimester Abortion Life in Fetus," p. 166.

80 Ibid.

81 Effenberger, "Minnesota Investigates Case of Babies Allowed to Die," p. 4.

82 McClinton, "Witnesses Claim Aborted Fetus Could Have Been Saved," p. 8.

83 Barbara J. Culliton, "Edelin Trial: Jury Not Persuaded by Scientists for the Defense," *Science* 187 (March 7, 1975): 814-816.

[84] Cyril H. Wecht, "A Comparison of Two Abortion-Related Legal Inquiries," *Journal of Legal Medicine* (September 1975): 44.

[85] Direct Examination of Ronald J. Cornelsen, California vs. Waddill, April 11, 1977, pp. 141-155.

[86] Statement of Ada B. Ryan, M.D. before the House Judiciary Committee with Reference to the Nomination of Nelson Rockefeller, November 25, 1974, p. 9.

[87] Michael Litchfield and Susan Kentish, *Babies For Burning* (London: Serpentine Press Ltd., 1974), p. 148.

[88] "Death of a Baby: Inquiry in Glascow," *British Medical Journal* 2 (June 14, 1969): 705.

Chapter 9

DEATH STATISTICS

[1] Joseph Wechsberg, ed., *The Murderers Among Us: The Wiesenthal Memoirs* (New York: McGraw-Hill Book Company, 1967), p. 98.

[2] Affidavit by Dieter Wisliceny, November 29, 1945, *Nazi Conspiracy and Aggression*, vol. 8 (Washington, D.C.: U.S. Government Printing Office, 1946), p. 610.

[3] Extract from the Affidavit of Defendant Brack, 14 October 1946, Describing Administrative Details and Procedure of the Euthanasia Program, *The Medical Case*, 1: 844.

[4] Peter Roger Breggin, "The Killing of Mental Patients," *Freedom*, June-July 1974, p. 6.

[5] Opening Statement of the Prosecution by Brigadier General Telford Taylor, 9 December 1946, *The Medical Case*, 1: 67.

[6] Fredric Wertham, *A Sign for Cain: An Exploration of Human Violence* (New York: The Macmillan Company; London: Collier-Macmillan Limited, 1966), p. 158.

[7] Raul Hilberg, *The Destruction of the European Jews* (Chicago, Ill.: Quadrangle Books, Inc., 1967), p. 256.

[8] Gerald Rietlinger, *The Final Solution: The Attempt to Exterminate the Jews of Europe 1939-1945*, 2nd rev. and aug. ed. (South Brunswick, New York: Thomas Yoseloff, 1968), p. 233.

[9] Hilberg, *Destruction of Jews*, p. 256.

[10] Central Commission for Investigation of German Crimes in Poland. German Crimes in Poland, Warsaw, 1946, cited by Elie A. Cohen, *Human Behaviour in the Concentration Camp*, trans. M. H. Braaksma (London: Jonathan Cape, 1954), p. 35.

[11] Olga Lengyel, *Five Chimneys: The Story of Auschwitz* (Chicago and New York: Ziff-Davis Publishing Company, 1947), pp. 68-69.

[12] G. M. Gilbert, *The Psychology of Dictatorship* (New York: The Ronald Press Company, 1950), p. 247.

[13] Lengyel, *Five Chimneys*, p. 70.

[14] Testimony by Rudolf Hoess, *Trial of the Major War Criminals Before the International Military Tribunal*, vol. 11 (Nuremberg, Germany, 1947), p. 415.

[15] G. M. Gilbert, *Nuremberg Diary* (New York: Farrar, Straus, and Company, 1947), pp. 249-250.

[16] Central Commission for Investigation of German Crimes in Poland, cited by Cohen, *Human Behaviour in Concentration Camp*, p. 20.

[17] Zdenek Lederer, *Ghetto Theresienstadt* (London, 1953), pp. 247-248, cited by Hilberg, *Destruction of Jews*, p. 283.

[18] Affidavit by Dr. Wilhelm Hottl, November 26, 1945, PS-2738; Affidavit by Wisliceny, November 29, 1945, *Nazi Conspiracy and Aggression*, pp. 606-621.

[19] Rietlinger, *The Final Solution*, p. 546.

[20] Ibid., p. 533.

[21] Edward Weinstock et al., "Legal Abortions in the United States Since the 1973 Supreme Court Decisions," *Family Planning Perspectives* 7 (January/February 1975): 29.

[22] Jane E. Hodgson, "Community Abortion Services: The Role of Organized Medicine," *Minnesota Medicine* 56 (March 1973): 241.

[23] Abner I. Weisman, "Abortion Is Not The Answer," *Journal of the American Medical Association* 217 (September 13, 1971): 1554.

[24] Bernard N. Nathanson, "Deeper Into Abortion," *New England Journal of Medicine* 291 (November 28, 1974): 1189.

[25] Arthur J. Snider, "Pro-Abortion Doctor Has Second Thoughts," *St. Louis Post-Dispatch*, January 9, 1975, p. 4-D.

[26] Bernard N. Nathanson, "Ambulatory Abortion: Experience with 26,000 Cases (July 1, 1970, to August 1, 1971)," *New England Journal of Medicine* 286 (February 24, 1972): 405.

[27] Charles Remsberg and Bonnie Remsberg, "Second Thoughts on Abortion from The Doctor Who Led the Crusade for It," *Good Housekeeping*, March 1976, p. 130.

[28] Ibid.

[29] Ellen Sullivan, Christopher Tietze, and Joy G. Dryfoos, "Legal Abortion in the United States, 1975-1976," *Family Planning Perspectives* 9 (May/June 1977): 127.

[30] Weinstock et al., "Legal Abortions Since Supreme Court Decisions," p. 23.

[31] Sullivan, Tietze, and Dryfoos, "Legal Abortion in the United States, 1975-1976," p. 116.

[32] Weinstock et al., "Legal Abortions Since Supreme Court Decisions," p. 23.

[33] Sullivan, Tietze and Dryfoos, "Legal Abortion in the United States, 1975-1976," p. 116.

[34] Weinstock et al., "Legal Abortions Since Supreme Court Decisions," p. 26.

[35] Ibid., p. 31.

[36] The Alan Guttmacher Institute, "The Unmet Need for Legal Abortion Services in the U.S.," *Family Planning Perspectives* 7 (September-October 1975): 227.

[37] "Abortions Reported Denied To Hundreds of Thousands," *St. Louis Post-Dispatch*, October 8, 1975, p. 13D.

[38] Lester R. Brown and Kathleen Newland, "Abortion Liberalization: A Worldwide Trend," A Worldwatch Institute Paper, 1976, p. 1.

[39] Ibid., pp. 2, 7.

Bibliography

DOCUMENTS

Doe v. Bolton, 410 U.S. 179 (1973).

International Military Tribunal. *Trial of the Major War Criminals Before the International Military Tribunal: Official Text.* 42 vols. Nuremberg, 1947-1949.

Kinter, Earl W., ed. *Trial of Alfons Klein and Others (The Hadamar Trial).* London: William Hodge and Company, 1949.

Nuernberg Military Tribunals. *Trials of War Criminals Before the Nuernberg Military Tribunals Under Control Council Law No. 10.* 15 vols. Washington, D.C., 1946-1949.

O'Donnell, D. A., and Atlee, W. L. "Report on Criminal Abortion." *Transactions of the American Medical Association* 22 (1871): 239-258.

Office of the United States Chief of Counsel for the Prosecution of Axis Criminality. *Nazi Conspiracy and Aggression.* 11 vols. Washington, D.C., 1946-1948.

Phillips, Raymond, ed. *Trial of Josef Kramer Defendant and Forty-Four Others (The Belsen Trial).* London: William Hodge and Company, 1949.

Roe v. Wade, 410 U.S. 113 (1973).

Storer, Horatio R.; Blatchford, Thomas W.; Hodge, Hugh L.; Barton, Edward H.; Lopez, A.; Pope, Charles A.; Brisbane, William Henry; and Semmes, A. J. "Report on Criminal Abortion." *Transactions of the American Medical Association* 12 (1859): 75-78.

The People of the State of California v. William Baxter Waddill, Jr., Transcripts of Preliminary Examination, In the Municipal Court of the West Orange County Judicial District, State of California, Case No. 77W2085, 11 April 1977, and 18 April 1977.

"Therapeutic Abortion." *Proceedings of the American Medical Association House of Delegates* (June 1967): 40-51.

"Therapeutic Abortion." *Proceedings of the American Medical Association House of Delegates* (June 1970): 221.

359

BOOKS

Arendt, Hannah. *Eichmann in Jerusalem: A Report on the Banality of Evil.* New York: The Viking Press, 1963.

Bates, Jerome E., and Zawadzki, Edward S. *Criminal Abortion: A Study in Medical Sociology.* Springfield, Ill.: Charles C. Thomas, 1964.

Binding, Karl, and Hoche, Alfred. *The Release of the Destruction of Life Devoid of Value.* Leipzig, Germany: Felix Meiner, 1920. Compiled by Robert L. Sassone. 900 N. Broadway, Santa Ana, Calif., 92701: A Life Quality Paperback, 1975.

Calderone, Mary S., ed. *Abortion in the United States.* New York: Hoeber-Harper, 1958.

Cohen, Elie A. *Human Behaviour in the Concentration Camp.* Translated by M. H. Braaksma. London: Jonathan Cape, 1954.

Denes, Magda. *In Necessity and Sorrow: Life and Death in an Abortion Hospital.* New York: Basic Books, Inc., 1976.

Dicks, Henry V. *Licensed Mass Murder: A Socio-Psychological Study of Some SS Killers.* New York: Basic Books Inc., 1972.

Francke, Linda Bird. *The Ambivalence of Abortion.* New York: Random House, 1978.

Friedman, Filip. *This Was Oswiecim: The Story of a Murder Camp.* Translated by Joseph Leftwich. London: The United Jewish Relief Appeal, 1946.

Fromm, Erich. *The Anatomy of Human Destructiveness.* New York: Holt, Rinehart and Winston, 1973.

Garrison, Fielding H. *An Introduction to the History of Medicine.* 4th ed. Reprint. Philadelphia and London: W. B. Saunders Company, 1929.

Gasman, Daniel. *The Scientific Origins of National Socialism: Social Darwinism in Ernst Haeckel and the German Monist League.* New York: American Elsevier Publishing Company, Inc., 1971.

Gilbert, G. M. *Nuremberg Diary.* New York: Farrar, Straus and Company, 1947.

_____. *The Psychology of Dictatorship.* New York: The Ronald Press Company, 1950.

Group for the Advancement of Psychiatry. *The Right to Abortion: A Psychiatric View.* New York: Charles Scribner's Sons, 1970.

Haeckel, Ernst. *The History of Creation: Or The Development of the Earth and Its Inhabitants by the Action of Natural Causes.* Translated by E. Ray Lankester, vel. 1. 4th ed. New York: D. Appleton & Co., 1892.

_____. *The Riddle of the Universe: At The Close Of The Nineteenth Century.* Translated by Joseph McCabe. New York and London: Harper & Brothers, 1900.

_____. *The Wonders of Life: A Popular Study of Biological*

Philosophy. Translated by Joseph McCabe. London: Watts and Co., 1904.

Hall, Robert E., ed. *Abortion in a Changing World.* 2 vols. New York and London: Columbia University Press, 1970.

Harsch, Joseph C. *Pattern of Conquest.* New York: Doubleday, Doran and Co., Inc., 1941.

Hilberg, Raul. *The Destruction of the European Jews.* Chicago: Quadrangle Books, Inc., 1967.

Hilgers, Thomas W., and Horan, Dennis J., eds. *Abortion and Social Justice.* New York: Sheed & Ward, 1972.

Jewish Black Book Committee. *The Black Book: The Nazi Crime Against the Jewish People.* New York: Duell, Sloan and Pearce, 1946.

Kogon, Eugen. *The Theory and Practice of Hell: The German Concentration Camps and the System Behind Them.* Translated by Heinz Norden. New York: Farrar, Straus & Company, Inc., 1950.

Kraus, Ota, and Kulka, Erich. *The Death Factory: Document on Auschwitz.* Translated by Stephen Jolly. New York: Pergamon Press, 1966.

Lader, Lawrence. *Abortion.* Indianapolis: Bobbs-Merrill Company, Inc., 1966.

Lengyel, Olga. *Five Chimneys: The Story of Auschwitz.* Chicago and New York: Ziff-Davis Publishing Company, 1947.

Levin, Nora. *The Holocaust: The Destruction of European Jewry 1933-1945.* New York: Schocken Books, 1973.

Lingens-Reiner, Ella. *Prisoners of Fear.* London: Victor Gollancz Ltd., 1948.

Litchfield, Michael, and Kentish, Susan. *Babies For Burning.* London: Serpentine Press, Ltd., 1974.

Major, Ralph H. *A History of Medicine.* 2 vols. Springfield, Ill.: Charles C. Thomas, 1954.

Mannes, Marya. *Last Rights: A Case for the Good Death.* New York: William Morrow and Company, Inc., 1973.

Milgram, Stanley. *Obedience to Authority: An Experimental View.* New York: Harper & Row, 1974.

Mitscherlich, Alexander, and Mielke, Fred. *Doctors of Infamy: The Story of the Nazi Medical Crimes.* Translated by Heinz Norden. New York: Henry Schuman, 1949.

Mohr, James C. *Abortion in America: The Origins and Evolution of National Policy, 1800-1900.* New York: Oxford University Press, 1978.

Mosse, George L., ed. *Nazi Culture: Intellectual, Cultural and Social Life in the Third Reich.* Translated by Salvator Attanasio and others. New York: Grosset & Dunlap, Universal Library, 1968.

Nathanson, Bernard, N., with Ostling, Richard N. *Aborting Amer-*

ica. Garden City, New York: Doubleday & Company, Inc., 1979.

Nilsson, Lennart; Ingelman-Sundberg, Axel; and Wirsen, Claes. *A Child Is Born: The Drama of Life Before Birth.* Translated by Britt Wirsen, Claes Wirsen, and Annabelle MacMilan. New York: Dell Publishing Co., Inc. 1966.

Nyiszli, Miklos. *Auschwitz: A Doctor's Eyewitness Account.* Translated by Tibere Kremer and Richard Seaver. New York: Frederick Fell, Inc., 1960.

Pearl, Gisella. *I Was A Doctor In Auschwitz.* New York: International Universities Press, 1948.

Planned Parenthood of New York City, Inc. *Abortion: A Woman's Guide.* New York: Abelard-Schuman, 1973.

Proceedings of a Conference of the National Committee on Maternal Health. *The Abortion Problem.* Baltimore: Williams and Wilkins Company, 1944.

Ramsey, Paul. *The Ethics of Fetal Research.* New Haven and London: Yale University Press, 1975.

Rietlinger, Gerald. *The Final Solution: The Attempt to Exterminate the Jews of Europe 1939-1945.* 2d and aug. ed. South Brunswick: Thomas Yoseloff, 1968.

Rongy, Abraham J. *Abortion: Legal or Illegal?* New York: Vanguard Press, 1933.

Rugh, Roberts; Shettles, Landrum B.; with Einhorn, Richard N. *From Conception to Birth: The Drama of Life's Beginnings.* New York, Evanston, San Francisco, and London: Harper & Row, Publishers, 1971.

Russell, O. Ruth. *Freedom to Die: Moral and Legal Aspects of Euthanasia.* New York: Human Sciences Press, 1975.

Sarvis, Betty, and Rodman, Hyman. *The Abortion Controversy.* New York and London: Columbia University Press, 1973.

Schreiber, Bernhard. *The Men Behind Hitler: A German Warning to the World.* Translated by H. R. Martindale. Les Mureau, France: La Haye-Mureaux, n. d.

Sereny, Gitta. *Into That Darkness: From Mercy Killing to Mass Murder.* London: Andre Deutsch Limited, 1974.

Shryock, Richard H. *Medicine in America: Historical Essays.* Baltimore: Johns Hopkins Press, 1966.

Steiner, Jean-Francois. *Treblinka.* Translated by Helen Weaver. New York: Simon and Schuster, 1967.

Sweeney, William J., with Stern, Barbara Lang. *Woman's Doctor: A Year in the Life of an Obstetrician-Gynecologist.* New York: William Morrow & Company, Inc., 1973.

Taussig, Frederick J. *Abortion Spontaneous and Induced: Medical and Social Aspects.* Saint Louis: C. V. Mosby Company, 1936.

Wechsberg, Joseph, ed. *The Murderers Among Us: The Wiesenthal Memoirs.* New York: McGraw-Hill Book Company, 1967.

Wertham, Fredric. *A Sign for Cain: An Exploration of Human Violence.* New York: The Macmillan Company; London: Collier-Macmillan Limited, 1966.

Willke, Dr. J. C. & Mrs. *Handbook on Abortion.* rev. ed. Cincinnati: Hayes Publishing Co., Inc., 1976.

ARTICLES AND PERIODICALS

"Aborted Hurler's Twin is Delivered with Normal One." *Medical World News,* 15 May 1978, p. 12.

"Abortion and Race Hygiene." *Journal of the American Medical Association* 105 (July 20, 1935): 212-213.

"Abortion: The Doctor's Dilemma." *Modern Medicine* 35 (April 24, 1967): 12-13.

"Abortions Reported Denied to Hundreds of Thousands." *Saint Louis Post-Dispatch,* 8 October 1975, p. 13D.

Adam, Peter A. J.; Raiha, Niels; Rahiala, Eeva-Liisa; and Kekomaki, Martti. "Oxidation of Glucose and D-B-Oh-Butyrate by the Early Human Fetal Brain." *Acta Paediatrica Scandinavica* 64 (January 1975): 17-24.

Alexander, Leo. "Destructive and Self-Destructive Trends in Criminalized Society: A Study of Totalitarianism." *Journal of Criminal Law and Criminology* 39 (January-February 1949): 553-564.

_____. "Medical Science Under Dictatorship." *New England Journal of Medicine* 241 (July 14, 1949): 39-47.

_____. "The Molding of Personality Under Dictatorship: The Importance of the Destructive Drives in the Socio-Psychological Structure of Nazism." *Journal of Criminal Law and Criminology* 40 (May-June 1949): 3-27.

_____. "War Crimes: Their Social-Psychological Aspects." *American Journal of Psychiatry* 105 (September 1948): 170-177.

"AMA Policy on Therapeutic Abortion." *Journal of the American Medical Association* 201 (August 14, 1967): 544.

"A Statement on Abortion by One Hundred Professors of Obstetrics." *American Journal of Obstetrics and Gynecology* 112 (April 1, 1972): 992-998.

"Attack on the Law Concerning Abortion." *Journal of the American Medical Association* 96 (February 14, 1931): 541-542.

"Avoiding Tough Abortion Complication: A Live Baby." *Medical World News,* 14 November 1977, p. 83.

Ballard, Charles A., and Ballard, Francis E. "Four Years' Experience with Mid-Trimester Abortion by Amnioinfusion." *American Journal of Obstetrics and Gynecology* 114 (November 1, 1972): 575-581.

Benjamin, Robert B. "Abortion or Compulsory Pregnancy?" *Minnesota Medicine* 52 (March 1969): 457.

Berg, Paul. "Battle Lines in a Moral and Legal Dispute." *Sunday Pictures — Saint Louis Post-Dispatch*, 20 May 1973, pp. 1-15.
_____. "The Story of How the Jews Fought Back." *Sunday Pictures — Saint Louis Post-Dispatch*, 11 November 1973, pp. 32-39.

Berkowitz, Gila. "Desperate Measures." *Medical Dimensions*, October 1975, p. 9.

Bloch, Harry. "The Berlin Correspondence in the JAMA During the Hitler Regime." *Bulletin of the History of Medicine* 47 (May/June 1973): 297-305.

Boland, John. "Chicago Firm Offers Embryos, Human Organ 'Paper Weights.'" *The Wanderer*, 10 June 1976, p. 1.

"British Doctor Tells of Mercy Killings." *Saint Louis Post-Dispatch*, 8 November 1974, p. 14A.

Brown, Norman K.; Bulger, Roger J.; Laws, E. Harold; and Thompson, Donovan J. "The Preservation of Life." *Journal of the American Medical Association* 211 (January 5, 1970): 76-82.

Burkman, Ronald T.; Athenza, Milagros F.; King, Theodore M.; and Burnett, Lonnie S. "The Management of Midtrimester Abortion Failures by Vaginal Evacuation." *Obstetrics and Gynecology* 49 (February 1977): 233-236.

"Changes in the Penal Code." *Journal of the American Medical Association* 101 (September 23, 1933): 1011.

Char, Walter F., and McDermott, John F. "Abortions and Acute Identity Crisis in Nurses." *American Journal of Psychiatry* 128 (February 1972): 952-957.

Colen, B. D. "Hospital Got Cash for Fetuses." *Washington Post*, 29 February 1976, pp. B1, B11.

Collins, Thomas. "Fetuses in Street: 'Horrible,'" New York *Daily News*, 7 August 1975.

"Congress of the European Society of Mental Hygiene." *Journal of the American Medical Association* 111 (December 24, 1938): 2404-2405.

"Criteria for the Interruption of Pregnancy." *Journal of the American Medical Association* 88 (February 19, 1927): 582-583.

"Criteria for the Interruption of Pregnancy." *Journal of the American Medical Association* 102 (January 13, 1934): 144.

Crowley, Ralph M., and Laidlaw, Robert W. "Psychiatric Opinion Regarding Abortion: Preliminary Report of a Survey." *American Journal of Psychiatry* 124 (October 1967): 559-562.

Danon, Ardis Hyland. "Organizing an Abortion Service." *Nursing Outlook* 21 (July 1973): 460-464.

"Death of a Baby: Inquiry in Glascow." *British Medical Journal* 2 (June 14, 1969): 704-705.

Dillett, Pamela. "Inside an Abortion Clinic." *National Observer*, 15 February 1975, pp. 1, 18.

Dillon, Thomas F.; Phillips, Louise Lang; Risk, Abraham; Horiguchi, Terusada; Mohajer-Shojai, Ezatolah; and Mootabar, Hamid. "The Efficacy of Prostaglandin F_2a in Second-Trimester Abortion: Coagulation and Hormonal Aspects." *American Journal of Obstetrics and Gynecology* 118 (March 1, 1974): 688-699.

Dudar, Helen. "Abortion for the Asking." *Saturday Review: The Society,* April 1973, pp. 30-35.

Duff, Raymond S., and Campbell, A. G. M. "Moral and Ethical Dilemmas in the Special-Care Nursery." *New England Journal of Medicine* 289 (October 25, 1973): 890-894.

Eastman, Nicholson J. "Induced Abortion and Contraception: A Consideration of Ethical Philosophy in Obstetrics." *Obstetrical and Gynecological Survey* 22 (February 1967): 3-11.

Edwards, T. Keith. "What It's Like To Do An Abortion." *West Virginia Medical Journal* 71 (May 1975): 122-123.

"Eugenics in Germany." *Journal of the American Medical Association* 101 (July 22, 1933): 294-295.

Galen, Robert S.; Chauhan, Prem; Wietzner, Howard; and Navarro, Carlos. "Fetal Pathology and Mechanism of Fetal Death in Saline-Induced Abortion: A Study of 143 Gestations and Critical Review of the Literature." *American Journal of Obstetrics and Gynecology* 120 (October 1, 1974): 347-355.

Gaylin, Willard. "Harvesting the Dead: The Potential for Recycling Human Bodies." *Harper's Magazine,* September 1974, pp. 23-30.

Glueck, Helen I.; Flessa, Herbert C.; Kisker, C. Thomas; and Stander, Richard W. "Hypertonic Saline-Induced Abortion: Correlation of Fetal Death With Disseminated Intravascular Coagulation." *Journal of the American Medical Association* 225 (July 2, 1973): 28-31.

Goldsmith, Sadja; Kaltreider, Nancy B.; and Margolis, Alan J. "Second Trimester Abortion by Dilation and Extraction (D & E): Surgical Techniques and Psychological Reactions." Paper presented at the Annual Meeting of the Association of Planned Parenthood Physicians, 13-14 October 1977, in Atlanta, Georgia, pp. 1-14.

Gustafson, James M. "Mongolism, Parental Desires, and the Right to Life." *Perspectives in Biology and Medicine* 16 (Summer 1973): 529-557.

Guttmacher, Alan F. "The Law That Doctors Often Break." *Redbook Magazine,* August 1959, p. 96.

Hall, Elizabeth, with Cameron, Paul. "Our Failing Reverence for Life." *Psychology Today,* April 1976, pp. 104-113.

Hammond, Howard. "Therapeutic Abortion: Ten Years' Experience With Hospital Committee Control." *American Journal of Obstetrics and Gynecology* 89 (June 1, 1964): 349-355.

Harrison, Barbara Grizzuti. "Now that Abortion is Legal." *McCall's,* November 1973, pp. 64-74.

Herczeg, Janos; Resch, Bela A.; and Szontagh, Ferenc E. "On the Time of Fetal Survival of Abortuses Induced by Hypertonic Saline or Prostaglandin F_2a." *American Journal of Obstetrics and Gynecology* 118 (April 15, 1974): 1154-1155.

"Hereditary Transmission and Natural Selection." *Journal of the American Medical Association* 76 (May 21, 1921): 1415-1416.

Hern, Warren M., and Corrigan, Billie. "What About Us? Staff Reactions to the D & E Procedure." Paper presented at the Annual Meeting of the Association of Planned Parenthood Physicians, 26 October 1978, in San Diego, California, pp. 1-9.

Hodari, A. Alberto; Peralta, Jose; Quiroga, Pablo J.; and Gerbi, Enrique B. "Dilatation and Curettage for Second-Trimester Abortion." *American Journal of Obstetrics and Gynecology* 127 (April 15, 1977): 850-854.

"Indications for Abortion and the Law." *Journal of the American Medical Association* 96 (May 23, 1931): 1810-1811.

"Interruption of Pregnancy from Eugenic Indications." *Journal of the American Medical Association* 86 (February 27, 1926): 639-640.

Kady, John T. "Fetus Burning Is Halted." *Daily Standard* (Celina, Ohio), 18 May 1978, p. 3.

Kane, Francis J.; Feldman, Michael; Jain, Susheila; and Lipton, Morris A. "Emotional Reactions in Abortion Services Personnel." *Archives of General Psychiatry* 28 (March 1973): 409-411.

Karman, Harvey. "The Paramedic Abortionist." *Clinical Obstetrics and Gynecology* 15 (June 1972): 379-387.

Kerenyi, Thomas D.; Mandelman, Nathan; and Sherman, David H. "Five Thousand Consecutive Saline Inductions." *American Journal of Obstetrics and Gynecology* 116 (July 1, 1973): 593-600.

Kerslake, Dorothea, and Casey, Donn. "Abortion Induced by Means of the Uterine Aspirator." *Obstetrics and Gynecology* 30 (July 1967): 35-45.

Kibel, Howard D. "Staff Reactions to Abortion: A Psychiatrist's View." *Obstetrics and Gynecology* 39 (January 1972): 128-133.

Kilby-Kelberg, Sally. "The Abortion." *Medical Dimensions,* May 1974, pp. 35-36.

"King of the Abortionists." *Newsweek,* 17 February 1969, p. 92

Kopelman, J. Joshua, and Douglas, Gordon W. "Abortions by Resident Physicians in a Municipal Hospital Center." *American Journal of Obstetrics and Gynecology* 111 (November 1, 1971): 666-671.

Kummer, Jerome M. "Abortion: The Rearguard in Birth Control." *Journal of Reproductive Medicine* 5 (October 1970): 71-74.

Laros, Russel K.; Collins, Jack; Penner, John A.; Hage, Marvin L.;

and Smith, Samuel. "Coagulation Changes in Saline-Induced Abortion." *American Journal of Obstetrics and Gynecology* 116 (May 15, 1973): 277-285.

Lauersen, Niels H.; Wilson, Kathleen H.; Beling, Carl G.; and Fuchs, Fritz. "Comparison of Prostaglandin F_2a and Hypertonic Saline for Induction of Midtrimester Abortion." *American Journal of Obstetrics and Gynecology* 120 (December 1, 1974): 875-889.

Laws, E. Harold; Bulger, Roger J.; Boyce, Thomas R.; Thompson, Donovan J.; and Brown, Norman K. "Views on Euthanasia." *Journal of Medical Education* 46 (June 1971): 540-542.

Lebensohn, Zigmond M. "Abortion, Psychiatry, and the Quality of Life." *American Journal of Psychiatry* 128 (February 1972): 946-951.

Lindheim, Barbara L., and Cotterill, Maureen A. "Training in Induced Abortion by Obstetrics and Gynecology Residency Programs." *Family Planning Perspectives* 10 (January/February 1978): 24-28.

Lipper, Steven, and Feigenbaum, W. Morton. "Obsessive-Compulsive Neurosis After Viewing the Fetus During Therapeutic Abortion." *American Journal of Psychotherapy* 30 (October 1976): 666-674.

Mandel, Mark D. "An Operational and Planning Staffing Model for First and Second Trimester Abortion Services." *American Journal of Public Health* 64 (August 1974): 753-764.

McDermott, John F., and Char, Walter F. "Abortion Repeal in Hawaii: An Unexpected Crisis in Patient Care." *American Journal of Orthopsychiatry* 41 (July 1971): 620-626.

McLaughlin, Herbert. "Clinic Design Emphasizes Restraint to Minimize Patients' Tensions." *Modern Hospital* (September 1973): 74-75.

"MDs Shun 16th Week D & E as Reminder of Destroyed Fetus." *Medical Tribune*, 25 January 1978, p. 9.

"Meeting of the Prussian Council on Health." *Journal of the American Medical Association*, 99 (August 20, 1932): 666.

"Mercy Death Law Ready for Albany." *New York Times*, 14 February 1939, p. 2.

"Mid-Trimester Abortion Life in Fetus." *Ob-Gyn Collected Letters of the International Correspondence Society of Obstetricians and Gynecologists* 15 (November 1, 1974): 163-167.

Miller, Jane. "Fetal Tissue Disposed of Here Just as Other Specimens Are." *Lincoln Journal-Star*, 11 June 1978.

"Modern Medicine Poll on Sociomedical Issues: Abortion-Homosexual Practices-Marihuana." *Modern Medicine* 37 (November 3, 1969): 18-24.

Nathanson, Bernard N. "Deeper Into Abortion." *New England Journal of Medicine* 291 (November 28, 1974): 1189-1190.

Nemy, Enid. "Even Now, Helping With Abortions Is Traumatic Shock for Some Nurses." *New York Times*, 1 February 1972, p. 32.

"New Decisions on Sterilization and Castration." *Journal of the American Medical Association* 104 (June 8, 1935): 2109-2110.

"Nurses Are Reacting Against Abortions." *Saint Louis Review*, 6 November 1970, p. 2.

"Panelists' Views on Killing Child Not Recommendation." *Pediatric News*, April 1977, p. 32.

Peretz, A.; Grunstein, S.; Brandes, J. M.; and Paldi, E. "Evacuation of the Gravid Uterus by Negative Pressure." *American Journal of Obstetrics and Gynecology* 98 (May 1, 1967): 18-22.

Podhoretz, Norman. "Beyond ZPG." *Commentary*, May 1972, pp. 6-8.

"Problems of Heredity." *Journal of the American Medical Association* 105 (September 28, 1935): 1051-1052.

"Protection to Posterity in Relation to Social Politics." *Journal of the American Medical Association* 78 (February 11, 1922): 447-448.

Quay, Eugene. "Justifiable Abortion — Medical and Legal Foundations." *Georgetown Law Journal* 49 (1961): 395-538.

Ratner, Herbert. "Editor's Comments." *Child and Family* 12 (1973): 285-286.

Remsberg, Charles, and Remsberg, Bonnie. "Second Thoughts on Abortion From the Doctor Who Led the Crusade For It." *Good Housekeeping*, March 1976, pp. 69, 130-134.

"Reports Abortion Fetuses Put in Disposer Are Probed." *Omaha World-Herald*, 12 June 1978.

Resch, Bela A.; Papp, Julius G.; Szontagh, Ferenc E.; and Szekeres, Laszlo. "Comparison of Spontaneous Contraction Rates of In Situ and Isolated Fetal Hearts in Early Pregnancy." *American Journal of Obstetrics and Gynecology* 118 (January 1, 1974): 73-76.

Rooks, Judith Bourne, and Cates, Willard. "Emotional Impact of D & E vs. Instillation." *Family Planning Perspectives* 9 (November/December 1977): 276-277.

Rosen, Harold. "Psychiatric Implications of Abortion: A Case Study in Social Hypocrisy." *Western Reserve Law Review* 17 (1965): 435-464.

Rosen, Norma. "Between Guilt and Gratification: Abortion Doctors Reveal Their Feelings." *New York Times Magazine*, 17 April 1977, pp. 70-80.

Rosencher, Henri. "Medicine in Dachau." *British Medical Journal* 2 (December 21, 1946): 953-955.

Sackett, Walter W. "I've Let Hundreds of Patients Die. Shouldn't You?" *Medical Economics* 50 (April 2, 1973): 92-97.

"Saline Proves Safe for Late Abortions." *Medical World News*, 10 May 1974, p. 22.

Selzer, Richard. "What I Saw At The Abortion." *Esquire*, January 1976, pp. 66-67.

Shainess, Natalie. "Abortion: Inalienable Right." *New York State Journal of Medicine* 72 (July 1, 1972): 1772-1775.

_____. "Abortion Is No Man's Business." *Psychology Today*, May 1970, pp. 18-22, 74-76.

_____. "Abortion: Social, Psychiatric, and Psychoanalytic Perspectives." *New York State Journal of Medicine* 68 (December 1, 1968): 3070-3073.

Shaw, Anthony. "Dilemmas of 'Informed Consent' In Children." *New England Journal of Medicine* 289 (October 25, 1973): 885-890.

Sherman, David H. "Salting Out: Experience in 9,000 Cases." *Journal of Reproductive Medicine* 14 (June 1975): 241-243.

Stroh, George, and Hinman, Alan R. "Reported Live Births Following Induced Abortion: Two and One-Half Years' Experience in Upstate New York." *American Journal of Obstetrics and Gynecology* 126 (September 1, 1976): 83-90.

Sturgis, Somers H. "Alan Guttmacher, M. D.— A Life Fulfilled." *New England Journal of Medicine* 290 (May 9, 1974): 1085.

Sullivan, Ellen; Tietze, Christopher; and Dryfoos, Joy G. "Legal Abortion in the United States, 1975-1976." *Family Planning Perspectives* 9 (May/June 1977): 116-129.

"The Abortion Profiteers." *Chicago Sun-Times*. Special Reprint. 1978, pp. 1-48.

"The Attitude of Women Physicians Toward the Abortion Question." *Journal of the American Medical Association* 98 (April 30, 1932): 1580.

"The Congress of Gynecology." *Journal of the American Medical Association* 102 (January 6, 1934): 56-57.

"The Session of the League of German Medical Societies." *Journal of the American Medical Association* 85 (October 17, 1925): 1237-1238.

"Two-Minute Abortion is Here — Are We Ready?" *Medical World News*, 12 May 1972, pp. 15-17.

"Use of Disposal Sparks Abortion Fireworks." *Omaha World-Herald*, 11 June 1978.

Vojta, M. "A Critical View of Vacuum Aspiration: A New Method For the Termination of Pregnancy (Suction Evacuation)." *Obstetrics and Gynecology* 30 (July 1967): 28-34.

Walker, William B., and Hulka, J. F. "Attitudes and Practices of North Carolina Obstetricians: The Impact of the North Carolina Abortion Act of 1967." *Southern Medical Journal* 64 (April 1971): 441-445.

Wang, Jack; Roufa, Arnold; Moore, Thomas J.; Tovell, Harold M. M.; and Pierson, Richard N. "Body Composition Studies in the Human Fetus After Intra-Amniotic Injection of Hypertonic Saline." *American Journal of Obstetrics and Gynecology* 117 (September 1, 1973): 57-63.

Watson, James D. "Children From the Laboratory." *Prism*, May 1973, pp. 12-14, 33-34.

Weisman, Abner I. "Abortion Is Not The Answer." *Journal of the American Medical Association* 217 (September 13, 1971): 1553-1554.

Williams, Robert H. "Our Role in the Generation, Modification, and Termination of Life." *Archives of Internal Medicine* 124 (August 1969): 215-237.

Wolf, Sanford R.; Sasaki, Tom T.; and Cushner, Irving M. "Assumption of Attitudes Toward Abortion During Physician Education." *Obstetrics and Gynecology* 37 (January 1971): 141-144.

Yaloff, Beverly; Wade, Margot; and Burlingame, Mildred. "Nursing Care in an Abortion Unit." *Clinical Obstetrics and Gynecology* 14 (March 1971): 67-84.

Zahourek, Rothlyn. "Therapeutic Abortion and Cultural Shock." *Nursing Forum* 10 (1971): 8-17.

Index

Should Christians Mix in Politics?
YES!

There are at least three compelling reasons Christians must be involved in politics and government. First, as citizens of the nation-state, Christians have the same civic duties all citizens have: to serve on juries, to pay taxes, to vote, to support candidates they think are best qualified.

Second, as citizens of the Kingdom of God they are to bring God's standards of righteousness and justice to bear on the kingdoms of this world.

Third, Christians have an obligation to bring transcendent moral values into the public debate.

The real issue for Christians is not whether they should be involved in politics or contend for laws that affect moral behavior. The question is how.

CHARLES COLSON

with Ellen Santilli Vaughn

KINGDOMS IN CONFLICT

Harper Paperbacks

Harper & Row, Publishers, New York
Grand Rapids, Philadelphia, St. Louis, San Francisco
London, Singapore, Sydney, Tokyo, Toronto

Harper Paperbacks a division of Harper & Row, Publishers, Inc.
10 East 53rd Street, New York, N.Y. 10022

This book is published by arrangement with Zondervan
Publishing House.

Unless otherwise noted, Scripture references are taken from
the *Holy Bible: New International Version* (North American
Edition), copyright © 1973, 1978, 1984 by the International
Bible Society. Used by permission of Zondervan Bible
Publishers.

First Harper Paperbacks printing: October, 1990

Printed in the United States of America

HARPER PAPERBACKS and colophon are trademarks of
Harper & Row, Publishers, Inc.

10 9 8 7 6 5 4 3 2 1

CONTENTS

vi ═══ Contents

To those who serve in "the little platoons"
around the world, faithfully evidencing
the love and justice of the Kingdom of God
in the midst of the kingdoms of this world

KINGDOMS
IN
CONFLICT

Prologue

March 24, 1998

General Brent Slocum's T-shirt stuck to his sweaty back and powerful, heaving shoulders as he grinned at his twenty-nine-year-old opponent. His adjutant's urgent breathing filled the small handball court.

"Gonna make it through the last point, Rob?" the general asked. It was a pleasure, at fifty-four, to whip a younger man.

Suddenly there was a pounding on the door. "General," another aide shouted from outside. "Command Center on the line, sir."

Slocum hesitated. He wanted to finish the game. The pounding resumed.

"All right, Sloan," the general bawled. "I heard you. Those boys better have something worth my

1

time." Someone was forever using the channels. He wondered whether anybody could get through if a real emergency command—like war—was needed.

The youthful voice on the other end of the mobile communications line was shaking, probably scared half to death to be speaking to the chairman of the Joint Chiefs of Staff. "It's the White House signal agency calling, sir. Shall I patch it in?"

"Of course," Slocum grunted. Almost instantly he heard a second voice, crisp and precise.

"General Slocum, POTUS has asked you to come immediately, sir. The diplomatic entrance. Enter through the south gate. Can I give an affirmative, sir?"

"Of course," he grunted again, then tossed the receiver in his aide's direction as he headed for the locker room. The White House? Six in the morning? Why on earth do they use an acronym for every last living thing in this city, Slocum grumbled to himself, including the President of the United States?

Eight minutes later he strode in full-dress uniform toward his waiting car. From Fort Myer to the White House was a ten-minute drive without traffic. His driver, the Army's best, had practiced many times. Fortunately, the city was just coming to life. Most of the streets were gray and deserted.

The general sat back as his limousine raced toward its destination, his thoughts swirling. He had seen the president only a few times since becoming chairman in January. Never had he entered the White House outside regular hours. Something hot was up. He ran through the possibilities.

It might be Mexico. The Sandinista-backed guerrillas had killed thirty-three in a bomb blast in Aca-

pulco last Friday. Slocum still didn't have an op.
plan ready to seal the border; he'd be in trouble if
the old man wanted that.

The Middle East? That very morning, before
leaving for the handball court, Slocum had glanced
over a report of two new Soviet divisions moving
into Iran.

Or perhaps, though less likely, it was Britain.
Nobody had anticipated the vehemence of the Kin-
nock government when they discovered two Posei-
don subs in their waters in violation of Britain's
nuclear-free policy.

Go to the Residence, he had been ordered. Whatever it was, it was important.

The blue-jacketed White House policeman saluted and waved the general's car through the heavy
black-steel gates and up the long curved driveway
that cut across the South Lawn of the White House.
Slocum counted five limousines, all larger than his,
at the door. The secretary of defense . . . the secretary
of state. . . . Getting out of the car, he stood for a moment and gazed up at the light scum of late snow
clinging to the gutters of the Residence. *This could
be war,* he thought.

"Right this way, sir," announced a young marine. He steered the general through the oval-shaped
Diplomatic Receiving Room and up the flight of marble steps to the Great Center Hall. From there the
general followed him toward another flight of stairs
carpeted in thick red pile. They led, he knew, to the
family quarters, although he had never been above
the first floor.

At the head of the stairs stood a secret-service

agent, a plug in one ear. He glanced at the general and then seemed to look through him. The agent's suit sagged as though he'd worn it for a week. It annoyed Slocum. After a life in the military, sloppy civilian dress was difficult to accept.

His marine escort clicked his heels softly and announced, "The Lincoln Sitting Room, sir." He nodded to the door of the study directly off the president's bedroom. The secret-service agent leaned to one side and swung the door open, never taking his eyes off the stairway.

Larry Parrish, the sandy-haired, ivy-league White House chief of staff, was the only one to nod at Slocum as he entered. The others were preoccupied in knots of uneasy conversation. Parrish waved the general into a hard-backed antique chair, then caught President Hopkins's eye.

"Everyone's here," he said.

The small room, which had once served Abraham Lincoln as an office, was crowded with antiques; this morning it seemed even more crowded by the egos of the handful of powerful men the president had summoned. Parrish had taken their measure long ago, however, and he somehow managed to make these egos work together for whatever goals the president chose. He knew people, he knew the system, and he had a finely tuned political sense for what would fly on the 6:00 news. "I'm a technician," he would say with a smile when pressed about his role in the government. He thought of that now as he surveyed the men before him.

Though the general was the most recent of the president's top appointments, Parrish had known

Brent Slocum through a decade of Washington receptions. The general was the best sort of military man: politically unimaginative, but quick to seize the main issues. Neither a paper pusher nor a cowboy, he had just the kind of solid, capable confidence to command any situation.

Seated next to Slocum was Alexander Hartwell, the secretary of defense, revered as the nastiest infighter in Washington's brutal bureaucracy. Parrish had often thought he was glad Hartwell was *their* s.o.b. He would make a formidable enemy.

A veteran of twenty years in the House, Hartwell had worked the deals reconciling the Christian right to the Republican hard-liners that laid the foundation for Hopkins's election. For his reward Hartwell had demanded and been given Defense. He sometimes acted, however, as if he had been given the White House. Parrish worked hard to stay one jump ahead of Hartwell—and to remind him who was president.

Next to Hartwell was Secretary of State Henry Lovelace. Parrish suspected Henry was out of his depth, and so did a lot of other people who referred to him privately as Secretary Love. Lovelace owed his job to his friendship with the president, dating back to college days. The president was comfortable with him, and his weaknesses were compensated for by the strength of Alan Davies, the national security advisor. It was doubtful anyway whether Davies could have worked with a strong counterpart at State.

Davies, whose wispy appearance, blank stare, and ubiquitous bow tie belied his power, crouched in the room's one overstuffed chair. He always reminded Parrish of a time bomb, staring and ticking.

Davies read everything and forgot nothing. The president had come to rely on him during his fourteen months in the White House. Almost dangerously so, Parrish thought.

Finally, slumped on a rosewood chair purchased by Mary Todd Lincoln, was the professorial attorney general, Hyman Levin. How the man could talk! He kept the right-wingers happy, crusading with the vigor of the recently converted. Fortunately, though, he was a realist who knew how to talk on one line and compromise on another.

Any one of the five men, with the possible exception of Lovelace, would have dominated another setting. But bluster as they would, in the end they did the president's bidding.

How Hopkins managed this trick Parrish had not quite figured out. Part of it, he sometimes mused, was physical. The president looked like the president: tall, with a magnificent silver mane, a jutting jaw that suggested strength to men, and sparkling blue eyes that charmed women. And he sounded like God Almighty, his thunderclap voice rising out of some lower register.

Mostly, though, Parrish had begun to believe that the president dominated them by sheer goodness. After surviving decades of politics, Parrish didn't believe goodness had anything to do with effective leadership. But Hopkins was different. He radiated something that made you feel morally small after being around him.

Despite these natural assets, Shelby Hopkins had come late to political life. For over twenty years he had been a professor of history and later academic dean at Baylor University. He had entered the political arena in the eighties when evangelical Christians came out of nowhere to become a major force in national politics.

Hopkins had been nominated to run for governor of Texas chiefly because Republican political consultants thought he looked and sounded good on television. To the surprise of many, he had governed imaginatively and circumspectly, coming to national prominence through his handling of the Dallas AIDS riots, which had put him on the network news every night for two weeks. When the Republican hard-liners patched things up with the Christian right after the big split in 1992, Hopkins was a natural candidate for president.

Parrish's thoughts were interrupted now as the president looked up from some papers, smiled briefly, and looked at each of the men. "Gentlemen, let's get started. Sorry to call you in so early this morning. I appreciate your promptness." There was just a trace of Texas in his voice.

"I've asked you here to the Residence because if we were seen at this hour in the west wing, the press would be onto things in nothing flat. We can't have that.

"We seem to have a little trouble brewing in Israel. You all know that the Knesset has been paralyzed for some time, with neither the Likud nor the Labor parties able to get a stable majority to form a government."

Hopkins held up the black-leather notebook engraved with gold letters, *For the President's eyes only,* and continued.

"But this morning's intelligence summary suggests that the logjam is breaking. Both parties have been bargaining with small fringe parties, as you know. Our sources say that the Likud party is very close to striking a deal with the Tehiya party. In fact, since it's midafternoon in Israel now, they may have already reached an agreement. I talked this over with Alan earlier this morning and decided we'd better get to work on it right away."

Parrish scribbled notes furiously. This was the first indication of what had stirred the president. Was it truly an emergency? The difference between the two chief Israeli parties appeared minuscule, especially in their attitudes toward the Arab world. So far as the U.S. was concerned, it made little difference which actually gained power.

At the president's invitation Alan Davies leaned forward and, consulting a red notebook that looked like the president's but without the lettering, told them more than anyone could possibly want to know at 6:30 in the morning about the tiny fanatical religious party known as Tehiya.

The leader was Yosef Tzuria, an Albanian refugee who favored driving all Arabs out of the occupied territories. Tzuria also believed that God had given Israel title to all land west of the Euphrates River—territory inconveniently known as Iraq, Lebanon, and Syria. But—Parrish almost missed the emphasis because of Davies's monotone—Tzuria's big scheme was religious. He wanted to blow up the Dome of the Rock, the sacred Muslim shrine in Jerusalem, and build a temple in its place.

Davies concluded his briefing with a quote from

Tzuria: "'We must establish a permanent place of prayer on the mount. It is a desecration of God to enter the mount under the authority of an Arab guard.'

"I might add," Davies said dryly, "that they're quite serious. They're being bankrolled by some big industrialists in Israel, along with a fundamentalist group in Texas, which, we gather, has handed them at least twenty-five million dollars. They've got men in training." A trace of a smile curved his lips. "Not only commandos, but priests. They're in training to perform Jewish sacrificial rites."

Priests? Sacrificial rites? Parrish searched the faces of the other men. Did they understand the significance here? He didn't. Nor could he decipher the strange, excited light in the president's eyes.

"I hate to sound uninformed," Parrish said finally, "but so what?"

"So what?" the president echoed slowly. "*So what?* This could mean war!"

"The Likud party isn't going to let some marginal crowd of fanatics carry them into war," Parrish said. "Anyway, it sounds to me like their big thing is religion, not politics."

"Yes, that's right, Larry," the president said, nodding his silvery head. "That's just the problem. They take the Old Testament prophecies very seriously. And on the question of whether Likud would allow them to carry the nation into the war, that's why I called you together. This morning's briefing says, and Alan tells me the sources are impeccable, that Tzuria and the Likud leader, Moshe Arens, are in negotiations right now. And Arens has tentatively

agreed to look the other way when Tzuria's commandos blow up the Dome of the Rock. What they've
yet to agree on is whether Arens will promise to
declare Israeli sovereignty over the whole Temple
Mount. It looks as though it could actually happen.
The Jewish Temple could be rebuilt."

"And that would mean war," added Attorney
General Levin. "The Arabs are very religious too, you
know—they have always said they are prepared to
die before any Jew will pray on the Mount."

Parrish shifted uncomfortably. His own Epis-
copalian background differed considerably from the
president's Southern Baptist roots, and though this
had never created any strain between them, Parrish
felt out of his depth when it came to the finer nuances
of the religious world.

"I'm sorry, Mr. President," he said apologetically. "Maybe everyone else understands this, but
I'm not with it. Could you bear with me here until
someone explains about the Temple? I must have
missed that briefing." He saw to his relief that at least
Hartwell and Slocum were in the same boat he was,
for Slocum nodded at his request and Hartwell was
wearing a tight, bemused smile.

"Maybe I can get Hyman to brief us on that,
Larry. He was quite a Levitical scholar up at Yale,
you know. Now since his conversion he knows even
more than he used to. Explain it, will you Hy?" The
president and his attorney general grinned at each
other.

This suggestion did not set Parrish at ease. He
knew of Levin's conversion to Christianity, but what
in heaven's name was a Levitical scholar? And the

glances exchanged by Levin and the president, as if they shared some secret fraternity ritual, made him feel like an outsider.

Levin had a high choirboy voice and held his chin up slightly when he talked. He loved the chance to lecture.

"I suppose you know, Larry, that the ancient Israelites worshiped in a Temple built by Solomon in Jerusalem. By the time of King Hezekiah, in 715 B.C., worship was allowed nowhere else. That Temple was destroyed, however, by Babylonian armies in 586 B.C. Then came the Babylonian captivity, after which the returning Jews built a second Temple. That was later replaced by an elaborate monument for King Herod." Levin grinned. "You have heard of King Herod?"

Parrish nodded.

"Good," continued Levin in a high, ironic tone. "But the main fact you need to know is that in A.D. 70 the Jews revolted against Rome, and the Romans retaliated by destroying their Temple. It was never rebuilt. The Muslims erected a mosque over the ruins centuries later. During the Crusades the Christians gained control and turned it into a church, but in recent centuries it has reverted to the Arabs. Today it is the Dome of the Rock, one of the holiest Muslim shrines. They would view its desecration as an unspeakable outrage.

"Now that, Larry, poses quite a problem. Because the devout Jew cannot just forget the Temple. They consider the site sacred. The Temple originally built there contained the Holy of Holies where no one could set foot—except the high priest, once a year—without desecrating God's holy name. So the Muslim control of that spot is . . . a desecration of all that is sacred to them."

"So somebody gets desecrated no matter what," Parrish interjected.

"Very good, Larry. Furthermore, the Jew cannot fulfill the Old Testament sacrificial laws unless a Temple is rebuilt on that site. Promises of Messiah's return to a new Temple are found in Scripture; there and only there does He wish to make His residence. So for the devout Jew a rebuilt Temple is more important than the renewal of the state of Israel."

"But . . . they have synagogues," Parrish said.

"A synagogue is not the Temple. A synagogue is a house of prayer. But you cannot do the blood sacrifices there."

Parrish's face twisted into a combination of pain and disbelief. "Blood sacrifices?"

"Yes, a sheep, a goat, a bull. Killed on the altar and burned on the perpetual fire."

"What in the world—"

"There is one more thing I should add," Levin interrupted him. "To the devout Christian who pays attention to prophecy, the rebuilding of the ancient Temple will set the stage for the last great act of history. It will signal Armageddon. That explains why Christian groups are funding the Tehiya. The Temple will pave the way for Christ's triumphant return."

Levin leaned back, pleased with his presentation. The president looked inquiringly at Parrish.

"Does it make sense now, Larry? Obviously, while these reports are frightening, there's some ex-

citement that comes with them too. You can't help
but wonder if these could be events we've all waited
for.''

Parrish felt a sudden tightening in his stomach
as he remembered former President Frank's charges
in the '96 campaign that Hopkins would try to make
Bible prophecy self-fulfilling and bring on Armageddon. Never before had it crossed Parrish's mind that
those accusations were anything but hysteria.

Brent Slocum struggled to accommodate his six-
foot-three frame to the undersized antique chair. His
head was spinning, particularly with the attorney
general's last words. He had visited Israel several
times, but to observe Israeli defenses on the Golan
Heights, not mosques in Jerusalem. He was a man of
war, comfortable talking about supply operations and
air support. Not Armageddon.

He glanced at Hartwell. He knew that behind his
narrowed eyes and high forehead the secretary of
defense was computing fast. Slocum didn't particularly like Hartwell, but he did expect him to talk in
terms that made some sense.

Hartwell didn't disappoint him. ''So the gist of
it is, Mr. President, Armageddon or no Armageddon,
we need to head off this deal. It's explosive. Why
would Arens even entertain it? He must know all this
better than we do.''

Davies leaned forward and answered before
Hopkins could respond.

''Arens is an old fool,'' he said flatly. ''He'd do
anything to regain power. And this issue, strange as
it sounds to us, is really quite popular within certain

powerful segments of the Israeli population."

"Not with Arens!" Slocum blurted. "I know the man. He doesn't have a religious bone in his body."

"Right," Davies said. "But he's a politician who knows how to play religious issues."

"If he's a politician," Hartwell sneered, "then he ought to know that Israel's existence depends on the good opinion of the United States. If this cockamamy scheme is as serious as you seem to think, then why don't we get him on the phone and tell him to forget it? No ifs, ands, or buts."

"Now hold on," Secretary Lovelace interjected. "That's no way to treat our ally."

"What if he says no?" Parrish asked, looking up from his note taking. "Could you back it up?"

"With a bullet, if necessary," Hartwell said. "We have agents who would find it a pleasure."

Hopkins shook his head violently, and Parrish quickly interjected, "Such matters are never discussed in the president's presence."

Slocum grabbed onto a possibility that made some sense to him. "I can have the Delta Force in the area ready to go in twelve hours, sir."

"Hold on, now," said Parrish. "If I understand it correctly, the question isn't military in nature. We could drop an atom bomb on Jerusalem, if it came to that. The question is, could we back it up politically? Do you really think we can dictate policy to Israel, our only reliable ally in the Middle East? You think the Israel lobby would give us room to maneuver? And Arens knows just how much leeway we have."

"Come off it, Larry," said Hartwell. "We can

make Arens come around if we're willing to get rough."

President Hopkins had moved from his chair to the window overlooking the South Lawn, but hadn't said a word. It was unusual for him not to take part in the discussion; he enjoyed a spirited debate. But this morning he seemed far away, his eyes fixed on some distant point.

"Gentlemen," he said finally, "we must keep in mind the very real possibility that this situation is beyond us all." The words hung suspended in the air for a long, awkward moment. Only Levin nodded.

Hartwell shook his head with annoyance and reflexively reached into his jacket pocket for a cigarette. Then he remembered that no one smoked in the White House anymore.

"Mr. President," he said angrily, "whatever cosmic forces may be involved here, Tzuria must be stopped. There's nothing more dangerous than allowing religious fanaticism to replace reasoned political judgment."

"Are you talking about me or Tzuria?" the president asked coldly. Being called a religious zealot during the campaign had stung Hopkins. He had run on the platform "Return America to God" and left no doubt where he stood, but the fanatic label always annoyed him.

"No, Mr. President, of course not. I'm talking about Tzuria. He's the menace."

"Good," said Hopkins, putting on his half-circle reading glasses and picking up a well-worn brown-leather Bible from a table beside Davies's chair. "At the risk of appearing fanatical, I'd like to read you all a passage from Ezekiel. It was written five centuries before the birth of Christ." He flipped a few pages until he located his text. "Listen to this: 'My dwelling place will be with them; I will be their God, and they will be my people. Then the nations will know that I the Lord make Israel holy, *when my sanctuary is among them forever.*'

"Ezekiel tells us that Gog, the nation that will lead all the other powers of darkness against Israel, will come out of the north. Biblical scholars have been saying for generations that Gog must be Russia. What other powerful nation is to the north of Israel? None. But it didn't seem to make sense before the Russian revolution, when Russia was a Christian country. Now that Russia has become communistic and atheistic, it does. Now that Russia has set itself against God, it fits the description of Gog perfectly."

President Hopkins put down the Bible, removed his glasses, and ran a hand through his hair. He stared into the eyes of each man one by one. Slocum felt self-conscious. Parrish, who usually had his head down, taking notes, stared back up at Hopkins.

"I ran my campaign on the Bible," Hopkins said, "and I intend to run this nation on the Bible. Let's keep in mind while we make our plans that God has already made His."

Then the president smiled and broke the tension. "Now let's get down to business. We've talked enough. You know the situation. I want strategy options out of all of you by noon. Keep the subject as mysterious as possible to your aides. I don't want any leaks. Repeat—no leaks."

Turning to Parrish, he asked, "Larry, one key

question. Is there any hint of this in the press? Do they know about the Arens-Tzuria deal at all?"

"Not to my knowledge," said Parrish. "I'll check, but I don't think there's been anything in the wind."

"Good," the president said tersely. "In fact, just to be sure we keep it that way, steer them a little. Put out a story, Larry. Something from, you know, 'informed sources.' Say there will be a labor—left-wing coalition. Or whatever you think is best. We must buy some time here."

The president sat down, took off his watch, and wound it. "Anything else?" he asked. There was no response. "Then at the risk of again appearing to be a religious zealot, may I suggest that before you leave to prepare your recommendations, we invoke God's blessings upon us and upon this nation. Henry, will you lead us in prayer?"

Slocum watched in horror as the secretary of state stood up, turned around, and knelt before his chair. The president and Parrish followed suit. So did Levin. Davies, with an annoyed look on his face, got slowly onto his knees.

Brave enough to have won a Silver Star in Vietnam, Slocum was not sure he had the courage for this. He looked over at Hartwell who sat obstinately in his chair, his eyes on the floor, his chin on his fist.

But Slocum was a soldier, and a soldier followed his commander-in-chief. Awkward though it felt, he turned his long body around and knelt.

Secretary Lovelace began to pray in a deep, passionate voice. "We humble ourselves before You, the one true God, who governs the affairs of this beloved nation. We serve You only because You have granted us this privilege and authority, and so we ask You, dear Father, to lead us. We seek Your will. Whatever all this means, give us the eyes to see and the ears to hear. Have it Your way, not ours, and forgive us the sin that would make us blind to Your truth. . . ."

8:45 A.M., the White House

Each day at 8:00 A.M. the senior aides to the president gathered around a giant mahogany table in the Roosevelt Room, the windowless conference chamber just across from the Oval Office. This morning Parrish's eyes had been drawn to the famous painting on the north wall, Teddy Roosevelt charging up San Juan Hill. The chief of staff had sighed inwardly, wondering exactly what they were charging into with the Israel situation.

Now, over an hour later, Parrish sat, hardly listening, as several self-important aides held forth on a variety of matters—the latest nomination to the Supreme Court; the plan to abolish the Department of Education; and the drive in the Senate for welfare reform. At the moment James Shepherd, head of the Budget Office, was off on his usual tirade about agencies refusing to cooperate with the 10-percent across-the-board budget cut.

A master at disguising his true feelings behind an impassive mask, Parrish stared soberly at Shepherd as his mind churned. One mishandled crisis, especially in Israel, could destroy a popular president's ratings overnight. And as volatile as the Middle East was, one incident there could escalate into a major situation. As concerned as he was about that, however, he was more concerned about another matter. He was beginning to worry about the president.

Parrish had joined Hopkins's team late in the campaign after backing another candidate. Nevertheless, until this morning he felt he knew the president better than his own brother. He still remembered that first interview during the campaign when Hopkins had been feeling out possible talent for his team; within thirty minutes the two men had been talking with the freedom of old acquaintances.

Once in the White House, they enjoyed complete rapport on political matters. Perhaps, Parrish was prepared to admit, that had been easy because so many events had broken in their favor. Oil prices had dropped, curbing the runaway inflation of the early nineties. A cure for AIDS had been announced, without warning, and had given the nation a huge psychological lift. Still, it seemed that the two men understood each other's intentions intuitively through a peculiar type of political telepathy.

Parrish at first thought he might be uncomfortable with Hopkins's up-front religiosity, but he wasn't. Hopkins was so decent and open. He was a good man. *You don't meet many people like that*, Parrish often thought, *especially not in Washington*. Yet there was nothing holier-than-thou about the president. A less sincere man would never have gotten away with such White House piety.

Even the daily prayer and Bible readings at staff meetings had been accepted respectfully. Parrish himself had opened this morning's session with a reading from Psalm 90. The practice had grown out of the president's acceptance speech at the Dallas convention when he had pledged to 100 million Americans watching on TV that he would begin every day on his knees and require the same of his key advisors.

It was a popular promise. People had been fed up with the waves of change sweeping the nation in the early nineties. Not only was prayer outlawed in schools, but in all public places, before football games and commencements, and in all public buildings. Even the Senate chaplaincy had been abandoned. A series of ACLU-sponsored cases had reshaped American geography: Bethlehem, Pennsylvania, was forced to change its name, as was Corpus Christi, Texas. St. Louis was narrowly spared by a five-four decision that held that the word *saint* no longer held a specifically sacred connotation. America's population was declining due to soaring abortions. Drug dealers' armed gangs controlled many public schools.

Hopkins had stood rock-solid against all that, and on that basis he had been elected. But now, for the first time, Parrish was not so sure about the president's motives. He didn't understand the currents moving in Hopkins's mind on the Israeli situation. He had left the president just an hour before, staring into the big brown Bible open before him. Parrish told himself that it was perfectly reasonable for a president to draw strength from the Bible at such a time. What bothered him was that Hopkins didn't seem to be reading his Bible for strength. He seemed to be looking for directions.

10:00 A.M., the Pentagon

Once General Brent Slocum was back at the Pentagon, the praying and Bible reading seemed so distant and strange that he almost wondered whether he had imagined the scene at the White House. Relieved to be in familiar territory among a group of uniformed brass, he watched the secretary of defense pace back and forth behind his desk like the pendulum of a tightly wound clock swinging in double time. Shirtsleeves rolled up, tie loosened, collar open, Hartwell punctuated his lecture with readings from intelligence reports clutched in his left hand. His right hand held a cigarette, which he rubbed out whenever it burned down to a stub, only to light another. Ashes floated like dirty snow onto the navy-blue carpet, the desk, and Hartwell's beautifully tailored pants.

He talked as quickly as he walked, a practice he had developed during his twenty years as a congressman.

This former representative from Wisconsin was the unlikeliest member of the cabinet, as profane as the president was pious. A party loyalist since the early sixties, he had stuck staunchly with the party regulars when they fought off the Christian New Right's attempt to take over the precinct caucuses in 1988. But that fight led to the Christian walkout from the '92 convention and their running their own candidate in the general election. As a result of the split, the Democrats won in a record landslide.

The Republican recovery owed much to Hartwell. Always a realist, he had worked tirelessly for a reconciliation before the 1996 election, even to the renaming of the party. Though the words almost choked him, Alexander Hartwell now belonged to the Christian Republican party.

These were not traits to endear Hartwell to a man like Slocum, who distrusted politicians. But the secretary of defense had other more attractive qualities. He was a formidable debater, quick with the facts or, if necessary, his mesmeric personality. He knew how the government worked—and had it down cold—and could store more facts about the budget in his head than an IBM computer.

Now he was jabbing his cigarette in the air like a weapon, lecturing them on the immediate action required. "Arens must be ordered to drop Tzuria like a piece of pork. If not, we will withdraw all support, military or otherwise. The subject is nonnegotiable." Stopping his pacing for a moment, he glared at his audience. "Anybody disagree?"

Slocum shook his head and the others followed suit. Hartwell made sense. They should do all they could to persuade Arens to desist.

General Curt Oliver of Central Intelligence, who sat beside Slocum, had delivered actual transcripts of the Arens-Tzuria meetings. They showed Arens as depressingly querulous and erratic, while Tzuria had the constancy of a hungry predator. Tzuria offered to deliver the votes the Likud needed to form a government, but there was a price. Arens must look the other way when the commandos took out the Dome of the Rock; then he must claim Israeli sovereignty over the site. Tzuria would do the rest. They would move so fast the Arabs wouldn't have time to react. Marble slabs had been precut. The Temple could be up within thirty days. The Soviets, Tzuria argued, would hold back since the rock was strategically worthless.

By now Slocum understood what had earlier sounded like an old adventure movie. On reaching his Pentagon office after the early White House meeting, he had called in a young captain who he knew to be highly religious. "What do you know about the Temple Mount?" Slocum had asked. Captain Bryce had confirmed just what President Hopkins had said, and more. The Temple must be rebuilt within the next generation, according to prophecy, Bryce said. As far as he knew, all born-again Christians believed it because the Bible taught it.

Hartwell was waiting for some verbal response. Slocum cleared his throat. "Mr. Secretary, I confirm your objectives. But I think we need to optionalize contingencies. What if Arens refuses to listen to us? What then? This thing could slip out of gear in a hurry."

"Refuse to listen?" Hartwell snapped. "Come off it, General. Absolutely not. We own him. Three of his Knesset members work for us. Oliver here signs their paychecks." Hartwell gestured toward the deputy director of the CIA. "We say the word, and Arens and his nasty little party dry up and disappear."

"Yes, sir," Slocum said. "I'm sure that's right. However, it seems optimal to prepare for all contingencies. People do strange things when religion gets involved. Also Arens might think he can call our bluff. He knows that this administration will never abandon Israel."

Hartwell flushed. He took a long drag on his cigarette. "General," he said scornfully, "I think I know where this administration stands. The abandonment of Israel is not at stake. The abandonment of Moshe Arens is more to the point."

"Yes, sir," said Slocum. "But the Israelis have been known to confuse the two. And they have a track record of maximizing independence. I'd propose we optionalize the possibility—however infinitesimal—that they ignore our counsel."

Hartwell fumed, stared at Slocum, blew smoke. He detested Slocum's Pentagonese but knew the general was right. The president's loyalty to Israel was a matter of faith, and the Israelis would play that for all they could.

"What do you propose then, General?" Hartwell asked, lighting another cigarette and leaning on the back of his overstuffed, shiny-blue leather desk chair.

"The marines, sir. We have an LPH with the Sixth Fleet that could be off the coast in a little under twenty-four hours. It's up to T/O requirements—and ready . . . one battalion . . . good troops. We'd be able to put twenty choppers with six hundred men into Jerusalem thirty minutes after lift-off. The Israelis wouldn't know how to react, especially if we told them we were on an antiterrorist maneuver. It's now 7:00 P.M. in Tel Aviv. My men could have the Dome of the Rock sealed by this time tomorrow."

Hartwell smiled but didn't interrupt.

"Of course, sir," Slocum continued. "I don't have an op. plan approved by the chiefs. We haven't even contemplated . . . that is, no one ever figured on defending a mosque in Jerusalem."

"Wasn't part of the war games, eh General?" Hartwell burst into laughter, which started a coughing spasm. His assistant, Frank Flaherty, was instantly out of his seat, slapping his boss on the back.

"You've got to quit smoking," Flaherty said mechanically. He'd been saying it for nearly twenty years.

Drying his eyes with a rumpled handkerchief, Hartwell said, "Sorry, General. Just the thought of American marines—probably Christians—defending an Arab mosque against our closest allies, the Jews—" With that he started laughing and coughing again. "Hopkins'll have kittens."

Slocum's military operation was both bold and simple, and thus likely to succeed. Nobody had a better idea, and they kicked it around, discussing logistics. But their conversation lacked energy, drifting to a halt whenever they moved from the military to the political situation. None of them could imagine the president authorizing the marines to invade Jerusalem.

As he thought of this ridiculous limitation on his power, Alexander Hartwell gradually warmed into a fury. He slammed his fist on the desk, jumped to his feet, and began to pace again.

"Something has to move him," he muttered. "Something has to make it too hot for him. Not State. The little pip-squeaks there will be wringing their hands all through afternoon tea. Nobody has the guts for this kind of crisis. Congress'll go berserk."

The others stopped talking, watching Hartwell

pace from one end of the room to the other.

Suddenly he whirled around and stabbed a finger at the general. "Slocum, what did you make of Parrish? Where is he in all this?"

"Sir?"

"Could we use Parrish? He seems to know the inside of the president's skull. Do you think he'd work with us?"

Slocum found the very idea of outflanking the president offensive. "Parrish is the president's man. He might agree with us, but I don't believe he'd scheme against his own boss."

Hartwell scowled but passed over the implicit warning. "You're right, I suppose. But we need some way . . ." He paused, his gaze fixed on the vivid colors of his desk pad, etched with the giant seal of the secretary of defense.

A smile twitched the corners of his lips. He muttered, "Of course, of course. Why hasn't anyone thought of this until now? Yes, we'll have to." He looked up at his assistant. "Frank, that's it."

After twenty years Flaherty knew enough to say, "Yes, sir."

"Get the story to the press. Leak it fast, and make sure they go after it full speed ahead. But be careful." He grinned widely. "If Hopkins ever found out it would be my—that is, all of our necks, right on the chopping block."

Slocum sat stiffly, as though coming to attention. "Sir, the president gave us strict instructions not to allow this story out."

"Yes, he did, didn't he, General? That's why I want it kept in this room. If it gets out who's re-

sponsible, you'll go down with me. Clear enough?"
He was on his feet, leaning across the desk, staring
directly at Slocum; then he sat down slowly. "General, I appreciate that this may go against your grain.
But this is a case when following protocol may not
be in the best interest of the commanding officer.
When the enemy's aiming a gun at your commander's
head, you just shove him into a foxhole. You don't
wait to say, 'sir!' Am I right?"

"Yes, sir," Slocum said grudgingly.

"That's all we're gonna do," said Hartwell with
a smile. "Give our commander a little shove into the
foxhole. You see?"

Slocum said nothing.

Hartwell was on his feet again, pacing behind
his desk, his attention back to the leak. "I can't believe this story hasn't broken yet anyway. Well, no
... it's a religious thing, so the press probably
wouldn't even understand. And the Israelis know
how to keep things quiet. I wish we did as well."

He pointed a nicotine-stained finger at his assistant. "Okay, Frank, move on it. Call Stuart or Marvin. No, they're too well plugged in. Call Nolan. He'll
buy it in a minute. And let it all out: 'Arens is dealing
with the Devil ... would constitute the worst offense
against Arab rights in thirty years of occupation ...
fanatical religious elements are gaining control of
Israeli foreign policy.' Just make sure we're well under cover—'informed sources,' you know. Once we
point the press in the right direction, they'll scare
themselves half to death without our help. But it
needs to move fast."

"Yes, sir." Flaherty never looked up from his notes.

"But the Arabs will be tipped off too," General Oliver added. "And that may force Arens's hand. Tzuria may strike before the marines are in position."

"No, no. Think it through, gentlemen. The Israelis can't move except by surprise. This'll create confusion for them, and it'll force Hopkins to intervene. Otherwise he'd appear weak." Hartwell licked his lips. He was obviously pleased with himself.

"General." He wheeled around and jabbed his finger at Slocum. "Order the marines to head due east, full steam ahead. Put the Sixth Fleet on standby alert, and have your battle plan ready to issue as soon as possible. That means in the next hour."

Hartwell took one long satisfied look at the military men arrayed before him and chuckled. "From the Halls of Montezuma to the Dome of the Rock, eh? All right. Get to it."

Slocum felt a sudden sense of exhilaration as he marched out of the secretary's spacious office. He couldn't quite remember feeling the same way in years. Not since Vietnam when he had led his troops through a particularly bloody firefight. His two waiting aides with braided epaulets draped from their shoulders joined him, and the three men walked briskly to the escalators that would take them down to the War Room in the Pentagon basement. Devising strategy in international affairs was heady business. Someday this would all be in the history books, no doubt. Slocum tightened his lips, thrust his shoulders back, and began walking faster.

Late afternoon, the White House Press Room

At 2:30 in the afternoon Hartwell's leak exploded in the middle of an otherwise routine Washington day. First, Nolan was on Cable News with the bizarre story. Then the wire services ran their versions, crediting "informed sources," that U.S. policymakers were working day and night to head off a militant Tehiya party takeover of the Israeli government; intelligence experts considered war in the Middle East a real possibility.

A separate story, pulled up on short notice out of the files, told the history and objectives of the Tehiya party, including their financial links to American groups who shared their belief that these were the "last days" and that the Arab-Israeli standoff would be broken only by violent confrontation. The Tehiya rallying cry was "they must go," referring to the Arabs.

Reporters began to congregate in the White House Press Room, first reading the story on computer monitors in the little cubicles lining the back of the room, then rushing to phone their editors.

By 3:00 P.M. the Associated Press cited unconfirmed reports that the U.S. Sixth Fleet had been ordered to the eastern Mediterranean. The Pentagon press office issued a flat denial. But only a half hour later there were reports from naval headquarters in Naples, Italy, that all leaves had been cancelled.

That triggered a flood of dispatches from Middle East correspondents eager to catch up. These included wild and vitriolic quotations from various leaders of the Tehiya; of the Waqf, the Jordanian-backed Muslim group that controlled the Temple Mount; and others.

At 4:15, ABC broke into daytime programming with a brief report. The other networks were on the air by 4:25.

The Christian Broadcasting Company interrupted its regular programming for what they called their "Last Things Report." This included continuous live satellite coverage of the Dome of the Rock, using the site as the backdrop for their news set. The host, an Australian named Sydney Halford, interviewed several Bible scholars, evangelists, and a retired Navy admiral. The White House and Pentagon telephone numbers flashed across the screen at five-minute intervals, and Halford urged everyone who wanted to hasten the return of Christ to call and express unqualified support for Israel.

By 5:00 P.M. the White House switchboard was overloaded, and the signal agency was called in to help.

As the network evening-news deadline drew near, Press Secretary Dolores Lawrence pleaded with Larry Parrish for some kind of release. The White House Press Room was like a den of underfed animals, she said. Parrish told her tersely to stick with "no comment." Finally, after she had interrupted him three times, Parrish checked with the president and then sent Davies down with a written statement reaffirming the government's faith in Israel's democratic processes and stating that no unusual military maneuvers were being called for or contemplated.

5:00 P.M., the Oval Office

It was clear to Larry Parrish that Hopkins was angry and flustered. An ordinary observer would not have recognized this; Hopkins had his reading glasses on and was perusing reports as though he were reading birthday cards. But his chief of staff had learned the signs. When the president was angry, he would take off his watch, chafe the inside of his wrist, and then put the watch back on—sometimes four or five times in a row. Today his watch was on and off incessantly.

"Larry," the president said in a voice that should have been accompanied by lightning bolts, "I want to know who did it. You find out. I don't care what means you have to take. Well, you know what I mean. I don't want Nixon's plumbers or Reagan's polygraphs. Nothing dirty, understand. But spare no effort. This kind of thing can destroy us. It has us up against the wall right now."

"Yes, sir," Parrish said.

The president took off his glasses, tossed them onto the desk, and rubbed his hands through his hair. "I don't know, Larry. What do we do next? Wait and see what Arens says to Ambassador Walker? This is the first time I've really felt what I've read so often of other presidents: to have the responsibility for the world and yet so little power to do anything. I don't think I've ever prayed like I have today."

"You have the option papers from Hartwell and Davies, sir," Parrish said crisply. "They both want to see you, quite urgently. They're rather insistent. Also, Dolores is begging you to make a statement.''

The president was silent for a moment, then said softly, "Larry, I read those option papers. And frankly, I just couldn't believe it. I ran on a platform of military strength, it's true, but not against our allies. And certainly not against Israel. I don't know what's gotten into those men. I can't see any point in talking to them right now. It'd just disturb me.''

The president flipped through a few of the reports on his desk, indicating that the subject was closed for the moment. "Did you see this report on phone traffic between Jerusalem and the U.S.? It says a lot of money—millions—is being offered to Tzuria. From Arizona, Texas, California, Florida, Alaska mainly. Some from people we know: the Temple Foundation, the international Christian embassy, the Thromos, the Merchessens. But what I found interesting is that a lot of big money is coming from the oil men, especially in Alaska.''

"Davies has a theory on that, Mr. President,'' Parrish said. "He thinks some of the big oil companies would like nothing better than an Arab-Israeli war to send oil prices soaring again. The oil crowd could be stirring this thing up.''

Hopkins peered over his reading glasses. "Yes, yes, I suppose. We'll watch that. You call Hy Levin and tell him to alert the FBI. Christians and Zionists have pure motives, but those oil boys, well, that's another story.'' Then Hopkins gestured with his left hand, as if he were brushing away an annoying insect, and reached across the desk for his Bible. Parrish had never seen Hopkins so preoccupied.

"You know, Larry, I never thought of it before, but isn't there a prophecy of that in Luke? Yes. Here. Listen to this. 'It was the same in the days of Lot. People were eating and drinking, buying and selling, planting and building. But the day Lot left Sodom, fire and sulfur rained down from heaven and destroyed them all. It will be just like this on the day the Son of Man is revealed.' That's Luke 17:28. You see, people will keep right on doing business up to the very moment of Christ's return." The president smiled, the first break in his gloom all afternoon. "Can you imagine the looks on the faces of those oil boys?"

The president paused, looking up as though he were trying to see through the ceiling. "You know, Larry, I can't help thinking—this really could be *the time.* The generation that saw the Jews return to their homeland is about to pass. It almost has to happen soon. All that is left is for the Temple to be built. That's the last big sign before—"

Parrish stood to his feet as though facing a firing squad. "Mr. President, I feel it's my duty to beg you not to pursue such thoughts. The people of the United States didn't elect you to be their . . ." Parrish groped for the right term. "To be their crystal-ball gazer. They elected you to protect and defend the Constitution of the United States."

Hopkins looked at Parrish, deep disappointment in his eyes. "Larry, you sound like somebody from the *Washington Post.* I made my position perfectly clear during the campaign. Didn't we say we would seek God's will? That God is the ultimate defender of this nation and its Constitution? That's why we were elected."

"Sir, I understand that. But you're the president, and as such, you have clear duties. You took an oath of office—"

Hopkins cut him off. "Larry, you called me a crystal-ball gazer. But that's the farthest thing from what I'm doing. Don't you believe that Ezekiel was a prophet inspired by God? We can't just close our ears to those words and pretend they're irrelevant to this situation."

"No, sir. But when you're in this room, you represent all the people—Christian, Jew, Muslim, atheist. You can't let one view of Bible prophecy influence you. Your job is to protect the nation—and everyone's religious views. I mean, we're talking about war and peace, Mr. President, not church."

The president took off his watch. "Larry, I'm truly disappointed. It sounds to me like you've been blinded by people who want to keep God out of anything that truly matters. The way separation of church and state has been used is just a cover-up for secularization. I'm not trying to impose my view on anyone. It's not my view, Larry. It's what God has to say so clearly in the Bible. I do want to bring the wisdom of God into the conduct of our affairs. And if the wisdom of the Bible doesn't have anything to say about Israel, I guess I don't know a thing about the Bible."

Parrish was about to respond, but the president's phone beeped gently and a light flashed. Hopkins punched the speaker button hard.

"Sir," said his secretary's gentle voice, "Mr. Davies insists he must see you right away."

*   *   *

Alan Davies strode into the office two minutes later, his normally bland face glistening with perspiration, his bow tie askew. The president seemed glad for an excuse to break off the discussion with Parrish.

"What happened to you, Alan?" the president said jovially.

"Those vultures." Davies gestured in the direction of the Press Room. "They're after red meat. I couldn't get out. They were clawing me with questions."

"Tell me about it," the president said dryly. "And if you have any information about who leaked this business, I want to know."

"Yes, Mr. President," said Davies. "That's not my concern at the moment, however." He pulled a Queen Anne side chair up to the president's massive mahogany desk and began talking even before he sat down. "Ambassador Walker visited Arens an hour ago at his residence, conveyed your concern, and got no satisfactory response. Nothing. The old coot just sat there and said, 'You tell your president that Israel has never had a better friend than Shelby Hopkins.' That's the same thing they've been telling every president since Truman. Now, Mr. President, we need a tough note from you that I can telefax to Tel Aviv. It can be handed to Arens at 8:00 A.M. their time. I have a draft here, sir."

Hopkins put on his reading glasses and took the

sheet from Davies. His lips hardened as he quickly scanned it.

"Paragraph three will have to go. I will not threaten any kind of military action against Israel." Hopkins swept his pen angrily across the center of the page.

"You must, sir. It's all they'll listen to," Davies insisted.

"That goes against my deepest convictions." Hopkins glared over his glasses. "And this could be leaked and destroy my credibility. Furthermore, it's unnecessary. Moshe Arens is a friend and a reasonable man."

Davies started to protest, but Hopkins held up his left index finger and kept scratching on the paper, mumbling to himself as he wrote. "There. That's more like it." He leaned back and read through his revisions, then spun the piece of paper across the polished desktop.

"Will that do, Alan?"

Parrish knew Davies was steaming. Hopkins wrote well, often drafting his own speeches, but Davies wasn't looking for subtlety. He wanted a sledgehammer.

Davies also knew, however, how far Hopkins could be pushed. He shrugged slightly. "It may work, Mr. President. I'll have it typed up and returned at once for your signature." He inserted the paper into a green folder and left immediately.

"Larry," the president said, "I want you to handle Hartwell and Slocum for me. Tell them I've read their papers and I'm weighing the whole thing. Hold their hands a little and let them know they're important. Tell them . . . tell them I fully understand their feelings about Tzuria.

"Call me if anything important happens tonight. But only important matters, please. I'll trust your judgment. I'm going to be in the Lincoln sitting room after dinner. I want time to think and pray some more . . . and I may call Dean Roberts."

"Who's that, sir?"

"Dean Roberts? He's a great old man I've known for many years, a theologian of sorts. He's been president of the Mid-South Seminary for decades. A real saint. I've looked to him for wisdom often when I've been at my wits' end. When my oldest daughter was divorced, I must have called him a dozen times."

As Parrish began gathering up his papers, the president said, "Larry, I'm sorry I lost my temper with you. This has been a trying day, but that's no excuse."

"No problem, Mr. President. I probably had it coming."

"Oh, and one more thing, Larry. When you talk to Hartwell, see if you can find out where this leak came from."

7:00 P.M., the White House Situation Room

Parrish had a strong suspicion who had leaked the story, but he needed to confirm it and find out whether any other secrets were about to hit the fan. He descended the narrow staircase in the West Wing, moved past the basement security desk, then followed the long corridor toward the White House staff dining room. Beyond that he came to an unmarked door and entered the Situation Room, the Security Council nerve center.

Designed for use in World War II, the Situation Room bore little resemblance to its Hollywood counterparts. There were no flashing lights or electronic displays. It was merely a large room with open-office furnishings, strangely silent except for the gentle, steady hum of computers. Men and women moved about in tightly controlled frenzy, transporting the paper that continuously spit from printers.

Parrish entered the nondescript conference room in the center. On one wall was a blackboard, on another a global map, and on a third, a giant video screen used for conferences with the national military command center in the Pentagon. Parrish had chosen to talk to Hartwell and Slocum from here because it was absolutely secure. Soviet listening devices at their hilltop embassy in Washington could pick up most transmissions in the city, but this room was surrounded by an impenetrable electronic shield.

At precisely 7:00 Hartwell and Slocum appeared, full size, on the video screen. With stereo sound, the simulation was so real that participants soon forgot they were five miles apart. A puff of smoke trailing from Hartwell's mouth drifted lazily across the screen. When he realized the video was on, he stared directly at Parrish.

"I don't want to talk with you," he snapped. "I want to talk to the president. We need action. Tell him I must talk to him. We have critical new intelligence."

Parrish deliberately spoke in a soft tone, almost

too soft to hear. "The president understands the situation fully. He asked me to update you. He wants you to be fully informed at all times of our initiatives." He paused to let that sink in and then continued. "A very strong note signed by the president will be delivered to Arens first thing in the morning. We believe that once he realizes our displeasure, he'll reject Tzuria's offer."

"What're you guys smoking over there?" Hartwell exploded. "That's bull and you know it, Parrish. Words aren't going to stop Arens. We need action."

Parrish calculated quickly and decided to risk a slight evasion. "We'll know what we need soon. It's 4:00 A.M. in Jerusalem. In a few hours we'll have Arens's response. We can then proceed to other options as necessary." Hartwell began to interrupt, but Parrish raised his voice just enough to continue. "The president has read your option paper and has it fully in mind."

"What's that mean?" Hartwell asked sarcastically. "He's thinking about it? Don't run that White House we-know-it-all stuff at me, Parrish. Come tomorrow, we'll be in a dogfight. I guarantee it. You tell the president the task force'll be sixty miles off the coast, the Second Battalion Eighth Marines ready to go by tomorrow morning, seventeen hundred hours Jerusalem time."

"And we have an airtight op. plan," Slocum added. "We can secure the Temple Mount in thirty minutes from lift-off."

Parrish deliberately looked down at his fingernails until he had his anger under control. "Who authorized that?" he asked softly but forcefully.

"No authorization was necessary," Hartwell said. "Those are routine precautions—"

"Routine, my foot," Parrish snapped. "Hartwell, I know what you're up to. The president doesn't... yet. I haven't told him. But you should know you can't keep secrets from me."

"What are you talking about, Larry?"

"You know what I'm talking about. The leak. What a clumsy move." Watching closely, Parrish thought he saw Slocum flinch.

"Are you accusing me of leaking sensitive military secrets? Because if so—"

"Not me, Al." Parrish raised his hands in a gesture of peace. He knew Hartwell would like nothing better than a shouting match that blurred the issue. "No accusations here. Just mind me from now on. And listen to what I'm saying. You don't get your way with this president by pushing him into a corner. He'll push you right back. This leak has made a bad situation worse. It's distracting him. And it's fired up his fundamentalist brothers too. They've been calling him all day. So don't try anything with those ships and guns. I'm giving you the word right now: the policy of the United States government is that we will not interfere in the domestic affairs of our ally, the sovereign state of Israel. Period. Until you hear differently from here."

Hartwell blew a cloud of smoke over his right shoulder. "I know all that stuff the State Department puts out. By tomorrow the president will be more than grateful that we're ready for action when we have to be. So remember that, Larry, when tomorrow morning comes.

"Now look," Hartwell continued, narrowing his brown eyes slightly. "We've got something new. If the president won't talk to me, you better get this to him. You know we have a man in Arens's inner circle. And we now have absolute intelligence that the decision is made. There will be a deal; Arens will go along fully with Tzuria. And Arens doesn't for a moment believe that Hopkins will lift a finger. In fact, he believes that Hopkins is sympathetic with them." He paused, waiting for a reaction.

"Go on," Parrish said.

"So they'll move on the mosque. We don't know when, but soon. The Arabs will respond. Their honor's at stake. And the Russians, God forbid, may come in. I insist that you inform the president of this. As commander-in-chief, he must know."

"You're saying," Parrish repeated after taking a deep breath, "that the Arens-Tzuria deal is confirmed. You expect the mosque to be invaded shortly. Is that correct?"

"That's it."

"I'll inform him immediately," Parrish said. "I'll phone him from here. Call Alan Davies if anything changes." He punched a button and the screen went blank.

Parrish wanted to get outdoors and clear his head with some fresh air; he wanted to see his wife and kids. He had eaten only a sandwich for lunch—hours ago—yet he felt uncomfortably bloated. He reached for a telephone, but the operator couldn't put his call through. The president was still on the phone with Dean Roberts, she explained.

7:25 P.M., the Lincoln Sitting Room

"Dean, slow down, if you don't mind. I'm taking notes." The president was seated in a yellow brocade easy chair with the phone cradled against his ear. An open Bible lay on the table next to him.

"The first principle, if I might summarize, is that we must stand with the Jews, Genesis 12:3 . . . yes, yes . . ." He scribbled a sentence on a yellow legal pad propped against his right knee. "And it doesn't matter whether the Israeli government truly believes or whether they're nonbelieving militant nationalists. The point is that Israel today is the biblical nation to which Jesus returns."

At that point the door swung open. The Secret Service would admit only his wife or Parrish without advance permission, so Hopkins scarcely looked up.

"And point two, God has been kind to America because America has been kind to the Jews." The president motioned for Parrish to sit down. "And you say it is clear in Ezekiel and Daniel that the attack will come on Israel from Russia."

Parrish stared at the deep pile carpet. His stomach was beginning to churn. This conversation on top of the information Hartwell had just given him was making the ache in his stomach a dull, dead weight.

"So you believe the 1967 war was a signal—of sorts, that is—that God was declaring Israel's military victory over Jerusalem? I see. I see. I hadn't really thought about that before." Again Hopkins motioned for Parrish to sit down.

"Then point number four is that the Jews must redeem the land. Is that the word, Dean? Redeem? ...I see...I see. So rebuilding the Temple would be the final step, along with preaching the gospel to all the world....Well, we are certainly doing that with all our satellites and radio antennas."

He was writing furiously now. "Yes....Oh, I think I know all that pretty well. The rapture and the tribulation...and yes, right, Armageddon. Which would be just about the end of the story, right? I mean as far as *these* events are concerned." Hopkins was beaming, nodding his head at Parrish. "Well, Dean, I can't tell you how much this has helped me. I'm familiar with all this from my own reading and Bible study, of course, but you've given me a succinct summary. This puts it together step by step....Yes, Dean, you do that. Pray that God will give me wisdom.... I understand. Yes, call me if you have any leading of any kind. God bless you, Dean."

Parrish wished he could disappear before the president put down the receiver.

"That was my old friend, Dean Roberts," the president explained. "A brilliant mind. At eighty-three he's still razor sharp."

"Yes, sir," Parrish said.

The enthusiasm on Hopkins's face drained away slowly as he confronted his aide's grim expression. "Larry, don't 'yessir' me. Say what's on your mind."

"I don't know what's on my mind, Mr. President. Frankly, sir, you're scaring me to death."

"You mean that, don't you, Larry?" The president stood, half turned away, then whirled back to face him. "I didn't think anything could ruffle you. Tell me why."

"I don't know how to explain it, if you can't see it for yourself, sir," Parrish replied. "You're responsible for hundreds of millions of lives, including mine, including my wife and kids. And you seem to be guiding us by some obscure, kooky theory about the end of the world."

"What if the obscure, kooky theory happens to be true?"

"I'm happy to leave that decision up to God. The end of the world is His business. Our business here in the White House is to *prevent* the end of the world."

"Well, according to my theology, Larry, the end of the world—"

Parrish interrupted, something he never would have done had he not been deeply distressed. "Your theology is irrelevant right now! You weren't elected to be the nation's theologian."

Hopkins was visibly shocked by his aide's words. He turned and walked over to the window and looked out across the South Lawn at the Washington monument, floodlit against the darkened sky. "Larry, you remember what I said in the campaign: 'America needs a president who will speak for God as well as for the American people'? The people voted for me and for that. So maybe in a sense they did elect me their theologian."

"You know better than that, sir. Not five percent of them know what the word *theology* means. They elected you because you were moral and upright, have one wife, nice kids, and speak soothingly on TV. And they were fed up to here with anti-family, anti-God, anti-everything except the orca whale. So they decided to trust you, Shelby." Parrish had never before called the president by his first name. "They trust you. You can't betray them."

"But I only avoid that if I keep trust with God."

"Then keep us out of a war! Surely God did not put you here to cheer on the Israelis while they blunder into World War Three. Hartwell has information that Tzuria and Arens have reached an agreement. If we don't stop them with our marines, they'll destroy the mosque, probably within the next twenty-four hours. We have to move militarily or there'll be war."

"No," Hopkins said vehemently. "I will not lift a hand against God's chosen people."

"Then you shouldn't have taken that oath last year, Mr. President. You didn't promise you'd defend us against anybody but God's chosen people. You said you'd defend the Constitution—period. And by the way," Parrish said, looking at his watch, "the fleet will be off the coast of Israel in about twelve hours."

"Who ordered that?" Hopkins demanded, taking off his watch to chafe the inside of his wrist.

"Hartwell said it was a routine precaution."

"Routine, my foot."

"That's what I said. But at least it keeps your options open."

Hopkins accepted that with a grunt and dropped into the yellow chair again, stretching out his legs and running his fingers through his hair. "By the way, did you learn anything about the leak?"

Parrish hesitated. "Nothing solid, sir. But I suspect Hartwell was behind it."

The president accepted that too with a grunt, his mind obviously elsewhere. Parrish wondered whether he should leave.

"The truth is, Larry, I'm not sure what to think," Hopkins said gloomily. "You're talking political sense. And my Christian friends are talking another kind of sense. It's almost as though two worlds are colliding here, and I'm in the middle. I wouldn't say this to anyone but you, but maybe I just don't belong in this place."

For the first time, Parrish saw a hint of weakness in Hopkins's eyes, an almost pleading look.

"Larry . . ." The president's voice was tentative, hesitant. "Larry, how did we ever get into this mess?"

He sat forward, took a deep breath as if drawing on hidden reserves, and smiled. "Well, I guess we've done what we can for tonight. Arens will get my letter shortly. And the fleet, you say, is moving. Why don't you go home and spend some time with your family, Larry. It's been a long, frustrating day. Let's pray tomorrow is better."

3:00 A.M., Georgetown

The phone woke Parrish—the special secure phone. It rang five times while he tried to straighten the confusing shapes in his head; he was always slow to awaken. Finally his wife sat up in bed and turned on the light.

"Why don't you answer it?" she asked.

He picked up the receiver and heard Alan Davies's monotone. "Larry, the Soviets have put their Middle East forces on alert." He sounded as though he were reporting the daily amount of rainfall. "We received the first reports half an hour ago. I waited for confirmation before I called you."

"Thanks, Alan. What do you suggest?"

"The problem is to know what they're thinking. My best guess is that they're responding to our ships heading toward Israel. They've probably misinterpreted that as a sign of hostility."

By this time Parrish had fumbled a small notepad out of a drawer and was scribbling notes. His heart was pounding, and he had to force the edge out of his voice. The two men talked tersely for five minutes about possible options. When they finished, Parrish called the president.

Hopkins answered on the first ring; his voice sounded fresh and awake.

"Mr. President," Parrish began, "I must inform you that the Soviets have put their Middle East forces on alert." He waited through the silence, suddenly remembering that Hopkins had assigned the Soviets a role in biblical prophecy. Was the president hearing echoes of eternity in the news?

But the response was commonplace. "What are the Russians up to, then?"

"That's guesswork at this point, Mr. President. Davies's guess is that they've misinterpreted our fleet's movement toward Israel."

"Well, then, the first thing to do is to set their ambassador at ease, don't you think? Have Davies call their ambassador and tell him that our movements ought not to be misinterpreted as aggressive. Don't you think that's a good idea?"

"Yes, sir, I do. In fact, that was one thing Davies suggested."

"Then let's do it. What else did Davies have in mind?"

"He thought we should put our forces on alert in response. Just in case the Soviets have something aggressive in mind themselves. We want to be ready to respond."

"Yes, we surely do," the president said. "But might that too be misunderstood by the Soviets?"

"It could be," Parrish admitted. "We could cover that in our call too."

"Which assumes, doesn't it, that they believe what we say. Which, if they trust us as much as we trust them, isn't very likely. But we can't be caught with our pants down. Let's go on alert. And have Davies get on that call immediately. Anything else, Larry?"

"No, sir."

"No word on a response from Arens, is there?"

"Nothing so far."

"Well, let's all meet at 6:00 A.M. Make it the Oval Office—it doesn't matter now. Hartwell, Slocum, Lovelace, Davies, you, and me.... Larry, are you still scared? I've been praying for you and your family."

"Thank you, sir. No, I guess I'm not scared," he lied.

"Well, good. The Lord has been speaking to me,

telling me there is no need to be afraid. When this is all over, we're going to praise Him for the magnificent wonders He has wrought. Be of good courage. That's the Lord's message to us both."

7:15 A.M., the Oval Office

Alexander Hartwell stood before the president's desk and pounded on it with his fist. The cigarette in his hand trailed ashes across the carpet—the first cigarette in the Oval Office in fourteen months, Parrish thought as he watched in horrified astonishment.

"Mr. President!" Hartwell was almost shouting. "The marines are ready. They'll be in the air within sixty seconds if you say the word. I'm telling you, our information is absolutely certain. Tzuria has the okay from Arens. He'll move on the mosque if we don't get there first. And the Soviets have their blood up. You've got to move!" Hartwell punctuated his last words with two desk-shuddering blows.

The president stood to majestic height. "Hartwell, that's enough," he said in a splendid, controlled bass. "Go sit down. You've had your say."

To Parrish's surprise, Hartwell obeyed. As he sat down, he glanced at his cigarette as though surprised to find it in his hand. Parrish picked up a cup and saucer, and shoved it toward him. Hartwell ground out the cigarette.

"Now I'd like to hear what the rest of you think," the president said, sitting down again. "Come along," he urged, as his invitation was greeted by silence. "What are our options?"

Lovelace finally spoke. "Mr. President, I think the reason we're all sitting here like slugs is we've probably said what we have to say."

It was the first time Parrish had ever heard Lovelace say anything in one sentence. And Lovelace was right. They had been in the Oval Office since sunrise; they had talked themselves out. Everyone except Lovelace favored immediate military action, reasoning that there was no point in having a CIA if they couldn't trust information it said was firm. Lovelace wanted to wait for a definite response from Arens. But the president's note had been given to the Israeli leader almost eight hours before, and there was still no reply. Arens was holed up in his office and had put off the American ambassador repeatedly.

"Nobody wants to say anything else? That's amazing, isn't it? Who would have thought it? Silence from this group." Hopkins smiled wanly. "I'll tell you what I've decided then. I can't in conscience move our troops, with all the risks that entails, until I've heard from Arens. If he won't talk to our ambassador, I guess he'll have to talk to me. Alan, get Arens on the phone for me."

Hartwell exploded again, jumping to his feet. "That'll take time, and we don't have time. Let's at least get our men in the air. We can always recall them."

"No, no, I'm not ready to raise a hand against Israel," the president said decisively.

Davies got up and walked briskly out of the room.

Then the president began to talk, the music of

Texas in his voice, something that happened when he reached for his full eloquence. Using his big hands like a television evangelist, he tried pulling his listeners into his point of view, changing the shape of things by massaging the air. He took them back to the Christian Republican convention, recalling his acceptance speech and his promise to undergird his government in prayer. He told of the campaign, of the statement they had repeated from one end of the country to the other.

It is the plight of politicians, Parrish thought, to believe that words still make a difference when events are racing past them. Speeches like this one had gotten Hopkins to the White House. No wonder, when he didn't know what to do, he talked.

The president spoke of the meaning of Israel, how it embodied the hopes the Jews kept through the millennia. He quoted the Bible from memory. He recited America's enduring commitments, suggesting that America's great blessings were linked to its protection of the Jews. On and on and on he went. He could not seem to stop.

Suddenly the door burst open. "Mr. President," Davies announced, "the Dome of the Rock has been destroyed. One minute ago Israeli commandos blew it up!"

Hopkins, interrupted midsentence, stood with mouth open. Hartwell began to swear.

After a brief stunned silence, Slocum asked, "Any casualties?"

"Definitely. Hundreds of worshipers were in and around the mosque. There were Arab militants all around it too. How many, we don't know yet. Israeli troops are trying to seal the area.''

Parrish stood and walked to a wall cabinet. He opened the doors, switched on the large television set inside, and flipped across several channels. The morning talk shows were blathering on, still unaware of the event. But the picture on the Christian Broadcasting Company channel looked like something straight out of hell. Two broadcasting voices were talking on top of each other. The picture seemed out of focus or full of dust.

"That's the mosque," President Hopkins said in a low voice.

Out of the dust appeared two tiny blurred objects. The camera zoomed in on them. They were trucks. When they stopped, small dark particles seemed to scatter from them.

"They're deploying their men," said Slocum. "Throwing up a perimeter, I would guess."

"Extraordinary," murmured Lovelace. "I assume this is live?"

"Alan," said the president softly, "you weren't able to get Arens on the telephone?"

"No, sir."

They watched the picture for another minute. No more movement was discernible. Both broadcasting voices had stopped; the background sound was now a choir singing "The Battle Hymn of the Republic."

"What do you suggest we do, Alan?" the president asked.

Parrish thought he saw just a flicker of the earlier

how-did-we-get-into-this-mess look cross Hopkins's grim face.

"I think we'd better try to get General Secretary Kalganov on the telephone," Davies said.

The president nodded and turned to his desk.*

---

*Although this story is fictional, certain quotations attributed to Israeli and U.S. political and religious leaders have been taken from actual public statements; material regarding the takeover of the Temple Mount is also taken from public records.

PART

I

NEED FOR THE KINGDOM

ONE

Kingdoms in Conflict

> Men never do evil so completely and
> cheerfully as when they do it from
> religious conviction.
>
> —Blaise Pascal

> Without Christian culture and Christian
> hope, the modern world would come to
> resemble a half-derelict fun-fair, gone
> nasty and poverty-racked, one enormous
> Atlantic City.
>
> —Russell Kirk

"How did we get into this mess?" Our fictional president's anguished query echoes a cry heard across our country. For while this story of a decent, moral leader who lets the world slip to the brink of Armageddon would have seemed outrageous fiction just a few years ago, for millions today a similar scenario looms as a terrifying possibility. Equally disturbing to many is the realization that if this nightmare came true, millions of others would welcome it as a long-awaited consummation of human history.

These tensions run deep. On one side are those who believe that religion provides the details for political agenda. On the other are those who see any religious involvement in the public arena as dangerous. Not since the Crusades have religious passions and prejudices posed such a worldwide threat—if not through a religious zealot or confused idealist whose finger is on the nuclear trigger, then certainly by destroying the tolerance and trust essential for maintaining peace and concord among peoples.

Middle East terrorists, many religiously motivated, have spread panic throughout Europe and the United States. Ireland, Sri Lanka, India, and Indonesia are grim examples of nations deeply torn by sectarian strife. Jews, Muslims, and Christians alike endure horrendous persecution under oppressive Marxist regimes. In the West, church-state confrontations are multiplying. As one prominent sociologist observed, this strife "has little to do with whether the state espouses a leftist or rightist political philosophy";[1] the fires rage amid a variety of political systems.

Diverse as they may seem, these tensions all arise from one basic cause: confusion and conflict over the respective spheres of the religious and the political. What Augustine called the City of God and the city of man are locked in a worldwide, frequently bitter struggle for influence and power.

Nowhere has this conflict been more hotly debated than in America. Throughout most of its history, the U.S. has enjoyed uncommon harmony between church and state. The role of each was regarded as essential, with religion providing the moral foundation upon which democratic institutions could function. As recently as 1954 the Supreme Court explicitly rejected the contention that government should be neutral toward religion. Justice William O. Douglas stated that "we are a religious people whose institutions presuppose a Supreme Being."[2] But only nine years later, barbed wire was flung up on the "wall of separation" between the two as the court reversed itself in its landmark school-prayer decision. Though the expulsion of formal prayer from the schoolroom did not impede people's ability to talk to God wherever they wished, the decision reflected the shifting public consensus about the role of religiously based values in public life. It set off major tremors along long-dormant fault lines in America's political landscape.

At the same time the works of such writers as Camus and Sartre were enjoying enormous popularity on American college campuses. These existentialists argued that since there is no God, life has no intrinsic meaning. Meaning and purpose must be boldly created through an individual's actions, whatever they may be.

This relativistic view of truth perpetuated a subculture whose password was "do your own thing"— which for many meant a comfortable spiral of easy sex and hard drugs. Personal autonomy was elevated at the expense of community responsibility. Even as many pursued these new freedoms in search of fresh utopias, some acknowledged the void left by the vacuum of values. Pop icons like Andy Warhol spoke for the mood of a generation: "When I got my first TV set," he said, "I stopped caring so much about having close relationships . . . you can only be hurt if you care a lot."[3]

Liberal theologians eagerly adapted to the powerful trends of the day. Bishop Robinson's book *Honest to God*, published the same year as the school-prayer decision, gave birth to the God Is Dead Movement, popularized on the cover of *Time* magazine.

By the seventies, classical Judeo-Christian values were toppling as the fault line groaned almost daily. Religion was fast becoming an irrelevant, even an unwanted intruder in politics and public affairs. The Supreme Court often practiced what one dissenting justice in the school-prayer case had warned against: a "brooding and pervasive devotion to the secular and a passive or even active hostility to the religious."[4]

Roe v. Wade, the 1973 decision legalizing abortion, was the final blow for traditionalists. Not only was it seen as a rejection of America's commitment to the sanctity of life, but as a repudiation of moral values as a factor in court decisions. For the first time the justices excluded moral and philosophical arguments from their determination.

Roe v. Wade triggered a counterreaction, sending tremors from another direction. Determined to preserve moral values in the public sphere, conservative church members who had long disdained politics began organizing furiously; the Pro-Life Movement spread quickly across the country. By 1976 evangelicals were flexing their muscles behind a "born-again" presidential candidate. In 1979 a group of conservative Christian leaders met privately in Washington; the result was the Moral Majority and the Christian New Right. Within only six years this movement became one of the most formidable forces in American politics, registering millions of voters, raising vast war chests for select candidates, and crusading for its "moral agenda" with the fervor of old-time, circuit-riding preachers.

In 1984 the fault line broke wide open with a presidential campaign that resembled a holy crusade more than an election.

First, the Democratic candidate for vice-president, Geraldine Ferraro, questioned whether President Reagan was "a good Christian" because of his policies toward the poor.[5] Days later, the Catholic archbishop of New York challenged Mrs. Ferraro's faith because of her support for pro-choice legislation. At the Republican convention President Reagan told 17,000 foot-stomping partisans that "without God democracy will not and cannot long endure."[6] His Democratic challenger, former Vice-President Mondale, said that faith is intensely personal, should never be mixed up with politics, and that Reagan was "trying to transform policy debates into theological disputes."[7] Governor Cuomo of New York gave a widely heralded address at Notre Dame, in which he stated that as a Catholic he could personally oppose abortion, yet support it as governor as a "prudential political judgment," since he was following the will of the majority.[8]

In thousands of precincts across the country, fundamentalist ministers organized voter-registration campaigns, equating conservative political positions with the Christian faith. New Right spokesmen trumpeted the call for God, country, and their hand-picked candidates, and compared abortion clinics to the Nazi holocaust.

Civil libertarians reacted with near hysteria.

Some labeled Jerry Falwell an American version of the Ayatollah Khomeni. People of the American Way, a group organized to counter the Moral Majority, launched a slick media campaign attaching the Nazi slur to the religious right.

Never had religion become such a central issue in a presidential campaign; never had the church itself been so dangerously polarized.

The fissures that broke open in 1984 remain wide and deep today. On one side are certain segments of the Christian church, religious conservatives who are determined to regain lost ground and restore traditional values. "America needs a president who will speak for God," proclaimed one leader. Whether out of frustration or sincere theological conviction, the Christian New Right has become politicized, attempting to take dominion over culture through legislation and court decisions.

Those on the other side are no less militant. Believing Christian political activists will cram religious values down the nation's unwilling throat, they heatedly assert that faith is a private matter and has no bearing on public life. The *New York Times*, for example, accused Ronald Reagan of being "primitive" when he publicly referred to his faith: "You don't have to be a secular humanist to take offense at that display of what, in America, should be private piety."[9]

The real tragedy is that both sides are so deeply entrenched that neither can listen to the other. Invective and name calling have replaced dialogue. Nothing less than obliteration of the enemy will suffice; either Christianize or secularize America. Many citizens feel that they must choose sides; either enlist with Norman Lear and People of the American Way, or join up with the Moral Majority (now the Liberty Federation) and the Christian New Right.

No matter how we got to this point, the fact is that both extremes—those who want to eliminate religion from political life as well as those who want religion to dominate politics—have overreacted and overreached. Theologian Richard John Neuhaus does not overstate the case when he argues that this confrontation can be "severely damaging, if not fatal, to the American democratic experiment." Furthermore, both exclusivist arguments are wrong.

There is another way, however. It's a path of reason and civility that recognizes the proper and necessary roles of both the political and the religious. Each respective role is, as I hope this book will demonstrate, indispensable to the health of society.

Wise men and women have long recognized the need for the transcendent authority of religion to give society its legitimacy and essential cohesion. One of the most vigorous arguments was made by Cicero, who maintained that religion is "indispensable to private morals and public order . . . and no man of sense will attack it."[10] Augustine argued that the essence of public harmony could be found only in justice, the source of which is divine. "In the absence of justice," he asked, "what is sovereignty but organized brigandage?"[11]

In the West the primary civilizing force was Christianity. According to historian Christopher Dawson, Christianity provided a transcendent spiritual end which gave Western culture its dynamic purpose. It furnished the soul for Western civilization and provided its moral legitimization; or, as was stated somewhat wistfully in the *London Times* recently, "The firm principles which could mediate between the individual and society to provide both with a sense of proportion and responsibility in order to inform behavior."[12]

The American experiment in limited government was founded on this essential premise; its success depended on a transcendent reference point and a religious consensus. John Adams wrote, "Our constitution was made only for a moral and religious people. It is wholly inadequate for the government of any other."[13] Tocqueville credited much of America's remarkable success to its religious nature; it was later called a nation with "the soul of a church."[14]

Today, increasing numbers of thinkers, even those who reject orthodox faith, agree that a religious-value consensus is essential for justice and concord. Polish dissident Adam Michnik, who describes himself as a "pagan," applauds the church for resisting tyranny. Religion, he says, is "the key source of encouragement for those who seek to broaden civil liberties."[15] To disregard the historic Western consensus about the role of religion in culture is to ignore the foundation of our civilization.

But men and women need more than a religious value system. They need civic structures to prevent chaos and provide order. Religion is not intended or equipped to do this; when it has tried, it has brought grief on itself and the political institutions it has attempted to control. An independent state is crucial to the commonweal.

Both the City of God and the city of man are vital to society—and they must remain in delicate balance. "All human history and culture," one historian observed, "may be viewed as the interplay of the competing values of these ... two cities";[16] and wherever they are out of balance, the public good suffers.

This is why today's conflict is so dangerous. It would be a Pyrrhic victory indeed should either side win unconditionally. Victory for either would mean defeat for both.

*   *   *

I have brooded over this dilemma since the mid-seventies. My concerns deepened each year as the conflict intensified between the body politic and the body spiritual. A variety of questions plagued me: To what extent can Christians affect public policy? Is there a responsible Christian political role? In a pluralistic society, is it right to seek to influence or impose Christian values? How are the rights of the nonreligious protected? Are there mutual interests for both the religious and the secular? Is it possible to find common ground? What does the experience of history say to us today? What would God have us understand about this torn and alienated world—or, considering the mess we've made, has He given up on us?

Friends urged me to write on the subject since I've been on both sides—first, as a non-Christian White House official, and now as a concerned Christian citizen. But the task always appeared too daunting. I couldn't sort out all the questions raised in the blistering American debate. Both sides seemed hopelessly intractable.

Oddly enough, it was on a visit to India in the fall of 1985 that I came to the unmistakable conviction that I must write this book.

At a friend's home in New Delhi, I listened to shocking stories of conflict between Indian Christians and their society. One young man who was converted to Christ after reading Christian tracts had been forced to leave his rural village by his outraged family. Another man who had been preaching on the street was cornered and beaten by an angry crowd. Many others, after converting to Christianity, had been tried by civil authorities.

The same day I was in New Delhi, opposition leader Charan Singh called upon Prime Minister Gandhi to "stamp out" all Christian missionaries lest their converts in certain states seek political independence.[17] Why, I wondered, is there such hostility to one faith in this Hindu culture that believes all roads lead to heaven? They should be the most tolerant of all. What is it about the Judeo-Christian message that makes it so offensive? Ironically, the Indians may understand the heart of the gospel—that Christ is King, with all that portends—better than many in the "Christian" West.

Later that day as my flight lifted off for Bombay, I looked down on New Delhi, which was shrouded in a dense smog from the open cooking fires of its crowded streets. Then, as we broke through to the blue sky above, it was as though the clouds surrounding these issues also broke open for me. I began to see the struggle in America—and around the world—

more clearly than ever before.

So it was high in the skies between New Delhi and Bombay that I first wrote, "The kingdoms are in conflict, both vying for ultimate allegiance. Not just in America, but around the world. By his nature man is irresistibly religious—and he is political. Unless the two can coexist, mankind will continue in turmoil. Tragically, we have lost sight of both the nature of man and the nature of God and His rule over the world."

To put it simply, humanists—using that term in its best sense—fail to understand humanity and Christians fail to understand the message of Christ.

Men and women have always been spiritual beings. But modern culture, in its zeal to eliminate divisive influences and create a self-sufficient, "enlightened" society, has ignored this fundamental truth. Along with denying God, today's social visionaries have denied man's intrinsic need for God. At the same time, Christianity has become a pale shadow of the radical Kingdom its Founder announced.

The shock waves that threaten the very foundations of our culture today, then, emanate from society's failure to understand man's need for God and the Christians' failure to accurately present Christ's message of the Kingdom of God. So before we can hope to deal with the modern religious-political conflict, we must take what at first may seem to be a digression. But bear with me. For until we understand the true nature of man and the true nature of Christ's message, we cannot hope to understand the story of President Hopkins and why we are in the mess we are in today—or, more importantly, the way out.

The place to begin, then, is with human nature itself. We'll start with a man who embraced the spirit of the twentieth century and lived it to its logical conclusion.

After the Feast

*Our Nada who art in nada, nada be thy
name thy kingdom nada thy will be nada
in nada as it is in nada. Give us this nada
our daily nada and nada us our nada as
we nada our nadas and nada us not into
nada but deliver us from nada; pues nada.
Hail nothing full of nothing, nothing is
with thee.*

> —*"A Clean, Well-Lighted Place"*

The last party went on that entire summer. Papa
had come to Spain to relive memories from earlier,
happier days. He delighted in the rough red Spanish
wines, the fresh flowers of the countryside, the uproar of the *fiera*. He ran with the bulls in Pamplona
and crisscrossed the country following his favorite
bullfighters, hanging over the edge of the ring in his
barrera seat, tanned and squinting in the sun and
dust, cheering the skill of the matadors. He loved the
moment of death: the immense bull, thrusting and
dancing with the slim figure of the matador; the glit-
tering sword raised high in the air above the deadly
horns; and finally the blade plunging deep between
the animal's shoulders. Sometimes, when the bull
could not be killed with the sword, the matador used
a short knife, or *puntillo*. "I love to see the puntillo

used," Papa would say happily. "It is exactly like turning off an electric light bulb."[1]

After the bullfights came the midnight feasts with the matadors and a variety of guests. American college coeds who had hesitantly approached Papa for his autograph suddenly found themselves swept into the party, mingling with Hollywood stars and Papa's old friends from the Spanish Civil War. They clustered around him, toasting his health, laughing at his stories.

That summer of 1960 was Papa's last happy time before the depression set in. It was as if he had gathered all his forces—the friends, the wine, the feasts, the women, the bullfights—for one final tribute to the things that had filled his life so well over the years. The highlight was his sixtieth birthday party, a grand event designed to make up for all the birthdays that had slipped by while he was pursuing lions on safari, marlin off Key West, or lime daiquiris at his favorite Havana bar. Even if the passing of years was no great pleasure for Papa, the fact that he had survived to sixty was cause for celebration.

Guests arrived from the corners of Spain, from Paris, Washington, and Venice. The party began at noon on July 21 at a friend's seaside estate in Malaga. Mary, Papa's wife, had imported champagne from Paris, Chinese food from London, a shooting booth from a traveling carnival, fireworks and flamenco dancers from Valencia. An enthusiastic Spanish orchestra played on the balcony.

Papa declared it the best party ever. He danced through the house, a champagne glass in one hand, shotgun in the other. As the evening spilled on, he entertained guests by shooting cigarettes from the pursed—and presumably drunken—lips of two guests, the Maharajah of Cooch Behar and Antonio Ordonez, Spain's premier bullfighter. When the fireworks erupted, cheers resounded through the estate, and Papa led his guests in the *riau-riau*, the festive dance of the bullfights.

Evening spiraled into dawn, and at noon the next day the last guest staggered home. Before going to bed Papa plunged into the ocean, swimming in long, steady strokes parallel to the shore. A friend swam beside him. As they emerged from the water, Papa said with a sigh, "What I enjoyed most is that these old friends still care enough to come so far. The thing about old friends now is that there are so few of them."

Papa had made hundreds of friends over the years, collected everywhere he had lived and worked. He had lost many as well, abruptly cutting ties with those who disappointed him by being weak or dishonest. With his grizzled white beard, barrel chest, and baggy clothes, he was a man's man who in his fame had become almost a caricature of himself: the world traveler equally at home in Spain, France, Italy, Cuba, Idaho; the mighty big-game hunter of African lion, elephant, kudu. He had collected many women as trophies as well and had married four of them.

Papa started collecting adventures early. Born in Illinois in 1899 into a staunchly religious home, he had escaped during World War I to drive ambulances for the Italian Army. He was nineteen and relished the sweat, the blood, the spectacle of it all. Later a critic would write that he had been born twice—once in Oak Park, then born again to the reality of death on the Italian battlefields of Fossalata.

A few days after he volunteered for frontline duty, an Austrian mortar landed almost on top of him. The man it did hit disintegrated. Papa was severely wounded. He felt life begin to slip from his body "like you'd pull a silk handkerchief out of a pocket by one corner."

But he survived, even carrying a wounded comrade to safety, and spent half a year convalescing in Italian hospitals and back home in the States. (As the years went by, his wounds would continue. Plate glass sliced his head in Paris; a car crash crushed him in London; two plane crashes in Africa left him wounded and burned; boating accidents off the coast of Cuba resulted in concussions.)

After recovering from his war wounds, Papa became a journalist, writing crime stories in Chicago and feature stories in Toronto. He married and decided that Paris was the best place to refine his craft. For first and foremost Papa was a writer. Journalism had given him clean declarative sentences and the beginnings of a style; Paris was to provide a feast of experience that would last the rest of his life.

Papa wrote in cafés of the city. Using a stubby pencil and a small notebook, sipping a *café au lait*, he transformed his experiences into stories. When a story was done, he leaned back and splurged on a carafe of crisp white wine and a dozen oysters fresh from the sea, feeling empty and happy as if he had just made love.

Paris in the twenties had become a haven for

writers and artists, and Papa was friends with many of them: Pablo Picasso, James Joyce, Gertrude Stein, Ezra Pound, F. Scott Fitzgerald. From these fellow expatriates, Papa learned how to write dialogue and refine his style. Of their philosophy he learned little, for the prevailing mood already matched his own. Papa had long since given up on the orthodox faith taught in his childhood—what he called "that ton of [manure] we are all fed when we are young." God was irrelevant, if He existed at all. The measure of a man's life was what he did—his experiences, actions, his courage in the face of death. Life was a wine glass to be filled to the brim and relished.

Papa's books of short stories and first novel brought him recognition, success, and granted him the freedom to pursue what suited him best: writing hard, loving hard, eating and drinking well, war, the hunt, and the bullfight.

When the writing flourished, he exuded a vitality, a sense of keen enjoyment that others could not help but admire.

But beneath that fulfillment was a vacuum that sometimes sucked him under. All his life Papa suffered bouts of depression—he called it "Black Ass." As long as there was another fiesta, another party, another good day's work ahead of him, the depression eventually lifted.

But in the end, when he had nothing with which to fill his life, it didn't.

By 1961 Papa had high blood pressure and diabetes. He was overweight and tired of dieting. His liver was corroded from alcohol. He was no longer able to function like a man's man. He had mental problems.

After all, Papa told a friend, "What does a man care about? Staying healthy. Working good. Eating and drinking with his friends. Enjoying himself in bed. I haven't any of them—none of them." Maybe the time had come, he thought.

Papa felt he had already died. After watching the failure, years earlier, of a once-great matador, he had said, "The worst death for anyone is to lose the center of his being, the thing he really is. Retirement is the filthiest word in the language. Whether by choice or by fate, to retire from what you do—and what you do makes you what you are—is to back up into the grave."

For even as he had danced with death over the years—he called it "that old whore"—he believed that when it came time to take her upstairs, that was his choice and his right. What else could a man control in his life if not the time and means of his death? His own father had killed himself years earlier.

If God existed, He might be fair reason to reject the whore; but if not, nothing made much difference after all. Papa had given up on God long before. Taking his life would prove he was master of his own fate.

What interested him most was how to do it. Dying, he said, was easy; it meant "no more worries." But a real man would die "intelligently, the way you would sell a position you were defending . . . as expensively as possible, trying to make it the most expensive position ever sold."

*　　　*　　　*

Papa woke up early that Sunday morning, put on his red robe, and padded down the carpeted stairway of his Idaho home, which faced the magnificent Sawtooth Mountains. His wife knew he wanted to make his assignation, so she had locked his hunting guns in the basement. But she had left the keys on the window ledge above the kitchen sink. Perhaps she felt she had no real right to keep Papa from his choice.

He got the keys, went down the basement stairs, and unlocked the dark storage room. He chose a custom-made twelve-gauge Boss shotgun, inlaid with silver, which he had used for years to shoot pigeons. It was his favorite gun—not just a firearm, but a near-sacred object. He selected ammunition, locked the door, and climbed back up to the bright living room.

In the front foyer, a five-by-seven entryway walled with oak, he pushed a shell into each barrel and carefully lowered the gun butt to the floor. He stooped slightly, took a deep breath, and placed the cold metal inside his mouth. Then he tripped both triggers.

Thus did Ernest Hemingway give in to death's seduction. His work and his pleasures were gone; his once-full life had emptied. With no God, it was up to him to assert control over the one thing he still could—his own death.

His immediate legacy was the ruin of blood, bones, teeth, and hair that his wife found blasted onto the foyer walls that sunny morning, July 2, 1961. The legacy of his writing and his philosophy lives on.

In one sense Ernest Hemingway is the quintessential twentieth-century man. Born the year before the century began, he experienced its rapid advance of technology and depersonalization, its growing faith in science and government, and its declining belief in orthodox religion.

The week after the shotgun blast heard throughout the literary world, *Time* magazine reflected,

> Though he was leery of metaphysical systems, Hemingway was really on a metaphysical quest...a tenacious observer of the crisis in belief and values which is the central crisis of Western civilization.... Hemingway's "ingenuous nihilism" was early set, but...[if] life was a short day's journey from nothingness to nothingness, there still had to be some meaning to the "performance en route." In Hemingway's view, the universal moral standard was nonexistent...[so] he invented the Code Hero, the code being what we have instead of God.[2]

Hemingway was never far from his characters. He extended the drama of his books and stories into the stream of his own life—or vice versa: "The characters Hemingway creates drink everything, see everything, feel everything, do everything. Life to them is a chain of varied links, each different, each exciting and uniquely interesting, and the last link is the largest and most interesting of all, the link of death."[3]

And why not? If Hemingway and his existential friends who frequented the cafés of Paris were correct, their code is reasonable and even heroic. If this life is merely a glass to fill, when the glass is emptied, why not smash it against the living-room wall?

As Hemingway's friend Jean-Paul Sartre put it, "On a shattered and deserted stage, without script, director, prompter, or audience, the actor is free to improvise his own part."[4]

This view sounds both reasonable and romantic in literature or discussions in cafés and coffee bars. But the prospect in real life is stark. Among those who "tie a lamp to the masthead and steer by that" when "the stars are quenched in heaven,"[5] few take their existential belief to the ultimate conclusion. For this comfortless doctrine shreds the very fibers and design of the human psyche.

We need more. And most of us—deep down—cannot deny it. There is a core of truth buried in every heart, a truth that we can't escape.

Papa Hemingway thought he had when he consciously resisted it. The man in the next chapter knew he couldn't.

THREE

Crossing the Rubicon

*The heart has its own reasons which
Reason does not know; a thousand things
declare it. I say the heart loves the
universal Being naturally, and itself
naturally, according to its obedience to
either; and it hardens against one or the
other, as it pleases.... The heart has
reasons which Reason can never know.*
                              —Blaise Pascal

The rumpled middle-aged man checked the lock on the solid-iron security door of his apartment, then headed toward his office at Cable News Network's Beirut Bureau. Cool Mediterranean breezes rippled the dust of the street as he rounded the corner from his cul-de-sac and turned onto Rue Bliss.[1]

The dark expressive eyes held concern. Late last night there had been shooting between rival Muslim and Christian militia along the Green Line, the barrier dividing East from West Beirut. There had also been reports of scattered shooting in the mountains. *I hope the camera crew's okay,* he thought. He had sent them to the front in the south with a local guide.

He was also thinking about yesterday's surprising announcement. The leaders of Lebanon's major political factions had agreed to meet the following

Monday in Switzerland for a reconciliation conference. *Doubt if it'll make any difference,* he thought. *Reconciliation seems out of the question here.* Even the American-sponsored peace treaty between Lebanon and Israel was in danger of being cancelled. Syria was making headway in forcing Lebanon to end the agreement designed to keep the PLO out of an already chaotic Lebanon.

The light tap on his shoulder startled him. He turned and a short bearded man in his early twenties pushed a green handgun into his stomach, propelling him toward a small gray car pulling up to the curb. The back door gaped open. He didn't struggle when his assailant shoved him into the back seat and jumped in behind him.

"Close eyes. Close eyes," the man shouted, waving the revolver as the car sped away. "You see, I kill."

Life in Beirut before that clear March morning in 1984 had been exhilarating for Jerry Levin and his wife Sis. They had seen his assignment as Middle East bureau chief as a new adventure and had not been disappointed. Though the fifty-one-year-old newsman regularly put in fourteen- and fifteen-hour days reporting on the political situation, he relished the challenge of trying to unravel the enigma of Lebanon.

For her part, Sis had willingly interrupted her classes at the University of Chicago's divinity school and enrolled in the Near East School of Theology in Beirut. Typical of her enthusiasm, she had plunged into Arabic lessons, found the local Episcopal church, and made friends with the neighbors in their apartment building. Sis had already received several elegant invitations for teas and soirees, all neatly lettered with the disarming clause, "situation permitting."

Once the seaside Paris of the Mediterranean, Beirut was now a maze of gun emplacements, armed checkpoints, and patrolling militiamen. The civil war that began in 1975, the Israeli invasion of 1982, and the increasingly provocative rule by the Christian minority that had spurred the Shiite Muslim and Druze takeover of West Beirut just a few weeks earlier had all created chaos. No individual or military presence had been strong, willing, or able enough to impose order. Bombings, political assassinations, and kidnappings were the norm.

Jerry Levin was just one more victim.

Jerry and his colleagues at CNN had talked about the possibility of kidnapping. You couldn't live in Beirut with its almost daily "situations" without at least having it cross your mind. Now, the gun digging into his back was a sharp reminder that he had underestimated the reality. Jerry Levin was scared.

His captors had blindfolded him, but once they reached their destination, he could vaguely make out the shapes of shadowy figures who shoved guns up under the blindfold. They accused him of being a CIA agent, an Israeli spy, or a defender of the American foreign policy designed to eliminate them and their political goals. After several hours of inquisition they gagged him, wrapped him in heavy packing tape, and threw him in the back of a truck.

Jerry used all his senses to try to track their route. They had left Beirut and were climbing mountain roads that eventually stretched into level highways. They must have driven about two and a half hours. Jerry had studied maps of the area; he guessed they were in the Bekaa Valley, northeast of Beirut, somewhere near its main city, Baalbeck, and that his kidnappers were militant Shiite Muslims who favored the establishment of an Iranian-styled theocratic republic in Lebanon. He was correct on both counts.

When they stopped, he was led into a building and shoved into a room. There they shackled his right arm and leg to a radiator. Then they left. Jerry waited, listened. He was alone.

He lifted his blindfold and blinked, not so much from the light—the blindfold wasn't that impenetrable—as the reality of the situation. The room was tiny and bare except for the narrow foam-rubber mattress he was sitting on. The one small window had been painted over. His arm and leg were secured to the wall by a bicycle-length chain that stretched only enough for him to sit or lie on his left side. He turned and with his free hand carefully scratched a tiny mark on the dingy wall. Day one.

The days passed in a blur of monotony and fear. Once a day his guards led him to the bathroom next door. That was the outer limit of his world for months. Otherwise, he was alone in his small room.

At first Jerry willed himself to think only pleasant thoughts. He blotted out his situation by reliving his first meeting with Sis. He saw her smile at him across the ballroom of an elegant opera party in Alabama. He pictured family and friends. He created long lists of major-league baseball teams and players. It took three days to mentally list every opera he had ever seen—all ninety-eight of them. He envisioned resplendent scenes from his favorites, playing out such roles as Floristan, the political prisoner in Beethoven's *Fidelio*. Chained to the wall in the depths of a dungeon, he sang, "God! This is miserably dark. How horrible the silence, here in my lonely cell." At the end of the aria Floristan's wife, Leonore, came to save him. "I see her. An angel. She leads me to freedom and heavenly life." Jerry imagined Sis rescuing him from his Lebanese prison.

All his escape routes led back to his prison. The labyrinth of his memories could take him only so far. The bicycle chain held him fast to dismal reality.

He lost weight. His back and left shoulder ached from the cramped position. Then the scary thing happened: he began talking to himself. That worried him. *I'm going crazy*, he thought. *But if I don't talk to myself, I'll go crazy anyway.*

What if he talked to someone besides himself? People had been talking to something they called God for several thousand years and hadn't gone crazy. Rabbis did it. Priests did it. Lots of different kinds of people did it. Maybe he could too.

No.

He had no right to talk to God unless he believed in God. He couldn't talk to someone who didn't exist. "If one-millionth of one percent of me doubted, then—I reasoned—I really would not be talking to God; but I would be doing what I was afraid would happen after all—be talking to myself. So I would go crazy anyway."

Jerry had long been an atheist, or perhaps an agnostic. It was a toss-up. His Jewishness was more a cultural than religious force in his life, but he had long since dismissed Christianity as irrelevant. Sis was a Christian, and though he respected the strength of her faith, it held no appeal for him. To him Christianity called up childhood memories of neighbors' rural country churches in Michigan, musty smells, faded lace doilies—a quaint, American-Gothic experience that had little to do with his fast-paced urbane life. And besides, what about the Christian persecution of Jews, the Inquisition, the atrocities committed in the name of Christ?

Hunched on his foam-rubber mattress, Jerry remembered as best he could the scene from Dostoyevski's *Brothers Karamazov* in which the story is told of a village in Spain during the Inquisition. As he recalled it, Christ Himself returns to the town and begins preaching the gospel. The Grand Inquisitor has Christ thrown into prison, then sentences Him to be burned at the stake. "We can't survive on these teachings," says the Inquisitor. "What you're saying is seditious as far as the church is concerned." Then he pauses and suddenly orders that Jesus be released. "Say all you want," he concludes. "It won't make any difference anyway."

I keep coming back to choices, Jerry thought. Believe God or don't believe. Reject Jesus for His followers' perversions of the faith He taught, or accept Him as the Son of God because of His incredible "extrahuman" life and teachings. Days went by.

Jerry's mental struggle continued.

"It was a cosmic Catch-22, definitely not something to be fooled with. Ten days after my meditating began, on April 10, 1984, I approached and then crossed a kind of spiritual Rubicon, a diminishing point in time, a shrinking thousandth, then millionth of a second, on one side of which I did not believe and then on the other side I did."

When he crossed that line, things began to make sense. For example, he had always thought of Jesus' teaching about forgiveness as incredibly tacky, wimpy, and weak-kneed. Now, in his solitary cell, Jerry saw that "the bully with the gun is the wimp. The man who says go ahead and shoot is not." His first prayer was for Sis and his family. Then these words came out: "God, please forgive men like these—like I'm doing now—because they are in part responsible for bringing me to You and Your Son." He learned to forgive his captors even as he saw more clearly their bitter rage and desperation.

The hostile, bitter men who were holding him had actually done God's work. God had used their bondage to get his attention. *After all*, he thought, *why else would a middle-aged grandfather be sitting in his underwear here in a bare little room in Lebanon, chained to a wall?*

Within a few months, Jerry was moved to a different house. There he was allowed to use the bathroom unaccompanied. When he was ready to leave, he had to tie his blindfold back on and knock on the door. Then his captors would lead him back to his room next door.

As the spring and summer passed, he heard the

knocks of other hostages being shuffled in and out of the bathroom. The terrorists must have rounded up more Americans for bargaining chips.

In July he understood for the first time why he was a hostage. Looking into the lens of a video camera, he was forced to read a statement written by his captors, appealing to Ted Turner, founder of Cable News Network, to urge the U.S. government to intercede with the government of Kuwait to free the prisoners there. "My life and freedom," said Jerry's message, depended on the "life and freedom of the prisoners in Kuwait."

The prisoners were seventeen Shiite Muslims convicted of bombing the United States and French embassies in Kuwait in December 1983. Six people had been killed, eighty others wounded. Three of the men had been sentenced to death, the others to long prison terms. Some of Jerry's kidnappers were relatives of these prisoners.

Jerry was certain the U.S. government would never make such a deal. Again he was faced with a choice. Should he try to escape? The youths guarding him had been careless with his chains on several occasions. Would it happen again? He needed to be ready.

The opportunity he had been praying for finally came on February 13, 1985. About midnight he worked his way out of the chain. He tied three thin blankets together and climbed through the window onto the balcony. He then secured the blankets on the railing and lowered himself to the ground. He couldn't let himself even think about the fact that he was free. He zigzagged down the mountain as fast as he could, tripping over loose stones, his heart pounding.

As he neared the bottom, a dog began to bark. The refrain was picked up by dozens of others. Then he heard voices in the dark. He threw himself under a parked truck. Guns fired into the air; lights pointed in his direction. They had caught him.

When he crawled out, however, he saw not his kidnappers, but Syrian soldiers. He began babbling in a mixture of English and French. The soldiers agreed to help, and within thirty-six hours Jerry Levin stepped off an airliner in Frankfurt, West Germany. He walked straight into Sis's waiting arms.

It was then he learned that for eleven and a half months Sis had been practicing what he was just learning. Praying passionately for him, she had traveled to the Middle East with a radical message of forgiveness and reconciliation. Behind the scenes she was helped by Christian, Muslim, and Jewish friends. One Muslim leader in Beirut had told her that never in a thousand years had so many people of different faiths worked together on behalf of one man.

"The irony," says Jerry Levin today, "is that they thought they were working for someone who was a godless man. They could not have known that the skeptic had become a reconciler himself.

"I am convinced now that none of us is ever really godless. I know now that He is always there for us whether or not we are there for Him."

FOUR

Faith and the Evidence

Now it is our preference that decides
against Christianity, not arguments.
                              —Friedrich Neitzsche

Experiences like Jerry Levin's are frequently described as foxhole conversions. Maybe so. My own conversion in the midst of Watergate certainly was greeted with skepticism. The cartoonists were busy for months with caricatures of Nixon's tough guy turned to God. But fourteen years later I can write that I, like Malcolm Muggeridge, am more certain of the existence of God than I am of my own.

I understand, however, how people can listen sympathetically to stories like Levin's or mine and still doubt. Just because we need God does not prove He exists. This was, of course, Sigmund Freud's central point: that religion perseveres because people need it. "A theological dogma might be refuted [to a person] a thousand times," he wrote, "provided, however, he had need of it, he again and again accepts it as true."[1]

The influential German philosopher Ludwig Feuerbach believed that God was made in the image of man, a creation of the human mind projecting man into the universe. And Karl Marx saw religion as nothing more than an opiate used by the powerful to tranquilize the exploited masses.

If these arguments are correct, then today's battle over the role of religion relates to the need for a psychological prop. If we create God for our individual needs and to civilize culture, then the secularist is right: religion is merely a personal illusion and has no place in political affairs.

But if there is strong objective evidence for the existence of God, if He is not a psychological prop but a fact, then we are dealing with the central truth of human existence. And if that is the case—if He exists—then God's role in human affairs, or religion's role in public life, is indeed the most crucial issue of this or any age.

So while it may seem an intrusion, please join me briefly as I relate a few of the evidences of God's existence and character that I have found convincing. For without such evidence, there is no point in your reading this book—or my writing it.

It was the very question of God's existence that created the most serious stumbling block to my own conversion. That August night in 1973 when my friend Tom Phillips first told me about Christ, I told him that I wanted no part of foxhole religion. And though later I tearfully called out to God, my mind still rebelled. I needed to know: Was this simply an escape from the trouble I was in? Was I having some sort of emotional breakdown? Or could Christianity be real? I needed evidence.

I started with the copy of *Mere Christianity* that Tom had given me. In C. S. Lewis's book I confronted powerful intellectual arguments for the truth of Christianity for the first time in my life.

The existence of God cannot be proved or disproved, of course, but the evidence can be rationally probed and weighed. Lewis does so compellingly, and he cites moral law as a key piece of evidence. Clearly it is not man who has perpetuated the precepts and values that have survived through centuries and across cultures. Indeed, he has done his best to destroy them. The nature of the law restrains man, and thus its very survival presupposes a stronger force behind it—God.

Or consider the most readily observable physical evidence, the nature of the universe. One cannot look at the stars, planets, and galaxies, millions of light years away, all fixed in perfect harmony, without asking who orders them.

For centuries it was accepted that God was behind the universe because otherwise "the origin and purpose of life [would be] inexplicable."[2] This traditional supposition was unchallenged until the eighteenth century's Age of Reason, when enlightenment thinkers announced with relief that the origins of the universe were now scientifically explainable. What we now call the "big bang theory" rendered the God hypothesis unnecessary.

Although this theory has captured the imagination of many, it leaves serious questions unanswered. Who or what made the big bang? What was there before it? And how in the big bang process—

a presumably random explosion—did planet earth achieve such a remarkable, finely developed state?* William Paley, the eighteenth-century English clergyman, told what has become a well-known parable on this point. A man walking through a field discovers first a stone, then an ornate gold watch. The stone, the man may reasonably conclude, has simply always been there, a sliver of mineral chipped from the earth by chance. But the watch, which has beauty, design, symmetry, and purpose, did not just happen. It had to have been made by an intelligent, purposeful Creator.

Some have asserted that the universe was self-generated. This violates, however, a primary law of logic: the law of noncontradiction that says the universe cannot be itself *and* the thing it creates at the same time.

Others simply state that the universe itself is self-existent and infinite; it has always been. Yet modern science has discovered no element in the universe that is self-existent.† Granted, the whole can be greater than the sum of the parts, but can it be of a different character altogether? Clearly not.

Nonetheless this is the view widely expressed

---

*The big bang thesis is not by itself antithetical to the Christian biblical view. Professor Owen Gingerich, noted Harvard astronomer, frequently lectures on the "strange convergence" between the biblical and modern scientific explanation of the universe's origin. He relates the scientific evidence for the so-called big bang event to the biblical affirmation that the universe flashed instantly into existence in a great showering of light. Gingerich believes, however, that science deals strictly with the question of "how," while the biblical account addresses the equally critical question of "who."

†A tentative theory exists today with respect to quantum physics that may raise questions about this conclusion.

today, most popularly by Carl Sagan, who proposes that "the Cosmos is all that is or ever was or ever will be."[3] That is simply another way of saying that the universe itself is transcendent. Though Sagan's films and books are widely used in schools as science, his argument is, in fact, only theory. It is also no more than an acknowledgment that we do not know how the universe began.

At one point or another even the most obstinate atheist or agnostic must deal with this question of first cause.

During the Watergate scandal, though a new Christian, I approached one of my colleagues to offer spiritual help. "No thanks," he replied. "I'm a rationalist." He tapped his head and said, "It's all in human will. I've thought it all through." He was a confirmed atheist and proud of it.

Since that time I've watched this man not only survive but recover remarkably. He served his prison term without apparent ill-effect, wrote memoirs, built a successful business, and kept his family intact. If anything, he appeared stronger for the ordeal.

Then, a few years ago, I learned that he was reading Christian literature. I wrote to him, and he replied that he was indeed seeking. "I'm now an agnostic," he wrote. "I can no longer be an atheist, for I cannot get by the question of the first cause— that is, how life began. The scientific rationales are simply irrational."

Even if modern scientific theories provided satisfactory explanations for the origin of the universe, however, the question of the origin of man would still be unanswered.

The prevailing view of Sagan and others is that a chance collision of atoms created life; subsequent mutations over thousands of years evolved into the extraordinarily complex creature we know as man.

If this is true, man is nothing more than an accident that started as slime or, as one theologian has put it, we are but grown up germs. Our intuitive moral sense rejects such a trashing of human dignity.

Interestingly enough, even modern scientific research is beginning to question some of its own theories. Given the laws of probability and even allowing for the oldest possible dating of the universe, they ask, has there been enough time for life to begin by random chance and for as utterly complicated a creature as man to evolve?*

_____

*A *Washington Post* article by Eugene F. Mallove, an astronautical engineer, science writer, and Voice of America broadcaster, noted that "some cosmologists are proposing that the universe has been perfectly 'designed' for life in a way that could not have happened 'by chance.'...There is an infinity of ways that the universe could have been set up that would have been more 'simple,' with fewer improbable coincidences....Of course in almost any of these 'simpler' universes, the odds for the development of anything as complicated as life—no matter how you imagined it—would be nil." Eugene F. Mallove, "The Universe as Happy Conspiracy: There are Too Many Coincidences for Life to Have Happened by Chance," *Washington Post* (October 27, 1985), B 1–2.

Actually such odds may indeed be nil. The French mathematician, Lecompte de Nouy, examined the laws of probability for a single molecule of high dissymmetry to be formed by the action of chance. De Nouy found that, on an average, the time needed to form one such molecule of our terrestrial globe would be about 10 to the 243 power billions of years.

"But," continued de Nouy ironically, "let us admit that no matter how small the chance it could happen, one molecule could be created by such astronomical odds of chance. However, one molecule is of no use. Hundreds of millions of identical ones are necessary. Thus we either admit the miracle or doubt the absolute truth of science." Quoted in "Is Science Moving Toward Belief in God?" Paul A. Fisher, *The Wanderer* (November 7, 1985).

Weighing the evidence, it is not unfair to suggest that it takes as much faith, if not more, to believe in random chance as it does to believe in a Creator. One can understand why no less a scientist than Albert Einstein, though not of an orthodox faith, felt "rapturous amazement at the harmony of natural law, which reveals an intelligence of such superiority that compared with it all the systematic thinking and acting of human beings is an utterly insignificant reflection." Einstein's belief in the harmony of the universe caused him to conclude, "God does not play dice with the cosmos."[4]

Scientific arguments also fail to take man's basic nature into account: we are imbued with a deep longing for a god. Even an obstinate unbeliever like philosopher Bertrand Russell wrote,

One is a ghost, floating through the world without any real contact. Even when one feels nearest to other people, something in one seems obstinately to belong to God, and to refuse to enter into any earthly communion—at least that is how I should express it if I thought there was a god. It is odd, isn't it? I care passionately for this world and many things and people in it, and yet . . . what is it all? There *must* be something more important, one feels, though I don't *believe* there is.[5]

When people try to suppress their essential nature, they must either admit the haunting desire for a god, as did Russell, or deal with the inner turmoil through their own means, often with disastrous consequences. Hemingway chose the latter course, as, for that matter, did Marx, Nietzsche, and Freud.

Near the end of their lives they were all bitter and lonely men. Nietzsche's insanity, many believe, was due as much to the despair of nihilism as to venereal disease. Freud could not be comforted after his daughter's death, as if he was grieving at the finality of life without God. In his last days Marx was consumed with hatred. All these men were simply reaping the logical consequences of their own philosophies.

But even should we concede that man just happened, and that he creates his own need for God, how do we explain his need for purpose? Consistent evidence points not only to man's deep spiritual longings, but to a purposeful nature in his desire for community, family, and work.

The great Russian novelist Fyodor Dostoyevski said that not to believe in God was to be condemned to a senseless universe. In *The House of the Dead* he wrote that if one wanted to utterly crush a man, one need only give him work of a completely irrational character, as the writer himself had discovered during his ten years in prison. "If he had to move a heap of earth from one place to another and back again— I believe the convict would hang himself . . . preferring rather to die than endure . . . such humiliation, shame and torture."[6]

Some of Hitler's henchmen at a Nazi concentration camp in Hungary must have read Dostoyevski. There, hundreds of Jewish prisoners survived in disease-infested barracks on little food and gruesome, backbreaking work.

Each day the prisoners were marched to the compound's giant factory, where tons of human waste and garbage were distilled into alcohol to be used as a fuel additive. Even worse than the nauseating odor of stewing sludge was the realization that they were fueling the Nazi war machine.

Then one day Allied aircraft blasted the area and destroyed the hated factory. The next morning several hundred inmates were herded to one end of its charred remains. Expecting orders to begin rebuilding, they were startled when the Nazi officer commanded them to shovel sand into carts and drag it to the other end of the plant.

The next day the process was repeated in reverse; they were ordered to move the huge pile of sand back to the other end of the compound. *A mistake has been made*, they thought. *Stupid swine.* Day after day they hauled the same pile of sand from one end of the camp to the other.

And then Dostoyevski's prediction came true. One old man began crying uncontrollably; the guards hauled him away. Another screamed until he was beaten into silence. Then a young man who had survived three years in the camp darted away from the group. The guards shouted for him to stop as he ran toward the electrified fence. The other prisoners cried out, but it was too late; there was a blinding flash and a terrible sizzling noise as smoke puffed from his smoldering flesh.

In the days that followed, dozens of the prisoners went mad and ran from their work, only to be shot by the guards or electrocuted by the fence. The commandant smugly remarked that there soon would be "no more need to use the crematoria."

The gruesome lesson is plain: Men will cling to

life with dogged resolve while working meaning-
fully, even if that work supports their hated captors. But purposeless labor soon snaps the mind.

You might argue that our need to work was acquired over centuries of evolution. But we must do
more than work just to survive; we must do work
that has a purpose. Evolution cannot explain this.
More plausible is the belief of Jews and Christians
that man is a reflection of the nature of a purposeful
Creator.

But for those who insist that God is created by
man, perhaps the most telling argument is to consider
the nature and character of the God revealed in the
Bible. If we were making up our own god, would we
create one with such harsh demands for justice, righteousness, service, and self-sacrifice as we find in the
biblical texts? (As someone has said, Moses didn't
come down from the mountain with the Ten Suggestions!)

Would Israel's powerful elite have concocted
such declarations as, "He defended the cause of the
poor and needy . . . Is that not what it means to know
me?"[7] Would the pious New Testament religious establishment have created a God who condemned
them for their own hypocrisy? Would even a zealous
disciple have invented a Messiah who called His
followers to sell all, give their possessions to the
poor, and follow Him to their deaths? The skeptic
who believes the Bible's human authors manufactured their God out of psychological need has not
read the Scriptures carefully.

But can we rely on the biblical accounts? you

may ask. When I first became a Christian, I certainly raised such questions. In fact, I began to study the Bible with a lawyer's skepticism. I suspected it was a compilation of ancient fables that had endured through the centuries because of its wisdom.

I made some startling discoveries, however. The original documents from which the Scriptures derive were rigorously examined for authenticity by early canonical councils. They demanded eyewitness accounts or apostolic authorship. Today, a growing body of historical evidence affirms the accuracy of the Scriptures. For example, the prophecy recorded in Psalm 22 explicitly details a crucifixion, with its piercing of the hands and feet, disjointing of the bones, dehydration. Crucifixion, however, was a means of execution unknown to Palestine until the Romans introduced it—several hundred years after the Psalms were written. So modern critics concluded the Psalms were written later, such "prophecies" perhaps even recorded after the fact. Then came the discovery of the Dead Sea Scrolls, which made possible the scientific dating of portions of the Psalms to hundreds of years before Christ.*

Modern technology and archeological discoveries are also adding substantial support to the his-

---

*Similarly, modern critics insisted there was no Hittite empire, since the only references to the Hittites were found in the Bible. But earlier this century the great Hittite civilization of ancient Asia Minor was discovered. Today no scholar would deny the authenticity of the Hittite civilization.

torical authenticity of Scripture.* As historian Paul Johnson has written, "A Christian with faith has nothing to fear from the facts."[8]

But sometimes personal experience offers the most convincing evidence. As I have written elsewhere, it was, ironically, the Watergate cover-up that left me convinced that the biblical accounts of the resurrection of Jesus Christ are historically reliable.

In my Watergate experience I saw the inability of men—powerful, highly motivated professionals—to hold together a conspiracy based on a lie. It was less than three weeks from the time that Mr. Nixon knew all the facts to the time that John Dean went to the prosecutors. Once that happened Mr. Nixon's presidency was doomed. The actual cover-up lasted less than a month. Yet Christ's powerless followers maintained to their grim deaths by execution that they had in fact seen Jesus Christ raised from the dead. There was no conspiracy, no passover plot. Men and women do not give up their comfort—and

---

*Researchers in Israel, for example, after subjecting the first five books of the Bible to exhaustive computer analysis, came to a different conclusion than expected.

The Torah, or Books of Moses, had long been assumed by skeptics to be the work of multiple authors. But Scripture scholar Moshe Katz and computer expert Menachem Wiener of the Israel Institute of Technology analyzed the book's material through sophisticated computer analysis. They discovered an intricate pattern of significant words concealed in the canon, spelled by letters separated at fixed intervals. Mr. Katz says that the statistical possibilities of such patterns happening by chance would be one to three million. The material suggests a single, inspired author—in fact it could not have been put together by human capabilities at all. Adds Mr. Wiener, "So we need a non-rational explanation. And ours is that the [Torah] was written by God through the hand of Moses." From an Associated Press news story in the *Washington Times* (July 18, 1986), D-5.

certainly not their lives—for what they know to be a lie.

Finally, many of the world's greatest philosophers and scientists have gone beyond deductive assent to the confidence that God exists because they have experienced Him. Were Augustine, Aquinas, Luther, Newton, and the great social reformers of the nineteenth century victims of infantile wish fulfillment? Did some psychological whim motivate St. Francis or George Fox to expend their lives in protest against economic elitism? Was Louis Pasteur, who labored against great physical handicaps to achieve scientific breakthroughs to benefit man, simply mistaken in his motivation to do so for the glory of God?

What is it that motivates people, both Christian and nonbeliever, to do works of mercy? The goodness of the human heart? Hardly. Man's basic nature, as we shall see in the next chapter, suggests just the reverse. Rather, love for others, like the need for purpose, is implanted in the hearts and minds of men and women—even those who don't acknowledge it—by a loving and purposeful Creator.

Faith requires no surrender of the intellect. It is not blind, unthinking, and irrational. Nor is it simply a psychological crutch. For me, the objective evidence for God's existence is more convincing than any case I argued as an attorney.

But most rebellion against God is not intellectual. I have met few genuine atheists who would argue passionately that there can be no God. Instead, the preponderance of objections are moral and personal. Before his eventual conversion, when philosopher Mortimer Adler was pressed on his reluctance to become a Christian, he replied,

> That's a great gulf between the mind and the heart. I was on the edge of becoming a Christian several times, but didn't do it. I said that if one is born a Christian, one can be light-hearted about living up to Christianity, but if one converts by a clear conscious act of will, one had better be prepared to live a truly Christian life. So you ask yourself, are you prepared to give up all your vices and the weaknesses of the flesh?[9]

It is on the moral level that the most intense battle is being fought for the hearts of modern men and women. If Hemingway and the twentieth-century skeptics are right—if God is dead or irrelevant—then the prospect for true harmony and justice is grim.

Sometimes children understand this profound truth better than adults. Several years ago my son Chris and I were discussing the evidences for God. As I argued that if there were no God, it would be impossible to account for moral law, my grandson Charlie, then four, interrupted.

"But Grandpa," he said, "there is a God." I nodded, assuring him I agreed.

"See, if there wasn't a God, Grandpa," he continued, "people couldn't love each other."

Charlie is right. Only the overarching presence and provision of God assures that both Christian and non-Christian enjoy human dignity and a means to escape our naturally sinful condition. Without His presence, we could not long survive together on this planet.

FIVE

Neither Ape nor Angel

> They that deny God destroy man's
> nobility; for certainly, man is akin to the
> beasts by his body; and if he be not of kin
> to God by his spirit, he is a base and
> ignoble creature.
>
> —Francis Bacon

In Aleksandr Solzhenitsyn's masterful novel *The Cancer Ward*, a young, cancerous political prisoner named Oleg finds momentary escape from the hospital's horrors in an attractive nurse, Zoya.[1] One day Oleg volunteers to help Zoya with her reports. Reading from patient records, Oleg notices hardly any deaths in the hospital.

"I see they don't allow them to die here," he says. "They manage to discharge them in time."

"What else can they do?" responds Zoya. "Judge for yourself. If it is obvious a patient is beyond help and there is nothing left for him but to live out the few last weeks or months, why should he take up a bed?...People who could be cured are kept waiting...."

Days later, one of Oleg's gravely ill friends is told he is being released from the hospital. The man struggles to dress, weakly bids adieu to his comrades, and sets out for the streets. The best he can hope for is an empty bench where he can lie down and wait to die.

This account may be cruel, but it is not illogical.

The Soviet system is committed to the eradication of any vital practice of religion. God is officially dead there. But the death of God ultimately spells the death of what it means to be truly human. For if worth is not God-given, it must be established by man. And atheistic philosophies, such as the Soviet system, treat man as an object whose value is determined solely by his usefulness to society. Why not, then, subject him to whatever will achieve the government's objectives: oppression, torture, genocide? In utilitarian terms, sending terminal patients out to die is not inhumane, but eminently sensible. Why waste a bed on someone who will not survive?

Now contrast *The Cancer Ward* with the wards of Mother Teresa. For years this faithful nun has provided shelter and help for the homeless, the sick, the poor; for AIDS patients dying in pain, afraid and alone. Sometimes she is criticized: "Why care for those who are doomed anyway?" But she explains, "They are created by God; they deserve to die with dignity." Christianity can never be utilitarian; it holds every human being as precious because human beings are created in the image of God.

To understand the unique nature of this Judeo-Christian view, we need only compare the ancient Hebrew law codes in the Old Testament with, say, the Assyrian laws of Hammurabi, another Middle Eastern legal code from the same period. Historian

Paul Johnson has noted that the Assyrian code made the rights of property ultimate, while "the Hebrew [laws] emphasized the essential rights and obligations of man, and their laws were framed with deliberate respect for moral values."[2]

Jesus continued—and expanded—the Old Testament law. He constantly affirmed the dignity and worth of the lowest members of first-century society—women, children, Gentiles, tax-collectors, lepers.

Today's clamor for human rights is ironic. Much of the activism emanates from those who claim no belief in God. But consider what many who have had a major influence on modern thinking believed.

Karl Marx, for example, thought man a victim of economic forces. Sigmund Freud believed all was lost in the dark web of the psyche. B. F. Skinner insisted that freedom was an illusion and dignity a lost cause. More extreme philosophers get downright angry at the snobbery of speciesists—those of us who see man as the highest species—and assert that man enjoys no special standing in the universe. A prominent bioethicist writes:

We can no longer base our ethics on the idea that human beings are a special form of creation, singled out from all other animals, and alone possessing an immortal soul. Once the religious mumbo-jumbo has been stripped away, we may continue to see normal members of our species as possessing greater capacities ... than members of any other species; but we will not regard as sacrosanct the life of each and every member of our species.... Species membership alone ... is not morally relevant.[3]

In this light, human dignity and human rights are tenuous assertions. If man is merely a fortuitous collection of molecules in a meaningless cosmos, why should he have any inherent rights?

Spinoza once observed that man builds his kingdoms in accord with his concept of God.[4] The rise of atheism in the twentieth century has thus provided unlimited license for tyrants. If there is no morally binding standard above the state, it becomes god and human beings mere beasts of bureaucratic burden. A government cannot be truly just without affirming the intrinsic value of human life.

The Judeo-Christian ethic does more than affirm human dignity, however; it also insists that we are inclined to do evil. Man is more than a beast, but he is not an angel. This dual nature is not properly understood apart from what theologians call *original sin*.

No modern parable portrays man's sinful nature more powerfully than Nobel prize-winning author William Golding's novel *The Lord of the Flies*, in which a planeload of English schoolboys is wrecked on a tropical island.[5] Good British subjects that they are, they attempt to organize themselves into an orderly society while awaiting rescue.

But darker urges soon grip the boys. The veneer of civilization melts away, and many of them revert to savagery, first as a game, then in deadly earnest.

One of them wounds a boar. Suddenly, "the desire to squeeze and hurt was overmastering." Soon the boys are chanting with ritualistic fervor, "Kill the pig! Cut his throat! Bash him in!"

A sow is caught and killed in a primitive sacrifice, the head cut off and placed on a post, allegedly to assuage the "beast" some of the boys have encountered. Great black and iridescent green flies buzz insistently around the severed head. The boys' "chieftain" giggles as he rubs his bloodied hands on the next boy's face.

The young savages soon turn on a fat, asthmatic, bespectacled lad nicknamed Piggy, who retains more civility than they care to have on their island. "Which is better," Piggy asks plaintively as they advance on him, "to have rules and agree, or to hunt and kill?"

Moments later, Piggy is knocked off a cliff. His skull cracks open, his arms and legs twitching. Eventually the pounding waves suck his body into the sea.

Piggy's friend Ralph collapses in a spasm of grief. "With filthy body, matted hair, and unwiped nose, Ralph wept for the end of innocence, the darkness of man's heart, and the fall through the air of the true, wise friend called Piggy."

Later, when the group is rescued, a shocked naval officer asks how such savagery could have happened. "I should have thought that a pack of British boys—you're all British, aren't you?—would have been able to put up a better show than that—I mean . . ."

Civilization, empire, education, all of the trappings of human progress had clothed these young innocents. Now, their faces smeared with blood, their consciences apparently inoperative, they bear the guilt of the death of two playmates.

When William Golding was awarded the Nobel Prize for Literature in 1983, the Swedish Academy declared that his novels "illuminate the human condition in the world today." They reflect as well what Golding described as "an attempt to trace the defects of society back to the defects of human nature. The shape of a society must depend on the ethical nature of the individual and not on any political system, however apparently logical or respectable."[6]

Golding's views sound grimly anachronistic in a culture constantly heralding man's ability to achieve utopia through modern science, education, and technology. This notion was given impetus by, among others, Jean-Jacques Rousseau, the Enlightenment writer who insisted that human misery was rooted in the structures of society. Change the structures and you change the man, he said.

Rousseau looked to primitive human experience as a rosy time of innocence free of socially induced vices. From the beginning of man's history, however, we see not guilelessness, but betrayal and evil. After the account of the Garden of Eden the Bible tells the story of the first four people on the planet—and before long, one of them killed his brother. This first murder was committed long before urban blight and social deprivations. There were—and are—no noble savages.

Human nature has not changed since Cain. This is vividly illustrated in the memoirs of Cuban poet Armando Valladares, *Against All Hope*, in which he recounts his twenty-two-year imprisonment by Fidel Castro for speaking out "against Communism because it went against my religious beliefs and some of my more idealistic notions of the world.'" For such treason, Valladares was thrown into the man-made hell of a Cuban prison. He was given showers of human urine and excrement by sadistic guards. During an escape attempt he broke three bones in his leg and was captured and brought back to his cell. "Guards . . . stripped us again," he writes.

> They were armed with thick twisted electric cables and truncheons. Suddenly, everything was a whirl—my head spun around in terrible vertigo. . . . The beatings felt as if they were branding me with a red-hot branding iron, but then I suddenly experienced the most intense, unbearable, and brutal pain of my life. One of the guards had jumped with all his weight on my broken, throbbing leg.[8]

One cannot read this and explain the torture, the sadism, and the evil only in terms of godless political systems. The problem is human nature. The only progress between Cain and the Communist jailers of Armando Valladares has been the technological sophistication of cruelty.

Given the wealth of such examples today, why is it so difficult for modern man to acknowledge the inherent evil in the human heart? Why is sin an outmoded term, used only by Bible-thumping preachers, born-again zealots, or the titillating covers of paperback thrillers?

English historian Paul Johnson contends that the great obstacle to modern belief in human sin began with the loss of belief in individual responsibility. Coupled with the ascendancy of Freud's theories and

Marxist ideologies, collectivism encouraged the belief that "society could be collectively guilty in creating conditions which made crime and vice inevitable. But personal guilt-feelings were an illusion to be dispelled. None of us was individually guilty; we were all guilty."[9]

This misreading of the nature of man, which resulted in the denial of personal responsibility, was institutionalized into various social reforms in the sixties; these contributed markedly to the social pathologies of American inner cities. Charles Murray of the Manhattan Institute for Policy Research has noted: "What many of these reforms shared (in varying ways and degrees) was an assumption that people are not in control of their own behavior and should not properly be held responsible for the consequences of their actions. The economic system is to blame; the social environment is to blame; perhaps accidents and conceivably genetics are to blame."[10]

Any effort to encourage individual initiative and responsibility among America's urban poor was derided as "blaming the victim." Blaming the system rather than the "victim" further eradicated individual responsibility and dignity. As Polish philosopher Leszek Kolakowski wrote: "I remember seeing on American television a young man who was convicted of brutally raping a child, a little girl; his comment was, 'Everybody makes mistakes.' And so, we now know who raped the child; 'everybody,' that is, nobody."[11]

This elimination of individual responsibility has encouraged the corresponding utopian belief in man's collective perfectibility. While Christian teaching emphasizes that each person has worth and responsibility before God, utopianism argues that salvation can only be achieved collectively. Mao Tse-tung could assert, therefore, that "our God is none other than the masses of the Chinese people."[12] And in the name of that god, millions of Chinese people were deprived of their lives.

Utopianism always spells disaster because "the utopian holds that, if the goal is goodness and perfection, then the use of force is justified," as Thomas Molnar writes.[13] In contrast, the Christian realization that perfection eludes us in this life resists the tyranny and bloodshed of the dictator who promises a brave new world.

Thus, twentieth-century men and women have inherited a stark dilemma. With God dead or ill, they are stripped of their source of dignity and reduced to sophisticated beasts. At the same time, society denies individual sin, blaming all social ills on environment, and illogically assumes human perfectibility.

Both propositions run counter to the evidence of history. Man is neither ape nor angel. And as Jerry Levin and countless others have experienced, deep down inside we know we are created. We desperately long to know the Power beyond us and discover a transcendent purpose for living. We long as well to shed the guilt of sin, to be free people, forgiven in the sight of the God we know is there.

Many search for Him through bizarre spiritual journeys, attested to by the popularity of Eastern religions and tabloid psychics, reincarnation, Beverly Hills gurus, crystals, cosmic energy, seaweed, and channeling. Such counterfeits only intensify frustration—and lessen belief in any God at all. And sometimes the end of the journey is gruesome and shocking, like the piles of bodies at Jonestown.

Diverted from the one source that can provide meaning and a sense of worth and responsibility, modern men and women are left to thrash about for themselves. Their frustration inevitably deepens into despair. For some, like Hemingway, who accept the logic of this age, the despair turns to tragedy; for millions of others it fosters a brooding sense of alienation and helplessness.

And so we come full circle, back to where we began. For it is this pervasive sense of impotence that has paved the way for the emergence of political saviors and the all-powerful state that promise salvation through changed structures. Before we discuss our situation today, though, we need to make one more stop. Having looked at the nature of man, we must now look at the nature of the two kingdoms in which he lives.

We can do this by stepping back to a time that bears a striking parallel to our day: Palestine in the first century, where a volatile population eagerly awaited the long-expected political Messiah who would deliver them.

PART

II

ARRIVAL
OF THE
KINGDOM

SIX

King Without a Country

My kingdom is not of this world.
—Jesus Christ

Two thousand years ago Palestine was (as it is today) a land in turmoil, its two and a half million inhabitants bitterly divided by religious, cultural, and language barriers. An unlikely mix of Jews, Greeks, and Syrians populated the coastal towns and fertile valleys of the ancient land, and tensions among them often erupted in bloody clashes. Rome did little to discourage this volatile bitterness. As long as the people's passions were spent on each other, they weren't being vented on their conquerors.

Among these disparate groups, the Jews alone had hope for the future, for they clung to the promise that a Messiah, sent from God, would one day come to set them free. According to their Scriptures, this savior would bring swift judgment to Israel's oppressors and triumphantly reestablish the mighty throne of the great King David. "The God of heaven will set up a kingdom that will never be destroyed," the prophecies said.

Some Jews were not content to wait and hope, however. Small groups of incendiaries, known as Zealots, mapped political strategies for supremacy, including terrorist plots and assassinations. Rome responded with deadly force.

In the midst of this oppression and chaos, a rumor began to spread. It harked back thirty years to a time when stories had circulated about angelic visitations attending the birth of a peasant child named Jesus in the village of Bethlehem. The child had grown up in Nazareth, a dusty stopping place on the caravan route to Damascus, where He had learned the carpentry trade from His father. Now stories about this Jesus were igniting the countryside. Apparently He had abandoned His carpentry tools and was going about preaching a spiritual message and gradually amassing followers. There had even been reports that He had supernatural powers.

Early one Saturday morning Jesus returned to Nazareth to speak in the synagogue. His friends and relatives and neighbors gathered in great excitement. They had watched Him grow to manhood; they knew His parents, Mary and Joseph. So they were astonished at His air of authority as He strode to the center of the crowded stone room and was handed the book of the prophet Isaiah from the Torah shrine. He found the passage He wanted, then read the ancient prophecy: "The Spirit of the Lord is on me, because he has anointed me to preach good news to the poor. He has sent me to proclaim freedom for the prisoners and recovery of sight for the blind, to release the oppressed, to proclaim the year of the Lord's favor."[1]

Jesus handed the Scriptures back to the attendant and stared quietly at the rows of townspeople. "Today," He said slowly, "this scripture is fulfilled in your hearing."

At first there were gasps, then excited murmurings. Was Jesus claiming that their hopes were to be realized? Had the long-dreamed-of day of the Lord— the coming of Messiah—arrived?

Then one of the elders called out sarcastically, "Isn't this Joseph's son?" Others laughed. After all, this young man was merely a hometown boy, a carpenter and the son of a carpenter. What could He know of Messiah?

Jesus knew what they were thinking. "No prophet," He said steadily, "is accepted in his hometown." Then He reminded them of two stories they knew well from their heritage: During a great drought, the prophet Elijah had brought water not to the dying widows of Israel, but to a heathen widow; and his successor Elisha had ignored Jewish lepers and cleansed a Syrian instead.

His words were like a dash of cold water in the faces of the crowd. They expected liberation for the Jews and judgment for all others. Now this arrogant young man was extending the long-awaited promise of their liberation with one hand and insinuating their own judgment with the other.

The crowd surged forward and dragged Jesus out of the building, shoving Him to the brow of the hill on which the synagogue perched. But when they reached the edge, they discovered that in the confusion, Jesus had slipped away.

This humble message at the remote Nazareth synagogue was the inaugural address for Jesus' entire ministry. Through it He formally announced His messiahship and the rule of God in this world. As a result, human history was forever altered.

The Kingdom of God had come.

* * *

I've used this message of human liberation from the Gospel of Luke countless times as the centerpiece of my message to prisoners. "He has sent me to proclaim freedom for the prisoners . . . to release the oppressed. . . ." It speaks of men and women set free by the good news of the gospel. Not until I began to research this book did I understand its wider significance.

Of all the Scriptures Jesus might have read, He chose the one that unmistakably announced the coming of the Kingdom of God. Furthermore, the listening Jews understood that in this particular passage of Isaiah, the one speaking is the messenger—the Messiah who ushers in the Kingdom era. To those in that synagogue, Jesus' words could only mean that He was claiming to be the Messiah. And if that was true, the Kingdom of Heaven had become a present reality.

One reason I, like many others, missed this deeper meaning of Christ's radical declaration is that I had always read the term kingdom metaphorically. Like the Jews in that Nazareth synagogue, most of us think of kingdoms as geographic entities, physical realms with boundaries and defenses and treasuries. But the Kingdom of God is a rule, not a realm. It is the declaration of God's absolute sovereignty, of His total order of life in this world and the next.*

Throughout His ministry Jesus repeatedly returned to the Kingdom theme. In the Sermon on the Mount, He told His followers to "seek first his kingdom and his righteousness."[2] He consistently defined His work as ushering in the Kingdom of God. Almost all of His parables focused on the Kingdom in one aspect or another, while His miracles authenticated His message. In converting water to wine, calming storms, multiplying loaves and fishes, healing the sick, and raising the dead, Jesus was not working magic to gather crowds; nor was He showing His power to gain credibility. He was demonstrating the reality of His rule. By exercising dominion over every phase of earthly existence, He revealed that in fact the Kingdom of God had come.

The Jews of first-century Palestine missed Christ's message because they, like many today, were conditioned to look for salvation in political solutions. More than anything else they wanted to be set free of Roman rule. They longed for a military messiah who would stamp out their hated oppressors. It is not surprising, then, that support for the Zealots was widespread.

The Zealot political vision was too narrow, however; for Jesus to embrace it would have been to limit the Kingdom of God to Israel. Though, ironically,

---

*That this Kingdom is not of this world, as Jesus later explained, and that it is spiritual rather than temporal makes it no less authoritative; that it is a rule not a realm makes it no less an actual kingdom, nor its laws less binding than those of nations and states, any more than unseen physical laws are less binding than the laws of legislatures.

Jesus was later tried and convicted as a Zealot, He dashed the hopes of those whose narrow political expectations blinded them to His real message.

The same could be said of the Jewish hierarchy. They might have welcomed Jesus because of their messianic expectations. Instead, they jealously guarded their own arrogant, self-righteous interpretation of the Jewish law, as well as the limited autonomy the Romans had given them.

Palestine's factions were embroiled in a struggle over the political and religious future of a limited ethnic group confined and defined by geographic borders. In pointing to a far larger Kingdom, Jesus was a leader without a constituency. Even His closest followers had times of doubt.

Another reason that the Jews missed the full significance of the message of the Kingdom of God was that Jesus spoke about a Kingdom that had come and a Kingdom that was still to come—one Kingdom in two stages. This still confuses people today. Perhaps a contemporary analogy will make it clearer.

Probably the most significant event in Europe during World War II was D-Day, June 6, 1944, when the Allied armies stormed the beaches of Normandy. That attack guaranteed the eventual destruction of the Axis powers in Europe. Though the war continued with seeming uncertainties along the way, the outcome was in fact determined. But it wasn't until May 8, 1945—VE Day—that the results of the forces set in motion eleven months earlier were realized.

We can compare this two-stage process to the strategy of the Kingdom of God.

A holy God would not take dominion over a

sinful world. So He first sent His Son, Jesus Christ, to die on the cross to pay the debt for man's sin and thereby provide for men and women to be made holy and fit for God's rule. To extend our war analogy, Christ's death and resurrection—the D-Day of human history—assure His ultimate victory. But we are still on the beaches. The enemy has not yet been vanquished, and the fighting is still ugly. Christ's invasion has assured the ultimate outcome, however— victory for God and His people at some future date.

The second stage, which will take place when Christ returns, will assert God's rule over all the universe; His Kingdom will be visible without imperfection. At that time there will be a final judgment of all people, peace on earth, and the restoration of harmony unknown since Eden.

Many soldiers died to bring about the victory in Europe. But in the Kingdom of God, it was the death of the King that assured the victory. And this leads to the third reason that the Kingdom is often misunderstood: the nature of the King Himself.

What king would ever sacrifice himself for his people? Kings sacrifice their subjects, not themselves. What king would wash his servants' feet, as Jesus did, or freely befriend his lowest subjects? Potentates maintain the mystique of leadership by keeping a distance from those they rule. A certain grandeur seems to robe those who occupy high office.

I vividly recall a glimpse of this from my White House days. One brisk December night as I accompanied the president from the Oval Office in the West Wing of the White House to the Residence, Mr. Nixon was musing about what people wanted in their leaders. He slowed a moment, looking into the distance across the South Lawn, and said, "The people really want a leader a little bigger than themselves, don't they, Chuck?" I agreed. "I mean someone like de Gaulle," he continued. "There's a certain aloofness, a power that's exuded by great men that people feel and want to follow."

Jesus Christ exhibited none of this self-conscious aloofness. He served others first; He spoke to those to whom no one spoke; He dined with the lowest members of society; He touched the untouchables. He had no throne, no crown, no bevy of servants or armored guards. A borrowed manger and a borrowed tomb framed His earthly life.

Kings and presidents and prime ministers surround themselves with minions who rush ahead, swing the doors wide, and stand at attention as they wait for the great to pass. Jesus said that He Himself stands at the door and knocks, patiently waiting to enter our lives.

This was not the kind of messiah the Jews expected. The symbol of the tribe of Judah was a lion, majestic and powerful. The Jews waited for the descendant of this tribe—a man like David, the lion warrior of Judah, to come with chariots and armies. Instead, Christ came as "the Lamb of God." But lambs were for sacrifice. Where was the mighty warrior who would tear Rome to shreds?

Because of the nature of the King and the price He paid for His Kingdom, much is required of its citizens, and Jesus made these demands of the Kingdom clear.

Through the centuries, however, many of His followers have watered down His teaching, stripped away His demands for the building of a righteous society, and preached an insipid religion concerned only with personal benefits. This distorted view portrays Christianity not as the powerful source of spiritual rebirth and the mediating force for justice, mercy, and love in the world, but as the ultimate self-fulfillment plan. The gospel is not a release for the captives, but confidence for the shy. It is the spiritual equivalent of racy sports cars, designer clothes, and Gordon's Gin—a commodity to help one get more out of life.

As we've seen in a previous chapter, many humanists have failed to understand human nature. But many Christians have failed also—failed to understand the utterly radical nature of the central message of Christianity. Other great leaders have expounded creeds, philosophies, and mystical visions. Many are wise and moral, but they are only belief systems: rules to live by, value codes. Men and women require more than rules; they require what Jesus' message of the Kingdom uniquely provides: answers to their most basic needs.

What are these needs?

To know God. "The heart of man is restless until it finds its rest in Thee."[3] With these simple words Augustine expressed man's most primal yearning— the need to know God. In announcing His messiahship Jesus was saying that God's love and just rule had come to earth—in Him. Men and women would thereafter be able to find rest not in a law they could never hope to fulfill, but in the actual person of Jesus Christ.

To find salvation. But how does one come to a personal relationship with this Christ? That is the archetypal question asked by the apostle Paul's jailer: "What must I do to be saved?"[4]

Because we interpret it from our perspective and not God's, salvation has always been misunderstood. The Jew wanted salvation from his oppressor, the Roman centurion. Instead, Christ came to save him from a much greater oppressor—the sin within him.

Sin is essentially rebellion against the rule of God. This is why Jesus coupled the message of the Kingdom with the call to repent and believe. Faith and repentance, the opposite of rebellion, are the necessary human responses to the divine initiative of spiritual rebirth, resulting in salvation.

When Christ first used the term *born again,* it was not the evangelical cliché or secular slur it is today. He used it in a late-night conversation with Nicodemus, a member of the Jewish religious community, telling him it was the key to entering into the Kingdom of God. Imagine the shock of the religious elite when they heard Jesus' words: Salvation was not to be found in proud piety or scrupulous adherence to religious rules, but in a turning from evil and humble faith in One greater than oneself. Just as a person is born physically in a particular nation, so he or she is born spiritually by submitting to God's rule in His holy nation.

To find meaning. This relationship with God meets man's deepest psychological need. As we have already seen, human beings cannot live in a vacuum.

We are not a chance collision of atoms in an indifferent universe or islands amid cold currents of modern culture. We each have a personal purpose in history, which is to be found under the purposeful rule of God, as a beloved citizen of His Kingdom.

To find authority. Christianity is more than simply a relationship between man and God, however. The Kingdom of God embraces every aspect of life: ethical, spiritual, and temporal, and it determines the "pattern, purpose and dynamic by which God orders life of the heavenly polis in this world."[5]

In announcing this all-encompassing Kingdom, Jesus was not using a clever metaphor; He was expressing the literal theme of Jewish history—that God was King and the people were His subjects. This tradition dated back to the days of Abraham and the patriarchs, when God made His original covenant with the Jews to be His "holy nation."*

David, the first great king of the Jews, consolidated a visible kingdom for the people of God, but it was to be only a reflection of the ultimate rule of God, their true King. From David, the scepter passed to his son Solomon and on through a succession of rulers, some good, some bad, but all serving as a link between God and His subjects. Later, when the Jews were conquered and sent into exile, prophets prom-

---

*As R. C. Sproul notes, Americans, steeped in the tradition of democracy, find a monarchy, even with Christ on the throne, an alien concept. We think in terms of human rulers whose limitless lust for power is a constant peril to mankind. But God is not a mirror reflection of human rulers. He is God— and as such, is entitled to rule over all things. His character, as revealed in the Bible and in the person of Christ, reveals absolute justice, mercy, and love. R. C. Sproul, *If There Is a God, Why Are There Atheists?* (Minneapolis: Dimension Books, 1978), 137.

ised the coming of Messiah and the eventual establishment of the Kingdom of God. Christ was the fulfillment of that prophecy; He was the final king in David's royal line. But Jesus was not just a king for Israel; He was King for all people.

His message, then, assumes the ultimate authority man requires: God rules every aspect of what He has made. Life, death, relationships, and earthly kingdoms are all in His hands.

This totality of God's authority is a major reason many non-Christians resent Christianity, seeing it as an excuse for religious zealots to try to cram absolute orders from their God down others' throats. But when Christ commanded His followers to "seek first the kingdom of God," He was exhorting them to seek to be ruled by God and gratefully acknowledge His power and authority over them. That means that the Christian's goal is not to strive to rule, but *to be ruled*.

While God's rule *is* authoritarian, it is also *voluntary*. The Good News is that the price has been paid, and His Kingdom is open to all who desire admission.

SEVEN

Politics of the Kingdom

*If the joyful news of the rule of God is
proclaimed, if men humble themselves
and do justice to its claims, if evil is
overcome and men are made free for God,
then the Rule of God has already become
actual among them, then the Reign of God
is "in their midst."*

—Hedda Hartl

After a recent lecture on a college campus I was
asked, "Mr. Colson, how can you try to live by the
Sermon on the Mount and at the same time support
the use of military might?"

It's a fair question. Jesus teaches that we should
love our enemies, return good for evil. But is this
realistic in a world in which evil so often triumphs?
Can one forgive seventy times seven and still restrain
wrongdoers? Turn the other cheek to terrorism?

These dilemmas lead many to conclude that
either Jesus was not speaking literally or if He was,
one must live a monastic life to be a Christian. We
reach such conclusions, however, because we mis-
understand Jesus' teaching about the Kingdom.

When Jesus announced the Kingdom, He did indeed set forth radical standards by which its citizens are to live. He knew such a lifestyle would be both costly and complex, but it would witness the values of God's Kingdom even in the midst of the evil of this world. Christ was not suggesting, however, that the obedient Christian would be able to usher in the Kingdom of God on earth. Only Christ Himself would do that when He returns.

But for this period between the two stages—the announcement of the Kingdom and its final consummation—God has provided structures to restrain the evil of this world. The state is even ordained to wield the sword when necessary; and the Christian is commanded to obey the state and to respect its authority as God's instrument.

The Christian, therefore, follows two commandments: to live by Christ's teaching in the Sermon on the Mount, modeling the values of God's Kingdom—*the one yet to come in its fullness*—and at the same time to support government's role in preserving order as a witness to God's authority over the *present* kingdoms of this world. So while the Christian is not to return evil for evil (he must instead exercise forgiveness, breaking the cycle of evil), he may participate in the God-ordained structure that restrains the evil and chaos of the fallen world by the use of force.

*   *   *

In addition to the state, which preserves order, God has provided two other institutions for the ordering of society: the family for the propagation of life and the church for the proclamation of the Kingdom of God. Each of these three institutions has been established to fulfill a distinct role.

The family is the most basic unit of government. As the first community to which a person is attached and the first authority under which a person learns to live, the family establishes society's most basic values. Paul Johnson observed that the family "is an alternative to the state as a focus of loyalty and thus a humanizing force in society. Unlike the state, it upholds nonmaterial values—makes them paramount indeed."[1]

In most Eastern cultures the family remains the fundamental unit of society. In the West, however, relativism has encouraged the belief that family is a matter of convenience rather than convention. The traditional family has all but disintegrated in the inner city, where more than 50 percent of the children are born out of wedlock. And in the nation as a whole more than half the children are raised in one-parent families where that parent works.[2] Some school textbooks even describe the family as any voluntary grouping of people living together.[3] This attitude is reflected in our laws, our court decisions, our public mores—and in our crime rates.

The widely acclaimed seventeen-year study of Stanton Samenow and Samuel Yochelson concluded that crime is not the result of environment or poverty, but of wrong moral choices.[4] Harvard professors James Wilson and Richard Herrnstein concluded in 1985 that such moral choices are determined by moral conscience, which is shaped early in life and most profoundly by the family. Without the lessons the family alone can teach, commitment to God and duty to fellow man become alien concepts.[5] Little wonder that many of today's youth have been lost to the streets.

Though it is not my purpose here to examine the issue of the modern family, the situation today merits a word of warning. The widespread loss of the God-ordained role of the family leads, as theologian Carl Henry has written, to the "deterioration of society and [the] eventual collapse of the nation."[6] The humanizing force of the family can never be replaced by political or bureaucratic means.

The *state* was instituted by God to restrain sin and promote a just social order. One of the most common misconceptions in Western political thought is that the role of government is determined solely by the will of the people. When Pilate questioned Jesus on the eve of His execution, Christ told the governor that he would not even hold his office or political authority if it had not been granted him by God. The apostle Paul spoke of civil authority as "God's servant, an agent of wrath to bring punishment on the wrongdoer."[7] Peter used similar language, saying that governments were set by God to "punish those who do wrong and to commend those who do right."[8]

Government originated as an ordinance of God. It is, in one sense, God's response to the nature of the people themselves. Man "can adapt himself somehow to anything his imagination can cope with ... but he cannot deal with chaos."[9] While it cannot redeem the world or be used as a tool to establish the Kingdom of God, civil government does set the boundaries for human behavior. The state is not a remedy for sin, but a means to restrain it. Its limited task is to promote "the good of the community in temporal concerns, the protection of life and property and the preservation of peace and order."[10]

When God established ancient Israel as a nation, His first order of business was the propagation of law, not just for religious purposes, but for the ordering of civil life. Even before the giving of the Ten Commandments there was great need for civil adjudication.

The biblical text records that "Moses took his seat to serve as judge for the people and they stood around him from morning till evening."[11] (Court dockets seemed to have been clogged from the very beginning.) Moses explained that "the people come to me to seek God's will. Whenever they have a dispute, it is brought to me, and I decide between the parties and inform them of God's decrees and laws."[12]

Thus the Israelite involved in a dispute looked not to the whim of a judge or to an arbitrary law but rather to a ruling based on divine laws. The judicial role was not a mechanism to advance the state's perception of social equilibrium, but to discern God's revealed law.

This is the origin of what we call the rule of law; it stands in stark contrast to modern moral relativism. Without transcendent norms, laws are either established by social elites or are merely bargains struck by competing forces in society. In the Judeo-Christian view, law is rooted in moral absolutes that do not vacillate with public taste or the whim of fashion.

Thus rooted, government can perform not only

the negative function of restraining evil, but the positive function of promoting a just social order so that people can live in harmony. The apostle Paul had this in mind when he urged his young colleague Timothy to pray "for kings and all those in authority, that we may live peaceful and quiet lives in all godliness and holiness."[13]

In the words of sociologist Robert Nisbet, man is engaged in a continual "quest for community."[14] It is important to remember, however, that the state is not itself that community. Anyone who has ever dealt with a government bureaucracy knows that it is rare enough to get a phone call through, let alone to cultivate warm fuzzy feelings for the mammoth machine of big government.

But the state can protect people's voluntary efforts to shape community by granting equal protection of the law, by upholding principles of justice so the weak and powerless are not exploited, and by guaranteeing liberty and providing security. In this way the government sustains a stable environment in which people can live, producing art, literature, music, and children. Or as C. S. Lewis alluded to it, they can partake of one of the primary benefits of democracy: the simple freedom to enjoy a cup of tea by the fire with one's family.

Christianity teaches, then, that the state serves a divinely appointed and divinely defined task, although it is not in itself divine. Its authority is legitimate, though limited.

The church is the community that administers and encourages the worship of God and meets the spiritual needs of God's people, including teaching, offering the sacraments, and the bearing of one another's burdens. "The primary purpose of the church in relation to the world is evangelization,"[15]—that is, to proclaim in word and deed the same gospel that Christ announced.

The church is not the actual Kingdom of God, but is to reflect the love, justice, and righteousness of God's Kingdom within society.* Though the church as a human institution often fails in this high calling, its most potent social weapon is its commitment to live out the Lord's command to love one's neighbor, the law of love. "In essence," writes historian Floyd Filson, "the program of the church disregarded the social divisions of society; it made the church a home for all classes; its democratic basis was a common worship and fellowship and mutual love."[16]

The church's transcendent vision holds the world accountable to something beyond itself. In doing so, its members serve as ambassadors, citizens of the heavenly Kingdom at work in this world. French theologian Jacques Ellul has well summarized the duty of those in the church:

The Christian who is involved in the material history of this world is involved in it as representing another order, another master (than the "prince of this world"), another claim (than that of the natural heart of man). . . . Thus he

---

*The church is, as one authority notes, "the community in which through its behavior and mission the reign of God becomes visible, serving as the precursor and avant-garde of the society that will be fulfillment of all hope." Stephen Charles Mott, *Biblical Ethics and Social Change* (New York: Oxford University Press, 1982), 106.

must plunge into social and political problems in order to
have an influence on the world, not in the hope of making
it a paradise, but simply in order to make it tolerable—
not in order to diminish the opposition between this world
and the Kingdom of God, but simply in order to modify
the opposition between the disorder of this world and the
order of preservation that God wills for it—not in order to
"bring in" the Kingdom of God, but in order that the gospel
may be proclaimed, that all men may really hear the good
news of salvation through the death and resurrection of
Christ.[17]

Thus, the church, while not the Kingdom of God,
is to live out the values of the Kingdom of God in
this world, resisting the ever-present temptation to
usher in the Kingdom of God by political means. Yet
this is the temptation to which the church, as we will
discuss more thoroughly in later chapters, has most
commonly succumbed, and certainly this is its greatest temptation today.

Pope John Paul II may well have had this concern
in mind when he addressed Latin American Catholics at Puebla, Mexico, in 1979:

The gospels make it clear that in Jesus' eyes anything
that would distort his mission as servant of the Lord was a
temptation. He did not accept the view of those who
confuse the things of God with attitudes that are purely
political. He rejects unequivocally any recourse to violence.
He offers his message of conversion to all, not excluding
even the tax collectors. The purpose of his mission
embraces far more than political order. It embraces the

salvation of the entire person through transforming and peace-giving love.[18]

Unlike the politics of the world, the politics of the Kingdom is the politics of "faith, hope and love: faith that confesses the Risen Savior, hope that looks for His appearing, love that is inflamed by His sacrifice on the cross."[19] The church "anticipates the form of the world to come and thus it transcends the social and political forms of this world."[20]

While Jesus did not come to establish a political kingdom, the announcement of the Kingdom had profound consequences for the political order.

When Jesus said to Pilate, "My kingdom is not of this earth," Pilate may have breathed a sigh of relief. He should have reconsidered. Which is more threatening to a ruler—an external foe with mighty but visible armies or an eternal king who rules the very souls of men and women? The latter can command the will and affections, demand absolute obedience, impart unlimited power to His subjects, and radically change their values and lives; His followers fear no earthly power and His Kingdom has no end. In the face of such a potentate, any mere political leader must shudder.

This is why the Kingdom of God has had such an astonishing effect upon the most powerful of human empires in every age. It is not a blueprint for some new social order; nor does it merely set the forces of radical cultural change in motion. Rather, God's Kingdom promises radical changes in human personalities.

This is the crucial point. While human politics is based on the premise that society must be changed in order to change people, in the politics of the Kingdom it is people who must be changed in order to change society.

Through men and women who recognize its authority and live by its ethical standards, the Kingdom of God invades the stream of history. It breaks the vicious and otherwise irreversible cycles of violence, injustice, and self-interest. In this way the Kingdom of God equips its citizens, as Augustine said, to be the best citizens in the kingdoms of man.

Such was certainly the case in early nineteenth-century England, when one man dared—against great personal and political odds—to represent the standards of the Kingdom of God for the good of his nation.

For the Good of the Nation

Things have come to a pretty pass when
religion is allowed to invade public life.
——Lord Melbourne (opposing
abolition of the slave trade)

Scudding clouds obscured the moon as the heavy schooner pitched forward in the dark waters. A lone sailor walked the deck on late watch; at the helm, three others held the wheel against the high seas. Below, the rest of the crew tossed in their hammocks, while in the main cabin the captain dipped his quill in a well of sepia ink and began the day's log. He squinted in the poor light from the tallow candle. "...1787...a fair wind today...five hundred miles off the coast of Africa...bound due east now for Jamaica with cargo...."

Packed into the dark hold beneath his feet was the ship's cargo—five hundred African men and women layered like fish packed in brine. Barely able to breathe in the air heavy with the stench of human waste and vomit, they lay chest to back, legs drawn into fetal position, feet resting on the heads of those in the next row.

Some had been taken prisoner during tribal wars; some had been jailed as petty criminals; and others had been unsuspecting dinner guests of Englishmen visiting their country. But all had been forcibly enslaved and held in a stockade on the African coast until sold to the highest bidder. That bidder was the captain in the cabin above.

Once purchased they had been branded and rowed to the schooner waiting offshore, their screams and cries ignored by the seamen who hoisted them aboard and chained them in the stinking hold. For the women, however, there was a further torture. The crew, diseased and ill-treated themselves, claimed the one sordid privilege of their trade—the pick of the slave women. Once under way, the ship had become half bedlam, half brothel.

Now, several weeks into the voyage, sixty slaves had already died. Fever had taken some. Others, driven insane by the horror of their lot, had been killed by the crew. Each morning when the lower decks were opened, several dead or near-dead bodies were thrown to the sharks trailing the ship.

The captain cursed as the bodies hit the choppy water. Each body overboard meant lost profits.

For those who survived the hellish three-month journey, an equally gruesome future awaited. They would be auctioned naked in the marketplace to planters who would work them to death on their Caribbean plantations. Never again would these African men and women see their homeland.

*　　　　*　　　　*

Thousands of miles to the north, in a country that profited richly from this human misery, another man sat at his desk. He too gazed into the flickering flame of his lamp, for the early morning darkness still filled his second floor library at Number 4 Old Palace Yard, London. Only his piercing blue eyes reflected the turmoil of his thoughts as he eyed the jumble of pamphlets on his cluttered desk.

He ran his hand through his wavy hair and opened his Bible to begin the day, as was his custom, with Scripture reading and prayer. But his thoughts kept returning to the pamphlets, grisly accounts of human flesh sold like mutton for the profit of his countrymen. No matter how he tried, William Wilberforce could not wipe these scenes from his mind.[1]

*   *   *

William Wilberforce was the only son of prosperous merchant parents. Though an average student at Cambridge, his quick wit had made him a favorite among his fellows, including William Pitt, with whom he shared an interest in politics. Often the two young men had spent their evenings in the gallery of the House of Commons watching the heated debates over the War of Independence in the colonies.

After graduation Wilberforce had run as a conservative for a seat in Parliament from his home county of Hull. Though only twenty-one at the time, the prominence of his family, his speaking ability, and a generous feast he sponsored for voters on election day carried the contest.

The London of 1780, when Wilberforce arrived to take his office, was described as "one vast casino" where the rich counted their profits through a fog of claret. Fortunes were lost and won over gaming tables, and duels of honor were the order of the day. The city's elegant private clubs welcomed young Wilberforce, and he happily concentrated on pursuing both political advancement and social pleasure.

High society revolved around romantic intrigue and adulterous affairs. An upper-class couple might not be seen together in public for weeks during the social season, for no popular hostess would invite a husband and wife to the same event.

The poor, of course, had no such opportunity to escape from one another. Crammed together in shabby dwellings, they were cogs grinding out a living in the Empire's emerging industrial machines. Pale children worked eighteen hours a day in cotton mills or coal mines to bring home a few shillings a month to parents who often wasted it on cheap gin.

Highwaymen were folk heroes. Newgate and other infamous prisons overflowed with debtors, murderers, rapists, and petty thieves—often children. The twelve-year-old who had stolen a loaf of bread might be hanged the same day as a celebrated highwayman, providing public entertainment.

In short, London was a city where unchecked passions and desires ran their course. Few raised their voices in opposition.

So it is not surprising that few argued against one of the nation's most bountiful sources of wealth—the slave trade. In fact, the trade was both a successful business and a national policy. Political alliances revolved around commitments to it. It be-

came known euphemistically as "the institution,"
the "pillar and support of British plantation industry
in the West Indies." In a celebrated case in England's
high court only four years earlier, slaves had been
deemed "goods and chattels."

Corruption in government was so widespread
that few members of Parliament thought twice about
accepting bribes for their votes. Planters and other
gentlemen involved in the slave trade paid three to
five thousand pounds to "buy" boroughs, which sent
their representatives to the House of Commons. The
same attitude reigned in the House of Lords. Their
political influence in Parliament grew until a large
bloc was controlled by the vested influence of the
slave trade.

The horrors of the trade were remote and unseen,
the cotton and sugar profits they yielded very tangible. So most consciences were not troubled about
the black men and women suffering far away on the
high seas or on remote plantations.

*   *   *

Early in 1784 Wilberforce's friend William Pitt
was elected prime minister at the age of twenty-four.
This inspired Wilberforce to make a big political
gamble. He surrendered his safe seat in Hull and
stood for election in Yorkshire, the largest and most
influential constituency in the country.

It was a grueling campaign; the outcome was
uncertain until the closing day when Wilberforce addressed a large rally. James Boswell, Samuel Johnson's celebrated biographer, stood in the cold rain
and watched the young candidate, barely five feet

tall, climb onto a table so the wet, bored crowd could see him. The power of his oratory, however, soon gripped them.

"I saw what seemed a mere shrimp mount upon the table," Boswell wrote, "but as I listened the shrimp grew and grew and became a whale."

Wilberforce was elected. As an intimate of the prime minister and as a man respected by both political parties, he seemed destined for power and prominence.

After the election, Wilberforce's mother invited him to take a tour of the Continent with his sister and several cousins. Subsequently, he happened to meet his old schoolmaster from Hull, Isaac Milner, and on impulse asked him to join the traveling party. That invitation was to change Wilberforce's life.

Isaac Milner was a large, jovial man with a mind as robust as his body. Called "an evangelical Dr. Johnson," Milner's forceful personality had contributed to the spread of Christian influence at Cambridge. Not unnaturally, then, he raised the matter of faith and religion to his former pupil as their carriage ran over the rutted roads between Nice and the Swiss Alps.

When Wilberforce treated the subject flippantly, Milner growled at his young companion's derisive wit and declared, "I am no match for you, but if you really want to discuss these subjects seriously, I will gladly enter on them with you." Provoked, Wilberforce eventually agreed to read the Bible.

The summer session of Parliament forced Wilberforce to make a break in his travels, and his visit to the social scene of London revealed subtle changes in his tastes. Parties he had once attended routinely now seemed "indecent." Letters to family and friends indicated his growing distaste for corruption he had scarcely noticed before.

When he and Milner continued their Continental tour in the fall of 1785, Wilberforce was no longer the same frivolous young man. In fact, the rest of the traveling party complained about his preoccupation when he and Milner studied a Greek New Testament in the coach.

Wilberforce returned to London in early November, but his travels had not rested him. Instead, he felt weary and confused. In need of counsel, he sought advice from John Newton.

Son of a sailor, Newton had been impressed into the Royal Navy when he was eleven. He deserted, was caught in West Africa, flogged, and placed into service on a slave ship. Eventually he became involved in the slave trade and in 1750 was given command of his own ship. On one especially stormy passage to the West Indies, however, Newton was converted to faith in Jesus Christ. He renounced slaving and expressed his wonder at the gift of salvation in his famous hymn, "Amazing Grace."

By the time Wilberforce knew of him, Newton was a clergyman in the Church of England, renowned for his outspokenness on spiritual matters. He counseled Wilberforce to follow Christ but not to abandon public office: "The Lord has raised you up to the good of His church and for the good of the nation." Wilberforce heeded his advice.

The responses of his old friends were predictable. Some thought his mind had snapped; others assumed he would now retreat from political life since religion could have little to do with politics. Many, however, were simply bewildered. How could a well-bred, educated young man with so much promise get caught up in a religious exuberance that appealed only to the common masses?

The reaction Wilberforce cared about most, however, was that of his friend Pitt. He wrote to the prime minister, telling him that though he would remain his faithful friend, he could "no more be so much of a party man as before." Pitt's understanding reply revealed the depth of their friendship, but after their first face-to-face discussion, Wilberforce wrote in his diary: "Pitt tried to reason me out of my convictions but soon found himself unable to combat their correctness, if Christianity was true. The fact is, he is so absorbed in politics, that he has never given himself time for due reflection on religion."

*　　*　　*

Thus Wilberforce arrived at that foggy Sunday morning in 1787 when he sat at his desk and stared out the window at the gray drizzle, thinking about his conversion and his calling. Had God saved him only to rescue his own soul from hell? He could not accept that. He could not be content with the comfort of life at Palace Yard and the stimulating debates of Parliament. If Christianity was true and meaningful, it must go deeper than that. It must not only save but serve. It must bring God's compassion to the oppressed as well as oppose the oppressors. And at the moment, all he could envision were loaded slave ships leaving the sun-baked coasts of Africa.

He turned back to the journal filled with his tiny, cramped writing and dipped his pen in the inkwell. "Almighty God has set before me two great objectives," he wrote, his heart suddenly pumping with passion. "The abolition of the slave trade and the reformation of manners."

With those words, an epic offensive was launched against a society pockmarked by decadence and the barbaric trafficking of human flesh that underwrote those excesses.

"As soon as ever I had arrived thus far in my investigation of the slave trade, so enormous, so dreadful, so irremediable did its wickedness appear that my own mind was completely made up for the abolition. A trade founded in iniquity and carried on as this was must be abolished."

Wilberforce knew the issue had to be faced head-on in Parliament. Throughout the damp fall of 1787 he worked late into the nights on his investigation, joined by others who saw in him a champion for their cause. There was Grenville Sharp, a hook-nosed attorney with a keen mind who was already well-known for his successful court case that had made slavery illegal in England itself—ironic in a time when the country's economic strength depended on slavery abroad. Another was Zachary Macaulay, a quiet, patient researcher who sifted through stacks of evidence to build damning indictments against the trade. A dedicated worker who took pen in hand at four o'clock every morning, he became a walking encyclopedia for the rest of the abolitionists. Whenever Wilberforce needed information, he would look for his quiet, heavy-browed friend and say, "Let us look it up in Macaulay."

Thomas Clarkson was another compatriot. The red-headed clergyman and brilliant essayist with a passion for justice and righteousness was Wilberforce's scout. He conducted exhausting—and dangerous—trips to the African coast. Once, needing some evidence from a particular sailor he knew by sight though not by name, Clarkson questioned dozen dozens of men from slave vessels in port after port until finally, after searching 317 ships, he found his man.

In February 1788, while working with these friends and others, Wilberforce suddenly fell gravely ill. Doctors predicted he would not live more than two weeks. Cheered by this news, the opposition party in Yorkshire made plans to regain his seat in Parliament. Wilberforce, however, recovered. And though not yet well enough to return to Parliament, in March he asked Pitt to introduce the abolition issue in the House for him. On the basis of their friendship, the prime minister agreed.

Lacking Wilberforce's passion but faithfully citing his facts, Pitt moved that a resolution be passed binding the House to discuss the slave trade in the next session. The motion provoked a lukewarm debate and was passed. Those with interest in the trade were not worried about a mere motion to discuss abolition.

Then another of Wilberforce's friends, Sir William Dolben, introduced a one-year experimental bill to regulate the number of slaves that could be transported per ship. After several members of Parliament visited a slave ship lying in a London port, the debates grew heated with cries for reform.

Now sensing a threat, the West Indian bloc rose up in opposition. Tales of cruelty in the slave trade were mere fiction, they said; it was the happiest day of an African's life when he was shipped away from the barbarities of his homeland. Besides, warned Lord Penrhyn ominously, the proposed measure would abolish the trade upon which "two thirds of the commerce of this country depends."

Angered by Penrhyn's hyperbole, Pitt himself grew passionate. Threatening to resign unless the bill was carried, he pushed Dolben's regulation through both houses in June of 1788.

The success of Dolben's bill awakened the slave traders to the possibility of real danger. By the time a recovered Wilberforce returned to the legislative scene, they were furious and ready to fight, shocked that politicians had the audacity to press for morally based reforms in the political arena.

"Humanity is a private feeling, not a public principle to act upon," sniffed the Earl of Abingdon.

Lord Melbourne angrily agreed. "Things have come to a pretty pass when religion is allowed to invade public life."

James Boswell, who had initially been astounded by Wilberforce's oratorical prowess, penned a bit of snide verse aptly reflecting the abuse heaped by Wilberforce's enemies:

> Go, W———— with narrow skull,
> Go home and preach away at Hull.
> No longer in the Senate cackle

In strains that suit the tabernacle;
I hate your little witling sneer,
Your pert and self-sufficient leer.
Mischief to trade sits on your lip,
Insects will gnaw the noblest ship
Go, W_____, begone, for shame,
Thou dwarf with big resounding name.

But Wilberforce and the band of abolitionists knew that a private faith that did not act in the face of oppression was no faith at all.

Wilberforce's first parliamentary speech for abolition shows the passion of his convictions as well as his characteristic humility:

When I consider the magnitude of the subject which I am to bring before the House—a subject, in which the interest, not of this country, nor of Europe alone, but of the whole world, and of posterity, are involved . . . it is impossible for me not to feel both terrified and concerned at my own inadequacy to such a task. But I march forward with a firmer step in the full assurance that my cause will bear me out . . . the total abolition of the slave trade. . . .

I mean not to accuse anyone, but to take the shame upon myself, in common, indeed, with the whole Parliament of Great Britain, for having suffered this horrid trade to be carried on under their authority. We are all guilty—we ought all to plead guilty, and not to exculpate ourselves by throwing the blame on others.

But the passionate advocacy of Wilberforce, Pitt, and others was not sufficient to deter the interests of commerce in the 1789 session. The House's vote spurred Wilberforce to gather further evidence that could not be ignored. He and his co-workers spent up to ten hours a day reading and abridging factual material, and in early 1791 he again filled the House of Commons with his thundering eloquence. "Never, never will we desist till we ... extinguish every trace of this bloody traffic, of which our posterity, looking back to the history of these enlightened times, will scarce believe that it has been suffered to exist so long a disgrace and dishonor to this country."

The opposition was equally determined. One member asserted, "Abolition would instantly annihilate a trade, which annually employs upwards of 5,500 sailors, upwards of 160 ships, and whose exports amount to £800,000 sterling; and would undoubtedly bring the West Indies trade to decay, whose exports and imports amount to upwards of £6,000,000 sterling, and which give employment in upwards of 160,000 tons of additional shipping, and sailors in proportion." He paused dramatically, pointed to the gallery where a number of his slave-trading constituents watched, and exclaimed, "These are my masters!"

Another member, citing the positive aspects of the trade, drew a chilling comparison: the slave trade "was not an amiable trade," he admitted, "but neither was the trade of a butcher ... and yet a mutton chop was, nevertheless, a very good thing."

Incensed, Wilberforce and other abolitionists fought a bitter two-day battle; members shouted and harangued as spectators and press relished the fray. But by the time votes were cast, "commerce clinked

its purse," as one observer commented, and Wilberforce was again defeated.

In 1792, when it became apparent that the fight
would be long, Henry Thornton suggested to Wilberforce that they gather and work at his home in
Clapham, a village four miles south of Westminster;
there they would be convenient to Parliament, yet
set apart. Thornton's home, Battersea Rise, a Queen
Anne house on the grassy Clapham Common, was a
lively household. As abolitionist friends came to live
or visit, Thornton added extra wings until eventually
Battersea Rise had thirty-four bedrooms as well as a
large, airy library designed by Prime Minister Pitt.
Here, in the heart of the house, many an intense
prayer meeting and discussion lasted late into the
night as the "cabinet councils" prepared for their
parliamentary battles.

Wilberforce took up part-time residence in
Thornton's home until his marriage in 1797, at which
time he moved to Broomfield, a smaller house on the
same property.

As the Clapham community analyzed their battle
in 1792, they were painfully aware that many of their
colleagues in Parliament were puppets, unable or
unwilling to stand against the powerful economic
forces of their day. So Wilberforce and his friends
decided to go to the people, believing, "It is on the
general impression and feeling of the nation we must
rely . . . so let the flame be fanned."

The abolitionists distributed thousands of pamphlets detailing the evils of slavery, spoke at public
meetings, and circulated petitions. The celebrated
poet William Cowper wrote "The Negro's Com-

plaint," a poem that was set to music and sung in many fashionable drawing rooms. Josiah Wedgewood, a master of fine china, designed a cameo that became the equivalent of a modern-day campaign button. It depicted a slave kneeling in bondage, whispering the plea that was to become famous: "Am I not a man and a brother?"

A boycott of slave-grown sugar was organized, a tactic even Wilberforce thought could not work. To his astonishment, it gained a following of some 300,000 people across England. Later in 1792 Wilberforce was able to bring to the House of Commons 519 petitions for the total abolition of the slave trade, signed by thousands of British subjects. This surging tide of public popularity along with Wilberforce's usual impassioned eloquence combined to profoundly disturb the House:

In the year 1788 in a ship in this trade, 650 persons were on board, out of whom 155 died. In another, 405 were on board, out of whom were lost 200. In another there were on board 402, out of whom 73 died. When captain Wilson was asked the causes of this mortality, he replied that the slaves had a fixed melancholy and dejection; that they wished to die; that they refused all sustenance, till they were beaten in order to compel them to eat; and that when they had been so beaten, they looked in the faces of the whites and said, piteously, "Soon we will be no more."

Even the vested economic interests of the West Indian bloc could not gloss over these appalling facts or ignore the public support the abolitionists were gaining. But again the slavers exercised their political muscle and the House moved that Wilberforce's motion be qualified by the word *gradually*. And so it was carried. Again the traders relaxed, knowing a bill could be indefinitely postponed by that seemingly innocuous word.

Though Wilberforce was wounded by yet another defeat, he had a glimmer of hope. For the first time the House had actually voted for an abolition motion; with the force of the people behind the cause, it would only be a matter of time.

That hope was soon smashed by events across the English Channel. The fall of the Bastille in 1789 had heralded the people's revolution in France. By 1792 all idealism vanished. The September massacres loosed a tide of bloodshed as the mob and the guillotine ruled France.

Fears of a similar revolt abounded in England until any type of public agitation for reform was suspiciously labeled "Jacobinic," after the radicals who had fanned the flames of France's Reign of Terror. This association and the ill-timed slave revolts in the West Indies stemmed the tide of public activism for abolition.

Sensing the shift in the public mood, the House of Commons rejected Wilberforce's motion. The attitude in the House of Lords was summed up by the member who declared flatly, "All abolitionists are Jacobins." Wilberforce saw his hopes wither and his cause lampooned in popular cartoons and ridiculed by critics.

Weary with grief and frustration, he often sat long into the night at his old oak desk, wondering whether he should abandon his hopeless campaign.

One night as he sat flipping through his Bible, a letter fluttered from between the pages.

Wilberforce stared at the shaky handwriting. The writer was dead. In fact, this letter was one of the last he had ever written. Wilberforce had read it dozens of times, but never had he needed its message as much as he did now.

My dear Sir,

Unless the Divine power has raised you up to be as Athanasius contra mundum,* I see not how you can go through your glorious enterprise in opposing that execrable villainy, which is the scandal of religion, of England, and of human nature. Unless God has raised you up for this very thing, you will be worn out by the opposition of men and devils, but if God be for you who can be against you? Are all of them together stronger than God? Oh, be not weary of well-doing. Go on in the name of God, and in the power of His might, till even American slavery, the vilest that ever saw the sun, shall vanish away before it. That He that has guided you from your youth up may continue to strengthen in this and all things, is the prayer of,

Your affectionate servant,
John Wesley

---

*This Latin phrase, which means "against the world," characterizes anyone who makes an unpopular moral stand against prevailing social opinions. Athanasius (c. A.D. 296–373) was an early church father who opposed many of the heresies of his time.

"Be not weary of well-doing." Wilberforce took a deep breath, carefully refolded the letter, and blew out the candle. He needed to get to bed; he had a long fight ahead of him.

Wilberforce's resolution returned and for the next several years he doggedly reintroduced, each year, the motion for abolition; and each year Parliament threw it out.

An abrupt reversal came early in 1796 after the fall of Robespierre in France and the resultant swing of public sentiment toward peace. Popular favor again began to swing toward Wilberforce, surprisingly reinforced by a majority vote in the House of Commons for his annual motion for abolition. Victory suddenly seemed within reach.

But the third reading of the bill took place on the night a long-awaited comic opera opened in London. A dozen supporters of abolition, supposing the bill would be voted in this time, skipped Parliament for the opera—and a grieving Wilberforce saw his bill defeated by just four votes.

And so it went—1797, 1798, 1799, 1800, 1801— the years passed with Wilberforce's motions thwarted and sabotaged by political pressures, compromise, personal illness, and the continuing war in France. By 1803, with the threat of imminent invasion by Napoleon's armies, the question of abolition was put aside for the more immediate concern of national security.

During those long years of struggle, however, Wilberforce and his friends never lost sight of their equally pressing objective: "the reformation of manners," or the effort to clean up society's blights. Several years before, backed by Pitt and others, Wilberforce had sent a proposal to King George III that Wilberforce hoped would capture public attention. He asked the king to reissue a "Proclamation for the Encouragement of Piety and Virtue and for the Preventing of Vice, Profaneness and Immorality." On June 1, 1787, the king issued the proclamation, citing his concern at the deluge of "every kind of vice which, to the scandal of our holy religion, and to the evil example of our loving subjects, have broken upon this nation."

Copies of the proclamation were distributed to magistrates in every county. Wilberforce mounted his horse and followed after them, calling on those in government and positions of leadership to set up societies to develop such a moral movement in Britain.

One prominent leader, Lord Fitzwilliam, laughed in Wilberforce's face. Of course there was much debauchery and little religion, he said, but after all, this was inevitable in a rich nation. "The only way to reform morals," he concluded, "is to ruin purses."

In many areas, however, the proclamation was received seriously. Magistrates held meetings to determine how to follow its guidelines, and long-ignored laws were dusted off and enforced.

The years of battle had welded Wilberforce and his Clapham group into a tight working unit; with five of them serving as members of Parliament, they exerted an increasingly strong moral pressure on the political arena of the day. They organized the Society for the Education of Africans, the Society for Bettering the Condition of the Poor, the Society for the Relief of Debtors, which over a five-year period obtained the release of 14,000 people from debtor's prisons. Various members were involved in prison reforms, establishing hospitals for the blind, helping war widows and distressed sailors. Zachary Macaulay, at one time a wealthy man, gave away all he had and died penniless. Derisively labeled "the saints," they bore the name gladly, considering such distinction a welcome reminder of their commitment not to political popularity but to biblical justice and righteousness.

* * *

As the abolitionists prepared for their fight in Parliament in 1804, the climate had changed. The scare tactics of Jacobin association would no longer stick, and public sentiment for abolition was growing.

The House of Commons voted for Wilberforce's motion by a majority of 124 to 49, but victory was short-lived. The slave traders were better represented in the House of Lords, which adjourned the bill until the next session.

In 1805 the House of Commons reversed itself, rejecting the bill by seven votes. A well-meaning clerk took Wilberforce aside. "Mr. Wilberforce," he said kindly, "you ought not to expect to carry a measure of this kind. You and I have seen enough of life to know that people are not induced to act upon what affects their interests by any abstract arguments."

Wilberforce stared steely-eyed back at him. "Mr.

Hatsell," he replied, "I do expect to carry it, and what is more, I feel assured I shall carry it speedily."

But Wilberforce went home in dismay, his heart torn by the notion of "abstract arguments" when thousands of men and women were suffering in the bonds of slavery. "I never felt so much on any parliamentary occasion," he wrote in his diary. "I could not sleep. . . . The poor Africans rushed into my mind, and the guilt of our wicked land."

Once more he went to Pitt to press for the cause, but his old friend seemed sluggish. Wilberforce pushed harder, reminding him of old promises. The prime minister finally agreed to sign a formal document for the cause, then delayed it for months. It was finally issued in September 1805. Four months later Pitt was dead.

Wilberforce felt his death keenly, sad that he had never seen the conversion of his dear friend. "I have a thousand times wished and hoped that he and I might confer freely on the most important of all subjects," he said. "But now the scene is closed—forever."

William Grenville became prime minister. He and Foreign Secretary Fox were both strong abolitionists. After discussing the matter with Wilberforce, Grenville reversed the pattern of the previous twenty years and introduced the bill into the House of Lords first. A bitter and emotional month-long fight ensued before the bill passed at four o'clock on the morning of February 4, 1807.

On February 22 the second reading was held in the House of Commons. Outside a soft snow fell. Inside candles threw flickering shadows on the cream-colored walls of the long room, filled to capacity but unusually quiet.

Lord Howick opened the debate with a nervous, disjointed speech that reflected the tension in the chambers. Then, one by one, members jumped to their feet to decry the evils of the slave trade and to praise the men who had worked so hard to end it. They hailed Wilberforce and praised the abolitionists.

As the debate came to its climax, Sir Samuel Romilly gave a passionate tribute to Wilberforce and his decades of labor, concluding, "When he should retire into the bosom of his happy and delighted family, when he should lay himself down on his bed, reflecting on the innumerable voices that would be raised in every quarter of the world to bless him; how much more pure and perfect felicity must he enjoy in the consciousness of having preserved so many millions of his fellow-creatures."

Stirred by Romilly's words, the entire House rose, cheering and applauding. Realizing that his long battle had come to an end, Wilberforce sat bent in his chair, his head in his hands, tears streaming down his face.

The motion carried, 283 to 16.

Late that night Wilberforce and his friends burst out of the stuffy chambers and onto the snow-covered streets. They frolicked like schoolboys, clapping one another on the back, their joy spilling over. Later, at Wilberforce's home, the old friends crowded into the library, recalling the weary years of battle and rejoicing for their African brothers and sisters.

Wilberforce, surely the most joyous of all, looked

into the lined face of his old friend Henry Thornton. Years of illness, defeat, and ridicule had taken their toll. Yet all of it was worth this moment.

"Well, Henry," Wilberforce said with joy in his eyes, "what do we abolish next?"*

---

*After the outlawing of the slave trade in 1807, Wilberforce fought another eighteen years for the total emancipation of existing slaves. Despite increasingly poor health, he continued as a leader of the cause in Parliament until his retirement in 1825. He also continued his work for reforms in the prisons, among the poor, and in the workplace. And on July 29, 1883, three days after the Bill for the Abolition of Slavery passed its second reading in the House of Commons, sounding the final death blow for slavery, Wilberforce died. "Thank God," he whispered before he slipped into a final coma, "that I should have lived to witness a day in which England was willing to give twenty millions sterling for the abolition of slavery!"

The Cross and the Crown

I die the king's good servant, but God's first.

> —Sir Thomas More

If I am faced with the choice between religion and my country . . . I will choose my fatherland.

> —Father Miguel d'Escoto,
> Nicaraguan Foreign
> Minister

Wilberforce's dogged campaign to rid the British empire of the slave trade shows what can happen when a citizen of the Kingdom of God challenges corrupt structures within the kingdoms of man. One excellent Wilberforce biography is aptly titled *God's Politician*, and truly he was, holding his country to God's standard of moral accountability.

The kind of conflict that Wilberforce and other activist Christians experience—between their Christian conscience and their political mandates—is unavoidable. Both church and state assert standards and values in society; both seek authority; both compete for allegiance. As members of both the religious and the political spheres, the Christian is bound to face conflict.

The conflict is particularly apparent in the Judeo-Christian tradition because of the assertion that the God of both the Old and New Testament Scriptures is King. That has been an offense to the proud and powerful since the beginning—and the reason Jews and Christians alike have been systematically persecuted.

The tension between the Kingdom of God and the kingdoms of man runs like an unbroken thread through the history of the past two thousand years. It began not long after Christ's birth. Herod, the Roman-appointed king over the Jews and as vicious a tyrant as ever lived, was gripped with fear when the Magi arrived from the East seeking the "King of the Jews." Though not a believer, Herod knew the ancient Jewish prophecies that a child would be born to reign over them, ushering in a Kingdom of peace and might.

Herod called the Magi to his ornate throne room. In what has become common practice in the centuries since, he tried to manipulate the religious leaders for political advantage. He told them to go find this King in Bethlehem so he too could worship Him.

The rest of the story is familiar. The Magi found Jesus but were warned in a dream to avoid Herod and return to the East. Jesus' parents, similarly warned, escaped with their son to Egypt—just ahead of Herod's marauding soldiers who massacred all the male children of Jesus' age in and near Bethlehem.

Herod didn't fear Jesus because he thought He would become a religious or political leader. He had suppressed such opponents before. Herod feared

Christ because He represented a Kingdom greater than his own.

Jesus was later executed for this same reason. Though He told Pilate His Kingdom was not of this world, the sign over His cross read "INRE"—King of the Jews. The executioner's sarcasm was double-edged.

His followers' faithfulness to Christ's announcement of His Kingdom led to their persecution as well. An enraged mob in Thessalonica threatened Paul and Silas, shouting, "These men who have caused trouble all over the world . . . are all defying Caesar's decrees, saying that there is another king, one called Jesus."[1] During the early centuries Christians were martyred not for religious reasons—Rome, after all, was a land of many gods—but because they refused to worship the emperor. Because they would not say, "We have no king but Caesar," the Roman government saw them as political subversives.

Christians who refused to offer incense before the statue of the emperor were flogged, stoned, imprisoned, condemned to the mines. Later, when Christianity was officially outlawed, they were tortured mercilessly and fed to the lions, to the delight of bloodthirsty crowds.*

---

*In the second half of the second century, Christians were systematically persecuted. This account of a massacre in the Rhone Valley is not atypical: "Many Christians were tortured in the stocks or in cells. Sanctus, a deacon from Vienna, had red-hot plates applied to his testicles—his poor body was one whole wound and bruise having lost the outward form of a man. Christians who were Roman citizens were beheaded. Others were forced through a gauntlet of whips into the amphitheater and then . . . given to the beasts. Severed heads and limbs of Christians were displayed, guarded for six days, then burned, the ashes being thrown into the Rhone. . . . One lady, Blandina,

With the conversion of Constantine, however, Christianity was legalized in A.D 313. This marked the end of persecution and ushered in a second phase in church-state relations.* In A.D. 381 Christianity became the official religion of Rome, and in an ironic turnabout, church leaders began exploiting their new-found power. As historian F. F. Bruce has written: "Christian leaders . . . exploit[ed] the influential favor they enjoyed even when it meant subordinating the cause of justice to the apparent interest of their religion . . . they were inclined to allow the secular power too much control in church affairs. . . . Where church leaders were able to exercise political as well as spiritual authority, they did not enjoy any marked immunity from the universally corrupting tendency of power."[2]

Even Augustine, the great church father who provided the classic definition of the roles of the City of God and the city of man, was beguiled by the lure of temporal power; after a wrenching internal strug-

---

was the worst treated of all, tortured from dawn until evening till her torturers were exhausted and marveled that the breath was still in her body. She was then scourged, roasted in the frying pan and finally put in the basket to be tossed to death by wild bulls." Paul Johnson, *History of Christianity* (New York: Atheneum, 1979) 72–73.

Many Christians went to their death praising their King, and such martyrdom became the church's most potent witness. Pagan Romans were convinced that Christ had taken away their pains. As has often been said, the church was built on the martyrs' blood.

*Historians have questioned Constantine's motives. Some believe it was an effort to save a dying empire, though one contemporary historian has come to a different conclusion. Christianity was practiced only by a small minority. Its universality, the message of Christ Himself, the reliability of written revelation as opposed to myths, began to attract pagan masses. Robin Lane Fox, *Pagans and Christians* (New York: Knopf, 1986).

gle he endorsed the suppression of heretics by the state.

Through succeeding centuries the church relied increasingly on the state to punish heresy. By the time of the Byzantine empire in the East, the state had become a theocracy with the church serving as its department of spiritual affairs. In the West both church and state jockeyed for control in an uneasy alliance. In the thirteenth century, for example, Frederick II, king of Sicily, was first excommunicated for not going on a crusade, then excommunicated for going on one without the Pope's permission. The state conquered territory, but the Pope distributed the land to the more faithful crusaders.

The consequences of this alliance were mixed. Certainly Christianity provided a civilizing influence on Western culture through art, music, literature, morality, and ultimately in government. One eminent historian concluded that "society developed only so fast as religion enlarged its sphere."[3] On the darker side, however, the excesses of the politicized church created horrors Augustine could not have imagined.

The church turned to military conquest through a series of "holy wars" that became more racial than religious. Jews, Muslims, and dark-skinned Christians were massacred alike. The goal was not to convert the populace, but to conquer it.

In the twelfth and thirteenth centuries a system was organized for adjudicating heresy. Like many well-intentioned reforms, however, the Inquisition simply produced a new set of horrors. Unrepentant heretics were cast out by a church tribunal, which regularly used torture, and were executed by the state.

The spiritual corruption of the church led to the Reformation of the sixteenth century, which produced several streams of church-state relations. One, believing the state to be essentially coercive and violent, rejected participation in any form of government. A second strand of Reformation thought dictated that the religion of a resident king or prince would be the church of the state. Thus, many kings became their own pope. A third principle encouraged church independence. Scottish church leaders like Samuel Rutherford revived the biblical view that God's law reigns over man and his kingdoms. This profoundly influenced the experiment in constitutional government then beginning in the New World.

A new phase of hostility between church and state began in the eighteenth century when waves of skepticism washed over the continent of Europe. Voltaire, one of the most influential philosophers of the day, was vehemently dedicated to the extirpation of what he called "this infamous superstition."

Religions had been assaulted before but always in the name of other religions. With the French Revolution, Tocqueville noted, "Passionate and persistent efforts were made to wean men away from the faith of their fathers. . . . Irreligion became an all-prevailing passion, fierce, intolerant and predatory."[4] For a time this all-prevailing passion was successful. Wrote Tocqueville: "The total rejection of any religious belief, so contrary to man's natural instincts and so destructive of his peace of mind, came to be regarded by the masses as desirable."[5] The

French Revolution was a conscious effort to replace the Kingdom of God with the kingdoms of man.

But the state must have some moral justification for its authority. Thus France's irreligion was soon replaced by a new faith—man's worship of man.

Against this backdrop Wilberforce and other heirs of John Wesley's Great Awakening in England brought the Christian conscience to bear on a society that was nominally Christian but engaged in vile practices. Their stand strengthened the church in England at the very moment it was under its most vicious assault.

Meanwhile, in the New World a radical experiment opened another chapter in church-state relations. There a group of gentlemen farmers, who were neither naïve about human nature nor pretentious about human society, were drawing up the American Constitution. By refusing to assign redemptive powers to the state or to allow coercive power to the church, the American experiment separated these two institutions for the first time since Constantine.

What might be considered the modern phase in church-state history has emerged in our century. It is an amalgam of elements from the previous eras. The rise of totalitarian regimes has brought back the kind of persecution the church experienced in early Rome; like Herod, modern dictators tolerate no other kings. In the West secularism has aggressively spread irreligion, turning Europe into a post-Christian culture and America into a battleground with orthodox religion in retreat.

Can we conclude from this cursory overview that the church and the state must inevitably be in con-

flict? To some extent the answer is yes. Dual allegiances always create tension. And in a sinful world
the struggle for power, which inevitably corrupts, is
unavoidable. When the church isn't being persecuted, it is being corrupted. So as much as anything
else, it is man's own nature that has created centuries
of conflict.

But every generation has an obligation to seek
anew a healthy relationship between church and
state. Both are reflections of man's nature; both have
a role to play. Christ's teaching clearly delineates
these roles.

Jesus was remarkably indifferent to those who
held political power. He had no desire to replace
Caesar or Pilate with His apostles Peter or John. He
gave civil authority its due, rebuking both the Zealots
and Peter for using the sword.

This infuriated the religious right of His day.
Eager to discredit Jesus, the Pharisees and Herodians
tried trapping Him over the question of allegiance to
political authority.

"Tell us," they asked, "is it right to pay taxes to
Caesar or not?"

The question put Jesus in the middle: if He said
no, He would be a threat to the Roman government;
if He said yes, He would lose the respect of the masses
who hated the Romans.

Jesus asked them for a coin. It was a Roman
denarius, the only coin that could be used to pay the
hated yearly poll tax. On one side was the image of
the Emperor Tiberius, around which were written

the words *Tiberius Caesar Augustus, son of the divine Augustus.*

"Whose portrait is this?" He asked, rubbing His finger over the raised features of the Roman ruler. "And whose inscription?"

"Caesar's," they replied impatiently.

"Give to Caesar what is Caesar's and to God what is God's," replied Jesus, handing the coin back to them. They stared at Him in stunned silence.

Not only had He eluded the trap, but He had put Caesar in his place. Christ might simply have said, "Give to Caesar what is Caesar's." That's all that was at issue. It was Caesar's image on the coin, and Caesar had authority over the state.

What made Him add the second phrase, "Give . . . to God what is God's"?

The answer, I believe, is found on the reverse face of the coin, which showed Tiberius's mother represented as the goddess of peace, along with the words *highest priest.* The blasphemous words commanded the worship of Caesar; they thus exceeded the state's authority.

Jesus' lesson was not lost on the early church. Government is to be respected, and its rule honored. "It is necessary to submit to the authorities," wrote the apostle Paul. "If you owe taxes, pay taxes."[6] But worship is reserved solely for God.

The distinction Christ made is clear; as discussed in chapter 7, both church and state have clear and distinct roles ordained by God. The issue is how to apply these teachings to each institution in today's volatile world.

"Christ did not give the keys of the Kingdom to

Caesar nor the sword to Peter," writes a contemporary scholar.[7] In God's provision the state is not to seize authority over ecclesiastical or spiritual matters, nor is the church to seek authority over political matters. Yet the constant temptation of each is to encroach upon the other.

Governments, with rare exceptions, seek to expand their power beyond the mandate to restrain evil, preserve order, and promote justice. Most often they do this by venturing into religious or moral areas. The reason is twofold: the state needs religious legitimization for its policies and an independent church is the one structure that rivals the state's claim for ultimate allegiance.

A contemporary example, though admittedly extreme, is the Soviet Union and its Act of 1918 on separation of church and state. This sounds benign enough, but what the Soviets decreed, reinforced in the 1929 law and in subsequent constitutions, is that churches may conduct worship services when licensed by the government but may not give to the poor, carry on education, or teach religion outside of church. State publishing houses in turn cannot publish religious literature; schools cannot teach religion but must actively teach atheism; and the government has embarked on a campaign to discourage orthodox religious participation and aggressively promote atheism.[8]

So while the edifice of the church is retained, it is a hollow structure; the work of the people of God, which is the true church, is forbidden. Yet in officially promoting atheism, the state is offering its own substitute religion to legitimate its own structure.*

Encroachment upon faith in the West is usually not as dramatic as it has been in modern totalitarian states. It begins in minor ways, such as a county zoning commission barring Bible studies in homes, suppers in church basements, or religious activities on public property. And even when it appears that the state is accommodating religious viewpoints, its action may well be a Trojan horse. Though my opinion is perhaps a minority one, I believe the much-debated issue of prayer in schools in a case in point.

Children or teachers who want to pray in schools should have the same rights of free expression and the same access to public facilities any other group has. But organized prayer, even if voluntary, is another matter. The issue is who does the organizing. If it is the school board, Caesar is being given a spiritual function; admittedly a small crack in the door, but a crack nonetheless. I for one don't want my grandchildren reciting prayers determined by government officials. And in actual practice they would be so watered down as to be of no effect except perhaps to water down my grandchildren's growing faith.

Whenever the state has presumed on God's role, whether in ancient Rome or modern America, the first liberty, freedom of conscience, suffers.

On the other side of the coin, the church, whose principal function is to proclaim the Good News and

---

*Oscar Cullman has written, "According to the Jewish, as to the early Christian, outlook the totalitarian state is precisely the classic form of the Devil's manifestation on earth." Oscar Cullman, *The State in the New Testament* (New York: Scribner's, 1956), 74.

witness the values of the Kingdom of God, must resist the tempting illusion that it can usher in that Kingdom through political means.* Jesus provided the best example for the church in His wilderness confrontation with Satan when the Devil tempted Jesus to worship him and thus take dominion over the kingdoms of this world.

No small temptation. With that kind of power, Christ could enforce the Sermon on the Mount; love and justice could reign. He might have reasoned that if He didn't accept, someone else would. This rationalization is popular today, right up through the highest councils of government: compromise to stay in power because there you can do more for the common good.

And think of the popularity Jesus could have gained. After all, the people wanted a Messiah who would vanquish their oppressors. But Jesus understood His mission, and it could not be accomplished by taking over the kingdoms of the world in a political coup.

Yet the most consistent heresy of the church has been to succumb to the very temptation Christ explicitly denied. In the Middle Ages this produced bloody crusades and inquisitions; in modern times it has fostered a type of utopianism expressed in a stanza from one of William Blake's most famous poems:

---

*James Schall reminds us that "if there is any constant temptation of the history of Christianity, from reaction to Christ's rejection of Jewish zealotism on to current debates about the relation of Marxism to the Kingdom of God, it is the pressure to make religion a formula for refashioning political and economic structures." James Schall, "The Altar as the Throne," in *Churches on the Wrong Road*, (Chicago: Regnery/Gateway, 1986), 227.

> I will not cease from mental flight,
> Nor shall my sword sleep in my hand,
> Till we have built Jerusalem,
> In England's green and pleasant land."⁹*

This century's social-gospel movement echoed Blake's sentiments, dissolving Christian orthodoxy into a campaign to eliminate every social injustice through governmental means. Objectives became political and economic to the detriment of the spiritual. The reformers' well-intentioned efforts were shattered as social programs failed to produce the promised utopia, leaving observers to conclude, "Things are no better. Where is your God now?"

Utopianism is often articulated today in contemporary Christian circles; it crosses political lines, from the liberation theologians to the New Right and to the mainline church leaders. As one bishop confided to Richard Neuhaus, "The mission of the church is to build the kingdom of God on earth, and the means of the mission is politics."¹⁰

Such preoccupation with the political diverts the church from its primary mission. This was evi-

---

*The problem is, as historian Christopher Dawson observed, "There are quite a number of different Jerusalems. . . . There is the Muscovite Jerusalem which has no temple, there is Herr Hitler's Jerusalem which has no Jews, and there is the Jerusalem of the social reformers which is all suburbs. But none of these are Blake's Jerusalem, still less [the Kingdom of God]." Christopher Dawson, "Religion and Politics," *Catholicism in Crisis*, (June 1985), 8.

All these New Jerusalems are earthly cities established by the will and power of man. And if we believe that the Kingdom of Heaven can be established by political or economic measures, then we can hardly object to the claims of such a state to embrace the whole of life and to demand the total submission of the individual will and conscience.

dent in the comment of an American lay missionary who described liberation theology as "a concern for man and the world as opposed to the concern of the traditional church for the salvation of man's soul."[11] All Christian political movements run this risk.

They run another risk too, particularly those on the political right where many want to impose Christian values on society by force of law. Some, such as those in the theonomist movement, even want to reinstate Old Testament civil codes, ignoring Christ's teaching in the parable of the wheat and the tares in which He warns that we live with both good (the wheat) and evil (the tares), and cannot root out the tares. Only God is able to do that and He will—when the Kingdom comes in its final glory.

It is on this point that the church most frequently has stumbled in its understanding of the Kingdom of God. Oscar Cullman writes: "In the course of history the church has always assumed a false attitude toward the state when it has forgotten that the present time is already fulfillment, but not yet consummation."[12]* Even if Christians advocating dominion gained power, they would be doomed to failure. As Martin Luther once wrote, "It is out of the question

---

*Cullman amplifies his point: "The church's task with regard to the state which is posed for all time is thus clear. First, it must loyally give the state everything necessary to its existence. It has to oppose anarchy and all zealotism within its own ranks. Second, it has to fulfill the office of watchmen over the state. That means it must remain in principle critical towards every state and be ready to warn it against transgression of its legitimate limits. Third, it must deny to the state which exceeds its limits, whatever such a state demands that lies within the province of religion-ideological excess; and in its preaching, the church must courageously describe this excess as opposition to God." Cullman, *The State in the New Testament*, 90–91.

that there should be a Christian government even over one land . . . since the wicked always outnumber the good. Hence a man who would venture to govern . . . with the gospel would be like a shepherd who should place in one fold wolves, lions, eagles and sheep together and let them freely mingle."[13]

It was perhaps because he realized this truth—that the world cannot be ruled by spiritual structures and that the church has long abused power—that John Paul I at his inauguration in 1978 refused to be crowned with the papal tiara, the vestigial symbol of the claim to temporal power. John Paul II followed his example. These dramatic gestures renounced a centuries-old tradition that has contributed to the darkest moments for the church.

But while the church must avoid utopianism and diversion from its transcendent mission, it is not to ignore the political scene. To the contrary, as will be explored in later chapters, its members, who are also citizens of the world, have a duty, as Carl Henry puts it, "to work through civil authority for the advancement of justice and human good." They may provide "critical illumination, personal example and vocational leadership."[14] Wilberforce is a prime example. There are proper ways as well for the institutional church to provide society with its moral vision and hold government to moral account.*

---

*Some Christian traditions similarly believe that they can best model Kingdom values not by involvement in politics but by the establishment of alternative communities in which they live out the teachings of the Kingdom. In its proper form, this is not a withdrawal from the world or abandonment of Christian responsibility; nor is it a privatization of Christian values as with those who profess to believe but live as if they do not. It is

Through the individual Christian's involvement in politics, as we will discuss later, the standards of civic righteousness can be influenced by the standards of righteousness of the Kingdom of God. Such an influence is what theologians call common grace (as distinguished from God's special grace that offers citizenship in the Kingdom of God to all who desire admission). Common grace is God's provision for the welfare of all His created beings, both those who believe in Him and those who don't.

The critical dynamic in the church-state tension is separation of institutional authority. Religion and politics can't be separated—they inevitably overlap—but the institutions of church and state must preserve their separate and distinct roles. In this regard, the American experiment merits closer examination.

America is not the New Jerusalem or a "city upon a hill," though some of its founders harbored that vision. Nor are Americans God's chosen people. The Kingdom of God is universal, bound by neither race nor nation. But Abraham Lincoln used an interesting phrase; Americans, he said, were the "almost chosen people."[15] If there is any justification for that term— not theologically but historically—it is because in the hammering out of a new republic, the combination of wisdom, reason, and providence produced

instead a different strategy to the same end of providing a witness in the kingdoms of man of the values of the Kingdom of God. While I do not agree with the generally negative view of government held by such groups, I respect the faithfulness by which they live their convictions.

a church-state relationship that uniquely respected the differing roles of each.

The basis of this radical idea came from the partial convergence of at least two conflicting ideologies: confidence in the eighteenth-century Enlightenment belief that both public and private virtue were possible without religion; and a reaction against the excesses of the state church in Europe. The first view was held by the Deists among America's founders, while the second particularly motivated the avowed Christians among them.

These men and women believed that Christ had given the church its own structures and charter, and the state, ordained in God's providence for the maintenance of public order, was not to tamper with it. The church was ordained principally for the conversion of men and women—conversion grounded in individual conscience wrought by the supernatural work of a sovereign God upon the soul. So the state could neither successfully establish nor destroy the church, since it could not rule conscience nor transform people's hearts and souls.*

Thus two typically mortal enemies, the Enlightenment and the Christian faith, found a patch of common ground on American soil. Both agreed (for different reasons) that the new government should

---

*The comment of Baptist minister Isaac Backus is representative: "Nothing can be a true religion but a voluntary obedience unto his revealed will, of which each rational soul has an equal right to judge for himself, every person has an unalienable right to act in all religious affairs according to the full persuasion of his own mind." "A Declaration of the Rights of the Inhabitants of the State of Massachusetts-Bay in New England," in Edwin S. Gaustad, ed., *A Documentary History of Religion in America, Vol. 1* (Grand Rapids, Mich.: Eerdmans, 1982), 268.

neither establish nor interfere with the church.* It was this reasoning that led to the adoption of the First Amendment, expressly to protect the individual's right to freedom of conscience and expression, and to prevent the establishment of a state church.

But contrary to the belief of many today, this separation of church and state did not mean that America was to be a nation free of religious influence. From the very beginning the American Revolution itself was seen by many as a rebellion fueled by the conviction that man is a creature of God, and his political life is conditioned by that truth. As James Madison insisted, "This duty [homage to the Creator] is precedent, both in order of time and degree of obligation, to the claims of civil society. Before any man can be considered as a member of civil society, he must be considered as a subject of the governor of the universe."[16] A nation under God was no idle phrase.

Nor did the separation of church and state mean religion and politics could be separated or religious values removed from the public arena. For one's political life is an expression of values, and religion,

---

*One phrase in James Madison's "Memorial and Remonstrance," presented to the Commonwealth of Virginia in 1785, succinctly sums up the thinking of our Founding Fathers: "...that Religion or the duty which we owe to our Creator and the manner of discharging it, can be directed only by reason and conviction, not by force or violence. The Religion then of every man must be left to the conviction and conscience of every man; and it is the right of every man to exercise it as these may dictate." "James Madison's Memorial and Remonstrance, 1785," in Gaustad, ed., A Documentary History of Religion in America: Vol. I, 262.

by definition, most profoundly influences values.*

The Founding Fathers were well aware that the form of limited government they were adopting could only succeed if there was an underlying consensus of values shared by the populace. I am always reminded of this when I visit the House of Representatives. A beautiful fresco on the upper walls of the chamber itself contains the portraits of history's great lawmakers. Standing at the speaker's desk and looking straight ahead over the main entrance, one's eyes meet the piercing eyes of the first figure in the series: Moses, the one who recorded the Law from the original Lawgiver.

John Adams eloquently acknowledged the understanding of our constitutional framers when in 1798 he wrote: "We have no government armed in power capable of contending with human passions unbridled by morality and religion. . . . Our constitution was made only for a moral and religious people. It is wholly inadequate for the government of any other."[17]

Many of these original American visionaries believed that Christian citizens would actively bring their religious values to the public forum. George Washington faintly echoed Augustine when he asserted, "Of all the dispositions and habits which lead to a political prosperity, religion and morality are indispensable supports. In vain would that man claim that tribute of patriotism, who should labor to

_____

*The concept of a "wall of separation," a phrase incidentally first used by Jefferson fifteen years after the Constitution was adopted, applied to institutions of church and state, not religious and political values.

subvert these great pillars of human happiness."[18]

Thus, when laws were passed reflecting the consensus of Christian values in the land, no one panicked supposing that the Christian religion was being "established" or that a sectarian morality was being imposed on an unwilling people. The point of the First Amendment was that such convictions could only become the law of the land if a majority of citizens could be persuaded (without coercion), whether they shared the religious foundation or not, of the merits of a particular proposition.

Today's widespread relegation of religion to merely something people do only in the privacy of their homes or churches would have been unimaginable to the founders of the republic—even those who personally repudiated orthodox Christian faith. Though America has drifted far from the vision of its founders, this system continues to offer one of the world's most hopeful models in an otherwise contentious history of conflict.

The record of the centuries should not cause despair, however. Tension between church and state is inherent and inevitable. Indeed, it is perhaps the outworking of one of God's great mysteries, part of the dynamic by which He governs His universe. For from the constant tension—the chafing back and forth—a certain equilibrium is achieved.

To maintain this balance the church and the state must fulfill their respective roles. One cannot survive without the other; yet neither can do the work of the other. Both operate under God's rule, each in a different relationship to that rule.

Certainly one thing is clear. When they fail in their appointed tasks—that is, when the church fails to be the visible manifestation of the Kingdom of God and the state fails to maintain justice and concord— civic order collapses. The consequences can be cat- astrophic, as the tumultuous events described in the next two chapters demonstrate.

PART
III

ABSENCE OF THE KINGDOM

TEN

Roots of War
(Part I)

> In Germany they came first for the
> Communists, and I didn't speak up
> because I wasn't a Communist. Then they
> came for the Jews, and I didn't speak up
> because I wasn't a Jew. Then they came
> for the trade unionists, and I didn't speak
> up because I wasn't a trade unionist. Then
> they came for the Catholics, and I didn't
> speak up because I was a Protestant. Then
> they came for me, and by that time no one
> was left to speak up.
>
> —Martin Niemoller

One match flared, illuminating a single face
above the collar of a brown shirt. He was a middle-
aged man with a paunch and a face scarred by innumerable street battles.[1]

The man held the match to a fuel-soaked torch,
which leaped into flame. Quickly he held the torch

This account is based on historical records and quotations from the major
figures. In an effort to recreate the historical environment, however, some
dialogue has been invented, along with some minor characters. The main
characters, their activities, and their views, are as accurate as it is possible
to make them.

to another and then another. In a matter of minutes hundreds were alight, their flickering red glare glazing the street crowded with men dressed in brown shirts and dark pants.

They formed into ranks and began their march through the city. Singing, shouting in triumph, swaggering as though they owned the world, thousands marched, filling the widest streets of Berlin and lighting its ancient walls with their smoking torches. They swept under the Brandenburg Gate and down the Wilhelmstrasse. When they passed the chancellery, they became strangely agitated. The tramping of their steps grew louder and the men strained their necks looking upward.

"Sieg Heil, Sieg Heil." Their cries echoed from the buildings at the sight of their leader.

Above them, at a window, Adolf Hitler fondly looked down. After years in the political wilderness, that very day, January 30, 1933, he had been named Chancellor of Germany.

February 1, 1933, Berlin

A tall, blond young man, well-dressed and carrying himself with aloof self-confidence, stepped out of the heavy black car that had pulled up in front of the German Broadcasting Company on the busy Potsdamerstrasse. As he entered the building, a younger man in a neat but frayed jacket hustled up to greet him enthusiastically.

"Dr. Bonhoeffer! Please come in. Let me take your coat. It is indeed a pleasure for the former student to welcome his professor. You have your script?"

Dietrich Bonhoeffer tapped his chest. "It is here."

"You have it memorized?" the younger asked, his eyes widening. "Are you sure? This is a live broadcast, you know."

Bonhoeffer's cold, patrician face broke into an amused smile. "No, Herr Schmidt, I have the script here, in my pocket." He reached inside his suitcoat and pulled out a sheaf of typed pages.

"Oh, excuse me, Doctor." Schmidt murmured with a look of embarrassed pleasure. "I know you are brilliant, but . . . one can be too brilliant.

"You know the time limit," the younger man added as he led Bonhoeffer upstairs to the broadcast room. "I'm sure I don't have to tell you it is very strict." Bonhoeffer nodded. He had worked out the length of his speech with his usual precision.

Schmidt took a seat before the microphone and glanced at his watch. "We have a little time," he said. "Would you like to smoke?" Bonhoeffer declined.

Then, with an effort at casualness, Schmidt said, "I hope you won't mind if I say that I was quite surprised at your choice of the subject, 'The Younger Generation's Changed View of the Concept of Führer.' Most of the theologians who come here speak on very dry material. But you have chosen just the topic people want to discuss. Tell me, were you inspired by the parade in the Wilhelmstrasse last night?"

"Inspired?" Bonhoeffer seemed suddenly to notice the younger man. "What do you mean, 'inspired'?"

At this invitation, the words poured out of Schmidt. "People say that Hitler is just one more politician, but I don't think so. Somehow, Dr. Bonhoeffer, I feel he is a different kind of man, a man who knows the soul of Germany. I am sure you must know what I mean. The old people cannot stop living in the past. But they will learn. This man may be the leader we in the younger generation have been seeking. That is what I meant by 'inspired.' That march seemed to signal that he had touched some secret chord in our hearts."

Bonhoeffer appeared aloof, almost bored, when in fact he was intensely interested. "What do you think he will do now that he has power, Herr Schmidt? He has been very evasive in laying out his plans."

"But that is exactly what I mean! He is not just another politician, with one promise or another. He offers himself. We have had so many years of these weak politicians. They act as though Germany's defeat and betrayal is simply a fact that must be accepted. If that is realism, we should get rid of realism! We don't need just another political program; we need a complete transformation of the nation. You can only get that from a leader you trust completely. Our soul was meant to be forged into unity! Don't you think so?"

"I doubt Hitler will last long in power," said Bonhoeffer coolly. "He seems strong because he has not had to be responsible. Now he will have to make the usual compromises." As he spoke, Bonhoeffer fingered a signet ring on his left hand. "Nor, Herr Schmidt, do I completely agree with you about the need for a leader. It is, of course, a very appealing idea. We are so tired of politics. We would naturally like to give it all over to a leader in the way that a child can turn over some difficult struggle to his father. But we cannot just hand over authority to our leaders and consider that the end of our responsibility. I think that is what Herr Hitler would like us to do. But the government can only do, and should only be called on to do certain things. It cannot replace God."

Schmidt was silent for a few moments. When he spoke, he weighed his words carefully. "For years godless Communists have had the run of the streets. You have seen the fights, real battles, as though Berlin were in a war zone. The national economy is devastated. People lack food, jobs. Money has become worthless. Nobody goes to church any more. Now Herr Hitler has at last barred the Communists from meeting, something none of our 'leaders' had the courage to do. He will save us from Bolshevism. This is leadership. This will lead the German people to greatness."

"Be careful that such leadership does not lead you to disaster," Bonhoeffer said quietly.

Schmidt stood up. "Did you bring the extra copy of your script, Dr. Bonhoeffer? I should take it to the director now."

"Why does he need it?"

"It's a new directive. Everything should go across his desk."

Bonhoeffer reached into his suitcoat pocket and

pulled out a second copy of his script. Schmidt took it away. Shortly after he returned, Bonhoeffer went on the air.

Bonhoeffer, who spoke rapidly in normal conversation, delivered his radio address slowly and deliberately. He described the development of Adolf Hitler's "Führerprinzip," or "leadership principle," through which discipline and dignity would be restored by vesting authority in a single leader. This idea was tremendously attractive to young Germans who had known only the chaos of the last fifteen years. At many points in his address it seemed that Bonhoeffer was embracing the Führer principle. But at the end his words grew ominous as he warned against placing blind faith in any authority.

"For should the leader allow himself to succumb to the wishes of those he leads, who will always seek to turn him into an idol," he concluded, "then the leader will gradually become the image of 'mis-leader.' This is the leader who makes an idol of himself and his office, thus mocking God."

When he finished, Bonhoeffer glanced at his watch, stood and shook hands with Schmidt, and left the broadcasting room. As he was putting on his overcoat on the ground floor, Schmidt came down the stairs hurriedly.

"Dr. Bonhoeffer," he called. "Just a moment. . . . The director said I ought to tell you . . . just so you would not be surprised . . . that unfortunately the last few sentences of your address were not broadcast. It seems you went slightly over the time allotted."

Bonhoeffer's blue eyes were icy behind his rimless glasses. "What do you mean? They turned off the microphone?"

Schmidt smiled. "I'm so sorry, Doctor. But you know radio is very precise."

February 27, 1933

While at a party in his honor at the apartment of Joseph Goebbels, Adolf Hitler received a call telling him that the ornate, gilded Reichstag building was in flames. The Reichstag was the historic German parliament building. "It's the Communists!" the Führer shouted. Then he stalked out into the frigid night where the buildings were silhouetted against an orange sky.

Shortly thereafter, Hitler convened a meeting in Hermann Göring's nearby office. Cabinet ministers filed in, talking excitedly. Finally Rudolf Diels, head of the Secret Police, was ushered in to report on the initial investigation. Diels said that a Dutchman named van der Lubbe had been arrested and had confessed to lighting the fire as a protest.

Both Göring and Hitler began shouting simultaneously. "This is the beginning of a Communist uprising! Now we'll show them! Anyone who stands in our way will be mowed down!"

Diels interrupted them. The idea of an uprising was nonsense; his spies all said no Communist move was coming. Undoubtedly van der Lubbe had acted alone.

Hitler ignored Diels. "This is a cunning and well-prepared plot! But they have reckoned without us and without the German people! In their rat holes, from which they are now trying to crawl, they cannot hear the jubilation of the masses!" He ranted until Diels and everyone else fell silent.

By morning truckloads of hurriedly deputized brownshirts were breaking down doors and arresting Communists throughout the nation. Four thousand suspects were sent to newly organized concentration camps. Hitler, claiming a national emergency and demanding instantaneous action, convinced the government to suspend all constitutional rights. News broadcasts proclaimed that Hitler had miraculously saved Germany from a Communist insurrection.

In this frenzied atmosphere Adolf Hitler won his first bare majority in the March 5 elections.*

April 1, 1933

The first splash of morning light struck the front door of the small hardware store as three young brownshirts, laughing and joking, began fixing a large poster to the front window. The proprietor, who was sweeping the sidewalk, came over to ask what they were doing. After a short, noisy argument he retreated into his store. He could be seen from time to time peering out the door.

The sign announced, in six-inch letters visible from across the street, that the proprietor was a Jew and requested that shoppers not patronize his busi-

---

*It is generally accepted now that the fire was set by the Nazis to give them pretext for destroying the Communist political organization.

ness. A few curious passersby gathered on the sidewalk and watched the stormtroopers post the signs on several other storefronts.

A man dressed in dark blue working clothes came down the sidewalk and walked up to the door of the hardware store, not noticing the signs or the small crowd. Before he could enter the store, one of the brownshirts politely stopped him and explained that a national boycott of all Jewish businesses had been called by Adolf Hitler. The man looked up and around, startled to see the spectators, and hurried off. The crowd chuckled.

After three days the boycott ended. Hitler had learned what he wanted to know: no one would stand up for the Jews.

On the same day the boycott was launched, a group known as the German Christians held their first national rally. Included in their number were some widely respected theologians and church leaders. Their chosen name, which placed more emphasis on *German* than *Christian*, expressed their belief that German experiences and culture had given them a unique understanding of God.

The German Christians wanted to harmonize the church in Germany with Hitler's political movement, which was, to them, more than politics; it was the revival of hope and the force of destiny for their nation. Many of them believed the Germans were God's chosen people and Hitler the new messiah. The national revival was more vital than anything they had ever found in their faith.

July 1933

In six months Hitler had accomplished an almost unbelievable consolidation of power. He had, thanks to the Reichstag fire, imprisoned all known Communists. He had convinced the members of the Reichstag parliament to virtually suspend its own powers. He had outlawed all significant opposition parties and imprisoned many of their leaders. He had taken over, by force, all labor unions and removed all Jews from the civil service.

More significantly, however, he had done all this without arousing any substantial resistance. In January he had been head of a minority party, little liked or trusted. By July, thanks to his skillful manipulation, the majority of German citizens had fallen under his spell. Germans talked excitedly of the renewal of their country. It was no longer only his swaggering, heel-clicking brownshirts who cheered Hitler to the skies. Ordinary men and women, laborers and tradesmen, businessmen and housewives went into hysterical chants of "Heil Hitler!" when he passed through the streets, his motorcade swathed in red and black Nazi flags. He had given them hope again.

William Shirer, an American correspondent in Berlin, wrote in his diary: "I'm beginning to comprehend, I think, some of the reasons for Hitler's astounding success. Borrowing a chapter from the Roman church, he is restoring pageantry and color and mysticism to the drab lives of twentieth-century Germans. This morning's opening meeting...had something of the mysticism and religious fervor of

an Easter or Christmas Mass in a great Gothic cathedral."

The pageant Shirer had viewed was played dozens of times in every part of Germany: an immense
hall packed with citizens and soldiers . . . a sea of red
and black Nazi standards swaying overhead . . . a
giant golden eagle glaring down from an upper balcony . . . an orchestra playing solemn symphonic music.

The orchestra stops. A hush falls over the
strangely orderly crowd and thousands of people
crane their necks to see. Then a stately patriotic an-
them begins and from far in the back, walking slowly
down the wide central aisle, comes the Führer.

Thousands of arms snap stiffly out in salute.
Thousands of eyes focus on Hitler's pale, grave face.
Behind him march his closest aides—faces and
names that will go down in history, recorded in
blood—Göring, Goebbels, Hess, Himmler. They take
their places on the raised dais under huge lights.
Above them is the huge Nazi Blood Flag, stained with
the blood of Nazis killed in the Munich Beer Hall
Putsch.

Finally the Führer himself rises to speak. Beginning in a low, velvety voice, which makes the audience unconsciously lean forward to hear, he speaks
of his love for Germany and his long struggle to restore its dignity. He describes his own humble beginnings, his injuries as a foot soldier in World War
I, and the terrible injuries Germany has suffered as
a result of that war. Gradually his pitch increases
until he reaches a screaming crescendo. But his au-

dience does not think his rasping shouts excessive. They are screaming with him.

July 14, 1933

By now Hitler had only one significant source of opposition. Not the journalists, political parties, universities, or labor unions; all these he had almost completely converted to Nazism in less than six months. Instead, opposition came from a most unexpected source: the church.

Two thirds of the German population— 45,000,000 people—were Protestants, primarily Lutherans, who traditionally kept their noses entirely out of politics. As a group, they were known as the German Evangelical Church. They were conservative, rural, and patriotic, and had Hitler been content to leave them alone, they undoubtedly would have supported him almost unanimously at this stage. But Hitler would allow no independent source of authority in his resurrected Germany. Everyone must answer to a single leader, the Führer. Every institution must serve the aims of the Fatherland, including the church.

Publicly, in the beginning, Hitler gave the appearance of being a religious man. A nominal Catholic, he sometimes displayed a tattered Bible and spoke of its inspiration in his life. Officially, his party platform called, rather ambiguously, for religious freedom and supported "positive Christianity." In private, however, he expressed his utter contempt for the church, particularly for the Protestants. He expected their pastors to knuckle under easily to his schemes for remolding the church, his main source of opposition. "They will betray anything for the sake of their miserable little jobs and incomes."

Early on he had negotiated an agreement with Rome that removed Roman Catholic opposition to his regime. Eager to support the spirit of the times, the twenty-eight main Protestant denominations voluntarily began work on a new constitution that would unite them under one leader according to the "Führer principle."

But Hitler was impatient; he did not want to wait for the church bureaucracy. He decided to push an obscure, obsequious naval chaplain, Ludwig Müller, into leadership of the newly united Protestant church. Despite the Führer's prestigious support, however, Muller was defeated in a May 27 election.

Hitler refused to meet the elected bishop. Instead, radio and press propaganda poured out favorable material about Müller. Then in late June Nazi government officials invaded church offices, forcibly taking over administrative positions. Müller proclaimed himself national bishop-elect.

The new officials ordered services of praise and thanksgiving for this takeover. Every church in Germany was to be decorated with Nazi flags and a proclamation read from the pulpit, stating that "all those who are concerned ... feel deeply thankful that the state should have assumed, in addition to all its tremendous tasks, the great load and burden of reorganizing the church."

But while all Germany was being wooed to Hitler, a stubborn resistance was taking root within the church itself: the Young Reformation Movement.

Martin Niemoller, Hans Jacobi, and Dietrich Bonhoeffer were among its first members. They were apolitical, and their meetings often included a resolution of loyalty to the government and, sometimes, to Adolf Hitler. But they also valued the church's independence and rejected any attempt to blend a religion of Germany with the religion of Jesus Christ.

On July 14, 1933, Hitler surprised everyone by calling a special church election to be held nine days later on July 23. The German Christians were given complete access to the state-run radio and newspapers; the Young Reformation hastily organized a slate of candidates and began feverish campaigning. Over the weekend leaflets were written and duplicated.

On Monday, July 17, the Gestapo invaded the Young Reformation offices and confiscated all 620,000 campaign leaflets.

July 17, 1933

The cramped offices of the Young Reformers, which just two days earlier had been a hive of activity, were ominously silent. Martin Niemoller, whose rounded face and cleft chin gave him the appearance of perpetual boyhood, paced around Bonhoeffer, Jacobi, and a young man wearing the brown shirt and Nazi armband of the SA.

"I don't see any point in appealing to underlings," Niemoller said stubbornly. "You might as well appeal to the stones in the street. I would rather go directly to Hitler. If he knew what was being done, he would put a stop to it. But I am sure they all lie to him."

"How do we get to Hitler?" Jacobi asked.

"Perhaps through President Hindenburg," said Niemoller. "We have contacts there, and he has always been sympathetic."

Bonhoeffer's impatience would have been invisible to anyone who did not recognize his mannerism of fiddling with the ring on his left hand. "That is a fine idea, Martin," he said, "but the elections are Sunday. If we have no literature we might as well go home. What else can we do, stand in the street and yell our slogans? We must go to the Gestapo now!"

The discussion seesawed until Niemoller shrugged his large shoulders and smiled. "All right, go then," he said. "But at least take Henke with you." He pointed to the young storm trooper, a hybrid rare but not unknown—a staunch Nazi who was also a Young Reformer. "They may respect his uniform more than they respect yours."

Jacobi vetoed this. "Martin, I think not. Maybe these will count as much as Henke's swastikas." He indicated the two Iron Crosses he wore, won in World War I. "At any rate, for every SA member we can produce, the German Christians can show fifty."

At Gestapo headquarters on the Albrechtstrasse, Jacobi and Bonhoeffer's demand to see Rudolf Diels, the Gestapo chief, met with opposition by several underlings. They persisted. Finally a rude, overbearing officer ushered them into Diels's presence.

To their surprise, the Gestapo chief politely invited them to sit down and said that he certainly hoped he could be of help to them. It was really not his department, but he would do what he could. He noticed Jacobi's decorations and asked about his service in the war.

But the initial cordiality was mere display. When he heard their complaint, Diels did not budge an inch.

"It seems clear to me, Pastors, that you are in the wrong. You have published scurrilous literature. You have taken a slogan that cannot be proper, 'The Program of the Evangelical Church.' You are fortunate not to have been arrested yourselves." He stood up and held out his hand, as though that closed the matter.

Neither Bonhoeffer nor Jacobi moved.

"The Führer made the explicit promise that this election would be free and secret," Bonhoeffer said. "He wanted to settle the political quarrels of our church through a fair election. Do you think confiscating all of one party's literature can be considered fair treatment? It is certainly a violation of the Führer's words."

Diels slowly took his seat again.

"Pastor, I have heard the Führer's words. He appointed me to safeguard them. He did not give you that responsibility. My officers have been very lenient with you. If it were up to me I would send you to the concentration camp now. In fact I am thinking of it. Why don't you simply leave now and go prepare your next sermon?"

"You have not answered my question," Bonhoeffer pressed him. "The state has promised a free election. How can this be considered free?"

The Gestapo leader leaned back in his chair and looked Bonhoeffer over while absentmindedly brushing off his jacket. He forced a smile. "You do not really have much respect for the state, do you, Pastor?"

"I have enough respect for the state to protest when it does wrong," Bonhoeffer snapped back.

After another silence, Diels asked, "What do you want me to do? There is a court injunction against you. Do you want me to ignore it? That would be contrary to the law."

Jacobi spoke up. "The injunction is against our slogan, not against our literature."

"But the slogan is all over your literature."

"Not all of it."

Diels agreed, finally, to let them have their literature back. The pastors, in turn, agreed to change their slogan from "Evangelical Church" to "Gospel and Church."

The parting was stiff and unfriendly; no one was satisfied.

"I assure you, Pastors," Diels said, "that I am still considering whether you are safe outside this building or whether you would be better off in the KZ.* If a single pamphlet appears, under your names or anyone else's, that insults the German Christians or that uses some slogan similar to the one you have agreed to discard, I will certainly send for you. Do not think that I lack the power to put you anywhere I want to, or that I will hesitate again."

That weekend Hitler was in Bayreuth for the annual Wagner Festival. During an interval in the program, he broadcast a message calling for the German people, in support of all he had done, to elect

---

*Concentration camps.

those forces that "as exemplified by the German Christians, have deliberately chosen to take their stand within the National Socialist State."

For Martin Niemoller that address was a lightning bolt. As a former U-boat captain from World War I and an ardent German patriot, he had supported Hitler. Now he heard, in disbelief, a state official telling the church whom to elect as their spiritual representatives. Niemoller would never trust Hitler again.

For others, however, the address proved that as popular as Hitler was, he could sway most church members to support anything he wanted. When the votes were tallied the next day, the German Christians had over 70 percent. Even in Niemoller's parish they took half the vote. Now, by "legal" means, the Nazis took over key positions in the church.

September 1933

In September the new governing body of the German Evangelical Church met. It became known as the Brown Synod because most of the delegates wore the brown shirts of the SA. They elected Hitler's man, Müller, their bishop and passed the much-debated Aryan Paragraph, outlawing all Jews or persons married to Jews from church office. They also passed a ruling that all pastors take a loyalty oath to Hitler and his government.

Dietrich Bonhoeffer urged vehemently that all dissenting pastors resign from the church. Instead, protest formed under a new organization, the Pastors' Emergency League, led by the tireless Martin Niemoller. Within a week 2,300 pastors had signed its pledge to be bound in their preaching "only by Holy Scripture and the Confessions of the Reformation." By the end of the year members would total 6,000, approximately the same number as the German Christians.

October 17, 1933, London

Dietrich Bonhoeffer stood at the window of his new London vicarage, thoughtfully smoking a cigarette. Though located in the south London suburb of Forest Hill, the large Victorian house was surrounded by a forest of trees. He watched the dying leaves being whipped away by a strong wind and shivered in the wet English air. The room behind him, one of two he would occupy, was bare and inhospitable; clearly mice had been its most frequent residents. His furniture and his piano had yet to arrive from Germany.

Bonhoeffer had come to London to pastor two tiny German-speaking congregations and to place some distance between himself and the church struggle in Germany. Still under thirty years of age, yet often consulted for his wisdom, Bonhoeffer needed time to think and pray. He was deeply concerned with the Jewish question, and he was frustrated by the gap between his own uncompromising stand and the views of others who still thought accommodation with Hitler possible.*

Just three days before Hitler had announced that

---

*Often in his meditations in those days he turned to the Sermon on the Mount. A few years later his thoughts would coalesce into his book *The Cost of Discipleship*.

Germany was resigning from the League of Nations. Germans, for whom the League was a symbol of their World War I defeat, had rejoiced as though at a stunning martial victory. Even Martin Niemoller, to Bonhoeffer's horror, had sent Hitler a congratulatory telegram.

The Germany he had left rang with the marching and singing of tanned, fit bands of children, the Hitler Youth. Hitler was obviously preparing to violate the Versailles Treaty, which limited the size and armaments of Germany's army. Yet few Germans, including his comrades in the church struggle, saw any danger. They were stirred by their love for their nation and their faith in its God-given destiny.

Sadly, the people in England were equally unaware of the danger. They did not understand the degree to which Hitler had transformed the German nation, particularly the young people, into passionate believers. They wanted Bonhoeffer to explain what was happening in Germany, but their attention span was short. The Christians he had spoken with could not even distinguish between the German Christians and those who opposed them.

London was to give Bonhoeffer a chance to develop perspective from a distance. Yet he longed for the battle he had deliberately left. He spent hours on the phone and found excuses for returning to Berlin frequently.

November 12, 1933, Berlin

Martin Niemoller was a popular preacher and the services in his newly built church in the affluent suburb of Dahlem were generally full. But this Sunday many people, including the usual Gestapo plainclothesmen, came early and waited with particular expectation. Yesterday church officials had informed Niemoller and two other leaders of the Pastors' Emergency League that they were suspended from their pastorates. Later in the day the suspension had been cancelled; some said because Hitler had ordered it.

Niemoller was very different from the introspective Bonhoeffer. Blunt to a fault, he never kept his thoughts to himself. His critics called him unreasonable and unbending.

This Sunday marked the four-hundred-and-fiftieth anniversary of Martin Luther's birth. The German Christians claimed Luther as their hero. To them the bluff, courageous, uncompromising reformer embodied the true German character. What would Niemoller say to that?

He began by welcoming this "1933 picture of Luther, which represents him as a fighter." Clearly battle lines were being drawn in the German church today. It was proper to ask, which side of the battle would Luther be on if he were here?

Niemoller acknowledged with a warm smile that behind all the German Christians' discussion of the "Luther spirit" lay a genuine admiration for Luther's "naïve unconcern, for his intrepid courage, for his tenacious steadfastness, for his straightforward and unflinching will, for his profound tenderness." Many Germans felt, said Niemoller, that Germany and its church desperately needed more of this Luther spirit if they were to renew themselves.

"But here is a grave error," Niemoller said, his

clear voice ringing over the quiet congregation, "the substitution of a human hero for the message God sent through him. What a strange paradox it would be if the Devil used Luther's four hundred and fiftieth birthday to fill German minds with the delusion that they needed not the grace of God, but the courage of Martin Luther! Luther's message was always that no human qualities or human works could bring salvation—only the goodness of God."

Now Niemoller applied this to practical political issues. "One can even hear that our whole nation would do the will of God if only it had purified its species and its race!" Luther himself, Niemoller said, would certainly have fought such ideas.

"There is absolutely no sense in talking of Luther and celebrating his memory within the Protestant church if we stop at Luther's image and do not look at Him to whom Luther pointed." And Luther pointed, Niemoller reminded his listeners, to a Jew, the rabbi of Nazareth.

The next evening, as though in confirmation of Niemoller's words, 20,000 German Christians, including bishops and church officials in full regalia, gathered in the Berlin Sports Palace, a massive new building, symbolic of the Nazi resurgence in its raw modernistic architecture.

Joachim Hossenfelder, head of the German Christians and a Berlin pastor, presided in his Nazi uniform. After the usual parade of swastika-bedecked flags, a fanfare of trumpets and throaty chorus of "Now Thank We All Our God," Hossenfelder announced that in his diocese the Aryan paragraph, dismissing all Jews from church office, was being put into effect immediately. He also announced that Niemoller and other leaders of the Pastors' Emergency League would be suspended, since their activities were entirely foreign to the true spirit of Germany. At each announcement the crowd erupted into a resounding cheer.

The main speaker of the evening was a senior Nazi official who demanded that everything un-German be purged from the church. His final admonition was that the Bible be reexamined for non-German elements: "liberation from the Old Testament, with its Jewish money morality and these stories of cattle-dealers and pimps." It also meant purging the New Testament of its Jewish elements, especially the unheroic theology of the apostle Paul with his "inferiority complex." A proud, heroic Jesus must replace the model of a "suffering servant."

His speech was interrupted again and again by applause. Not one of the bishops or church leaders stood to disagree. Instead, when the speaker had finished, resolutions were enthusiastically passed supporting his words and calling for Jewish Christians to be forced into "ghetto churches."

In the days that followed, the reports in the press of the Sports Palace rally shocked many. The Emergency League printed a protest to be read from their pulpits the next Sunday, but the proclamation was confiscated and fifty pastors who read it were dismissed from their churches.

Bishop Müller, terrified that he might lose his position as head of the national church, resigned from the German Christians. He also rescinded the

Aryan paragraph. At the same time, he published vol-
leys of orders, some illegal, some self-contradictory.
He secretly arranged for the transfer of all church
youth work to the leadership of the Hitler Youth. He
then reinstated the Aryan paragraph and published
the Muzzling Decrees, which forbade the discussion
of all church issues by pastors, on pain of dismissal.
Most church leaders lost all confidence in him.

In January Hitler intervened. He had hoped that
Müller would unite the entire church behind the
Nazi program, but Müller had failed. Now the Führer
himself would meet with the leadership of the German Evangelical Church.

January 25, 1934, Berlin

Martin Niemoller and a group of his fellow bishops waited quietly in the Reich Chancellery watching
the black-uniformed SS officers marching back and
forth. One of the bishops nudged Niemoller as a Nazi
official passed carrying a scarlet briefcase under his
arm. Niemoller recognized fat, baby-faced Hermann
Göring. Truly they were near the seat of power!

Finally they were ushered into the Führer's office. Hitler rose from behind his desk and came forward to greet them. Seen closely, he was less than
superhuman. He was not tall; his complexion was
pale, his face almost undernourished. Only his frigid
blue eyes betrayed the real man.

Hitler was about to begin the discussion when
Göring burst into the room. He clicked his heels, gave
the Nazi salute, and breathlessly launched into a dia-
tribe accusing Bishop Niemoller of conspiring

against Hitler. As Göring read from a paper, Niemoller recognized some of his own words, a direct quote from an innocent jest he had made less than an hour before in a telephone conversation with one of his fellow pastors from the Emergency League. The slightly garbled version presented by Göring made it sound as though Niemoller had been gloating about political maneuverings that would outsmart Hitler, the master politician.

Hitler's face flushed and he began to lecture the pastors angrily, pacing the room while they stood before him. Hitler's entire manner made them feel like criminals.

"Do you think you can pull such outrageous, backstairs politics with me? You underestimate me if you do. I am sick of being treated this way, by the church leaders of all people. What have I done to you? Only tried to make peace between all your warring factions. Peace in the church and peace with the state! And this is my reward! You obstruct me at every point and sabotage every move!"

Hitler raved on. The bishops were dumbfounded and Niemoller was horrified. The thought of a treason trial crossed his mind. How would he answer these complaints? *If only Hitler would stop his horrid tirade*, Niemoller thought. *Dear God, let him stop.*

When Hitler finally did stop, Niemoller stepped to the front of the group and tried to explain calmly that the comments had been made during a private conversation with his secretary and were a perfectly innocent joke. Niemoller went on to explain that the struggle for the church was by no means aimed against the Third Reich; it was for the sake of the

nation. As a pastor his concern was that the people
of Germany not be deluded or led astray.

"I will protect the German people," Hitler
shouted. "You take care of the church. You pastors
should worry about getting people to heaven and
leave this world to me."

The shaken clergymen timidly tried to soothe
Hitler's temper, assuring him that isolated expressions of political discontent indicated no overall dis-
loyalty. They suggested that Bishop Müller simply
lacked the mature qualities that a national bishop
needed. For their part they were tremendously grateful for the Führer's efforts to make peace in the
church. The reason for their concern was the possibility of mixing false doctrines with the true
gospel.

At this the German Christian representatives
spoke up and said that as far as they were concerned
the whole controversy was purely church politics.

Hitler listened to their wrangling without apparent interest. He had already stated in his original
tirade that he would not remove Müller.

Surprisingly, in light of his anger, Hitler did
shake hands with the churchmen when they left. As
he came to Niemoller, the pastor looked into the
Führer's face and spoke directly and carefully. "A
moment ago, Herr Hitler, you told us that you would
take care of the German people. But as Christians and
men of the church we too have a responsibility for
the German people, laid upon us by God. Neither
you nor anyone else can take that away from us."

For a moment Hitler stared at him. Then he

touched Niemoller's hand and moved on without a word.

Outside, several of the clergymen accosted Niemoller. "How could you speak that way to the Führer? Don't you see that you have ruined it all?"

On the Monday after their meeting with Hitler, the Protestant bishops of Germany gathered for a meeting with National Bishop Müller. Shocked and frightened by Niemoller's behavior, they completely capitulated. They issued a statement of unconditional support for Hitler, the Third Reich, and Bishop Müller, and vowed to carry out any measures and directives he ordered.

Alarmed by Niemoller's radical leadership, two thousand members of the Pastors' Emergency League—almost a third of the group—resigned. Encouraged by this victory, Bishop Müller became more aggressive and dictatorial. He published a series of disciplinary measures, suspensions, dismissals, and retirements. He declared that from then on the church would not be governed by useless synods but by a centralized bureaucracy. He appointed a Nazi lawyer with lapsed church ties to head this administration.

March 13, 1934

Seeing Müller's tactics, several church leaders who had pledged loyalty began to backtrack. Two key bishops, Wurm and Meiser, met with Hitler to complain. This time Hitler was sharply belligerent.

"Christianity will disappear from Germany just

as it has in Russia," he told them. "The German race existed without Christianity for thousands of years before Christ and will continue to exist after Christianity has disappeared.

"The church must get used to the teachings about blood and race. Just as the Catholic Church couldn't prevent the earth from going around the sun, so the churches today cannot get rid of the indisputable facts connected with blood and race. If they can't recognize these, history will simply leave them behind."

Other Nazi leaders had expressed such views, but never the publicly pious Hitler. Shaken, the two bishops said if this was his view they could only look forward to being his most loyal opposition. Hitler flew into a rage.

"You are not my most loyal opposition, but traitors to the people, enemies of the Fatherland and the destroyers of Germany."

May 29, 1934, Barmen, Germany

They met in a large church in a modern industrial town: 139 delegates in all—half pastors, half laymen—representing eighteen different German denominations. A few wore Nazi uniforms; some were state officials. Some were frightened, others elated about the statement of faith they were about to draw up as the charter of the church's resistance.

The Barmen Declaration was not a political document, and it said not a word about Hitler or Müller. Rather, it set out the theological foundations of the church for which they were prepared to suffer, and it spoke strongly and directly against the false teachings of the German Christians. The clear implication was that Hitler's elevation of the German race was anti-Christian. God had not specially revealed Himself through the German nation, blood, race, or even Hitler.

Barmen also spelled out an understanding of church and state:

The Bible tells us that according to divine arrangement the state has the responsibility to provide for justice and peace in the yet unredeemed world, in which the church also stands. . . .

We repudiate the false teaching that the state can and should expand beyond its special responsibility to become the single and total order of human life, and also thereby fulfill the commission of the church.

We repudiate the false teaching that the church can and should expand beyond its special responsibilities to take on the characteristics, functions and dignities of the state, and thereby become itself an organ of the state.

The commission of the church, in which her freedom is founded, consists in this: in place of Christ and thus in the service of His own word and work, to extend through word and sacrament the message of the free grace of God to all people.

For their expression of faith, some of those present would lose their livelihood, be imprisoned or exiled. Others would lose their lives. A great many others, however, would fail the test.

One of the results of the Barmen meeting was the organization of a group that called themselves the Confessing Church. They represented the large number of Christians within the badly divided German Evangelical Church who most opposed the policies of Hitler. Among their numbers were Niemoller and Bonhoeffer.

A month after Barmen, Hitler murdered hundreds of militant, dissident Nazis in a bloody slaughter that became known as the Röhm Purge. Even the Confessing Church made no public protest—not even Niemoller. Most members expressed thankfulness that Hitler had restrained the more violent elements among his followers.

November 28, 1934, London

Winston Churchill stood before Parliament. He was an old man, a defanged lion, regarded sometimes with pity in the House of Commons. Even his own party would not give him a cabinet position. Still the old lion could roar.

Today his deep growl was asserting that "the strength of our national defenses, and especially of our air defense, is no longer adequate to secure... peace, safety, and freedom." Germany's air force, which according to the Versailles Treaty should not exist, "is rapidly approaching equality with our own" and would be fifty percent stronger by the end of 1936.

The MPs settled back into their seats with relief when Prime Minister Stanley Baldwin, another old but more amiable man, far better liked than Churchill, flatly contradicted him. Few noticed that Baldwin carefully hedged his cheery assessment of the future with the condition, "If Germany continues to execute her air program without acceleration." And while it was true that Churchill had exaggerated, it was also true that the Secret Service had told Baldwin of Hitler's plans to surpass Britain's air force by the fall of 1936.

March 10, 1935, Berlin

Outside a cold March wind swept the sky, but inside the old brick house the coal fire burned hot. Niemoller, his collar loosened, held his youngest son, Martin, on his knee. From the kitchen came the sounds of his wife washing dishes. Two of his older children were curled in chairs by a window, reading. Niemoller's eyes began to droop.

In the midst of this sleepy Sunday afternoon a knock came at the door. When the maid answered it, Niemoller heard a voice he did not recognize. She ushered in a slim, dark man in a heavy overcoat, who introduced himself as Pastor Schollen from a small church in the countryside about fifty miles from Berlin.

Schollen seemed frightened. He declined a cup of tea and sat fidgeting and glancing around nervously until Niemoller said impatiently, "Get on with it, man! What did you come about?"

Schollen fished in his wallet and brought out a small red card, which he tried to hand to Niemoller. Niemoller waved it away, smiling. He recognized it as the membership card for the Confessing Church.

"Yes, I knew you had joined, Pastor Schollen. I recognize your name."

"I came for counsel, Brother Niemoller. Did you read the statement aloud today?"

"Yes, of course. We had a meeting with the entire congregation in the parish hall. I not only read it, I demanded that everyone make clear where they stand. We took a vote and it was passed overwhelmingly."

Schollen fidgeted, looked down at his feet, then said, "I didn't read the statement this morning because the chief of police is in my congregation. He warned me against it, told me I could lose my position. And I did not feel certain that the tactics were correct." As an afterthought he added. "None of the pastors in my valley will read it. But I told them I would go and talk to you."

Niemoller's sleepiness was gone. "Pastor Schollen, you are not the only one lacking courage. But many pastors were not afraid this morning. They read the statement and hundreds more will read it next week."

"You don't think it is too severe?" Schollen asked. "Some of the pastors thought a more reasonable tone would be more honoring to those with different views. I mean, calling it 'a new religion making idols of blood, race, nation, honor, eternal Germany.' That's quite strong."

"It is nothing less than a new religion," Niemoller said. "A new religion with a different God. Do you know what they are teaching the Hitler Youth now? They are saying that just as Jesus went through three days in the grave, Hitler spent a year in prison. But Hitler's resurrection did not take him away from earth; he stayed here to save the German people. They are teaching that to our children now! Don't you know that?"

"One hears all kinds of things. But how do you know that it is the whole picture?"

"By the time you know the whole picture they will have taken down our crosses and put up swastikas. And you and I will be in the KZ!"

A tremor shook Schollen's body. Quietly he said, "They have already put Hitler's picture next to the crucifixes in our Catholic schoolrooms. One of the teachers told me."

"You see?" Niemoller said, striding to the window. "What is there to discuss?"

"But even Bodelschwingh, your old mentor, says we should wait," Schollen said. "They are talking to Hitler, and soon they will reach a reasonable solution. We are good Germans. We are thankful for what the government has done. Is it proper to be making proclamations against the government when discussions are continuing on a daily basis? I ask myself, how could I justify this to the Führer?"

"Justify yourself to the Lord Jesus!" Niemoller shouted.

"I will tell you something," Niemoller added in a lower tone. "Hitler is a coward, a coward and a bully. He will terrify you so long as you are willing to be terrified. We must stand up to him for the church of Jesus Christ. I beg of you!...Bodelschwingh, Meiser, Wurm...they think they will work out some sort of agreement with the beast. But the beast will swallow them up."

"I really must go, Pastor Niemoller," Schollen

said stiffly. He had heard what he needed to hear to make up his mind. He left quickly, not looking back.

That week seven hundred pastors were arrested before they went to church to read the statement passed by the Prussian synod, which was a regional faction of the Confessing Church. German Christians were dispatched to lead the services in their churches. In some Berlin churches the congregations walked out on these substitutes after singing "A Mighty Fortress Is Our God."

Niemoller was one of those arrested. The police were polite and released him after two days. From then on, Niemoller's prayers from the pulpit included prayers for pastors in prison, in concentration camps, or under house arrest. The Gestapo came and took notes.

On the same Sunday as the arrests, the most massive military parade in decades marched through Berlin, viewed by cheering, jubilant throngs estimated at half a million. Hitler had announced that all young men would be conscripted into the growing army.

September 15, 1935, Nuremburg

Every September in the Third Reich thousands gathered at the ancient city of Nuremburg for the Nazi Party convention. From all over the nation they came, the best and most loyal Nazi farmers, students, and workers. They stayed in carefully regimented tent camps and marched in precise formations to the vast field where rallies were held. The gigantic assemblies were masterpieces of emotional orchestration, building up to the moment each night when Hitler arrived.

The tiny specks of humanity in the darkened stadium welcomed their Führer in a frenzy of awe and worship. During his two years in office, unemployment, inflation, and poverty had magically disappeared. Germans now had clean streets, orderly cities, disciplined and enthusiastic young people. They remembered the disorder and decadence of only a few years ago and were grateful. Part of their pride was in the resurgent German army; it meant the shame of World War I was erased. Germany was strong and independent again.

When the wild cheering had quieted, Hitler began to speak in his quiet, fatherly tone. This year he had reassuring words for Christians: the Nazis would never intervene against Christianity or against either the Roman Catholic or Protestant churches. This came on top of his formation, two months before, of a new government department, the Ministry of Church Affairs.

Then Hitler's voice changed to a snarl as he turned to the subject of his most implacable hatred. He had summoned the Reichstag, the almost useless Parliament, to Nuremburg just for this. He asked them to unanimously pass two laws against Jews. One took away all their rights of German citizenship. The other forbade marriages between Germans and Jews. From now on, Jews had no rights in Germany.

September 23, 1935

"I can see no purpose in self-inflicted martyrdom," Bishop Meiser said to Martin Niemoller. The two men sat facing each other in a small hotel room, heatedly discussing the agenda for the gathering of the Free Synod at the Berlin-Steglitz church. This was the same body that had passed a strong antiheathenism resolution in March, but now they were greatly divided in spirit.

The radicals, led by Martin Niemoller, did not want to compromise with Hitler's new church ministry nor to approve the Nuremburg laws. Many others, such as Meiser, counseled moderation and conciliation.

"We are trying to bring peace to the church," said Meiser, "and this Jewish question can only make us seem like the greatest troublemakers in Germany."

"What does it matter how we look in Germany compared with how we look in heaven?" Niemoller replied forcefully. "We pray for our pastors when they are imprisoned. Why has no one prayed for the Jews?"

"But the business of a synod is the church. We cannot pronounce judgment on all the ills of society. Most especially we ought not to single out the one issue that the government is so sensitive about, with the foreign criticism filling the air. First things first."

"And what is the first thing you are referring to?" Niemoller asked.

"The very existence of a church free from interference!" Meiser said.

"And how are we free if we cannot pronounce judgment on the ills of society?" Niemoller asked wearily. "Tell me that."

*   *   *

The Free Synod ended with nothing resolved. True they had, over Bishop Meiser's opposition, asserted that everyone, including Jews, should be offered salvation. They had strongly censured congregations that refused baptism to Jews. But the matter of the general condition of Jews in Germany had been referred to a committee. The majority of pastors thought laws about Jews were a state matter. So long as the Jews' position in the church remained unrestricted, the church should not interfere.

Bonhoeffer was depressed. Back in Germany now and heading a new seminary for the Confessing Church, he had come to the conference along with several of his students, who were bitter. They were becoming an embattled minority within an embattled minority—the radical faction of the Confessing Church in a Germany that cared little about the disputes of a handful of pastors and bishops.

Only Niemoller still had fire in his eyes. As he looked out over the delegates, he issued a solemn warning: "We shall be obliged to say more," he said, "and it may be that our mouths will only be really opened when we have to undergo suffering ourselves."

December 1935

Hans Kerrl, the new government minister heading Hitler's Ministry of Church Affairs, had set up a church committee to resolve the disputes within the German Evangelical Church. He persuaded a widely reputed clergyman to chair it, and some of the foremost leaders of the Confessing Church agreed to cooperate—against Niemoller's adamant disapproval.

Kerrl declared all organizations of the Confessing Church illegal and gradually, firmly, began to tighten the noose around the necks of those who would not cooperate with his new committee. Pastors who belonged to an illegal organization were not paid their state-supported salaries. Seminarians from Bonhoeffer's seminary could not get pastoral appointments. Kerrl's bureaucratic harassment so blurred the issues—they were arguing not doctrine now but salaries and pensions and appointments—that most of the Confessing Church pastors found cooperation easier than defiance.

In the following months the great energetic unity of Barmen began to crack into a thousand fragments.

March 7, 1936, Norfolk, England

Lord Lothian's twelve guests gathered around the radio after dinner to listen to the BBC. Among them were the Astors—Waldorf, one of the richest men in the world, and his witty, beautiful wife, Nancy, who would later become the first woman to sit in Parliament; Thomas Jones, secretary to the British cabinet and a close friend of the prime minister; Thomas Inskip, a cabinet minister; and Arnold Toynbee, the famous historian. Their host, Lord Lothian, was himself one of the most eloquent and renowned statesmen in Britain.

All were weekending in the beauty and luxury of Lothian's ancient rose-red brick castle, Blickling Hall, with its deer park at one end and acres of grass and woodland at the other.

Tonight, however, their pleasure was interrupted by the dry authoritative tones of the newscaster announcing that earlier that day German troops had moved into the Rhineland. Hitler had offered twenty-five years of peace based on disarmament of both sides of the border. The peace proposal was, according to the French ambassador to Germany, "as though Hitler struck his adversary across the face and said, 'I bring you proposals for peace!'"

Lord Lothian, a broad-chested, handsome man in his fifties, flicked off the radio, loosened his tie, and sat back in a heavy leather chair. "I never thought I'd hear this group so quiet," he said. "Do you think war has begun?"

"If this means war," Nancy Astor said, "it will be because of the French, not the Germans. If the Germans want to march into their own backyard, I wish them well."

"What nonsense!" said someone from the other end of the room.

"I have a suggestion," said Thomas Jones with a twinkle in his eye. "We'll form a shadow cabinet and draw up a list of suggestions. I'll call up the prime minister tomorrow morning and tell him what we think."

Toynbee enthusiastically supported the idea. He himself had recently returned from a long meeting with Hitler. "I suppose that this may well be the only drawing room in all Britain containing two men who have had a long conversation with Herr Hitler," he said. "Lord Lothian, it seems to me that the essential question is one of motive. Do you think, based on your conversation with the man, as well as with Göring, Ribbrentrop, and so on, that Hitler is merely making the first of a series of expansionist movements? Or are you convinced as I am that Hitler really has no evil intentions? He certainly convinced me that he wants peace."

"Why don't we call up Winston and ask him to help us on that point?" Jones jested.

"Heavens, no!" Nancy Astor retorted. "If the real cabinet won't have him, why should the shadow?"

"Hear, hear!" said Lothian. "We can easily refer to Churchill's views on the Germans without his presence. To him the Germans are the Devil incarnate.

"Speaking of the German motives," said Lothian, folding his arms across his chest, "I would state firmly that the Germans are not fundamentally aggressive. They have been goaded into aggression by the Versailles Treaty and by the French policy of encirclement. A great nation with an ancient culture and history cannot reasonably be denied a position of equality in Europe. Yet the view of the French government, and incidentally some elements in our Foreign Office, is that they are a group of gangsters the likes of which the world has never seen."

"If we don't give them what they deserve," said Nancy Astor, "we'll have war, and we'll be the ones to blame when the entire continent is Bolshevik."

The debate carried late into the night, for this mannered, richly dressed crowd loved talking politics more than almost anything. In the morning, Jones telephoned Prime Minister Baldwin with their resolutions: the group "welcomed Hitler's declaration wholeheartedly" and thought he wanted "above all to be accepted by England as respectable"; therefore, the militarization of the Rhineland was to be treated as relatively insignificant. The chief thing was to seize on Hitler's peace proposals.

Nobody mentioned the military fact that was to be reinforced so strikingly in years to come. The Rhineland had been demilitarized at Versailles deliberately to make Germany vulnerable; without it, France and Britain lost any leverage short of war— for which the underarmed British and disorganized French were clearly unprepared.

In permitting the German troops to march into the Rhineland, both countries were betting that reason alone would persuade the Germans to behave in a civilized manner. And the elegant men and women at Blickling Hall believed in the power of reason.

August 3, 1936, Berlin

They sat in a circle, sober-faced and quiet. In the distance they could hear the popping of fireworks and the low murmur of sound from a crowd of happy Berliners enjoying the festivities of the Olympic games. Those sounds came from a different world than the one facing these leaders of the Confessing Church.

Bonhoeffer was there, as well as Niemoller and Jacobi—the young and the middle-aged, but not one of the older bishops.

Bonhoeffer was depressed. He was thinking of yesterday, spent at the games in Olympic Stadium. He had been happy and excited.

Warm summer sun had bathed the tanned,

happy crowds surrounding him. Children, their hair bleached white from hours in the sun, clutched their parents' hands and tried to see everything. *I do love my country*, Bonhoeffer had thought, *in spite of everything*.

Berlin was decorated and scrubbed clean for the games. White Olympic flags and red Nazi pennants hung from every lamppost. The ugly signs warning shoppers away from Jewish shops had disappeared overnight. Uniformed, heel-clicking troops still filled the streets, but they seemed like part of the parade.

With Bonhoeffer had been a seminarian named Schultz. Ordinarily a serious and rather dull fellow, the young man bubbled with enthusiasm. But his pleasure had turned to sadness during their parting conversation at the end of the day.

"Dr. Bonhoeffer . . . I must tell you," the young man had begun haltingly, "I am taking a parish in Hamburg. I could not refuse."

For a moment Bonhoeffer had been speechless. "Leaving the Confessing Church?"

"No, Dr. Bonhoeffer, please understand my deep respect and admiration for all that you stand for. I only think that I am called to be a pastor and there are no pastorates for those of us who will not co-operate. What is the good in preaching if you have no congregation? Where will this noncooperation lead us? We are no longer a recognized body; we have no government assistance; we cannot care for the souls in the armed forces or give religion lessons in the schools. What will become of the church if that continues? A heap of rubble!"

"Those are not your words," Bonhoeffer had instantly accused.

"No, you are right. They are Riehl's. He has convinced me that we must for the sake of Jesus Christ make use of the great opportunities the government is offering us rather than sticking to a path so narrow there is only space for one at a time."

Bonhoeffer had stared disbelievingly at him. "If you board the wrong train, Schultz, it is no use running along the corridor in the opposite direction."

Schultz's words had been like a knife. So all the teaching and all the community they had practiced at the seminary had been wasted on this man! And, Bonhoeffer wondered, on how many others? That was the question that pounded in him as he sat in the meeting. How many others?

Suddenly his reverie about the day before was broken by the words of Niemoller—"Why not read the whole memorandum, just as we sent it to Hitler?"

"We will certainly lose Meiser and others if we do that, Martin," said Jacobi. "They will say we should stick to the issues of the church and leave the politics to the state."

"The Jews are our issue!" Niemoller shot back. "And the concentration camps! We had the courage to write to Hitler. Why not read it to our congregations?"

Someone asked Bonhoeffer what he thought. He had difficulty raising himself out of his gloom.

"I think," he said slowly after a few moments of silence, "I think we must not worry what people think. We must be the church and speak as Christ. And the words of Proverbs, which some have quoted so often, remain relevant, 'Open your mouth for the dumb.' "

On August 23 only a few hundred pastors, out of perhaps 18,000, read the proclamation. The uncompromising Confessing Church was now very small.

July 1, 1937, Berlin

The symbol of defiant resistance to Hitler crouched on the floor in his bathrobe, pushing a toy car. His son, Martin, only a toddler, yelped with glee.

Niemoller had arrived home late the night before, exhausted from a tour of church meetings. His eyes and gaunt face showed the strain. The screws had tightened on the Confessing Church. In the past three weeks many of the resisting leaders had been arrested. But with every arrest Niemoller's drive seemed to grow.

Downstairs the doorbell rang. The maid came to tell him that two Gestapo agents were waiting in the living room. It had become a familiar routine.

Niemoller dressed hurriedly and went downstairs. The officers shook hands politely. They had a few questions to ask him. Would he please accompany them?

A trace of sadness crossed Niemoller's face. This once, on a Saturday, he would have liked to play with his son and talk to his wife. He went to tell Else what was happening. "They say it will be brief," he said. "But only God knows, my love."

Once he was seated in the black police van, he did not bother to look out the window. He knew too well the route to police headquarters. Exhaustion settled over him and he nearly slept.

At the Alexanderplatz they took him to a large room and left him. Several hours passed inside the bustling headquarters before a tall captain entered, called Niemoller's name, and coldly told him to follow.

The officer did not take the familiar route up the stairs to the interrogation rooms. Instead, he turned in the opposite direction and led the pastor outside to a black police van.

"Are you sure?" Niemoller asked the officer. "No one has talked to me yet."

The captain just nodded. Now Niemoller was strangely afraid, and this time he looked out the window. They were not retracing the route.

Eventually they reached Moabit prison, its ancient dark walls fringed with barbed wire. *You do not come here for questions*, Niemoller thought. *You come to stay.*

When they heard of Niemoller's imprisonment, many pastors felt ill-disguised satisfaction. They had, after all, warned him. Perhaps now he would not disturb them with his uncompromising speeches.

An earnest chaplain, visiting the Moabit prisoners, happened upon Niemoller. Somehow this chaplain had not heard the news of his arrest.

"But brother!" he said in shock, "What brings

you here? Why are you in prison?"

"And, brother, why are you not in prison?" Niemoller replied.

In succeeding months seven hundred pastors
were arrested. Most were released after a few days
or weeks behind bars. Some were sent to concentration camps. Yet the vast majority of the 18,000 German Evangelical Church pastors stayed well out of
trouble. The reputable Bishop Marahrens issued a
statement: "The National Socialist conception of life
is the national and political teaching that determines
and characterizes German manhood. As such, it is
obligatory upon German Christians also."

March 2, 1938, Moabit Prison, Berlin

It was the final day of Martin Niemoller's trial.
He sat in the courtroom, awaiting the judges' verdict,
dressed neatly in a dark suit, conservative wing collar, and black tie. He had lost weight but not spirit.
In the front row sat his Else and his eldest daughter,
Brigette. They had been apart for eight months. How
wonderful even to see their faces. Perhaps tonight
they would be together again.

He had been charged with "malicious and provocative criticism of the minister of Propaganda and
Public Enlightenment, Dr. Goebbels, of the Minister
of Education, Dr. Rust, and of the Minister of Justice,
Dr. Gurtner, of a kind calculated to undermine the
confidence of the people in their political leaders."
Another charge dealt with his reading from the pulpit
names of people the government had imprisoned.

Yet the prosecution had failed to bring out any convincing evidence of his guilt. Instead, a series of witnesses had endorsed him as a man of sterling character. Niemoller's spirits, so grim at the beginning of the trial, had been rising. Waiting for the judges to enter, he could not keep a smile from his face. He chatted and joked with his attorney and kept glancing at his wife's shining, hopeful face.

The presiding judge began to read, slowly. They had found him guilty!

As the fifteen typed pages of the judgment unfolded, however, it became clear that the conviction was merely a slap. Niemoller, the judge read, had been inspired by "completely honorable motives." He was a man of "unquestionable veracity, the type of person who has nothing whatsoever of the traitor in him." Nonetheless, he has violated the letter of the law and must be found guilty. He would be imprisoned for seven months and fined 2,000 marks. The eight months he had already served would apply, so he could be freed today. As the implication came home to him, Niemoller beamed. It was as good a verdict as he could have possibly hoped for—as good as an acquittal. So there were still honest men in Germany!

At last the judges were finished and he was able to grasp his wife's hand. "Pack our trunks," he said in her ear. "We'll have a holiday together."

"Will they really let you go?" Else asked, still uncertain of their good fortune.

"Pack our bags!" he said, looking into her eyes. "I'll be home in an hour or two."

*　　　　*　　　　*

Hitler had arranged to hear the Niemoller verdict immediately. He was furious. He remembered well meeting the pastor two years before when Niemoller had spoken so impudently.

Calling an immediate cabinet meeting, Hitler demanded a resolution that Niemoller be placed in a concentration camp.

"This man is my personal prisoner," Hitler shouted. "And that is the end of it!"

In the early hours of the morning, Martin Niemoller passed through the barbed wire of Sachsenhausen, a concentration camp of 30,000 prisoners.

ELEVEN

Roots of War
(Part II)

*For any government deliberately to deny
to their people what must be their plainest
and simplest right [to live in peace and
happiness without the nightmare of war]
would be to betray their trust, and to call
down upon their heads the condemnation
of all mankind.*

*I do not believe that such a government
anywhere exists among civilized peoples.
I am convinced that the aim of every
statesman worthy of the name, to
whatever country he belongs, must be the
happiness of the people for whom and to
whom he is responsible, and in that faith I
am sure that a way can and will be found
to free the world from the curse of
armaments and the fears that give rise to
them, and to open up a happier, and a
wiser future for mankind.*

 *—Prime Minister Neville Chamberlain,
  November 1937*

March 11, 1938, No. 10 Downing Street, London

Prime Minister Neville Chamberlain gave no impression of bending to his nearly seventy years. He was a tall, hawkliike man with a luxuriant mustache and a rather high opinion of himself. Perhaps he was entitled. No one in government worked harder than he.[1]

Chamberlain came from a peculiar background for a prime minister. Unlike a great many members of his cabinet, he had made a success of himself—first in running a hard-headed, family-owned manufacturing firm and later in politics—without benefit of a huge inheritance or elegant title. A further drawback might have been his religious affiliation. His family had long been Unitarians, who, because they rejected the deity of Christ, were ostracized from semiofficial Church of England channels. Yet it was that very affiliation that contributed so strongly to the Chamberlain family's dedication to public service; both his father and older brother were prominent in politics. Government was a natural vocation for those raised in Unitarian tradition, with its belief in the universal goodness of all men, growing out of a sense of duty to mankind and a deep-seated belief that reasonable, fair-minded men could work together to solve any difficulty.

Chamberlain had reached the pinnacle of power in his country, succeeding Baldwin without a struggle because no one else was comparably qualified. Now, well into his first year, he was warming to his

task with all sorts of ambitious improvements in
mind. If only he could keep the German issue in its
proper perspective and not let the war-lovers in
either country gain too much momentum.

The latter concern was on his mind today as he
greeted the German ambassador, Joachim von Ribbentrop, whom he had invited to this farewell lun-
cheon in the spacious inner rooms of his residence.
Ribbentrop was a ridiculous, strutting ninny with
cotton for a brain, but he was closely connected with
Hitler. What a pity, Chamberlain thought, that a great
nation is governed by such irrational men, driven by
such illogic. If he could only make them see sense!

Chamberlain, a private man whom most thought
cold and arrogant, tried to make small talk as he
escorted the German ambassador among the clusters
of men he was hosting; most were chatting informally
and shaking hands with an easy, confident charm, as
well they might. They were on the whole the most
powerful men of the most powerful empire in the
history of the world.

Feeling the pull of the leonine presence, Chamberlain looked over at Churchill sprawled in a chair
at the other end of the table. The prime minister
could never help feeling a little scornful of the man
who had never made the top rank despite his long
career in government and his rhetorical gift. They
had worked together on previous cabinets, but he
would never let Churchill serve under him. The man
was too emotional, drank too much, and his tirades
took up precious time. He rarely had his facts
straight. Churchill, Chamberlain thought, would
gladly fight Germany tomorrow, if only to give him-

self a chance to make saber-rattling speeches in the House.

The lunch went well, Chamberlain thought. With elaborately feigned politeness, Ribbentrop raised the issue of Chamberlain's "White Paper on Defense" given to the House five days before.

"Why do you talk of fighting?" Ribbentrop asked. "You say that you want peace and then you talk of fighting. The Führer is a man of peace, but he is also a man of strength, and this talk of fighting for democracy he can only see as pure aggressiveness."

Only a German could have read his talk as aggressive, Chamberlain groaned inwardly. But he answered patiently and logically that his policy had always been based on a willingness to defend his nation were it necessary. "I assume that Germany's policy is the same; that is the only legitimate reason for keeping armies and navies. You may remember that I also spoke of our earnest hopes for appeasement and then disarmament."

He was not sure his words made any impression on Ribbentrop, who immediately began speaking at great length on what a peace-loving man Hitler was. Fortunately Churchill held his tongue.

After lunch Chamberlain and Ribbentrop spent another twenty minutes together as the prime minister tried to drive home his one point: he wanted to solve any difficulties Germany might face as the result of the Versailles Treaty. If he repeated that message often enough it might make its way back to Berlin.

Yet Ribbentrop persisted in babbling on about the astonishing transformation of Germany, a miracle

to those who had known the bad years. "It is preposterous that the British public remains so utterly
ill-informed," he complained peevishly. "Yesterday
I met a mob of people shouting the most intolerable
insults about Pastor Niemoller's imprisonment. I am
sure they would be astonished to learn that there are
twice as many people in church today as there were
five years before, when Hitler came to power."

At last Chamberlain smilingly withdrew and returned to the drawing room where the other guests
lingered. He was handed some telegrams to read and
stopped short, bristling in disbelief. The telegrams
informed him that Hitler, that morning, had delivered an ultimatum to the Austrian Chancellor. Schuschnigg was to resign his office by 2:00 P.M. and turn
over the government to Seyss-Inquart, the Nazi Hitler
had forced into the government just a month before.
Hitler's troops were massed on the border, ready to
march if Schuschnigg refused. Schuschnigg begged
the British government for advice. All this had happened while he was chatting pleasantly about peace
with Ribbentrop.

Chamberlain quietly asked the German ambassador for "a private word" in his office downstairs,
along with Lord Halifax, England's foreign secretary.
Any attempts at friendliness had disappeared into
British frost as he read out the telegrams and stiffly
demanded an explanation. "I want you to understand
that this has the most serious implications for our
relations."

Ribbentrop smiled and said he personally knew
nothing about these negotiations. "Do you have any
confirmation of these reports? Because I know for a

fact that the Chancellor's discussions with Schuschnigg were conducted in a tremendously friendly
atmosphere. I was there personally. I must say that
I would think Schuschnigg's resignation would be a
very positive development and a hopeful sign for a
peaceful solution."

"This is intolerable behavior in a civilized nation," Halifax said, his voice loud and threatening.
He called it naked aggression.

Chamberlain admitted graciously that they had
no definite proof of aggression but said they had ample reasons for deep concern. "All we can ask is that
you convey to Herr Hitler our sincere and ardent wish
that he hold back from any rash act that would im-
peril our chances for a negotiated settlement."

After Ribbentrop left, Chamberlain sank into a
wing chair and cut short the overexcited Halifax. "If
you must, go and talk to Ribbentrop at the embassy."

Then he dictated a response to Schuschnigg,
which Halifax accepted with a pinched, reluctant
expression. "His Majesty's Government cannot take
responsibility of advising the chancellor to take any
course of action that might expose his country to
dangers against which His Majesty's Government are
unable to guarantee protection."

Afterward Chamberlain sat alone in his study
with his dark thoughts. He would not get off to the
country for a rest this weekend. His plans were
spoiled. His carefully drafted message to Hitler
would be buried under the necessary protests. It
meant more work for him—not positive work, but
preventive. Seeing Halifax in a rage had only reinforced the prime minister's conviction that he was

the only one cool enough to abide the Germans' irrational behavior and make them see reason.

Late that afternoon the Austrian government,
finding support from no other country, capitulated,
and the German army marched unopposed across
Austria's border.

Chamberlain wrote his sisters, his closest con-
fidantes, that he took comfort in the fact that the
Anschluss had taken place without any loss of life.

March 25, 1938, Cliveden

The house rose up ahead of them like a tiered
wedding cake, more of a monument than a home—
Cliveden, where for years Nancy Astor had gathered
the wittiest and wealthiest men and women in Britain for weekend parties. Hardly anyone of significance failed to turn up at Cliveden, even the king
and Gandhi. George Bernard Shaw was a frequent
guest, although he usually stayed in his room, writing.

Cliveden was a comfortable weekend retreat for
Prime Minister Chamberlain. Many of his cabinet
spent time there, and the ceaseless political talk was
so reliably conservative that the press had seized on
the idea of a "Cliveden set" that was supposed to be
darkly pro-German. Chamberlain found the idea
amusing; as though any Cliveden set determined *his*
foreign policy.

Today Nancy Astor, a short woman with a high-
cheeked face that had once been beautiful, met
Chamberlain and his wife at the door with one of her

usual greetings. "Hello, you old windbag. Your speech was so exquisitely balanced that no one had the slightest idea where you stood."

"Thank you," he said with a smile. "I intended that."

"If you were truly part of the Cliveden set you would let Herr Hitler know where you stand by singing 'Deutschland Uber Alles' to the House."

"I'll leave that to you, Nancy, in your next speech."

"No, no, those Nazis are not my friends. If they would stop locking up Christian Scientists they might be."

Nancy Astor was a devout Christian Scientist who always had Christian Science lecturers at her weekend gatherings. Lord Astor and Lord Lothian were Christian Scientists too. Their sympathetic view of Germany was strengthened by the Christian Science doctrine that man is good, that there is no evil that the mind cannot overcome. This Chamberlain was inclined to agree with, though he was quite irreligious himself.

As they bantered, waiting for the servants—there were dozens of them at Cliveden—to hustle in the Chamberlains' luggage, other guests began drifting into the vast dark paneled entrance hall with its elaborately carved wooden columns, suits of armor, and tapestries. Chamberlain knew most of the guests, except for an American couple and an odd-looking man whom he supposed was one of Nancy's ever-present Christian Science lecturers. Several people thanked him for the speech he had given in the House on Thursday. Sir Alexander Cadogan, his undersecretary of state for foreign affairs, took him aside and said that the nation had breathed a sigh of relief at stepping back from the brink.

"I don't believe we stepped back," Chamberlain said dryly. "I wanted us to avoid stepping over." He had declined before the House of Commons to guarantee that Britain would come to Czechoslovakia's aid if Germany invaded. Since Austria had been adopted into the Reich, Czechoslovakia was now vulnerable, half-surrounded by German armies.

"Yes, I liked what you said," Cadogan admitted, "about not letting others determine when we would fight."

"I have the sense," said Chamberlain, "that to draw a line in the dust is to dare Herr Hitler to cross it. I am not anxious to enter matches of daring with him. I want to convince him that he can get all that Germany is entitled to without having to fight."

The next morning Chamberlain rose early and went into the dining room where breakfast was laid out as a self-service buffet. Nancy Astor always provided every luxury and pleasure imaginable—except liquor; she was an absolute teetotaler. Nancy herself, as usual, would not join her guests until nearly noon; she was alone in her bedroom reading her Bible.

A light mist was falling as Chamberlain strolled out across the formal garden, past pieces of Italian statuary, and into one of the long lanes that led through Cliveden's forest, with views over the Thames. A solitary person, Chamberlain loved to walk. Often after a session of Parliament he would walk as many as six miles to calm himself.

He mused as he walked about the state of affairs with Germany. The subject nagged at him as though there were some detail he had neglected. Yet really things were going well. The whole country stood behind him.

But he saw clearly enough that this support might not last. Europe was an unstable mass, like snow on the mountains that even a loud shout might turn into an avalanche. He had to find the way to create stability, with little time to do it. He had to discover precisely what Germany wanted and how to get it for them. *If only we could sit down and reason together,* he thought. *I am sure we could ease the tensions overnight.*

His thoughts grew darker, for the future was so unknown and he was a man who liked to make tidy plans.

Churchill had made one of his magnificent bursts of oratory in response to Thursday's speech. Chamberlain could still hear that deep, robust voice booming out the warning like Pompeii's town crier.

"I have watched this famous island descending incontinently, fecklessly, the stairway which leads to a dark gulf. It is a fine broad stairway at the beginning, but after a bit the carpet ends. A little farther on there are only flagstones, and a little farther on still these break beneath your feet. . . ."

Yes, Chamberlain thought, *the warning is just. Except Winston's warmongering is likely to speed our journey down.*

On his return to the house he walked through a little cemetery. Cliveden had served as a hospital during the Great War, and those who had died of their wounds were buried here under a Union Jack. It was a beautiful, melancholy spot, all moss and shadows. Standing there, he thought of his cousin Norman, the only man he had ever been truly attached to, buried in France in a much vaster cemetery than this. Nothing matters more, he thought, than avoiding war; another generation of Normans must not die.

Suddenly his melancholy lifted. He would find a way to make a lasting peace.

September 12, 1938, London

Chamberlain sat by a large radio cabinet at No. 10 Downing listening fretfully to the man who held the world in the palm of his hand. It was the end of the greatest Nuremburg Party Congress yet—the first to celebrate the new, expanded Germany. Now, at the climax of the week, endless squadrons of Hitler Youth, Hitler Workers, SS, army, navy, and air force had converged to hear their Führer. All over the world, in Czechoslovakia, in France, in England, and in America, men and women listened in rapt fear to the crowd's roars of "Sieg Heil!"

Chamberlain was not afraid. He was distressed. The world held its breath waiting for the words of a lunatic! How foolish. How utterly mad! How could the lives of hundreds of millions, as well as his own reputation, hang on this?

He had written his sister: "I fully realize that if eventually things go wrong...there will be many, including Winston, who will say that the British government must bear the responsibility and that if only they had had the courage to tell Hitler now that, if he used force, we would at once declare war, that would have stopped him.''

Now, as the prime minister listened, Hitler began his assault on Czechoslovakia, working himself into his usual snarling frenzy. Thousands standing before him responded wildly. They were primed for battle, ready to die for the honor of Germany.

The world waited, expecting Hitler to declare war. But instead, he veered onto another subject.

Listening to the distant roar, Chamberlain let out an involuntary sigh. "Not so bad as I feared," he said to himself. "Distasteful, though."

September 24, 1938

Chamberlain was leaving Germany after his second visit with Adolf Hitler in ten days. On September 15 he had arrived at Hitler's Berghof headquarters for his first face-to-face encounter with the man who was shaking the world. At that time he had learned of Hitler's plans to proceed against Czechoslovakia.

Shocked at first, he had left feeling he had made an impression on the Führer. His only problem was convincing his own nation and France—as well as Czechoslovakia—to simply cede a large portion of Czechoslovakia to Nazi Germany, a portion that held large numbers of Czechs as well as Germans and also contained most of the border defenses that made Czechoslovakia a significant, if overmatched, opponent for the invading German army. Chamberlain had already made up his mind that such a price was worth paying for peace.

Now the prime minister felt betrayed. He had risked his political career for the proposals given at Berchtesgaden a few days earlier. He could not understand why the Führer, when he would receive all the territory he wanted through peaceful means, insisted on using force. An immediate takeover of Czechoslovakia by German troops would be looked on as sheer aggression. All this he had said to the Führer, but Hitler was adamant.

Now that he was setting off for London, however, the prime minister had recovered some of his equilibrium. The situation did not look so utterly hopeless. He was beginning to adjust to Hitler's demands. The immediate occupation would offend democratic sensibilities, but was it worth fighting a war over?

Back in London at 5:30 that afternoon Chamberlain spoke to the cabinet.

He spoke of Hitler's anxiousness to develop better relations with Great Britain, stressing that Czechoslovakia was the last territorial claim the Führer would make. "It would be a great tragedy if we lost this opportunity of reaching an understanding with Germany. I have now established an influence with Herr Hitler. I believe he trusts me and is willing to work with me."

But the cabinet raised so many objections that Chamberlain backed off on his recommendation that they advise the Czechs to accept Hitler's plans.

A few days later the Czechs, who were given the

German demands without any recommendations, rejected them in ringing terms.

Spetember 26, 1938, Cliveden

Charles Lindbergh, the brave, dashing pilot who ten years before had challenged the Atlantic and won, was one of the most famous men in the world. Tall, firm, resolute, he never doubted himself for a moment. Full of his own importance in a tortured way, he hated yet needed adulation.

But Lindbergh was more than a great pilot; he had become a high priest of a new technological era. People listened to him, particularly of late.

He had spent several weeks in Germany, warmly welcomed by the Nazis, even given a medal, and had come away tremendously impressed. The democracies seemed to him tired and decadent; in Germany he found a virile masculinity and spirited commitment that resonated in his own soul.

He had also been impressed by the German air force; so much so that wherever he went he preached that no one could stand against it.*

After the terrible kidnapping and death of their son, the Lindberghs had fled America for England; today they were guests at Nancy Astor's Cliveden weekend. Anne, Lindbergh's pretty, shy, intelligent, and adoring wife, soon faded into the background

---

*Lindbergh was wrong in his estimates of German air dominance. London was at the very limit of bomber range from Germany. Without bases in Holland or France it is doubtful the German air force could have done significant damage.

when Charles and the others held forth on the possibility of war.

"I am afraid this is the beginning of the end for
England," Lindbergh said sternly. "The old instincts
are being summoned up for war. People are talking
about 'dishonorable peace,' and so on. Nobody seems
to realize that England is in no condition to fight a
war."

"It's madness," Nancy Astor said in one of her
wild, stabbing protests. "War will destroy Western
civilization. Europe will be destroyed. Then certainly
Communism will spread, for it always feeds on death
like a vulture."

Lord Astor and Thomas Jones came into the
room looking glum and depressed; they too had been
discussing war. Jones's Welsh twinkle was gone; he
looked old and haggard. "I understand that Chamberlain has sent two messages to Hitler to be delivered before he speaks tonight. The first is a last plea
for more negotiations on the terms they had previously agreed on. If Hitler rejects that, he will be given
the second message, a warning that if he marches
into Czechoslovakia England will go to war."

"It's madness," Lady Astor said. "To destroy our
civilization with our eyes open to all that we are
doing."

"There are some things that are worth more than
life," Jones said stiffly.

"Unquestionably!" said Lindbergh. "But that is
not the case now. We would not be fighting to preserve something. Unless war is averted now there
will be no one left who knows the meaning of the
words *right* and *wrong*. This is no longer an affair of

national pride and laws of right and wrong. It is a case of our whole civilization going under."

"I must disagree with you," Lord Astor said, his back to the fireplace. "I have supported all the prime minister has done to appease the Germans. But by now we can see that they are bent on war. We shall have to fight them, and I think it would be better to stop them now before they grow any stronger."

"Your logic may be sound, but it ought to lead you in the opposite direction," said Lindbergh, pouncing eagerly. "If we must fight—and I am not so certain as you seem to be that Hitler is bent on war—then by all means buy as much time as possible. At the moment England's defenses are so weak as to be utterly incapable of defending the nation, let alone punishing Hitler."

Astor looked around him with sad, kind eyes, but the way he gripped the fireplace betrayed his tension. "I think you have it wrong. Germany is already arming at full speed; it would be years before we could even reach her pace. So every day we wait to fight, Germany grows stronger. Furthermore, if we keep backing down to every threat Hitler makes, we will soon have no friends to fight with us."

"But don't you think that before you go to war you must have some idea of victory? You cannot separate political decision from military strategy."

"Would you simply have us surrender?" Astor asked.

"No, but avoid war at any cost!" said Lindbergh.

There was an awkward pause. Jones glanced at his watch. "The speech is about to begin," he said.

"Unfortunately, the decision may be out of our hands."

The small troop gathered by the radio in the parlor included two German boys summering in England. Lady Astor had asked them to translate the speech.

Lord Astor turned on the radio and almost immediately the angry roar of the mob could be heard. It was a terrifying sound: animalistic, threatening, violent. First Goebbels spoke, his high, ranting voice interrupted by cheers, chants, and shouts. The German boys scribbled on pads of paper and shouted out brief summaries during the roaring of the crowd.

Then Hitler spoke, beginning with his usual calm and slowly catching fire as never before. His voice snarled, ripped, rasped, and cut. He returned repeatedly to "Benes." The Czech head of state, his name spoken like a curse, had become the fountain of all the hurt and harm that Germany had ever suffered.

"My patience is at an end," Hitler concluded. "The decision now lies in his hands. Peace or war . . . I have never been a coward. Now I go before my people as its first soldier. And behind me—this the world should know—there marches a different people from that of 1918. We are determined!"

Hitler had never spoken with such demonic fury. The crowd roared on and on into a single furious will, delirious with the delight of hatred.

"A terrifying speech," said Jones. "But no declaration of war. He spoke gratefully of the prime minister's efforts on behalf of peace. He also said that there would be no more territorial demands after this one."

"We have a little more time," Lindbergh said solemnly. "And with every extra day there is a little more hope."

Jones and Astor, more at ease now, were gradually swayed by Lindbergh's argument. If he was right, it would be necessary to face facts and avoid war at all costs. They agreed before they went to bed that they would dedicate the next few days to escorting Lindbergh into the highest governmental circles they could reach. And those at Cliveden had access to some very high circles indeed.

September 28, 1938, London

A darkness hung over London. Trenches were being dug in every park. Children were being herded into trains, evacuating the city that everyone expected would be annihilated in flames within the next twenty-four hours. Outside Parliament a grim, quiet crowd gathered. Hitler's deadline for Czechoslovakia to accept his ultimatum had been 2:00. It was 2:50 when Chamberlain began his speech to the House of Commons where the narrow benches were jammed.

There was not a wearier, more discouraged man in England than the prime minister. He had not given up trying. He had sent fresh appeals to Mussolini and Hitler, suggesting a five-party conference. But little hope now existed.

Last night he had addressed the nation on the BBC, his voice filled with despairing resignation, yet still incredulous that his efforts had been in vain and that death would soon rain down on his beloved nation.

"How horrible, fantastic, incredible it is that we should be digging trenches and trying on gas masks here because of a quarrel in a faraway country between people of whom we know nothing. . . .

"I have done all that one man can do to compose this quarrel. . . . I shall not give up the hope of a peaceful solution or abandon my efforts for peace as long as any chance for peace remains. . . . But at this moment I see nothing further that I can usefully do."

Wearily, dryly, he told the whole story in careful chronological detail: of all the British government had done, of the moments of apparent hope and the dashing of hopes, of last-minute appeals. He spoke for over an hour, building to only one conclusion. The certainty of war.

Then, with hardly anyone noticing, a piece of paper was handed into the House. It moved to several ministers before John Simon, the chancellor of the exchequer, waved it at Chamberlain. Deeply involved in his speech, the prime minister did not immediately notice.

Simon finally got his attention and Chamberlain quickly scanned the paper. He hesitated for a moment, then whispered to Simon, "Shall I tell them now?" Simon vigorously nodded yes.

When Chamberlain spoke again, life had flooded into his voice. "I have now been informed by Herr Hitler that he invites me to meet him at Munich tomorrow morning. He has also invited Signor Mussolini and Monsieur Daladier . . . I need not say what my answer will be."

Someone in the back of the hall shouted, "Thank God for the prime minister."

Chamberlain continued. "We are all patriots and there can be no honorable member of this House who did not feel his heart leap that the crisis has been once more postponed to give us once more an opportunity to try what reason and goodwill and discussion will do to settle a problem which is already within sight of settlement. . . ."

Again from the back a voice boomed out, "Thank God for the prime minister." Then all were on their feet, applauding, cheering, crying, throwing papers into the air. The great fear that had gripped them all was ecstatically released.

No one, or practically no one, thought about the fact that although Hitler had invited Italy, France, and Britain to meet with him, he had not invited Czechoslovakia.

September 30, 1938

"What is that noise?" Chamberlain asked.

It was morning. They had signed the agreement at 1: 30 A.M., and after that he had had to endure the conference with the Czechoslovakians, who had wept.

William Strang, a top foreign office representative, strode to the window of the Regina Palace and looked out. "The street is full of people," he said. "They want to see you. Why don't you step out onto the balcony for a moment?"

Chamberlain did and found himself bathed in a warm ovation. Leaving the hotel a few minutes later, he had to press through the large, happy crowd, bronzed by the sun and still in summer clothing. He could not help smiling.

Chamberlain sat in a flowered armchair in the same apartment where Hitler, unknown to the prime minister, had only the day before villified him to Mussolini. Today Hitler was gracious, though pale and subdued. They talked in generalities, and nothing the prime minister could say would make the Führer disagree with him.

"I trust that the Czechs will not be mad enough to reject our agreement," Chamberlain said. "But in case they do, I hope that you will do nothing which would diminish the high opinion in which you will be held throughout the world in consequence of yesterday's proceedings." Chamberlain glanced at Hitler while the translator interpreted his words. Seeing no resistance, he pressed on. "That is to say, I trust that there will be no bombardment of Prague or killing of women and children by attacks from the air."

Hitler smiled and raised his hand. "As a matter of principle," he said, "I intend to limit air action to frontline zones. I will always try to spare the civilian population and confine myself to military objectives. I hate the thought of little babies being killed by gas bombs."

Returning to the hotel, Chamberlain's car could only creep through the crowds. Men and women pressed forward from all directions, trying to shake his hand. Children threw flowers. Some women wept. All cheered.

Sitting down to lunch with Strang at the hotel, the prime minister proudly patted his breast pocket. "I've got it," he said, a visionary gleam in his narrow eyes. "It" was a brief communique that Hitler had agreed to sign. The central paragraph read, "We regard the agreement signed last night ... as symbolic of the desire of our two peoples never to go to war with one another again."

He had the same scrap of paper in his hands when he stood, exhausted and elated, at a large open window at No. 10 Downing Street. The street below could not take another body; the cheering made it impossible to hear another sound.

All day he had been cheered—in Germany, then arriving back in England at Heston airport, and on the road all the way to Buckingham Palace where he had met with the king to accept his congratulations. Now he raised his hands until the crowd quieted enough for him to be heard.

Waving the communique, he said, "My good friends, this is the second time in our history that there has come back from Germany to Downing Street peace with honor."

The crowd roared its approval at the historic phrase that the famous statesman Disraeli had used at his hero's welcome sixty years before.

"I believe it is peace for our time," he concluded.

October 5, 1938, London

Winston Churchill was one of the few in all of England who understood that government's first duty was not to avoid confrontations with evil but to restrain it. As a result he was an outcast, going against the tide of opinion. He stood solemnly before the House of Commons, knowing full well the immense enthusiasm supporting Chamberlain. Nevertheless, his deep bass reverberated, full of doom.

"All is over.... Silent mournful, abandoned, broken, Czechoslovakia recedes into the darkness. I do not begrudge our loyal, brave people ... the natural, spontaneous outburst of joy and relief when they learned that the hard ordeal would no longer be required of them at the moment.... But they should know the truth. They should know that there has been gross neglect and deficiency in our defenses. They should know that we have sustained a great defeat without a war, the consequences of which will travel far with us.... They should know that we have passed an awful milestone in our history ... the terrible words have for the time being been pronounced against the Western democracies: 'Thou art weighed in the balance and found wanting.' And do not suppose that this is the end. This is only the beginning of the reckoning."

November 9, 1938, Crystal Night

It was late afternoon when the truck lurched to a stop in front of the synagogue in the small German town. About thirty men got out, some in uniforms, others in street clothing. A red can of paint appeared and one of them began painting a huge red star on the synagogue. The others shouted insults.

A passerby, a woman carrying a bulging shopping bag, asked what the problem was. A uniformed officer explained. "The diplomat Rath, the one the Jews shot in Paris, has died. We are expressing our outrage. This is to happen all over Germany."

Just then two of the men who had run inside emerged dragging a man in a skull cap. "There's more in there," they shouted. "Go get them out." Others raced into the building. From inside came angry cries and the sharp sound of breaking glass. Shards of crystal rained down on the street from a second-story window.

The dozen or so men who still stood in the street were shouting insults at the Jewish man. Two of them held him on his knees, pressing his nose into the cobblestones. A small silent crowd had gathered, standing cautiously at a distance.

Eight more Jews were herded out, five men, one woman, and two young girls. The jeers of the men grew louder as these too were forced to kneel on the pavement. One of the men struggled against his captors. They lifted his head by the hair and banged it down on the stones. Once, twice, three times. Blood oozed between the cracks in the stones.

The woman with the shopping bag approached the knot of men holding the two girls. "Why don't you let me take these two away. They're just children."

"No, Fräulein, these are not children," one said. "They're Jews."

"What's the difference?" the woman demanded.

The man hesitated a moment. Then he pointed his chin down to the road. "You go away if you don't want to watch this. Those who interfere will only be hurt. You go away now."

When the woman hesitated, he spat out, "So you're a Jew-lover?"

She turned and crossed the street, where she continued to watch.

The Jews were formed into a rough circle; then the men took turns kicking them, yanking their hair, slapping their faces. The victims stared at their tormentors silently. They had stopped crying for mercy. One of their number already lay on the pavement, blood flowing from one of his ears.

From one of the broken windows above, a thread of smoke wandered skyward. One man pointed it out to the others. "It's burning," he cried with excitement. He seized the hair of the woman and whirled her violently around, jerking her head back. "Look you bloodsucker!" he screamed. "You Christ-killer, your synagogue is burning!"

Similar scenes were played out in almost every town in Germany.

November 10, 1938

The world was shaken from its post-Munich bliss. The night, which became known as Crystal Night because of the broken glass, sparked foreign protest. In Germany, however, the government an-

nounced that the extensive damage would be repaid
by appropriating Jewish bank accounts. The Jews,
after all, had provoked the spontaneous reaction.

Chamberlain was annoyed. He would probably
have to make a statement in the House; someone was
certain to raise the matter. This could well disrupt
further negotiations. But he did not refer to it in his
public speech that night in which he said, "Political
conditions in Europe are now settling down to quiet-
er times."

Charles Lindbergh wrote with bewilderment in
his diary: "They have undoubtedly had a difficult
Jewish problem, but why is it necessary to handle it
so unreasonably?"

In Germany the official church said not a word.
Only a tiny minority of Christians were brave enough
to offer public sympathy. One lonely Catholic priest,
Father Lichtenberg, led his Berlin congregation in
prayer for the persecuted non-Aryans. He was imprisoned and eventually died in confinement. In
Württemberg, Pastor von Jan used his sermon to warn
against such violent hatred, which he said condemned the German people in the sight of God. He
called for contrition, lest God allow Germany to reap
the harvest they had sown. Eleven days later a
screaming mob of about five hundred men dragged
him from a home Bible study and beat him for two
hours. He was then imprisoned.

Dietrich Bonhoeffer found himself staring again
and again at Psalm 74. He underlined verse 8: "They
burned every place where God was worshiped in the
land," and in the margin beside it wrote, "Nov. 11,
1938." Then he underlined the verse that followed,

putting an exclamation mark beside it: "We are given no miraculous signs; no prophets are left, and none of us knows how long this will be."

March 15, 1939

In the frozen dawn Hitler's armed column probed its way through the thick fog that lay on the Czechoslovakian border. The proud Czech border guards did not resist, but stood and watched the tanks rumble by. Just a few hours before they had received orders from Prague not to fight.

Hitler had, through a series of manipulations and ultimatums, convinced a fractured government not to put up a pointless and bloody battle against his invasion.

In London Chamberlain was stunned. Less than a month before he had written to his sisters: "I myself am going about with a lighter heart than I have had for many a long day. All the information I get seems to point in the direction of peace.... I believe we have at last got on top of the dictators."

The British cabinet, meeting in emergency session, decided to offer no military aid to the nation they had "guaranteed" at Munich. Chamberlain held sway when he said that although he did "bitterly regret what has now occurred," the country should not "on that account be deflected from our course.... The aim of this government is now, as it always has been, to substitute the method of discussion for the method of force in the settlement of differences."

Yet they could not keep this blindfold on much longer. A few days later Chamberlain reversed himself completely, speaking long and bitterly about Hitler's broken promises. Wearily he spoke of the implications he had just begun to see and wondered aloud, "Is this, in fact, a step in the direction of an attempt to dominate the world by force?"

July 7, 1939, New York

Dietrich Bonhoeffer leaned on the railing of the ship looking at the jagged silhouette of Manhattan skyscrapers against the night sky. Tomorrow at 12:30, they would sail. He had been in New York for nearly a month. A month filled with frustration, anxiety, and uncertainty.

He smiled to himself and thought of how he must have confused his American hosts. Ostensibly he had come to the United States at the invitation of several professors who had made hasty arrangements under the mistaken impression that he was about to be thrown into a concentration camp. But his entire stay had been a struggle to determine why he was there. Had he fled the coming struggle in Germany? Was he afraid of what he had to do? His hosts had tried so hard to help, had welcomed him so warmly, and all he had done was smoke an endless chain of cigarettes, speak obscure and contradicting pronouncements, and scribble illegible notes to himself.

A few days ago, while still wavering, he had written in his journal: "Today I read by chance in 2

Timothy 4, 'Make every effort to come before winter,' Paul's petition to Timothy. 'Come before winter'—otherwise it might be too late. That has been in my mind all day. . . . We cannot get away from it any more. Not because we are necessary, or because we are useful (to God?), but simply because that is where our life is. . . . It is nothing pious, more like some vital urge. But God acts not only by means of pious incentives, but also through such vital stimuli. 'Come before winter'—it is no misuse of Scripture, if I accept that as having been said to me. If God gives me grace for it."

Now, at last, on the verge of returning to the darkest corner of the earth, his mind was at ease. He had not known how deeply he loved Germany and loved the church in Germany until now.

September 1, 1939, Border between Poland and Germany

The early morning darkness was warm and beautiful, the clear sky filled with clusters of stars. On the roads from Berlin long convoys of trucks, troop transports, tanks, and artillery moved slowly toward Poland. But here at the border nothing moved.

Suddenly a flare of light flickered through the trees; almost immediately the boom of an artillery piece followed. As if in reply, hundreds of guns up and down the border began to thunder.

The invasion of Poland was launched. World War II had begun.

Afterword

When Germany invaded Holland and France in 1940, Chamberlain's government collapsed in ignominy. Churchill became prime minister, promising "blood, toil, tears and sweat." Exhausted and sick, Chamberlain died that same year when a besieged Britain was the only democracy left in Europe.

During the war, pressure eased somewhat on the Confessing Church in Germany; the government had other worries. Besides, the most troublesome pastors were either in the army or in concentration camps. Only scattered individuals in the church protested against the wholesale annihilation of Jews, gypsies, and the mentally retarded.

Dietrich Bonhoeffer evaded the draft and continued secret activities in the resistance. In 1943 he was arrested and, just before the surrender of Germany in May 1945, was executed for his part in an attempted assassination of Adolf Hitler.

Martin Niemoller narrowly escaped execution and emerged from seven years in the concentration camps to play a significant role in the reconstruction of Germany.

It would be an overstatement to suggest that Chamberlain's inability or unwillingness to see the nature of Hitler's evil was the cause of World War II. Like all major events of history, the war was the result of a combination of powerful forces. But it is unarguable that Chamberlain and many in Britain grossly misjudged the situation on the continent. Why?

First of all, there was great revulsion in England over the senseless butchery of trench warfare in the First World War. The country had little stomach to fight again. Chamberlain himself had lost a cousin, perhaps his closest friend, in France. He never stopped grieving.

A second factor was Chamberlain himself. He had grown up in a tight-knit Unitarian family. They rejected the Christian belief in man's innate sinfulness, preferring to place faith in the innate goodness and "reasonableness" of man. Influential Britons of all backgrounds were infected by such thinking. Faith in the social sciences, in intellectual solutions to moral problems, had never been higher than in the thirties. The flourishing of Christian Science within Nancy Astor's influential circle at Cliveden was symptomatic; Christian Scientists believe that all evil is an illusion that can be eliminated by the exercise of the mind. Chamberlain, who was close to many of the Cliveden group, lived among people to whom the harshness of human evil had ceased to seem real. Hitler gave Chamberlain more than adequate evidence that he was evil, unreasonable, and bent on war. Yet the prime minister could not, would not, see it. Well-meaning, honorable, quoting Shakespeare all the way, he earned a dreadful epitaph: "He could have stopped Hitler."

And finally, the church in England failed to provide an independent moral voice for the country. They too had difficulty discerning evil except in "outmoded" policies. Much of the clergy seized on the peace issue and promoted forums like the League of Nations with such indiscriminate fervor that they seemed to believe that God Himself spoke exclusively through international gatherings. Led by Bishop William Temple, they put more faith in progressive politics and economics than in God. Churchmen were so enamored with the fledgling ecumenical movement that, to Bonhoeffer's disgust, they refused to censure the German church even after German Christians had taken control. Though a few individuals were well informed about Germany, most Christian leaders in Britain failed to see the critical moral issues unfolding there. Even though men like Dietrich Bonhoeffer made a point of appealing to them, they failed to understand what the church struggle in Germany represented and thus failed to warn against it. The church, representing the Kingdom of God, was caught up in the trendy issues of the time, surrendering its influence as an independent moral voice.

This failure of both the state and the church contributed to the disaster that befell the world. Had they acted sooner to discharge their respective duties, the Holocaust might well have been avoided.

On the continent the circumstances were reversed. A power-hungry maniac who masterfully played upon the passions of the masses seized the German government. From the start Hitler was determined to exceed government's ordained and delegated role. For him the state was everything, and he was its god. The Communists and the Jews, his hated targets, could offer little organized resistance, and no one spoke in their defense. In the face of Hitler's enormous popularity, all the trusted institutions of modern society utterly failed to resist. The trade unions, the Parliament, the political parties, the universities, the associations of medical doctors, scientists, and intellectuals—all were completely under Hitler's power within six months. Only the church had the independence and the institutional power to stand between Hitler and absolute totalitarianism.

Oddly, the story of the German church struggle has all but disappeared from modern historical accounts. But in contemporary writings it was cited as the single outstanding example of resistance to Hitler. The *New York Times*, for instance, filed approximately 1000 separate news accounts of the German church struggle from 1933 to 1937. Martin Niemoller's name was a household word.

Nazi files clearly record that the church struggle was a constant thorn in the flesh to Hitler and his aides during their early years in power. This was hardly due to the church's political vision or sophistication; rather it was a credit to the church's reliance on an ultimate authority and vision quite apart from the political order to resist Hitler's blasphemous claims, even when his political popularity was soaring. The church's authority, deeply rooted in the lives of the German people, could not be erased by a simple directive from Berlin. It was the only institution in Germany that offered any enduring or meaningful resistance.

But it was not enough. Eventually alone, divided from within, with large numbers of its membership capitulating and even supporting Hitler's schemes, the church failed to hold the state to account.

The roots of World War II were in a sense theological. In England and in Germany, the state and the church failed to fulfill their God-ordained mandates. And whenever that happens, evil triumphs.

TWELVE

Year Zero

*What will we do as the earth is set loose
from its sun?*

—*Friedrich Nietzsche*

Six years after Hitler's troops marched into Poland, much of Europe lay in ruins. London, victim of German air power in the early years of the war, had been bombed incessantly; France, Italy, and the Netherlands had faced the cruelty of enemy occupation. The soil was red with the blood of their defenders. But it was Japan that had borne the full brunt of modern warfare: the atom bomb. Her will to fight was incinerated in the mushroom clouds that devastated Hiroshima and Nagasaki.

Sunday, September 2, 1945, as the sun climbed in the sky over Tokyo Bay, the decks of the battleship USS *Missouri* grew hot. The massive hulk of steel, the length of a football field, was the site of the formal surrender ceremony of the Axis powers to the Allies.[1]

General Jonathan Wainwright, commander of the American forces defeated in the Philippines, had been liberated only four days earlier after three years in a Manchurian prison camp; he and Percival, the British general who had surrendered Singapore, flanked General Douglas MacArthur, now supreme commander for the Allied powers. Fanning out behind them on either side were Allied admirals and generals from England, Canada, Australia, New Zealand, Russia, China, the Netherlands, and America.

In the center of the rows of khaki, medals, and ribbons stood a microphone, an old mess table covered with a thick green cloth, and two straight chairs. Surrounding them was the network of scaffolding erected for war correspondents and cameramen, now clinging to their perches, checking camera angles, and scribbling notes. The gun turrets and decks overhead were lined with sailors in sparkling white. Many held Kodaks, straining for a shot of General MacArthur.

High above it all, the Stars and Stripes snapped in the breeze, the same flag that had flown over the U.S. Capitol on the morning of December 7, 1941, when the Japanese had destroyed the American fleet in Pearl Harbor.

At 9:00 A.M., Commander Horace Byrd, the *Missouri*'s gunnery officer, cupped his hands to his mouth and shouted, "Attention all hands." The jubilant buzz of conversation quieted as the Japanese delegation approached the *Missouri*.

Eleven Japanese officials, wearing silk hats, ascots, and cutaways, climbed the ship's stairway, their faces expressionless. Several had been forced to participate in the ceremonies by the emperor himself; they had vowed to commit hara-kiri, as many of their

fellow officers already had, upon their return to Tokyo.

The ceremony began with an invocation by the
ship's chaplain, then the "Star Spangled Banner"
blared over the public-address system. General
MacArthur, wearing his familiar sun glasses and visored cap, walked briskly to the microphone. He
stood erect and confident, though his hand trem-
bled slightly as he held the sheet of notes before
him.

"We are gathered here, representative of the major warring powers," he said in a strong voice, "to
conclude a solemn agreement whereby peace may be
restored.... It is my earnest hope and indeed the
hope of all mankind that from this solemn occasion
a better world shall emerge out of the blood and
carnage of the past—a world founded upon faith and
understanding—a world dedicated to the dignity of
man and the fulfillment of his most cherished wish—
for freedom, tolerance and justice."

Two copies of the surrender agreement lay on
the table, one bound in leather for the Allies, the
other bound in canvas for the Japanese. Cameras
clicked everywhere as the signing began. Foreign
Minister Shigemitsu sat down and fumbled with
his hat and gloves, obviously bewildered. Mac-
Arthur's chief of staff showed him where to sign.
Then the other Japanese officials signed the agreement, as did the nine representatives of the Allied
powers. At eight minutes past nine, MacArthur sat
at the table and affixed his signature to the document.

"Let us pray that peace be now restored to the

world and that God will preserve it always," he announced. At that moment a steady drone in the clouds above the ship became a deafening roar, and an aerial pageant of 400 B-29s and 1,500 carrier planes swept across the sky and disappeared in the mists of Mount Fuji to the southwest.

World War II had ended.

At that dramatic moment General Douglas MacArthur spoke the first words of peace to a waiting world.

"Today the guns are silent . . . the skies no longer rain death . . . the seas bear only commerce . . . men everywhere walk upright in the sunlight. The entire world is quietly at peace. . . .

"A new era is upon us. Even the lesson of victory itself brings with it profound concern both for our future security and the survival of civilization. The destructiveness of the war potential, through progressive advances in scientific discovery, has in fact now reached a point which revises the traditional concept of war. . . .

"Men since the beginning of time have sought peace, [but] military alliances, balance of power, leagues of nations, all in turn failed, leaving the only path to be by way of the crucible of war.

"*We have had our last chance. If we do not now devise some greater and more equitable system, Armageddon will be at our door. The problem is basically theological and involves a spiritual recrudescence and improvement of human character. It must be of the spirit if we are able to save the flesh.*"

*   *   *

Nineteen forty-five, "Year Zero," as one historian labeled it,* was the year of promise. Old mistakes were not to be repeated.

Douglas MacArthur was one of the few who was in a position to fully understand that the challenge of this new beginning was not primarily political, military, or economic, but spiritual. The crisis was not one of organization or technology, but of character and ideas. He issued his prophetic challenge in light of two events that had already occurred, ominous portents that would shape the post-war world: the atom bomb and the accession to Stalin's demands.

The bomb MacArthur had seen. He knew that the devastating power of the atom bomb would forever change the rules of war, international politics, and the universe. Hiroshima's blackened ruins testified to the possibility of global annihilation and the ultimate destructive power of man over nature and humanity. The mushroom cloud of Armageddon would haunt future generations.

Catholic novelist Georges Bernanos, author of *The Diary of a Country Priest*, called the use of the bomb the "triumph of technique over reason."[2] Questions of justice, prudence, responsibility, and con-

---

*John Lukacs in his book *1945: Year Zero* (Garden City: Doubleday, 1978). Lukacs explains: "Nineteen forty-five was both Year Zero and Year One. Year Zero, Jahr Null—this is what a generation of Germans called the year 1945. Year One, Year I of the Atomic Age, this is how certain intellectuals, editorialists, scientists kept referring to that year, at least for awhile." Lukacs contends that the end of a united Germany was a much more important event in 1945 than the atomic bomb.

sequences were set aside in pursuit of a technique
to win the war. Though the bomb hastened the end
of the war, it would shape civilization's values for
the remainder of the century. Just as technique had
triumphed over reason, so expediency would
triumph over morality.

The second event that was to significantly shape
the post–World War II world was the Allied decision
to accede to Soviet demands for the return of all
Russian nationals. Thus, the West was amazingly
compliant; the singular goal was victory and that
meant keeping Stalin happy. In 1944 hundreds of
thousands who had come under Allied control during the liberation of Europe were sent back to the
Soviet Union.

Sir Patrick Dean, legal advisor for the British
foreign office, advised his superiors: "This is purely
a question for the Soviet authorities and does not
concern His Majesty's government. In due course, all
those with whom the Soviet authorities desire to deal
must be handed over to them, and we are not concerned with the fact that they may be shot or otherwise more harshly dealt with than they might be
under English law."[3]

Again, technique superseded reason and principle at the price of an estimated one and a half
million people. The forced repatriation served Stalin's death warrant on Croats, cossacks, and the other
Russians who had hoped to escape Communist rule.

MacArthur realized the peril the post-war world
faced. But his stirring words of warning that day in
Tokyo Bay were washed away in the waves of eu-
phoric relief that swept over victor and vanquished

alike. Instead of seeking spiritual renewal, which might have established a healthy balance between the religious and the political, the post-war generation was left to thrash about in a vacuum of values.

For at that point the modern mind had already been seized by the powerful ideas of an odd prophet—a syphilitic and eventually insane German who could see into the soul of our century from the middle of the last.

In 1889 Friedrich Nietzsche told a parable:

Have you not heard of the madman who lit a lamp in the bright morning and went to the marketplace crying ceaselessly, "I seek God! I seek God!" There were many among those standing there who didn't believe in God so he made them laugh. "Is God lost?" one of them said. "Has he gone astray like a child?" said another. "Or is he hiding? Has he gone on board ship and emigrated?" So they laughed and shouted to one another. The man sprang into their midst and looked daggers at them. "Where is God?" he cried. "I will tell you. We have killed him—you and I. We are all his killers! But how have we done this? How could we swallow up the sea? Who gave us the sponge to wipe away the horizon? What will we do as the earth is set loose from its sun?"[4]

Nietzsche's point was not that God does not exist, but that God has become irrelevant. Men and women may assert that God exists or that He does not, but it makes little difference either way. God is dead not because He doesn't exist, but because we live, play, procreate, govern, and die as though He doesn't.

The effect of this widespread notion can be seen in the despair that followed World War I, in the void that gave rise to fascism, in the militant atheism that has claimed countless lives in Russia and China, and in modern Western culture. The death of God has profound implications for individuals as well as for society and politics because it is the philosophic context in which modern governments operate.

In Western civilization God had traditionally played the role of legitimizing government. In classical and Christian political philosophy He was the author of natural law—that body of just and reasonable standards that guided human rulers and by which the ruled were bound to respect and obey those given charge over them. Even atheistic political philosophy acknowledged that the idea of God was useful: a little dose of religion would keep the masses quiet. As Napoleon said, "Religion is what keeps the poor from murdering the rich."[5]

But Nietzsche's atheism was the most radical the world had yet seen. While the old atheism had acknowledged the need for religion, the new atheism was political, activist, and jealous. One scholar observed that "atheism has become militant . . . insisting it must be believed. Atheism has felt the need to impose its views, to forbid competing visions."[6]

Nietzsche himself predicted the result of this new atheism on politics. "I am not man, I am dynamite . . . my truth is fearful; it is that in the past we called lies the truth—the devaluation of all values. . . . The concept of politics is completely taken up in a war of the spirits, all the structures of power are blown up into the air, for they are based on the lie.

There will be wars of a kind that have never happened on the earth."[7]

"The devaluation of all values" is what the death of God has meant to politics. Distinctions between right and wrong, justice and injustice have become meaningless. No objective guide is left to choose between "all men are created equal" and "the weak to the wall."

In Year Zero no one could have predicted the consequences that the void at the heart of the nations would produce. But philosopher Blaise Pascal had foreseen, three centuries earlier, the chilling consequences. He argued that in a spiritual vacuum, men can pursue only two options: first, to imagine that they are gods themselves, or second, to seek satisfaction in their senses. Unknowingly, he predicted the routes that would be followed in the East and West in the aftermath of World War II.

On the surface, however, when the USS *Missouri* sailed out of Tokyo Bay, there seemed every reason for hope. Plans were being laid for a great council of nations dedicated to the dignity of man and the end of war. It would be a brave new world in which the nations of the globe could unite to seek peace and justice.

*   *   *

The United Nations complex sits on sixteen acres of New York City's choicest real estate, bordering the East River and Manhattan. The lean, immense Secretariat building rises into the sky, the sun reflecting off its window walls. Bright flags of the nations of the world fly in the breezes off the river;

the most prominent is the blue and white UN flag, its two white reeds of olive branches surrounding the world.

A visitor is immediately struck by the grandeur of the building, stirred by the sight of dignitaries stepping out of black limousines to cross the massive plaza. He realizes that if this place represents the powers of the world, one might well want to see the place of worship, where the nations bow before the One under whose rule they govern.

The information personnel are bemused. "The chapel? We don't have a chapel. If there is one, I believe it's across the street."

The visitor darts across the thoroughfare, dodging New York's taxis, and successfully arrives at the opposite building's security-clearance desk.

"Well, there's a chapel here," responds the officer, "but it's not associated with the UN." He thumbs through a directory. "Oh, I see, all right, here it is. It's across the street—and tell them you're looking for the meditation room."

Again the visitor dashes across the pavement. An attendant tells him that the room is not open to the public; it's a "nonessential area," and there has been a personnel cutback. But a security guard will escort the visitor through long, crowded hallways and swinging glass doors. Again, there is the pervasive sense of weighty matters being discussed in the noble pursuit of world peace.

The guide pauses at an unmarked door. He unlocks it and gingerly pushes it open. The small room is devoid of people or decoration. The walls are stark white. There are no windows. A few wicker stools surround a large square rock at the center of the room. It is very quiet. But there is no altar, rug, vase, candle, or symbol of any type of religious worship.

Lights in the ceiling create bright spots of illumination on the front wall. One focuses on a piece of modern art: steel squares and ovals. Beyond the abstract shapes, there is nothing in those bright circles of light. They are focused on a void. And it is in that void that the visitor suddenly sees the soul of the brave new world.

THIRTEEN

Marxism and the Kingdom of God

*If you will not have God (and He is a
jealous God), you should pay your
respects to Hitler and Stalin.*

— T. S. Eliot

"God remains dead," wrote Nietzsche. "How
shall we, the murderers of all murderers, comfort
ourselves? Must not we ourselves become gods simply to seem worthy of it?"[1] With these words
Nietzsche was at once echoing Pascal's first option
that "men become gods themselves" and heralding
the creation of a new type of man—a heroic indi-
vidualist no longer bound to a traditional "slave"
morality, but creating his own rules. Such a "super-
man" would exercise the "will to power."

Today one-third of the world's population lives
in the viselike grip of states that are the product of
such gangster-statesmen who established governments that attempted to fill the vacuum of values
with secular ideology or the cult of personality. The
goal of these massive bureaucracies is to preside over
the death of God; their system for achieving it is most

often called Marxist Leninism. It carries out its policies with surgical efficiency, as millions of Christians and Jews who have passed through Communist
gulags would testify. If they could. But sometimes
the system performs with comic clumsiness, as I witnessed one night in Leningrad.

In February 1973 President Nixon had sent me
to the Soviet Union for follow-up negotiations to the
trade agreements Nixon and Leonid Brezhnev had
announced at their 1973 summit. My real job, however, was to pressure the Soviets into allowing more
Jews to emigrate. Their refusal to do so was imperiling trade legislation in the U.S. Congress.

After our official meetings in Moscow, my wife
Patty and I were escorted on a three-day visit to Leningrad, Russia's showcase city for Western visitors.

Leningrad takes on an eerie beauty in the filtered
light of the northern winter, its sprawling skyline a
dazzling mix of gilded, traditional onion domes and
the rich blue and pastel hues of French and Italian
provincial architecture. This splendid city is the
place where East and West have traditionally met—
and divided.

Like all Western visitors, Patty and I eagerly
walked the treasure-laden corridors of the Hermitage,
one of the world's greatest art repositories; saw the
famed Peter and Paul fortress, within whose massive
walls have been enacted many of the turbulent events
of Russian history; explored the palaces where czars
of the Imperial era lived in unrivaled splendor; and
visited the cathedrals of Leningrad, which reflect the
Russian culture. The ecclesiastical façade of one, the
Peter and Paul Lutheran Church, has been preserved,

but the interior has been converted into a gigantic
public swimming pool. Another, the spectacular Cathedral of Our Lady, is now a state museum exhibiting the history of religion and atheism.

The Soviet Foreign Ministry capped our visit
with an evening at the Kirov Ballet for a performance
of Tchaikovsky's *Swan Lake*. The Kirov is the crown
jewel of Leningrad. The Soviets spared nothing to
repair the heavy damage the building suffered during
World War II, restoring its nineteenth-century ele-
gance. During the renovation, which was completed
in 1970, nearly nine hundred pounds of gold were
used to gild the interior walls where five tiers of
balconies sweep around the huge horseshoe-shaped
hall like elegant ivory and gold rings, glistening in
the blaze of massive crystal chandeliers. The sight
took our breath away.

Our escort, a veteran U.S. Consulate officer,
seemed pleased as we were shown to our orchestra
center seats—thick, plush, sapphire-velvet chairs.

"This is very good for protocol," he whispered.

"Good for watching great ballet too," I replied.

His smile vanished. "Of course we may not see
Swan Lake," he said.

I thought he was joking. "Why not?" I asked,
prepared for a quip.

"Well, we know the Soviets respect your high
rank because you got these seats," he said. "And
often when American VIPs come they pull a switch
at the last minute and put on a dreadful atheistic
propaganda piece called *Creation of the World*. I've
seen it six times."

"But these people," I said, gesturing at the audience. "They're here to see *Swan Lake*. They'll be in an uproar."

"No, they won't," the consular officer replied with a smile. "This is Russia."

Sure enough, when the lights dimmed and the velvet curtain rose, it was not the opening strains of Tchaikovsky's masterpiece we heard, but the strident chords of *Creation of the World*. I watched the faces of the surrounding audience. Not a murmur, not a single expression of displeasure. Seventeen hundred people sat stoically in their seats.

It was a dreary evening indeed. The ballet was a parody on the Garden of Eden, where a buffoonlike character, God, contested with a vital, vigorous figure, Satan, for the soul of man. In the closing scene God retreated lamely, vanquished, leaving self-sufficient man living happily ever after in his earthly paradise.

The architect of this earthly paradise was Vladimir Ilyich Ulyanov, the son of Christian parents, known to history as Lenin.

Lenin, a single-minded radical, became the most successful revolutionary of the twentieth century. With the "will to power," he pursued and eliminated his enemies ruthlessly—liberals and socialists, rival Marxists, reluctant peasants and skeptical military officers, monarchists and capitalists, Jews and various other "class enemies." Above all, Lenin pursued and murdered Christians. He hated them. "There can be nothing more abominable than religion," he wrote.[2]

Lenin particularly hated seriously committed

Christians. Weak Christians he could manage, but serious Christians meant nothing but trouble for a Marxist-Leninist regime. They owed allegiance to the one power greater than the totalitarian Communist state. History has borne Lenin out on this point, if not on others.

The pattern of Communist persecution of Jews and Christians is remarkably ecumenical. It has fallen on orthodox believers in Russia, Romania, Bulgaria, and the Ukraine; Roman Catholics in the Baltic Republics, Poland, Hungary, Cuba, Vietnam, and Nicaragua; Lutherans in East Germany and Czechoslovakia; Reformed Christians in Hungary and Czechoslovakia; Pentecostals, Baptists, and other evangelicals in Eastern Europe, Latin America, and Asia; house church believers in China.

In 1980 twenty-eight Marxist regimes around the world were committed to a policy of atheism, repressing and persecuting Christianity to some degree. These nations contained approximately 250 million Christians—almost one of every five Christians in the world. Those twenty-eight nations have a total population of 1.48 billion—more than a third of the world's people.[3]

Consider just a few representative reports of that persecution around the world:

—In Vietnam seventeen evangelical pastors are in jail. Some 200 churches have been closed since 1975, the year the only Protestant seminary in the country was closed.
—In the Soviet Union criminal charges are filed against Nedezhda Mativkhina for allowing a group

of Christians to meet in her home. Mativkhina, a double amputee, has already served two terms in the gulag and now faces a third.[4]

—In Czechoslovakia and Hungary the police crack down on leaders of "basic communities" where Catholic adults and young people meet for Bible study and prayer.

—In China authorities "liberalize" rules covering Christians by banning Protestant house churches, restricting religious gatherings to licensed church buildings, and forbidding evangelism.*

—In Nicaragua dozens of Moravian pastors serving impoverished Miskito Indians on the country's Atlantic Coast are imprisoned and killed. Moravian communities are uprooted.

—In the Soviet Union dissident Anatoly Shcharansky is given 130 days in solitary for refusing to surrender his book of Psalms.

---

*It is much more difficult to obtain accurate statistics on religious belief in China than in the Soviet Union—though there is evidence of a flourishing house-church movement, a state-controlled national Protestant church, and continuing Catholic presence. Before Mao Tse-tung's takeover in 1949, Christians were a tiny minority. Both Protestant and Catholic missionaries, however, had established a robust presence, and the 80 percent of the Chinese people who followed various folk religions seemed relatively receptive to the gospel. Indeed, the Christian churches have grown steadily in Hong Kong, Taiwan, and Macao—Chinese areas free of Communist control.

If the churches in mainland China had grown at the same rate as those in Taiwan or Hong Kong, we could have expected the Christian population of China to be 90 million by 1980. The most optimistic private Western estimate of China's Christian population is 50 million. The official government figure is 1.8 million—a scant 200,000 more than the Christian population in 1900. Nicholas Piediscalzi, "China's New Policy on Religion," *Christian Century* (June 19–26, 1985), 613.

The Soviet Union has set the course that virtually all Marxist governments have followed. Before the 1917 revolution 83.4 percent of the people living in what is now the Soviet Union were identified as Christians—three quarters of them Russian Orthodox. Orthodox, Catholic, and Protestant Christians have suffered violent persecution since the revolution, except for a brief period during World War II when the regime needed the support of the churches. Since 1917, some 60 million Soviet citizens have been killed and 66 million have been sent to labor camps or imprisoned. At least half of these have been Christians.[5]

Activist theologian Reinhold Niebuhr once described Communism as "an organized evil which spreads terror and cruelty through the world."[6] And Aleksandr Solzhenitsyn, the great writer who came to faith while in prison, explains why Communists are so determined to destroy Christianity: "They flee from Christ like devils from the sign of the cross."[7]

*   *   *

Cardinal Joseph Mindszenty, the primate of Hungary, stood naked in his chilly cell in the secret-police headquarters at 60 Andrassy Street in Budapest, trembling with fear and cold as a furious agent of the state advanced on him with a rubber truncheon in one hand and a long knife in the other.

"I'll kill you," the man snarled, lashing the truncheon across the cardinal's back. "By morning I'll tear you to pieces and throw the remains of your corpse into the canal. We are the masters here now."

He prodded Mindszenty with the knife. The cardinal moved away. Another prod. And another. The cardinal moved and moved again. Soon he was running in circles. For several hours the agent drove the naked, middle-aged prelate unrelentingly around the cell like a horse in training.

It was late January 1949. Cardinal Mindszenty had been enduring such tortures since his arrest the day after Christmas. Every night his Communist interrogators demanded that he confess to crimes against the state, including the preposterous charge that he had conspired with the American government to restore a Hapsburg king to the throne of Hungary. Every night Cardinal Mindszenty refused to sign the confession.

During the day the cardinal sat on a filthy couch trying to recover from the night's tortures. If he drifted into sleep, one of the jailers who sat in the room prodded him awake. At night the cycle began again.

"I was being made to feel in my soul, my body, my nerves, and my bones the power of bolshevism which was taking over the country," he later wrote.

Although his jailers may not have known it, Cardinal Mindszenty embodied, in a sense, the sufferings of an entire nation. The events that led to his imprisonment paralleled the ideological imprisonment of the Hungarian churches. The Communists had consolidated their power the summer before, in 1948, and their first target had been the churches. Two days after the new regime took control, they secularized the nation's religious schools. Party boss Matyas Rakosi pressed church leaders to submit to government control over church affairs, including requirements that priests and ministers publicly support government policies.

Bishop Lajos Ordass, the ablest leader of the Lutheran Church, refused to cooperate and was arrested and imprisoned. Bishop Laszlo Ravasz, the independent-minded head of the Hungarian Reformed Church, was forced out and replaced by a complaint theologian who thought support for Marxist Leninism was obligatory for Christians.

The chief obstacle to the Communists' plans, however, was Cardinal Mindszenty. As Catholic primate, he was the leader of the largest denomination in Hungary, a stubborn man with a record of fierce opposition to tyrants. The Nazis had jailed him during World War II. Later, as Communist power grew in Hungary, he constantly protested their abuses of human rights.

Cardinal Mindszenty was especially offended by the government's demands that the church sign a formal treaty with the state. He had watched Lenin and Stalin subdue the Orthodox Church in the Soviet Union through a campaign of terrorism, judicial persecution, and subversion. He vowed that he would not allow the same thing to happen in Hungary.

The church-state agreement in the Soviet Union gave the state control over religious instruction, seminary education, and appointment of bishops. Bishops were called upon to give public support to government policies when their Communist masters wanted it, and all priests had to swear allegiance to the Communist government.

Significantly, the party ruthlessly forbade the church to evangelize or to provide services to the poor, elderly, sick, and needy. Thus, the church was barred from conducting any activities that would publicly testify to its members' allegiance to another King.

Party Chief Rakosi wanted to make the church in Hungary a puppet church like the one in the Soviet Union. Cardinal Mindszenty would have none of it. After months of bickering with the recalcitrant cardinal, Rakosi and his henchmen moved against the church leader.

The day after Christmas 1948, police occupied the cardinal's offices in Esztergom. Officers carrying submachine guns led Cardinal Mindszenty to a car and drove him to secret-police headquarters in Budapest. There he was subjected to torture.

Thirty-nine days after his arrest—beaten, confused, plagued with despair, and racked with fear and anxiety—the cardinal signed the confession the authorities wanted.

Later he told the harrowing account of those weeks of torture in his memoirs.[8] The mental and psychological pain were far worse than the physical deprivations and beatings, he wrote, and he was certain that the police had used drugs on him. He candidly admitted that the Communist torturers had shattered his personality, reducing him to a state where even the regime's most absurd charges began to seem plausible.

Certainly the man whom the Communists put on public trial for treason in February 1949 looked like a drugged, programed shell, reciting the lines of a memorized script. He was found guilty of treason and sentenced to life in prison.

Soon after Cardinal Mindszenty's trial, the government suppressed the Catholic Church in Hungary. Religious schools were abolished, religious instruction was outlawed, and religious orders were dissolved. Monks and nuns scattered into the population and were left to find what work they could.

In their place the government organized "peace priests" composed of ambitious collaborators and covert Communist agents. Soon these priests, many of whom led dissolute lives, controlled all the higher posts in the church. Catholics who wanted authentic pastoral care had to seek out priests who carried on their ministry in secret.

Eventually the regime got the agreement it wanted. The bishops agreed to support the government and its "peace priest" movement, and to tolerate state supervision of seminary training, clerical appointments, and other internal matters. In return, the government allowed the church to open eight schools and put the clergy on the state payroll.

The Reformed Church submitted to a similar agreement.

Thus the Communist rulers in Hungary have achieved what they consider "normal" relations with the church. Church authorities clear key appointments in advance with the government. Troublesome clerics are reassigned to the provinces. Bishops make regular expressions of support to the regime. When needed, priests and ministers read from their pulpits pastoral letters composed by the government Bureau of Religious Affairs.

*   *   *

Why is the conflict between the Christian church and the Marxist state so fundamental, ceaseless, and protracted?

Many in the secularized, tolerant West are offended by terms like "mortal enemies," preferring to see Communists as a particularly enthusiastic band of social reformers and the church as one of the many social institutions that must adapt to changing political circumstances. History, however, teaches a different lesson. Communism and Christianity are at odds for very good reasons.

First, Christianity and Communism are irreconcilable in their basic premises. The Christian believes that the dynamic of all history is spiritual, that its unfolding reveals God's dealings with men, that Jesus Christ is God in the flesh, and that at the end of history, He will reign over all the nations.

For Marxists, the material realm is all there is. God and the spiritual order are illusions. Mankind swims in the current of history, which progresses by economic forces from the decline of capitalism, through the dictatorship of the proletariat, to the earthly paradise of the classless society. Communists are materialists and determinists; individuals count for nothing, the collective or state for everything.

Lenin thought that those who believed in God were worse than fools. "Every man who occupies himself with the construction of a god, or merely even agrees to it, prostitutes himself in the worst way," he wrote. "For he occupies himself not with activity, but with self-contemplation and self-reflection, and tries thereby to deify his most unclean, most stupid, and most servile features and pettinesses."[9] Consequently, anyone who believes in God is not simply in error; he is mentally deranged. This is why believers in the Soviet Union are frequently judged insane and committed to mental institutions.

Second, Communism and Christianity clash because each is a religion and each is inherently expansive and evangelistic.

Marxists claim that their system is scientific, in contrast to the "superstition" of Christianity. But anyone who has visited Communist countries knows better. Marxist Leninism functions as a religion in the lives of the faithful. Communist "saints" and martyrs are revered, their utterances preserved in books and studied carefully. May Day marches and other public ceremonies are atheistic liturgies whereby unbelievers worship the superiority of unbelief.

Philosophically, Marxism is certainly a religion. It offers a comprehensive explanation of reality and claims to put adherents in touch with higher powers—namely, the inexorable laws of history. Its eschatology is millennial. At the end of the class struggle against capitalism lies the classless society where exploiters are banished, the state withers away, and man's natural goodness flows forth unobstructed. The laws of history will bring justice to the oppressed and wipe away every tear. It's a system that an atheist can put his faith in.

Lenin, Stalin, and Rakosi recognized that a renewed and purified Christianity was the only force that could move the masses as powerfully as the

Marxist ideal could. They attacked it as the enemy that it was and is.

Trotsky, Tito, Mao, Ho Chi Minh, Castro—and the Sandinistas of the eighties—all the tyrants who have followed Marx have believed substantially the same thing about Christianity.

Nothing has changed. Despite his shrewd public effort to picture himself as a benign and progressive reformer, Mikhail Gorbachev adheres to this same ideology. As recently as November 1986, he described the struggle with traditional religion as "decisive and uncompromising" and called for more aggressive atheistic education.[10]

Like Lenin, Gorbachev knows who his enemies are. The greatest obstacle to the Marxist ideal of total control is the Christian faith, which is not simply a set of intellectual beliefs or weekly worship services, but involves personal submission to a King whose culture is incompatible with Lenin's. The Christian church and the Marxist state may work out an accommodation for a time, but they will always be adversaries. The very nature of each makes any lasting accommodation impossible. They are the two great contenders for the soul of mankind.

The people of Jaworzyna had had enough. For years they had petitioned the party authorities in the Silesia region of Poland for permission to build a church. Their repeated applications were denied. The men on the church-building committee tried pulling strings with higher party officials in Crakow and Warsaw. No luck. When they angrily protested the refusal, the petty bureaucrats turned a deaf ear.

Now, other measures were required.

Months before, the authorities had issued a permit to build an auto-repair garage on a site near a highway. Now workers moved onto the site, erected a tall fence, and began to build the garage. The building progressed slowly over a period of two years, but no one paid much attention. The party authorities in Jaworzyna were busy men.

Then, on Sunday, February 5, 1978, the fence came down and the garage turned out to be a new church—its wide portals adorned with a picture of Our Lady of Częstochowa, the protector of Poland. Masses were celebrated until late in the evening; thousands of people came to worship and rejoice.

That spring, Cardinal Karol Wojtlya of Crakow came to Jaworzyna to dedicate the church. Soon afterward the authorities tried to close it, but hundreds of angry Poles organized a twenty-four-hour guard. The church building committee was taken to court and fined. Their clever lawyers tied the case up in procedural disputes.

Just before the May Day celebrations of the glorious triumph of Communism in Poland, the party authorities attempted to hid the church from the nearby highway by surrounding it with giant billboards bearing propaganda. The next morning the billboards lay on the ground, their messages celebrating the revolution ripped and shredded, their supports smashed. Even the cement footings had been ripped from the ground.

The wreckage lay outside the church for months. Many in Jaworzyna took it as a graphic symbol of the conflict in Poland between the church, which bears authority, and the state, which merely has power.

Joseph Stalin, who murdered millions during his twenty-nine-year reign as perhaps the most ruthless tyrant in history, once scoffed at a colleague who warned that the pope was likely to denounce one of Stalin's barbaric plans. "The pope!" sneered Stalin. "How many divisions does the pope have?"[11]

The pope's divisions were on display to the entire world in June 1979 when the former Cardinal Karol Wojtlya of Crakow, now John Paul II, visited his homeland. Ecstatic crowds gathered everywhere he went—200,000 in Warsaw, 500,000 at the shrine of the Black Madonna at Częstochowa, 1,000,000 in Crakow. Similar throngs were present at Gniezno, the first capital of Poland; at Wadowice, the pope's birthplace; and at Auschwitz and Birkenau, the sites of the infamous Nazi extermination camps. The world saw that the church possessed the soul of the Polish people and embodied the essence of Polish nationhood. By contrast, the Polish Communists who operated the machinery of the state were alien usurpers who did the bidding of Russian masters. Though he went out of his way to avoid a direct confrontation with the Communist regime, John Paul's message was widely understood by the restive Polish masses, and he lit a fuse during his triumphant nine-day visit to his homeland.

"Christ would never approve that man be considered merely as a means of production," he told workers in his old archdiocese in Mogila.[12]

At Częstochowa, he urged the government to honor "the cause of fundamental human rights, including the right to religious liberty."[13]

At Novy Targ, he told Poles to set a Christian example "even if it means risking danger."[14]

The long fuse that the pope lit exploded in July 1980 when workers at the Lenin shipyards at Gdansk went out on strike. Under the leadership of a Catholic electrician named Lech Walesa, the workers seized the shipyards and made a radical demand of the authorities: the right to organize free labor unions. Workers throughout the country walked off their jobs in sympathy. The Communist regime, discredited and despised, lost control.

By 1981 the Polish government was desperate. Millions of Poles, including many members of the Communist party, had joined the Solidarity movement. Lech Walesa was a household name around the world. Labor unrest was spreading from the cities to the rural areas. The economy was a shambles. The Red army maneuvered on Poland's eastern border. No one doubted that Soviet party boss Leonid Brezhnev would use his divisions if the pope's couldn't be curbed.

John Paul II announced that if Soviet tanks moved, he would return to stand with his countrymen. In desperation the government did the only thing it could do: it turned to the church. Cardinal Stefan Wyszynski, the primate of Poland, skillfully negotiated a deal among church, state, and Solidarity. The state would allow Solidarity freedom to organize and would loosen censorship in return for labor peace and an end to attacks on the fundamental legitimacy of the regime. The church would guarantee the arrangement.

That June, shortly after negotiating the agreement, Cardinal Wyszynski died at the age of eighty. He had been imprisoned by the Communist regime from 1953 to 1956. Now he received a state funeral that rivaled the funerals of Winston Churchill and Charles de Gaulle for national pomp. The nation went into official mourning. The state radio played only solemn religious music. Theaters closed. Flags flew at half-staff. The president of Poland and three deputy prime ministers came to the funeral to honor the cardinal. They stood with a quarter million other Poles in Victory Square in Warsaw under a forty-three-foot-high wooden cross that proclaimed the triumph of Christianity.

Later that year, in December 1981, a reorganized Polish government imposed martial law and drove the Solidarity movement underground. That Solidarity was a religious movement no one, least of all the Soviets, can deny. In November 1981, *Pravda* denounced "religious fanaticism" as a grave challenge to socialism; failure to contain it, *Pravda* said, was at the root of the problems in Poland.[15]

Neither does anyone doubt that the currents of discontent will break out anew in the years ahead. Three times in forty years the Polish people have risen against their government and its Russian masters, each uprising triggered by Christian outrage over the brutality of the regime, its indifference to human needs, its suppression of fundamental rights, and its incessant lying. Christianity possesses the hearts of the people and shapes the Polish culture. This was evidenced at the height of the Gdansk strike when Western newspapers published front-page photos showing strikers in the Gdansk shipyards kneeling to receive communion. Such a sight was a shock to jaded, secularized eyes. Union workers in other industrialized countries are often part of the anticlerical left. In Poland the Christian workers are loyal to the church against the state.

Why is the church so much stronger in Poland than almost anywhere else in the world, certainly stronger than in Hungary and elsewhere in Eastern Europe?

The election of a Polish pope is surely a factor. So is the fact that Christianity has been firmly established in Poland for a thousand years. But a primary reason is the church's long tradition of resistance to secular power.

From 1795 to 1918 the Polish nation was divided among the Prussian, Austrian, and Russian empires, and church authorities resisted all three. In 1874 the archbishop of Poznan was imprisoned for opposing Bismarck's program of requiring religious instruction in German. The czar's plans for forced Russification in eastern Poland ran into similar opposition. From 1918 to 1939, during the period of the First Republic, the church remained independent from the Polish republic. The church also resisted the Nazi regime and suffered greatly for it. A third of the Catholic clergy in Poland were executed by the Germans or died in concentration camps.

When the Communists imprisoned him in 1953, Cardinal Wyszynski reflected that of his seventeen seminary classmates, only he had thus far escaped being sent to German or Russian concentration camps. Cardinal Wyszynski confided a somewhat wry reflection to his diary: "Most of the priests and bishops with whom I worked had experienced prisons. Something would have been wrong if I had not experienced imprisonment. What was happening to me was very appropriate."[16]

A church with such a history, led by such tough-minded men, was ready for anything the new totalitarian state could devise. As Jacques Ellul, the French Protestant philosopher, has written, the "role of Cardinal Wyszynski after 1945 was to uphold the traditional church in the face of Communist power ...to pressure [it] from...surrendering ideologically. It thus was and is the force behind Solidarity and the most powerful force in Poland today."[17]

The Polish church is one of the few in Eastern Europe to have avoided entanglement with the state. Many other church bodies allowed themselves to become closely identified with secular authorities, and in doing so, the official church in these countries lost the people. They are today mere puppets of their Communist ruler.

Ellul points out this lesson, one that the church around the world needs to remember: "Collaboration with power, whether Communist or not, is always ruinous for the church. If the church exists, if it is to have legitimacy in the eyes of the people, it must always stand erect as a counter-power to political power."[18]

Cardinal Wyszynski understood this. In prison in 1953, alone but supremely confident, he wrote a prophetic comment in his diary: "Any form of government, no matter how ruthless, will slowly cool and wane as it runs up against difficulties that the bureaucrat cannot resolve without cooperation from the people. Somehow the people must be taken into account."[19]

When the time came to reach the people, the Polish state found the church already there. It had been there for centuries.

*   *   *

The struggle between church and state has lasted for centuries in Poland. In Nicaragua it began in the early seventies when the Catholic church opposed the right-wing tyranny of the dictator Anastasio Somoza. It continues today.

Jimmy Hassan wasn't surprised when the police came for him in October 1985.

He had become national director of Campus Crusade for Christ in Nicaragua in 1982, when the revolutionary Sandinista government started serious persecution of evangelicals. Because Hassan was a lawyer and a former judge, his connections in Managua afforded him some protection. But many of his friends and co-workers had been harassed. Hassan had known it would only be a matter of time until the police came for him.

An officer at the security police headquarters held up a copy of Campus Crusade's basic literature, a small booklet called "The Four Spiritual Laws."

"Is this yours?" he snarled.

Hassan admitted it was. The officer ripped it up. Several agents shoved him in a car and drove him to Campus Crusade's Managua headquarters. There they confiscated about 2000 "Four Spiritual Laws" booklets and hundreds of books, including New Testaments and Bibles.

The next stop was the shop that did Campus Crusade's printing. There the junta's agents confiscated 50,000 copies of "The Four Spiritual Laws." They threatened the printer with jail if he ever did any more work for Hassan or Campus Crusade.

The police then locked Hassan alone in a room at the Interior Ministry.

Hassan thought of his wife and three children. He thought of the Moravian pastors in the remote Atlantic provinces of Nicaragua who had been murdered by Sandinista gangs. He thought of his evangelistic work and the churches that were growing. People were being saved despite the persecution. It gave him satisfaction to know he was being held because the Marxist authorities hated Campus Crusade's success. But he wondered whether he would ever see his family again.

The security forces released him in late afternoon, and Hassan went home. At 11:00 P.M. the agents returned with a summons to report back to the Interior Ministry the next morning.

When he got there, he was taken to a room and interrogated.

"Who is your CIA controller?" they asked.

"How much did the CIA pay you to do this work in Managua?"

"What political party do you belong to?"

"Why don't you make statements supporting the Sandinistas?"

To all the accusations Hassan replied that he was not involved in politics, that he had nothing to do with the CIA, and that he only wanted to be left in peace to preach the gospel.

The interrogators threatened him with prison. They said he would be beaten if he did not confess. Hassan took these threats seriously, but he would not budge.

Then a tall man came into the room, took out a pistol, and held it to Hassan's head.

"You have one more chance to confess," one of the agents said. "Do it now. You are a paid American agent. Tell us about it. If you don't, you'll be killed."

"My only activity is to preach the gospel," Hassan replied.

The tall man pressed the pistol against Hassan's forehead. Hassan could feel the pressure increase as the man pressed his finger on the trigger. Harder. He pulled the trigger.

Hassan heard a click. . . . The gun was empty.

Hassan was released later that day with threats that he would be killed the next time they had to deal with him. Just before Christmas that year, the Hassan family escaped to Mexico. In exile, Jimmy spoke for other evangelicals of his country: "No matter what the threat, no matter what the conditions, no matter what the persecution, we will not stop preaching the gospel to the people of Nicaragua."[20]

In 1982, the year Jimmy Hassan took over Campus Crusade, Nicaragua's evangelicals were a minority in a Catholic country. Traditionally, they avoided politics. That meant the Protestants had little leverage in high places; most didn't know what was coming when a Marxist regime began to consolidate its power.[21]

In May the authorities began to confiscate evangelical churches, many of them in remote Atlantic provinces far from the capital and the inconvenient scrutiny of the Western press.

In August Interior Minister Borge told a mob that Protestants were collaborating with the CIA and the defeated Somoza regime.

"*Que se vayan, que se vayan.*" "Get them out. Get them out," chanted a mob of militants. They seized more Protestant churches.

At the same time the Sandinista government moved against the Catholic Church, which claims the loyalty of 80 percent of the Nicaraguan people. The revolutionary junta expelled two foreign priests who had worked with the poor for many years and accelerated a propaganda campaign against Catholic clergy and lay leaders who were critical of the regime. The Sandinistas also pressured the Catholic schools, replacing loyal Catholic teachers with Cuban-trained personnel indoctrinated in Marxist ideology. The schools were forced to adopt a new curriculum featuring crude Marxist propaganda.

Since 1982 harassment and persecution of evangelicals has continued. Officials of the Assemblies of God, the National Council of Evangelical Pastors, and other churches have been arrested and questioned. Moravian pastors working in Miskito Indian communities on Nicaragua's Atlantic Coast have been beaten and killed. Whole Miskito communities have been uprooted and resettled in areas under army control. Thousands have been murdered.

The visit of Pope John Paul II in 1983 was marked by open hostility between the Sandinista regime and the Catholic church. Government officials lined the ramp when the pope descended from his plane on his arrival in Managua. Ernesto Cardenal, a Catholic priest who continued to serve as a member of the revolutionary government despite a papal ruling that he step down, knelt to kiss the pope's ring. John Paul II angrily snatched it away, thus making dramatically clear to those watching his disapproval of priests serving in the Sandinista government.

The climax of the pope's visit came when he celebrated Mass in a public square in the center of Managua. The pope stood alone on a platform while Sandinista officials held back the huge, friendly crowd. Then they took over the front seats and, for the benefit of the grinding television cameras, shook their fists and screamed at the pope. Each time they did so he lifted his crucifix higher over his head.

The Sandinista officials were genuinely angry. John Paul II, a remarkable linguist, was conducting the Mass in the language of the Miskito Indians. Symbolically he was conveying a powerful truth: God offers grace to the people you killed. He was also indicting the Sandinistas. The crowd cheered; the protesters howled with rage. Much of the American media missed it altogether, expressing wonderment that the Pope would conduct mass in the language of a remote tribe.

In 1985 ten foreign priests were expelled from the country. In 1986 the junta expelled Fr. Bismark

Carballo and Bishop Pablo Vega, president of the Nicaraguan bishops' conference. Both men were persistent critics of the Sandinista regime.

While these acts of overt pressure resemble the oppression of Christians in Eastern Europe in the fifties, in reality, Nicaragua opens a new chapter in the history of conflict between the Christian church and the Marxist state.

Most Christians, including the Catholic bishops, welcomed the 1979 revolution that toppled the corrupt regime of Anastasio Somoza. Archbishop Miguel Obando y Bravo had been a persistent and effective critic of Somoza for a decade. In fact, the revolution probably would not have triumphed without the active support of the bishops and the great mass of clergy and lay leaders.

The Marxist Sandinistas were a minority in the broad coalition that made up the revolutionary government that took over in 1979. By 1980, however, the Sandinistas had forced most of their democratic colleagues out of the governing junta by using time-honored Marxist techniques: control of the army and ruthless, single-minded pursuit of their goals, unhampered by democratic procedure. But the Sandinistas could not subdue the church. It had wisely kept a distance from the state before the Sandinistas came to power. The people were with the church.

So a new strategy emerged: the Sandinistas dressed the Communist program in Christian language and raised the "peace priests" tactics of Lenin and Hungary's Rakosi to new heights.

Four Catholic priests hold cabinet office in the

Sandinista government. Sandinista officials speak of
the "Kingdom of God" coming through the revolution, and many Sandinistas passionately regard
themselves as members of *la iglesia popular* (the people's church) and followers of *el Dios de los pobres*
(the God of the Poor). Protestant sympathizers with
the Sandinista regime act through the Center for Promotion and Development. One of its leaders declared
in 1982 that "it is required that we as Christians
understand that biblical faith is inseparable from political militancy."[22]

The strategy was expounded by Daniel Ortega,
the junta leader, in his address at Managua airport
welcoming Pope John Paul II. The true Christians in
Nicaragua, he said, were "basing themselves on faith
corresponding to the revolution."[23]

A coalition of "revolutionary Christians," both
Catholic and Protestant, expressed the same sentiments in theological terms in 1980: "The only way
to love God, whom we do not see, is by contributing
to the advancement of this revolutionary process in
the most sensible and radical way possible," they
wrote. "Only then shall we be loving our brothers,
whom we do see. Therefore, we say that to be a Christian is to be a revolutionary."[24]

The vehicle for this congruence of Christianity
and revolutionary politics has been liberation theology, a movement that has come to equate partisan
political involvement with Christian commitment.
As the Protestant liberation theologian Jose Miguez
Bonino says, "Latin American theology becomes a
militant theology—a partisan theology, perhaps."[25]

"Our only solution is Marxism," says Fr. Ernesto

Cardenal, the Nicaraguan minister of culture and one of the four priests in the government. "The revolution and the Kingdom of heaven mentioned in the gospel are the same thing. A Christian should embrace Marxism if he wants to be with God and all men."[26] Or as a revolutionary poster put it, "Faith without revolution is dead."[27]

This line of thinking guts the gospel. If a Christian must embrace Marxism and revolution to do God's will, then something was lacking in the atonement and revelation of Jesus Christ.

One Sandinista pamphlet makes exactly that point. On the cover is a drawing of a young man in a beret, wearing a crucifix around his neck, carrying an automatic rifle in his left hand and a Molotov cocktail in his right. One section inside is titled "Jesus Christ Is Not Enough for Us." The text explains how the gospel must be supplemented by Marxism.

The paradoxical end to this hall of mirrors is the bizarre conclusion that Christians need Marxists far more than Marxists need Christians. In fact, Fr. Miguel D'Escoto, the Sandinista foreign minister, came to precisely that conclusion. Marxism, he said, is "one of the great blessings on the church. It has been the divine whip to bring it back."[28]

This new strategy is spreading throughout Latin America. It has been echoed in Cuba by the government's director of religious affairs who said, "Christians won't be free without socialism, and socialism won't be built on this continent without Christians."[29] This statement comes on the heels of the disclosure in Armando Valladares' memoirs that for twenty-five years, Christians have been beaten and imprisoned in Castro's own gulags.

Despite co-opting and oppression, however, Catholic as well as Protestant churches continue to resist the Sandinistas. For years, church authorities denounced and opposed the tyranny of the right. Now they denounce and oppose the tyranny of the left. They resisted pressures to do the conservatives' bidding for the sake of "order, stability, and tradition." Today they resist the left's demands to identify the gospel with "equality, justice, and peace." They demonstrate the first law of survival for the church under pressure from secular authorities: Do not legitimize tyranny. Remain aloof from the enticements and threats of the secular authority. Be faithful to God alone.

These stories of the church in Hungary, Poland, and Nicaragua are just a part of the picture. They are, however, representative of the raging conflict. With rare exceptions, the church has been driven underground or made a puppet of the state in Marxist-dominated countries. At no other time in human history has so much of the world come under the dark cloud of an oppressive regime consciously determined to eliminate religious influence from culture.

But we can be grateful that the Kingdom of God does not depend on the structures of man. Though a third of the world lives under tyranny and the official "religion" of atheism, the Kingdom of God remains visible. It is visible when leaders like Jimmy Hassan and John Paul II take their stand. It is visible when ordinary people refuse to compromise what is most precious in their lives.

That was the case in the little town of Garwolin, Poland, in March 1984.[30]

The government of Polish Prime Minister Jaruzelski had ordered crucifixes removed from classroom walls, just as they had been banned in factories, hospitals, and other public institutions. Catholic bishops attacked the ban that had stirred waves of anger and resentment all across Poland. Ultimately the government relented, insisting that the law remain on the books, but agreeing not to press for removal of the crucifixes, particularly in the schoolrooms.

But one zealous Communist school administrator in Garwolin decided that the law was the law. So one evening he had seven large crucifixes removed from lecture halls where they had hung since the school's founding in the twenties.

Days later, a group of parents entered the school and hung more crosses. The administrator promptly had these taken down as well.

The next day two-thirds of the school's six hundred students staged a sit-in. When heavily armed riot police arrived, the students were forced into the streets. Then they marched, crucifixes held high, to a nearby church where they were joined by twenty-five hundred other students from nearby schools for a morning of prayer in support of the protest. Soldiers surrounded the church. But the pictures from inside of students holding crosses

high above their heads flashed around the world.
So did the words of the priest who delivered the
message to the weeping congregation that morning.

"There is no Poland without a cross."

FOURTEEN

Conflict and Compromise in the West

It is bad to live under a prince who permits nothing, but much worse to live under one who permits everything.
—John Calvin

Before the War of the Crosses erupted in the streets of Poland in 1984, a similar battle had already been lost in the U.S. In 1980 the Supreme Court declared unconstitutional a Kentucky law requiring that the Ten Commandments be posted in public-school classrooms.[1]

In Poland the outcry against removal of the crucifixes led to mass defiance. The crucifixes were reinstated. But in Kentucky, when the offending commandments were taken down, the few holdouts, threatened with court action, soon capitulated.

What a repressive government could not force upon Poland was quietly accepted in an indifferent West. The Kentucky case is less important on its own merits than as a symbol of a growing movement in the courts that is narrowing the influence of religion in American life. Of the many cases, none has been more revealing—and bizarre—than one originating in the quiet Oklahoma town of Collinsville.

"Welcome to Collinsville," proclaims the sign marking the city limits where state highway 20 slices through this small Oklahoma town and slows down to fit the lifestyles of its three thousand citizens. Many of them are retired, enjoying Collinsville's grid of neat streets, the Crown Theater, Deb's Happytime Pizza, Collinsville Cablevision, and the Ranch House Café. Residents can choose from five feed-and-seed stores, eleven grocery stores, two funeral homes, and twenty-nine churches.

Collinsville's teenagers hold a somewhat dimmer view of its charms. "There's nothin' to do but get drunk and drag Main," says a young waitress at the Tastee Freez.

But in 1984 Collinsville became the focus of a national media spotlight when one of its citizens, thirty-six-year-old nurse Marian Guinn, sued her church for invasion of privacy.[2]

Marian Guinn was raised in Kansas as a southern Baptist. She married at eighteen and had a child at nineteen. Three other children followed, then a divorce. Guinn wanted to start over. In 1974 she moved to Collinsville, about twenty-five miles north of Tulsa, to live with her sister, Sue Hibbard.

Sue was active at the Collinsville Church of Christ, and Marian began attending the 110-member church with her sister. The members welcomed her. They baby-sat her children while she attended a high-school equivalency class; they provided food, clothing, and Christmas presents after Guinn moved

into her own small rented house; the elders drove
her to the hospital when her daughter had pneumonia. Later the church gave Guinn a car.

Guinn joined the church and was baptized. She
eventually enrolled in college, then nursing school,
and seemed to be getting her life together. But after
a few years Marian Guinn's church attendance began
to slip. Perhaps it was her school schedule; or maybe
it was her romance with Pat Sharpe, part owner of
Howland and Sharpe Pharmacy and former mayor of
Collinsville.

Sharpe, like Marian Guinn, was divorced, and
neighbors began to notice his blue-and-white Cadillac parked in her driveway late at night. In Collinsville their relationship was the juicy gossip item
it might not have been in New York or Los Angeles.
But to the Church of Christ leadership it was a spiritual problem. The elders felt that Guinn's relationship with Sharpe and lack of participation in the
church were evidence of spiritual wavering. During
the course of a conversation with one of the elders
on an unrelated matter, Pat Sharpe admitted he and
Marian were sleeping together.

In spite of the later assertion of Guinn's lawyer
that "he was a single man. She was a single lady.
And this is America," the Collinsville Church of
Christ adhered to a different standard: the biblical
law from the Old and New Testaments stating that
sexual relations outside of marriage—fornication—
is sin. They also abided by the biblical mandate that
the church has a distinct responsibility "not to associate with sexually immoral people"[3] and that re-

buking their sin must be public "so that the others may take warning."[4]

Church elders Ron Witten, Ted Moody, and Allen Cash met with Marian Guinn three times, praying with her and asking her to break off her relationship with Sharpe and return to the church's fellowship. Guinn tearfully refused. The elders said they would give her time to reconsider, but after a certain date they must make a public announcement urging the congregation to withdraw fellowship from her because of her lack of repentance. This was in accordance with the mandates of Matthew 18:15–17 and with the practices of the church.

At this point Guinn, a slight woman with large dark eyes, was angry and embarrassed. She scribbled a letter to the elders: "I do not want my name mentioned before the church except to tell them that I withdraw my membership immediately!" she wrote furiously. "I have never fully adopted your doctrine and never will! ... You have no right to get up and say anything against me in church. ... I have no choice but for all of us [herself and her children] to attend another church—another denomination where men do not set themselves up as judges for God. He does His own judging."

The elders maintained that the church was not some sort of club. Guinn had agreed to abide by its doctrine and adhere to scriptural mandates. She knew, or should have known, the consequences of her actions.

At the end of the Sunday-morning service on October 4, 1983, elder Ted Moody read a short letter to the congregation: "After much time spent in counseling, exhorting, encouraging, and prayer, we the elders of the Collinsville Church of Christ have no alternative but to lead in the withdrawing of fellowship from our sister in Christ, Marian Guinn."

Guinn accused the elders of libel. But to be libelous, the things being said have to be untrue, and Guinn acknowledged in court depositions that she was having an affair. She was content, therefore, to file a $1.3 million civil lawsuit against the church and its elders for invasion of privacy and emotional distress.

A Tulsa court took jurisdiction over the case, and in March 1984, a twelve-member jury sided with Guinn and awarded her $390,000 for her distress. One juror summed up their reasoning: "I don't see what right the church has to tell people how to live."

This is the kind of case that makes everyone mad.

Christians see within it a takeover of the church's realm by the state. After all, people don't join a church blindly, not knowing what is expected of them. And if the church can't hold its members to a biblical standard, what is it allowed to do? Become a Sunday-morning hymn-singing club? What right does the government have to prevent a church from maintaining standards of holiness, one of its primary purposes?

Meanwhile, many secularists view the elders' actions as the worst type of backwoods inquisition. Guinn's colorful Tulsa lawyer, Tommy Frasier, called the elders a "goon squad" and the "the ayatollahs of Collinsville."

"It doesn't matter if she was fornicating up and down the street," Frasier declared angrily. "It doesn't give [the church] the right to stick their noses in."

One doubts that the citizens of Collinsville would agree that Guinn or anyone else has an inherent right to fornicate up and down highway 20. But Frasier's words reflect what has become a cardinal rule of American life: the right to personal autonomy.

The Guinn ruling pushes the privatization of religion to the extreme, allowing government to restrict religion to an internal matter bearing no relationship to one's behavior. It also says that the church has lost its right to define its own rules for membership.* And as Richard Neuhaus has written, "When an institution that is voluntary in membership cannot define the conditions of belonging, that institution in fact ceases to exist."[5]

But the church's principal task, as we have seen earlier, is a spiritual one—to proclaim the Good News and to cultivate holy living among its members. If a church cannot do this, it no longer has a purpose for existing.

The Guinn case is just one of the latest of assaults in the conflict between Christians and the state that have narrowed the influence of religion in American life. Others have dealt with equally sensitive issues, like religious activity on public property. The Evansville, Indiana, case is one.

---

*The government has consistently held that people not discriminate even in private organizations; but if a policy applies equally to all, it is nondiscriminatory. The Church of Christ rules applied equally to all. Guinn willingly surrendered her right to privacy when she joined the church. And while in some churches she might have been allowed to quietly resign, the particular doctrine of the Church of Christ, to which Guinn subscribed, does not permit resignation.

At the Harper Elementary School in Evansville, teacher's aide Mary May and several Christian co-workers had met before classes every Tuesday morning since early 1981 for prayer, Bible reading, and discussion. Students were not allowed to participate. But in 1983 the principal told May and her seven fellow Christians that there were to be no more Tuesday-morning meetings—or they would all be fired.

Mary May eventually sued the board of education and the superintendent of schools, claiming that the school board had violated her First Amendment rights to free speech, free association, and the free exercise of religion. She also argued that other teachers and aides discussed politics, economics, and sports over their morning coffee before school; why couldn't she and her friends talk about God?

A school-board representative replied that impressionable elementary-school kids might see "her carry a Bible to and from a meeting in their school, even if it is before classes. To children, teachers are very strong authority figures." And, he added, school officials would be forced to make sure that no Bibles or other religious materials were left behind. "We don't want the children exposed to them," he concluded ominously.[6]

Even the right of religious organizations to insist that their employees adhere to their beliefs has been challenged, as in the much-publicized 1986 case of the Dayton Christian School. The Court ruled that it was "unlawful discriminatory practice" for any employer to refuse to hire an employee because of the religion or sex of that person.[7]

By this ruling, notes constitutional lawyer Wil-

liam Ball, St. John's Church, a Lutheran congregation, could not, solely on the basis of the applicant's
religion, refuse to hire a pastor who was of some other
religious faith; nor could St. Mary's Seminary, a Roman Catholic Church seminary, refuse to hire a
woman as an instructor solely on the ground of her
sex—in spite of the Canon Law of the Catholic
Church that would forbid use of female instructors
within the seminary.

A number of zoning cases have affected the right
of worship in private homes. In Colorado Springs,
minister Richard Blanche has been repeatedly cited
for holding religious meetings in his home in violation of a city zoning ordinance. In Fairhaven, Massachusetts, local zoning officials ruled that Bible
studies were home occupations and therefore prohibited under the town's property-use ordinances. In
Los Angeles, officials ruled that home-occupancy
regulations forbade orthodox Jews from holding
prayer meetings in their homes. As civil-liberties
lawyers could not help but note in a Stratford, Connecticut, case, prayer in home Bible studies is pen-
alized while Tupperware parties enjoy the full
protection of the Constitution.

More recent cases seem to reflect a determination
to strip even the thin veneer of religious signs and
symbols from culture.

During the spring of 1986 a last-minute decision
by the Los Angeles Board of Education took God off
the programs of area high-school commencements.
A lawsuit filed by an area atheist successfully barred
prayers, invocations, or religious observances from
graduation ceremonies. Even as local schools made

sure that offending prayers were removed from the programs, one principal noted, however, that students will, God forbid, occasionally mention Him during a speech. "If you happen to get a kid who's religious, they frequently thank God. That's all right. I'm not going to censor the kids' speeches."[8]

We can be grateful for that at least.

The height of hysteria was reached in a conflict involving the city seal of Zion, Illinois, which since 1902 has included a cross, dove, crown, scepter, and the words *God Reigns*. The emblem appears on the city's water tower, badges worn by public officials, and city vehicles.

Robert Sherman, director of the Illinois chapter of the American Atheists, though not a resident of Zion, was so offended by the seal on the water tower that he threatened to sue if it wasn't removed, describing the seal as the "most blatant abuse of religious symbols by a governmental unit in the history of mankind."[9]

But where religious symbols have been spared, it has been on grounds that offer little solace to the religious. The celebrated Pawtucket crèche decision is a case in point.

For forty years, one of the highlights for Pawtucket's predominantly Catholic citizenry was the annual Christmas display that included something for everyone: Santa Claus, reindeer, Christmas trees, and a crèche scene with baby Jesus, Mary and Joseph, and assorted barn animals.

The crèche was challenged, however, because it was paid for ($1,365, with another $20 a year to maintain it) by tax money; this was said to be an infringement on the separation of church and state.

In 1984 the Supreme Court, in a 5–4 decision, upheld the city's right to display the crèche—because, as Chief Justice Warren Burger expressed it, the crèche served a "legitimate secular purpose." After all, he noted, the crèche was merely "a neutral harbinger of the holiday season, useful for commercial purposes, but devoid of any inherent meaning."[10]

Burger's words are significant beyond the Pawtucket case: religion "devoid of any inherent meaning" defines that which is legally and culturally acceptable in contemporary culture.

A torrent of church-state cases, which have with rare exception been decided against the church, was unleashed by the landmark 1963 school-prayer case, *Abington School District v. Schempp.* Contrary to popular opinion, the most radical import of this case was not that public Bible reading or organized prayer could not be held in public schools, but the grounds on which the court made its decision. While acknowledging as historical fact that religion had been a crucial aspect of human experience, it for the first time held as conscious policy that the state must be indifferent toward all religion in any form.

This was a dramatic turnabout from the 1954 *Zorach v. Clauson* case, in which Justice William O. Douglas, a civil libertarian, explicitly upheld what had been the law from the nation's beginning. Douglas refused to "find in the Constitution a requirement that the government show a callous indifference to religious groups. That would be preferring those who believe in no religion over those who do believe."[11]

Two dissenting justices in *Abington* warned that "unilateral devotion to the concept of neutrality can lead to...not simply noninterference and noninvolvement with the religious which the Constitution commands, but a brooding and pervasive devotion to the secular and a passive, or even active, hostility to the religious."[12]

The dissenters were prophets. No phrase could more aptly summarize public life of the last two decades than this "brooding and pervasive devotion to the secular." Seven years after *Abington* the Court redefined religion. What had been in 1931 "obedience to the will of God" was now defined as "a sincere and meaningful belief which occupies in the life of its possessor a place parallel to that filled by God."[13] Thus by 1970 religious belief had become a belief in whatever one might fancy—from the Rockettes to Ramtha.

Then in 1973 came the case that aroused the deepest passions of all, *Roe v. Wade.*

Could *Roe v. Wade*—or the entire Pro-Choice Movement—have been imagined without the dominance of a "passive, or even active, hostility to the religious"? The right to life, guaranteed by the Constitution, had always been understood as a sacred right, a right that preexisted all governments, grounded in the relationship of the Creator with His creation. But as Richard Neuhaus observed, "for the first time...it was explicitly stated that it is possible to address these issues of ultimate importance without any reference to Judeo-Christian tradition.... For the first time in American jurisprudence, the Supreme Court explicitly excluded philosophy, ethics

and religion as factors in its deliberation."[14] And in
Roe v. Wade, the Court replaced the right to life and
its transcendent origins with a new right, the right
to privacy or individual autonomy—regardless of the
expense.

The Supreme Court has thus held that great
moral issues can be decided without reference to
transcendent values. The decision assumes that government's sole purpose is to protect individual,
personal values.

Why such a radical reversal—from a court explicitly approving religion's crucial public role to
one committed to its total privatization—in just nine
years? The dramatic change has been nothing short
of a judicial revolution, but the reasons for the revolution are not so much legal as political and cultural. Judges, after all, don't live in cocoons—they
go to church, listen to television, read magazines,
belong to clubs, and talk to their families over the
breakfast table.

To understand this cultural backdrop, however,
we must go back to 1945, Year Zero. After fifteen
years of depression and war, unemployment and ra-
tioning, Americans were determined to make up for
lost time—and as the years went on, times were good.

The nation's nuclear monopoly seemed to assure
security; for the first time in history nearly everyone
could afford their own home; millions of returning
veterans went to college on the GI bill; business
boomed. Eisenhower's 1956 reelection theme,
"Peace, Progress, and Prosperity," captured the
mood of the nation.

Admittedly, there were undercurrents of discontent. The Korean War had not been lost, but it hadn't been won either. The "beats," led by Jack Kerouac and Allen Ginsberg, had already "dropped out" of society. In *The Lonely Crowd*, sociologist David Riesman described how self-discipline and self-motivation were being replaced by peer pressure as the primary determinant of American character. And though church attendance was up, religion was, in the words of an eminent historian, "so empty and contentless, so conformist, so utilitarian, so sentimental, so individualistic, and so self-righteous."[15]

On the surface, however, these were the best of times. The sixties began with the same confidence. A handsome young president expressed America's bravado and promised the moon. "Let every nation know, whether it wishes us well or ill, that we shall pay any price, bear any burden, meet any hardship, support any friend, oppose any foe to assure the survival and the success of liberty."[16] The future held only opportunity.

Five years later a rapid-fire series of historical events had shaken Americans' faith in their political institutions. Our vigorous young heroes were dead with the assassinations of John Kennedy, Bobby Kennedy, and Martin Luther King, Jr. Streets across the country reeked of pot and tear gas as a new generation bombed buildings, did drugs, and dodged the draft. Once again society was adrift.

The nuclear monopoly was lost when an aggressive Soviet empire acquired the bomb. An unending war in Vietnam took thousands of lives—and network television brought the carnage into American living rooms each evening. A once-popular and powerful president was forced to give up his reelection bid. Just a few years later, a White House scandal shook the confidence of the nation—and caused a disgraced president to resign in ignomy.

At the same time, a destructive philosophic trend had gripped American intellectuals. The long fuse lit by the ideas of Nietzsche, Freud, and Darwin finally set off an explosion of relativism. All moral distinctions were equally valid and equally invalid since all were equally subjective.

A bland civil religion was no match for these powerful trends. Millions felt betrayed by their leaders and resentful that the establishment had any more claim to truth than they did. Sociologist Daniel Bell argues that "the ultimate support for any social system is the acceptance by the population of a moral justification of authority."[17] Now this support was removed and all authority questioned.

These developments were most obvious in the universities, which became both centers of political activism and defenders of relativism. But just as the influence of the university was expanding, it suddenly had very little to teach. The very idea of truth had been called into question as early as 1940, when Reinhold Niebuhr warned that America was a victim of "an education adrift in relativity that doubted all values, and a degraded science that shirked the spiritual issues."[18]

Universities responded by simply changing the goal of education. Where once the object of learning had been the discovery of truth, now each student must be allowed to decide truth for himself. Dogma, not ignorance, became the enemy.

The youth culture of the universities took what they were taught to heart, developing what scholar James Hitchcock calls "a visceral sense that all forms of established authority, all rules, all demands for obedience, were inherently illegitimate."[19]

Influenced by existential writers such as Jean-Paul Sartre and Albert Camus, the generation of the sixties made autonomy its god and sought meaning in the pleasures of easy sex and hard drugs. The consequences were felt not only in private standards of morality, but in the literature and art of the times. Take for example the work of Andy Warhol, who on his death in early 1987 was hailed by *Newsweek* as "the most famous American artist of our time."[20] Warhol was responsible for the rise of "pop art" in the early sixties, gaining international fame for his two hundred Campbell soup cans, an oil painting of row after row of those familiar red and white labels.

Inspired by the mass production techniques of industrial societies, pop art deliberately denied the distinctions between high culture and popular culture. Implicitly and explicitly it asserted relativism's principal tenet that all values are equal: The distinction between bad taste and good taste is elitist; all notions of bad and good are merely one class's way of snubbing another. There are no lasting values, no timeless truths, only artifacts of the moment.

Within such an aesthetic vision there can be no room for the eternal. Shortly before his death, Warhol remarked that he always thought his tombstone should be blank. Then as an afterthought he added, "Well, actually I'd like it to say 'figment.'"[21]

In place of MacArthur's spiritual recrudescence,

the post-war generation created figments: images devoid of meaning in place of objective truth. These figments set the stage for the "me decade" of the seventies and the acquisitive yuppieism of the eighties captured in one popular T-shirt and bumper-sticker slogan, "He who dies with the most toys wins."

Pascal's second option has thus become the route of western experience: Separated from God, men seek satisfaction in their senses. This is more than mindless hedonism; it is a world view in which, according to professor Allen Bloom, "the self has become the modern substitute for the soul."[22]

A 1985 study titled *Habits of the Heart* calls this attitude "utilitarian individualism," arguing that the two primary ways Americans attempt to order their lives are through "the dream of personal success" and "vivid personal feeling."[23] This was reinforced as those interviewed consistently defined their ultimate goals in terms of self-fulfillment or self-realization. Marriage was seen as an opportunity for personal development, work as a method of personal advancement, church as a means of personal fulfillment.

What this study reflects is simply the inevitable consequences of four decades of the steady erosion of absolute values. As a result we live with a massive case of schizophrenia. Outwardly, we are a religious people, but inwardly our religious beliefs make no difference in how we live. We are obsessed with self; we live, raise families, govern, and die as though God does not exist, just as Nietzsche predicted a century ago.

This cultural revolution, rendering God irrelevant, has permeated the Western media, the instrument that not only reflects, but often shapes societal attitudes. God is tolerated in the media only when He is bland enough to pose no threat. One national columnist, annoyed by what she regarded as religious zealots, wrote longingly of ancient Rome, where "the people regarded all the modes of worship as equally true, the intellectuals regarded them as equally false, and the politicians regarded them as equally useful. What a well-blessed time. . . . I think we could try to emulate the laid-back spirit it reveals."[24]

More often, however, the media reflect something less than this laid-back spirit and at times even seems infected with a "brooding and pervasive devotion to the secular—and . . . hostility to the religious," a view confining religion to a "neutral status, devoid of any inherent meaning."

One illustration was the coverage of the so-called Monkey Trial II, the December 1981 challenge to the Arkansas statute requiring that creationism be taught in schools alongside evolution. The following description of the two parties involved appeared on the front page of the December 21, 1981, *Washington Post*.[25] "The ACLU and the New York firm of Skadden Arps attacked the Arkansas law with a powerful case. Their brief is so good that there is talk of publishing it. Their witnesses gave brilliant little summaries of several fields of science, history of sciences, history and religious philosophy." Such was the enlightened plaintiff.

The witnesses defending creationism, however, were "impassioned believers, rebellious educators and scientific oddities. All but one of the creation scientists came from obscure colleges or Bible schools. The one who didn't said he believed diseases dropped from space, that evolution caused Nazism, and that insects may be more intelligent than humans but are hiding their abilities."

With whom were uninformed readers going to align themselves? The firm of Skadden Arps with its brilliant summaries or the backwoods idiots from no-name colleges who probably still make live animal sacrifices up in the hills when nobody is looking?

Though such a negative slant within news coverage appears regularly, the more common tactic is to ignore religion altogether. A few years ago the late theologian and Christian writer Francis Schaeffer approached PBS to air *How Shall We Then Live*, his film series presenting a view of history, creation, and the universe framed in the Judeo-Christian tradition. He was turned down cold; his series was "too religious."

In a slick manifesto called *Cosmos*, Carl Sagan artfully packaged his own creed: "The Cosmos is all there is, or was, or ever will be."[26] The Supreme Court's working definition of religion, "A sincere and meaningful belief which occupies in the life of its possessor a place parallel to that filled by God," would seem to identify Sagan's video treatment of the Cosmos (which he religiously capitalizes) as religious. But PBS and public-school classrooms regularly air *Cosmos*, while they shun Schaeffer's or any similar work.*

---

*In fairness it should be noted that some viewers believe there is a significant quality difference between the two film series. Still, that was not the basis of PBS's rejection of the Schaeffer series.

I've often encountered the same attitude in interviewers who suggest, just before we go on the air, that we steer away from religious topics. "Some people take offense, you know," said one. Another advised me it was against station policy to discuss religion on the air. Others say nothing; once we begin they simply steer the questions to the comparatively safer ground of prisons, criminal justice, or politics. They usually appear aghast when I bring the answers back to my experiences with Jesus Christ.

The print medium does the same thing. Over the years since I became a Christian, I have always deliberately explained that I have "accepted Jesus Christ." These words are invariably translated into "Colson's professed religious experience." I discovered that one major U.S. daily, as a matter of policy, will not print the two words *Jesus Christ* together; when combined, the editor says, it represents an editorial judgment.

Such reporting is not always a matter of hostility; it often reflects the reporter's lack of knowledge in spiritual matters. It can also be the result of the very nature of news itself. By definition, the media report events that are out of the ordinary—the bizarre, the hostile, the aberrant; otherwise news is not news. Thus, coverage of Christianity, when it occurs at all, is most often the outlandish exception rather than the norm practiced by millions of Christians daily.

Consider the sensational coverage in early 1987 of Rev. Carl Thitchener, a New York minister who distributed condoms to his congregation to dramatize

332 ≡≡≡ Charles Colson

the AIDS crisis. Camera crews obligingly descended
on his church; evening news broadcasts featured
Thitchener's parishioners braying the word *condoms*
as he somberly challenged them to repeat it after him.
The ludicrous scene made for an entertaining close-
out to the evening news, featured as a current event
in the church.

What the media failed to distinguish, however,
is that as a Unitarian Universalist, Thitchener is not
a Christian minister. His church rejects the divinity
of Christ. The media also overlooked several small
details about Thitchener's life and character. Consider, for example, his police record: "Subject: male,
Caucasian, 54.... Pled guilty to second degree assault, 1957. Convicted of exposing himself, 1958.
Convicted of drunk driving, 1975. Convicted of 'Parading naked in front of Brownies,' 1982. Convicted
of drunk driving, 1984."[27]

Such selective media focus is not the result of a
conscious antireligious policy but is indicative of a
pervasive cultural attitude, what G. K. Chesterton
described as "a taboo of tact or convention,
whereby we are free to say that a man does this or
that because of his nationality, or his profession, or
his place of residence, or his hobby, but not because
of his creed about the very cosmos in which he
lives."[28]

Harvard psychiatrist Robert Coles gives a
poignant illustration of this taboo. He found he
could write about almost any human motivation
without having its authenticity questioned. But
when he once wrote about a Civil-Rights worker
who risked his life "out of love for Jesus," people

around him considered the worker, and maybe Coles himself, to be phony.[29]*

The same disposition to dismiss religious influence pervades the field of education.

Paul Vitz, professor of psychology at New York University, examined sixty social-studies textbooks used by 87 percent of the nation's elementary-school children in a study done under the auspices of the U.S. Department of Education.[30] He looked for "primary" references to religious activity such as prayer, church attendance, or participation in religious ceremonies, as well as "secondary" references, such as citing the date when a church was built. What Vitz discovered was a "total absence of any primary religious text about typical contemporary American religious life"[31] and only a few secondary pictures and passages touching upon the religious. The few direct references to historic religion centered on Amish, Catholic, Jewish, and Mormon faiths, leaving a "very curious" deletion of characteristic Protestant religious life.[32]

Religion appeared to be relevant only in remote points in history. Pictures of pilgrims and the first Thanksgiving were bountiful—without any mention of to whom thanks was being given. One mother told Vitz that her son's social-studies book made no mention of religion as part of the pilgrims' life. Her son told her that "Thanksgiving was when the pilgrims gave thanks to the Indians." When the mother called the principal of her son's suburban New York City

---

*In short, orthodox faith is treated the way homosexuality once was: it is tolerated as long as it is practiced only by consenting adults and isn't flaunted in public.

school to point out that Thanksgiving originated when the pilgrims thanked God, the principal responded, "That's your opinion." He continued by saying that the schools could only teach what was in the books.[33]

Vitz concluded that the study suggests "a psychological motive behind the obvious censorship of religion present in these books. Those responsible for these books appear to have a deep-seated fear of any form of active contemporary Christianity, especially serious, committed Protestantism. This fear could have led the authors to deny and repress the importance of this kind of religion in American life."[34]*

This elimination of the transcendent from serious public discussion is merely a reflection of an underlying cultural revolution that has eliminated absolute values from public consciousness, thus ushering in an age of relativism. This has inevitably affected public policy, as in the court decisions discussed earlier, and it has turned our traditional

---

*In the midst of the controversy aroused by the Vitz study, Doubleday, a major publisher, announced its decision to write God back into school textbooks. "We made a decision long before Judge Hand's decision in Alabama that you can't leave religion out of textbooks," said Herb Adams, president of Doubleday's Laidlaw Educational Publishing division, which ranks among the nation's top ten textbook publishers. "The allegation that religion has been softpedaled in textbooks is true," he added. So by the end of the year Doubleday will have prepared a supplementary book that discusses the role of religion in the development of the country. It is being designed to go along with existing history and social-studies books. Many other textbooks will be fully rewritten and revised, said Adams, but it will be a "long, long process." Adams added that the reason religion had been omitted from textbooks in the past was that publishers wanted to "avoid controversy." Evangelical Press News Service (February 6, 1987).

notion of pluralism on its head.

Historically pluralism meant that conflicting and firmly held values could be voiced in public debate, and from such debates might emerge a consensus of values by which a community would be governed. But relativism, which insists that there are no objective truths, drives all values out of public debate, since in a pluralistic society they are "divisive." In an attempt to be neutral, we ignore all values. Columnist Joseph Sobran writes, "The prevailing notion is that the state should be neutral as to religion, and furthermore, that the best way to be neutral about it is to avoid all mention of it. By this sort of logic, nudism is the best compromise among different styles of dress. The secularist version of 'pluralism' amounts to theological nudism."[35]

This modern vision of pluralism has infiltrated nearly every branch and level of government, progressively institutionalizing the privatization of religious values. The absurd extreme to which this has taken us is illustrated by the New York law outlawing the use of children in pornography.[36] In its preamble the statute specifically states that it is not based on any moral or religious considerations. Only by making such a disclaimer did the bill's drafters believe it could withstand a court challenge that it was "religiously" motivated and thus unconstitutional.

Congressman Henry Hyde offers a personal perspective of what it means to run afoul of the secular need for control. In 1976 Congress passed the Hyde Amendment, which barred federal funding for abortion in the Medicaid program. Planned Parenthood, the American Civil Liberties Union, and other groups challenged the amendment's constitutionality, claiming that it "used the fist of government to smash the wall of separation between church and state by imposing a peculiarly religious view of when a human life begins." To prove their theory, the lawyers for these organizations asked to review Hyde's mail for expressions of religious sentiment. They also hired a private investigator who followed Hyde to a Mass for the unborn and took notes as the congressman read Scripture, took communion, and prayed. The investigator even recorded in his notebook the inscription on the cathedral's statue of St. Thomas: "I die the king's good servant, but God's first."

In an affidavit, the plaintiffs presented these observations to the court as proof of a religious conspiracy. They claimed that Hyde, as a devout Catholic, could not separate his religion from his politics and that the amendment was therefore unconstitutional. The judge threw out the affidavit, and Planned Parenthood and the ACLU finally lost their case in 1980 when the Supreme Court affirmed the amendment's constitutionality.

Though victorious, Hyde was infuriated by his opponents' tactics. "The anger I felt when they tried to disenfranchise me because of my religion stayed with me. These are dangerous people who make dangerous arguments. Some powerful members of the cultural elite in our country are so paralyzed by the fear that theistic notions might reassert themselves into the official activities of government that they will go to Gestapo lengths to inhibit such expression."[37]

This stripping away of religious import is not limited to the U.S. Europe has become a post-Christian culture in which the principal religious influence is visible in art treasures and cathedrals filled with tourists rather than worshipers. Church attendance is 4 percent in West Germany, East Germany, Scandinavia, and Austria. In France regular attendance at Mass is below 15 percent, while in Spain it has dropped to between 3 and 5 percent. And in England, site of the great nineteenth-century awakening and home of missionary movements, more people worship in mosques than in the Church of England. Regular church attendance is no more than 6 percent of the population.[38]

In fact, resistance to Christian influence has become overt. Donald Bloesch cites an official on ecclesiastic affairs in Sweden who boasted, "We are dismantling the church bit by bit and where necessary we are using economic means to do so." Denmark is presently refusing to renew the visas of evangelical missionaries, particularly from America. There are reports on the desecration of churches and Christian cemeteries in Sweden and West Germany.[39]

Perhaps one of the most fitting images of this spiritual apathy was captured years ago in Italian filmmaker Federico Fellini's award-winning film *La Dolce Vita*. The movie opens with a panorama of Rome's magnificent skyline, the grand dome of St. Peter's in the center. A helicopter carrying a large object appears in the distance. The camera zooms in;

the object is a statue of Christ being hauled away from a downtown square. The camera then focuses on a group of young sunbathers who, distracted from their pleasure by the whirring blades, laugh mockingly. Why shouldn't Jesus take the bus like everyone else? The helicopter flies on to discard its outdated cargo on a trashpile, and the youngsters return to their sun worship.

Fellini filmed his blasphemous scene in 1959, but it has proved prophetic.

Many believe that religious values and liberties have fallen victim to some sinister conspiracy in which the ACLU, humanist educators, and the media meet in darkened corridors of CBS headquarters to plot the demise of religion in America.

Admittedly, the ACLU has a powerful lobby, the media are unsympathetic, and skeptics dominate college campuses. But even if such forces were organized to consciously eradicate religious values they could do little to wipe out real Christianity.

Christian values are in retreat in the West today, primarily, I believe, because of the church itself. If Christianity has failed to stem the rising tides of relativism it is because the church in many instances has lost the convicting force of the gospel message. Earlier we argued that while humanists did not understand humans, Christians did not understand Christianity. This is surely evident in post–World War II Christianity, which has become a religion of private comfort and blessing that fills up whatever small holes in life that pleasure, money and success have left open, what Bonhoeffer called a "god of the gaps."[40]

Television's emergence as the dominant medium of communication gave birth to the slickly marketed health-wealth-and-success gospel rampant in today's church. As Donald Bloesch notes, "I believe that technology can be harnessed in the service of the gospel, but I recognize that such a venture entails the risk of accommodating the Christian message to technological values. Utility, i.e., practical efficacy and tangible results, rather than fidelity to truth then becomes the criterion for evaluating the program of the church."[41] When asked about his affluent lifestyle in the face of a needy world, one prominent evangelist explained, "I live in one of the finest homes. I drive one of the finest, safest cars, and if a newer, safer one were to pull up in front of my door, I'd go out and say, 'I want it,'... God designed life for believers to be an abundant life, ...God designed for you to live in the overflow."[42]

In addition to succumbing to this arrogant heresy, the church has allowed itself to become dangerously polarized into two camps: politicized and privatized views of faith. The problem is, neither view has anything to do with historic Christianity.

The politicization of the church in the sixties was largely the work of liberal mainline denominations whose bureaucracies issued weekly policy papers on social issues. They became so absorbed in social causes that they neglected the church's first mission and in the process suffered declining membership.* Just as their influence was waning, the political polarity was reversed, and the Christian New Right emerged as a potent force in American politics. They made the same mistake—equating the gospel with a particular partisan agenda. Many in the New Right appear ready to make politics the ultimate goal, putting politics ahead of spirituality.

Politicized religion simply reinforces the tendency toward civil religion, which was perhaps best articulated by Dwight Eisenhower who once said that American government makes no sense "unless it is founded in a deeply felt religious faith—and I don't care what it is."[43] What Eisenhower was referring to was nothing more than a generic religion—any brand will do, no-name is the best—to encourage civic duty.

On the other side is privatized faith, which divorces religious and spiritual beliefs from public actions. Like its politicized counterpart, privatized faith has a mixed heritage theologically and politically. In the nineteenth century, conservative evan-

---

*As James Wall observed in the liberal *Christian Century*:

Mainline religion . . . has failed to convince the public that there is a link between its politics and its theology because, perhaps unwittingly, it has allowed religion to be confined to what David Tracy has perceptively termed the "reservation of the spirit."

. . . the political left has had a morbid fear of religion encroaching on the secular realm. This fear leads, at its extreme, to legal action if a crèche shows up on city property. Such expressions of cultural religion hardly pose a threat to the separation of church and state, but the doctrine of the left is that "religion" must not lead the public debate. Instead, it must be on call to serve only when commanded by secular leaders.

Ironically, this view of religion imposes as rigid an attitude toward societal solutions as that found on the political right. Mainline religion has for too long taken this "closed" attitude for fear of appearing to impose religious solutions in a pluralistic culture.

gelicals led the abolition campaign and progressive
social reforms; in the early twentieth century, they
abandoned this commitment in reaction against
modernism and the so-called social gospel. Fundamentalists separated from the mainstream, leaving
the world's concerns behind so they could preach
the good news among the faithful.

All of this dramatically changed by the late seventies when Jerry Falwell led a fundamentalist
stampede back to center stage. Ironically, liberals
who had been so socially concerned were now, in
reaction perhaps, arguing that faith is a private matter. Perhaps it depends on which issues are identified
at any given moment as religious and moral.

This would seem the case in the 1984 presidential campaign. Democratic challenger Walter Mondale attacked President Reagan's public statements
that "without God, democracy will not and cannot
long endure" as "moral McCarthyism."[44]

Mondale's running mate, Geraldine Ferraro,
added, "Personal religious convictions have no place
in political campaigns or in dictating public policy."[45] In an interview with the *New York Times*, Ms.
Ferraro asserted that her faith was "very, very private."[46]

Governor Mario Cuomo of New York made the
most eloquent defense of this privately engaging but
publicly irrelevant faith during his much-publicized
speech at the University of Notre Dame in 1984. As
a practicing Catholic, he said, he subscribed to his
church's teachings on the question of abortion. But
as an officeholder in a secular society he could not
impose his views on anyone else. So far, so good.

Cuomo then went on to say that he was under no obligation to advocate the views of his church or to seek a public consensus based on those views (which he confesses to be the truth of God) until there is what he calls a "prudential judgment" that could justify such a course.[47] In other words, one is under no obligation to provide leadership on moral issues. Thus, Cuomo carried privatized faith to its ultimate conclusion when he asserted that he could, while agreeing with his church, nonetheless tolerate or even support pro-choice legislation. This clever but dangerous argument gives sophistry a bad name.

Those who fear the encroachment of religion in public life can relax. Neither politicized civil religion nor privatized religion is likely to impose itself on our governmental or social institutions, for in either case there is nothing to impose. The one holds the gospel hostage to a particular political agenda while the other is so private it refuses to have any impact on daily life in the public arena. Thus is the divided church impotent to reverse the tides of secularism.

In 1896 the Victorian-minded planners of St. John the Divine in New York City envisioned a great Episcopal cathedral that would bring glory to God. Nearly a century later, though the immense structure is still under construction, it is in use—in a way that its planners might well have regarded with dismay.[48]

St. John's Thanksgiving service has featured Japanese Shinto priests; Muslim Sufis perform biannually; Lenten services have focused on the ecological "passion of the earth" (one gathers that Christ's passion is passé). The cathedral has featured

"Christa," a huge crucifix with a female Christ, and St. John's pulpit welcomes everyone from the Rev. Jesse Jackson to Norman Mailer, rabbis, imams, Buddhist monks, secular politicians, atheist scientists, and during the feast of St. Francis in October 1985, an arkload of animals received blessings from the high altar, including a llama, an elephant, and a goose.

Logistical questions such as curbing your elephant within the cathedral notwithstanding, St. John the Divine seems to have ceased to be a house of the one God of the Scriptures, and has become instead a house of many gods. Novelist Kurt Vonnegut Jr. wrote for the cathedral's centennial brochure that "the Cathedral is to this atheist . . . a suitable monument to persons of all ages and classes. I go there often to be refreshed by a sense of nonsectarian community which has the best interests of the whole planet at heart."

Underneath the main altar are seven stone chambers housing the cathedral's artists-in-residence: two painters, three photographers, a sculptor, a calligrapher, a poet, a blacksmith, and a high-wire performer. I suppose every church should have its own trapeze artist.

Dean James Morton has encountered opposition. Some Episcopalians are concerned about the menorah, Islamic prayer rug, and Shinto vases that adorn the sanctuary altar along with the crucifix. But the dean responds, "This cathedral is a place for birth Episcopalians like me who feel constricted by the notion of excluding others. What happens here—the Sufi dances, the Buddhist prayers—are serious spiritual experiences. We make God a Minnie Mouse in stature when we say these experiences profane a Christian church.''

As *Newsweek* observed admiringly, ''The eclectic dean of St. John's seems to be reaching for a theology as high and wide as the cathedral he serves.''

Maybe so. Or perhaps his grand cathedral, like the United Nations meditation room, is a monument to no god at all—and thus, a fitting icon of twentieth-century Western culture.

FIFTEEN

The Naked Public Square

> The greatest question of our time is not
> communism versus individualism, not
> Europe versus America, not even the East
> versus the West; it is whether men can
> live without God.
>
> —Will Durant

A recent *Time* magazine cover story titled "Ethics" raised many disturbing issues: "What's wrong? Hypocrisy, betrayal and greed unsettle the nation's soul.... At a time of moral disarray, America seeks to rebuild a structure of values."[1]

Yet even in the midst of this long-overdue national soul-searching, the authors still hedged the issue. "Who is to decide what are the 'right' values?" wrote a professor of education. "Does ultimate moral authority lie with institutions such as church and state to codify and impose? Or, in a free society, are these matters of private conscience, with final choice belonging to the individual?"[2]

What such experts do not see is that by raising such questions, they are pointing to the answer. We live in a society in which all transcendent values have been removed and thus there is no moral standard by which anyone can say right is right and wrong is wrong. What we live in is, in the memorable image of Richard Neuhaus, a naked public square.

On the surface, a value-free society sounds liberal, progressive, and enlightened. It certainly sounded that way to the generations of the sixties and early seventies—probably many of the same people now wringing their hands on the pages of *Time*. But when the public square is naked, truth and values drift with the winds of public favor and there is nothing objective to govern how we are to live together. Why should we be shocked, then, by the inevitable consequences; why should we be surprised to discover that society yields what is planted?

Why are we surprised that crime soars steadily among juveniles when parents fail to set standards of right behavior in the home, when school teachers will not offer a moral opinion in the classroom, either out of fear of litigation or because they cannot "come from a position of what is right and wrong," as one New Jersey teacher put it?[3]

Why are we horrified at the growing consequences of sexual promiscuity—including a life-threatening epidemic—when sex is treated as casually as going out for a Frosty at Wendy's?

Why are we shocked at disclosures of religious leaders bilking their ministries of millions when they've been preaching a get-rich-quick gospel all along?

Why the wonderment over the fact that, for enough dollars or sexual favors, government employees and military personnel sell out their nation's secrets? As C. S. Lewis wrote forty years ago, "We laugh at honor and are shocked to find traitors in our midst."[4]

Why is it so surprising that Wall Street yuppies make fast millions on insider information or tax fraud? Without objective values, the community or one's neighbor has no superior claim over one's own desires.

Whether we like to hear it or not, we are reaping the consequences of the decades since World War II when we have, in Solzhenitsyn's words, "forgotten God." What we have left is the reign of relativism.

As discussed in an earlier chapter, humanity cannot survive without some form of law. "The truly naked public square is at best a transitional phenomenon," wrote Richard John Neuhaus. "It is a vacuum begging to be filled."[5] Excise belief in God and you are left with only two principals: the individual and the state. In this situation, however, there is no mediating structure to generate moral values and, therefore, no counterbalance to the inevitable ambitions of the state. "The naked public square cannot remain naked, the direction is toward the state-as-church, toward totalitarianism."[6]

As we have seen, this has already occurred in Marxist nations where the death of God has created a new form of messiah—the all-powerful state whose political ideology acquires the force of religion. The same is true, though not as extreme, in the West where traditional religious influences have been excluded from public debates either by law or Chesterton's "taboo of tact or convention." As a result, government is free to make its own ultimate judgments. Hence government ideology acquires the force of religion.

The removal of the transcendent sucks meaning from the law. Without an absolute standard of moral judgment backing government "morality," where is the protection for the minorities and the powerless? "When in our public life no legal prohibition can be articulated with a force of transcendent authority, then there are no rules rooted in ultimacies that can protect the poor, the powerless and the marginal, as indeed there are now no rules protecting the unborn, and only fragile inhibitions surrounding the aged and defective."[7]

With no ultimate reference point supporting it—no just cause for obedience—law can only be enforced by the bayonet. So the state seeks more and more coercive power.

But the most dangerous consequence of the naked public square is the loss of community.

A community is a gathering of people around shared values, a commitment to one another and to common ideals and aspirations that cannot be created by government. As Arthur Schlesinger observed, "We have forgotten that constitutions work only as they reflect an actual sense of community."[8]

Without commitment to community, individual responsibility quickly erodes. One vivid illustration of this was a Princeton student's protest after President Jimmy Carter proposed reinstating the draft registration in 1977. Newspapers across the country showed the young man defiantly carrying a placard proclaiming: "Nothing is worth dying for."

To many, these words seemed an affirmation of

life, the ultimate assertion of individual worth. What they fail to reckon with, however, is the reverse of that slogan: if nothing is worth dying for, is anything worth living for? A society that has no reference points beyond itself "increasingly becomes a merely contractual arrangement," says sociologist Peter Berger. The problem with that, he continues, is that human beings will not die for a social contract. And "unless people are prepared, if necessary, to die for it," a society cannot long survive.[9]

In these last twenty years of the twentieth century, we are sailing uncharted waters. Never before in the history of Western civilization has the public square been so devoid of transcendent values.

The notion of law rooted in transcendent truth, in God Himself, is not the invention of Christian fundamentalists calling naively for America to return to its Christian roots. The roots of American law are as much in the works of Cicero and Plato as in the Bible. But if fundamentalists are guilty of distorting American history, their critics are guilty of distorting the whole history of Western civilization.

Plato, in terms as religious as Moses or David, claimed that transcendent norms were the true foundations for civil law and order. He taught that "there exist divine moral laws, not easy to apprehend, but operating upon all mankind." He refuted the argument of some Sophists that there was no distinction between virtue and vice, and he affirmed that "God, not man, is the measure of all things."[10]

Cicero, to whom the American Founding Fathers looked for guidance, maintained that religion is indispensable to private morals and public order and that it alone provided the concord by which people could live together.[11] "True law," wrote Cicero, "is right reason in agreement with Nature; it is of universal application and everlasting; it summons to duty by its commands, and averts from wrong-doing by its prohibitions."

Augustine wrote *The City of God* to defend the role of Christianity as the essential element in preserving society, stating that what the pagans "did not have the strength to do out of love of country, the Christian God demands of [citizens] out of love of Himself. Thus, in a general breakdown of morality and of civic virtues, divine Authority intervened to impose frugal living, continence, friendship, justice and concord among citizens."[12] Augustine contended that without true justice emanating from a sovereign God there could never be the concord of which Cicero wrote.

During the French Revolution, Edmund Burke acknowledged that the attempt to build a secularized state was not so much irreverent as irrational. "We know, and it is our pride to know, that man is by his constitution a religious animal; that atheism is against, not only our reason, but our instincts; and that it cannot prevail long."[13]

Religion has always been a decisive factor in the shaping of the American experience. According to one modern scholar, it was the Founding Fathers' conviction that "republican government depends for its health on values that over the not-so-long run must come from religion."[14]

John Adams believed that the moral order of the

new nation depended on biblical religion. "If I were an atheist . . . I should believe that chance had ordered the Jews to preserve and propagate to all mankind the doctrine of a supreme, intelligent, wise, almighty sovereign of the universe, which I believe to be the great essential principle of all morality, and consequently of all civilization."[15]

Tocqueville, the shrewd observer of American democracy, maintained that "religion in America takes no direct part in the government of society, but it must be regarded as the first of their political institutions. . . . How is it possible that society should escape destruction if the moral tie is not strengthened in proportion as the political tie is relaxed? And what can be done with a people who are their own masters if they are not submissive to the Deity?"[16]

In considering such lessons from the past, historians Will and Ariel Durant cited the agnostic Joseph Renan, who in 1866 wrote, "What would we do without [Christianity]? . . . If rationalism wishes to govern the world without regard to the religious needs of the soul, the experience of the French Revolution is there to teach us the consequences of such a blunder." The Durants concluded, "There is no significant example in history before our time, of a society successfully maintaining moral life without the aid of religion."[17]

The supreme irony of our century is that in those nations that still enjoy the greatest human freedoms, this traditional role of religion is denigrated; while in nations that have fallen under the oppressor's yoke, the longing for the spiritual is keenest. In the West intellectuals widely disdain religion; in the

Soviet Union they cry out for its return.

In a wave of recent articles, three popular contemporary Soviet writers, Vasily Bykov, Viktor Astafyev, and Chinghiz Aytmatov, have blamed
Russia's moral degradation upon the decline of religion. "Who extinguished the light of goodness in
our soul? Who blew out the lamp of our conscience,
toppled it into a dark, deep pit in which we are grop-
ing, trying to find the bottom, a support and some
kind of guiding light to the future?" asks Astafyev,
a Christian, in *Our Contemporary*, a popular Moscow
journal.[18] Though a Muslim, Aytmatov centers his
writings on Christ, whom he admires as a greater
influence than Mohammed. He and his fellow writers
have boldly attacked Communism for creating "an
all-encompassing belief" that has plunged the Russian people into a moral abyss. Bykov, winner of
every Soviet literary award, declares there can be no
morality without faith.[19]

Yet our twentieth century has set itself apart as
the first to explicitly reject the wisdom of the ages
that religion is indispensable to the concord and justice of society.

Mankind now has three choices: to remain divorced from the transcendent; to construct a rational
order to preserve society without recourse to real or
imagined gods; or to establish the viable influence of
the Kingdom of God in the kingdoms of man.

The first option invites chaos and tyranny, as the
bloodshed, repression, and nihilism of this century
testify. We are then left with the second and third
choices. These opposing arguments were well presented by two of the great thinkers of the twentieth

century: the eminent journalist, Walter Lippmann, and Nobel laureate, Aleksandr Solzhenitsyn.

Before writing *A Preface to Morals*, Lippmann concluded that modern man could no longer embrace a simple religious faith. For Lippmann, the goal was to create a humanistic view in which "mankind, deprived of the great fictions, is to come to terms with the needs which created those fictions." For himself, Lippmann came to a rather fatalistic conclusion: "I take the humanistic view because, in the kind of world I happen to live in, I can do no other."[20] Lippmann thus set about to extract the ethical ideals of religious figures from their theological and historical context. Man in his own rational interest, he believed, could sustain a man-made religion. Some religion, even if it was a religion that denied religion, had to be followed.

On the other side of the spectrum from this religion of humanism stands Aleksandr Solzhenitsyn, a lonely and often outspoken prophet. In his 1978 Harvard commencement address, Solzhenitsyn listed a litany of woes facing the West: the loss of courage and will, the addiction to comfort, the abuse of freedom, the capitulation of intellectuals to fashionable ideas, the attitude of appeasement with evil.

The cause for all this was the humanistic view Lippmann had embraced. "The humanistic way of thinking," thundered Solzhenitsyn, "which had proclaimed itself as our guide, did not admit the existence of evil in man, nor did it see any task higher than the attainment of happiness on earth. It started modern western civilization on the dangerous trend of worshiping man and his material needs ... gaps were left open for evil, and its drafts blow freely today."

In American democracy, said Solzhenitsyn, rights "were granted on the ground that man is God's creature. That is, freedom was given to the individual conditionally, in the assumption of his constant religious responsibility."

Solzhenitsyn lamented that two hundred years ago, as the Constitution was being written, or even fifty years ago, when Walter Lippmann was trying to preserve the husk of Western virtue, "it would have seemed quite impossible... that an individual be granted boundless freedom with no purpose, simply for the satisfaction of his whims.... The West has finally achieved the rights of man, and even to excess, but man's sense of responsibility to God and society has grown dimmer and dimmer."[21] Like MacArthur, Solzhenitsyn was saying that nothing less than spiritual renewal could save Western civilization.

If we reject the nihilism that denies all meaning and hope, we must believe human society has purpose. We are forced to choose, therefore, belief in man, faith in faith, hope in hope, and the love of love; or we must look for a point beyond ourselves to steady our balance.

The view that man in his own rational interest can sustain a man-made religion is voiced regularly on op-ed pages, on television specials, even from church pulpits. It remains fashionable because it offers a positive view of human nature, filled with hopeful optimism about man's capacities. But it ignores the ringing testimony of a century filled with terror and depravity.

If the real benefits of the Judeo-Christian ethic and influence in secular society were understood, it would be anxiously sought out, even by those who *repudiate* the Christian faith. The influence of the Kingdom of God in the public arena is good for society as a whole.

PRESENCE
OF THE
KINGDOM

SIXTEEN

Benefits of the Kingdom

Although church and state stand separate,
the political order cannot be renewed
without theological virtues working upon
it. . . . It is from the church that we receive
our fundamental postulates of order,
justice and freedom, applying them to our
civil society.

—Russell Kirk

If Solzhenitsyn, MacArthur, and many of the great political philosophers since Cicero are right that society cannot survive without a vital religious influence, then where does this leave us? Will any religion or belief do?

No. As expressed earlier, I believe as a matter of faith *and* intellect that the Judeo-Christian religion must be that transcendent base. But—and I cannot emphasize this too strongly—even if I did not, I would still argue that Christianity is the only religious system that provides for *both* individual concerns and the ordering of a society with liberty and justice for all. A creed alone is not enough, nor is some external law code.

If Christianity were merely another creed, it

would have no superior claim over Hinduism and Buddhism, for example. Or if it were merely another prescriptive order for society, it would have no advantage over Islam. Instead, Christianity alone, as taught in Scripture and announced in the Kingdom context by Jesus Christ, provides both a transcendent moral influence and a transcendent ordering of society without the repressive theocratic system of Islam.

I have already stated that humanists fail to understand human nature just as Christians fail to understand Christianity. This is particularly true when it comes to the presence of the Kingdom of God in this world. Christians tend to see their faith as either a belief system or a religious palliative for all life's ills. Secularists see it, most often, through the pejorative pen or the selective lens of the media, which portray the Christian activist as a religious Archie Bunker—a Bible-thumping bigot condemning everyone, expounding simplistically on everything from evolution to gun control, and pushing heatedly to take over the government to cram his narrow-minded agenda down society's unwilling throat. Sadly, many in the church have perpetuated this stereotype with thoughtless rhetoric and posturing.

Yet none of this bears any resemblance to true Christianity. The Kingdom of God provides unique moral imperatives that can cause men and women to rise above their natural egoism to serve the greater good. God intends His people to do this; furthermore, He commands them to influence the world through their obedience to Him, not by taking over the world through the corridors of power.

No one can be coerced into true faith, and the last people who even ought to try to do so are Christians, either individually or as members of the institutional church. As the Westminster Confession states, "God alone is Lord of conscience."[1] This conviction lies at the heart of the agreement reached by America's Founding Fathers. For them, secularists and believers alike, freedom of conscience was the first liberty guaranteed by the Constitution. This means religious liberty for all—Jew, Muslim, Christian, Hindu, Buddhist, atheist, or California bird worshiper.

The Christian, knowing that the will of the majority cannot determine truth, seeks no preferential favor for his religion from government. His confidence, instead, is that truth is found in Christ alone—and this is so no matter how many people believe it, no matter whether those in power believe it. While this may sound exclusivistic, it is this very assurance that makes (or should make, when properly understood) the Christian the most vigorous defender of human liberty. And those who resent the exclusive claims of Christianity are practicing the same intolerance they profess to resent. The essence of pluralism is, after all, that each person respects the other's right to believe in an exclusive claim to truth.

If society's well-being depends on the presence of a healthy religious influence, then, it is crucial that Christians understand their responsibilities in the kingdoms of man as mandated by the Kingdom of God. It is equally imperative that the rest of society realize the benefits those responsibilities, when properly carried out, offer them.

We are a benefit-driven society. How will this move benefit us? we ask. What benefits come with this plan? What benefits does this company offer if I take the job? It should come as welcome news to the pragmatists of the world that the Kingdom of God offers benefits no society can afford to be without.

* * *

When I was serving time for my part in the Watergate conspiracy, Al Quie, a senior congressman, offered to serve the remainder of my prison sentence if authorities would release me so I could be with my then-troubled family. Al, who later became governor of Minnesota, was a respected political leader; I was a member of the disgraced Nixon staff and a convicted felon. Al and I had not even been friends until a few months earlier when we met in a prayer group. Why would a man like Al Quie make such an offer?

The answer? Al took seriously Jesus' words: "As I have loved you, so you must love one another."[2] This commandment is a central law of the Kingdom, and Al Quie was my first encounter with it.

This law of the Kingdom is what motivates Christians to serve the good of society. Certainly it motivated Christians of the nineteenth century when they spearheaded most of our nation's significant works of mercy and moral betterment. They founded hospitals, colleges, and schools; they organized welfare assistance and fed the hungry; they campaigned to end abuses ranging from dueling to slavery. Though much of this work has now been taken over by government agencies, Christians provided the original impetus. Today, Christians still contribute the bulk of resources for private charities of compassion.

This is not to say that all good deeds are done by Christians or that all Christians do good deeds. Sacrificial deeds are often done for other than religious motives, of course. But in those instances the actions depend on an individual's personal reasons. Motive is crucial. In one instance it is an individual choice—a choice that often wavers or falters. For the Christian it is a matter of obedience to God's commandments; it is not choice, but necessity.

It is, in fact, their dual citizenship that should, as Augustine believed, make Christians the best of citizens. Not because they are more patriotic or civic-minded, but because they do out of obedience to God that which others do only if they choose or if they are forced. And their very presence in society means the presence of a community of people who live by the Law behind the law.

Even as unreligious a figure as modern educator John Dewey recognized that "the church-going classes, those who have come under the influence of evangelical Christianity . . . form the backbone of philanthropic and social interest, of social reform through political action, of passivism, of popular education. They embody and express the spirit of kindly good will towards [those] in economic disadvantage."[3]

A recent Gallup poll confirms Dewey's observations. Forty-six percent of those in the United States who describe themselves as "highly spiritually committed" work among the poor, the infirm, or the elderly—twice as many as those describing themselves as "highly uncommitted" spiritually.[4]

To accomplish works of mercy and justice, however, Christians do not rely on government, but on their own penetration of society as "salt and light." This too is in obedience to a command of God that orders them to be the "salt of the earth" and "the light of the world"[5]—the great cultural commission of the Kingdom.* In Hebrew times salt was rubbed into meat to prevent it from spoiling. In the same way the citizen of the Kingdom is "rubbed in" to society as its preservative.

Citizens of the Kingdom, therefore, form what Edmund Burke called "the little platoons," mediating structures between the individual and government that carry out works of justice, mercy, and charity.[6]

The presence of Christians in society also helps break the endless cycle of evil and violence in the world. For example, the generations-old conflicts in Northern Ireland and the Middle East thrive on hatred and bigotry, the basest of human instincts, which in turn beget violence, which begets more violence. Only forgiveness and love can break this cycle, and only the Kingdom of God orders its citizens to take such radical steps. God commands His

---

*The Great Commission is Jesus' command to *preach the gospel.* "Therefore go and make disciples of all nations, baptizing them in the name of the Father and of the Son and of the Holy Spirit" (Matt. 28:19). The cultural commission, as I've called it, is to *do the gospel.* That is, to be salt and light, letting "your light shine before men, that they may see your good deeds and praise your Father in heaven" (Matt. 5:16).

people to forgive those who hurt or wrong them and to love their enemies.

Though "turning the other cheek" may sound like weakness or impractical idealism, in reality it takes raw courage and is the most powerful weapon for restoring civil tranquility—far surpassing any bayonet or legislation. No conquering army can destroy evil; at best it can suppress it. But as we will see dramatically illustrated in a later chapter, whenever men and women are reconciled by the Law of the Kingdom, evil is defeated.

In this and many other ways, the moral standards demanded of the citizen of the Kingdom of God inevitably affect the moral standards of the kingdoms of man. This is not well understood today because of the widespread view that private moral values have no bearing on public conduct. Scripture and history indicate otherwise, as do our own life experiences.[7]

Whether a politician cheats on his wife, for example, should have no bearing on his fitness for office, many say. But a broken vow is a broken vow and reveals a weakness of character. If a man or woman cannot be trusted with private moral decisions, how can he or she be trusted with moral decisions affecting the whole of society?

Moral values do affect character, and the influence of individual character has an impact on society. Not just with public officials, but in the lives of ordinary citizens. Nowhere is this more evident than in the area of criminal behavior.

Though for years conventional wisdom held that racial discrimination, economic deprivation, and environment were the chief causes of crime, leading criminologists and psychiatrists are now concluding that personal character is the single greatest determining factor in criminal behavior.

James Q. Wilson, Harvard law professor, after surveying American history and comparing religious activity with crime data during specified periods, discovered a startling correlation.

In the middle of the nineteenth century when rapid urbanization would normally lead one to expect increased crime, the level of crime actually fell. Interestingly, it was during that same period that a great spritual awakening occurred. Thus, Wilson explains, morality took hold just as industrialization began. From the mid-1800s to 1920, despite environmental, economic, and social pressures that should have made it rise, the crime rate decreased.

Conversely, during the "good" economic years of the twenties, crime began to rise. Because, says Wilson, "the educated classes began to repudiate moral uplift, and Freud's psychological theories came into vogue." People no longer believed in restraining a child's sinful impulses; they wanted to develop his "naturally good" personality.[8]

Even more surprising, crime did not rise, as sociologists expected, during the Great Depression when, it is estimated, that 34 million men, women, and children were without any income at all—28 percent of the population.[9] Tough times seem to develop strength of character and a tendency for the populace to pull together, whereas good times leave people free to seek self-interest and satisfaction, legally or otherwise. If this correlation is valid, the soaring crime rates in today's affluent, egocentric

Western culture are altogether understandable.

Correlation between religious values and public order was dramatically evident during a religious revival early in this century. The revival began in small Methodist churches in Wales and quickly spilled out into society. During New Year's week in 1905, for the first time ever there was not a single arrest for drunkenness in Swansea County, the police announced. In Cardiff the authorities reported a 40 percent decrease in the jail population while the tavern trade fell off dramatically. Prayer meetings sprang up in coal mines; stores reported stocks of Bibles sold out; dockets were cleared in criminal courts; and many police were unemployed. Stolen goods were returned to shocked store owners. One historian reported, "Cursing and profanity were so diminished that . . . a strike was provoked in the coal mines . . . so many men had given up using foul language that the pit ponies dragging the coal trucks in the mine tunnels did not understand what was being said to them and stood still, confused."[10] The revival soon spread throughout the British Isles and much of the English-speaking world. Church attendance rose, and in many areas, as in Wales, public morality was dramatically affected.

Men and women who profess allegiance to the Kingdom of God become models for the rest of society. The role of the City of God, as Augustine said, is "to inspire men and women to organize their communities in the image and likeness of the heavenly city."[11]

Nowhere in modern culture is this more crucial than in the area of the nature and origins of law. In the Kingdom of God, God is King and Lawgiver for all. This does not mean that the Old Testament's civic code should be passed by modern governments. What it does mean, as Plato and Cicero recognized, is that there are moral absolutes that must govern human behavior; there is a law rooted in truth upon which the laws of human society are based.

The presence of the Kingdom of God in society means the presence of a community of people whose lives testify to this Law behind the law. They eschew relativism, believe that some things are right, some are wrong, and adhere to universal ethical norms. The presence of such people in society, therefore, is a powerful bulwark to legal sanity.

But the Kingdom of God is more than just a model. It actually operates as a restraint on the kingdoms of man through its individuals and through its most visible manifestation, the church. For in our society the church is the chief institution with the moral authority to mediate between individuals and the government, to hold the state to account for its obligations to its citizens.

The American government was established with the understanding that such transcendent values would affect what otherwise is simply a social contract. When the state forgets or denies those values that were original conditions of the contract, in essence it abrogates its contract with its citizens. It is then that the church must take the initiative and call the state to account, for as Richard Neuhaus writes, the church is "the particular society within society that bears institutional witness to the transcendent purpose to which the society is held accountable."[12]

This is the point at which the conflict between the two kingdoms often becomes the greatest. Government by nature seeks power and will always attempt to generate its own moral legitimacy for its decisions. Inevitably, it resents any group that attempts to act as its conscience.

But as history demonstrates, and as we have already discussed, the result of government attempting to impose its own moral vision upon society or acting without the restraint of an independent conscience is tyranny. Contrary to today's popular illusion, the job of propagating moral vision belongs not to government but to other institutions of society, most notably the church. When the state oversteps the bounds of its authority, the church becomes, as we have seen in Poland, the one effective source of moral resistance. The church does this not for its own ends as an earthly institution, but for the common good.

This may well be the area most perplexing to Christians and secularists alike, for both sides are frequently confused about the right, and indeed in some cases the duty, of the church, as well as individuals within the church, to confront the state.

To understand, we must first examine what citizenship in the Kingdom really means. What must citizens of the Kingdom do to be true to their allegiances and bring the healthiest influence of the Kingdom of God to bear on the kingdoms of this world—to be true patriots in the best sense of the word?

SEVENTEEN

Christian Patriotism

Whatever makes men good Christians,
makes them good citizens.

—Daniel Webster

In the kingdoms of man, young people learn the basics of good citizenship in high-school civics courses. Immigrants attend special classes to learn their new country's laws and their civic responsibilities; they must pass a test to prove they understand their new citizenship and then must swear their allegiance. Good citizenship requires such basic duties as paying taxes, voting, serving in the military and on juries, and obeying the laws of the land.

In the Kingdom of God one learns the obligations of citizenship from the Scriptures, the ultimate source of basic Christian truth. Unfortunately, most people, churched or unchurched, are woefully ignorant in this area. Though 500 million Bibles are published in America each year—that's two for every man, woman, and child—over 100 million Americans confess they never open one. In a recent survey only 42 percent could name who gave the Sermon on the Mount.[1] (Some thought it was delivered by a person on horseback.)

If the average churchgoer is uninformed, however, one does not have to look far to understand why. Church leaders have treated us to a smorgasbord of trendy theologies, pop philosophies, and religious variants of egocentric cultural values.

Recently, for example, a group of church scholars met to discuss which of Christ's words in the gospels could be accepted as authentic. Their modern critical analysis was carried out by ballot. Slips of colored paper were distributed to the group: a red slip meant the statement was authentic; pink meant probably authentic; gray meant probably not; and black meant not authentic. After intense discussion of each of Jesus' statements, participants cast their votes with the appropriate card. The Beatitudes and the Sermon on the Mount took a beating in the balloting. "Blessed are the peacemakers" was voted down; "blessed are the meek" garnered a paltry six red and pinks out of thirty votes. In the end only three of the twelve assorted woes and blessings from Matthew and Luke survived.

Such theological tomfoolery might be dismissed as too ludicrous to worry about except that this pink-slip mentality pervades the church. Orthodoxy—adherence to the historic tenets of Christianity—is under intense assault. This has been true since the Enlightenment, of course, but not until this century have so many in the church seriously argued that truth can be determined by majority vote or that the gospel should accommodate the whims of culture.

I have heard it said that reinterpreting the gospel in the context of modern culture is enlightened and progressive. Maybe some find that so, but Joseph Sobran better expresses my feelings: "It can be exalting to belong to a church that is five hundred years behind the times and sublimely indifferent to fashion; it is mortifying to belong to a church that is five minutes behind the times, huffing and puffing to catch up."[12]

Christianity rests on the belief that God is the source of truth and that He does not alter it according to the spirit of the times. When Christians sever their ties to absolute truth, relativism reigns, and the church becomes merely a religious adaptation of the culture.

Donald Bloesch maintains that modern "secularism is preparing the way for a new collectivism." He points to a historical precedent we have already looked at in some detail, the church in Germany. It was the confessing orthodox church in Germany that rose up in resistance to Hitler while "the church most infiltrated by the liberal ideology, the Enlightenment, was quickest to succumb to the beguilement of national societies."[3] Enticed by secular ideology, they saw the state as a vehicle for advancing the church.

Bloesch also points to a current illustration. In South Africa, "it can be shown that of the three Reformed churches the most illiberal theologically is the most illiberal in racial attitudes, whereas the most consciously Calvinist is the most courageous in speaking out against racial injustice."[4]

The effect of preaching a false theology can be disastrous. Most attribute the fall of Jim and Tammy Bakker to greed, sexual indiscretion, or the corruption of power. These were, of course, serious contributing factors. But the root cause of their downfall was that for years the Bakkers had preached a false gospel of material advancement: If people would only trust God, He would shower blessings upon them and indulge them with all the material desires of their hearts—a religious adaptation of the prevailing "what's in it for me" mentality. Tragically, the Bakkers deluded themselves into believing their own false message. Taking a two-million-dollar-a-year salary, living in splendor, and indulging their every whim didn't seem wrong; it was "God's blessing." And millions of followers continued to support them, even after their fall, because they too wanted such blessings.

The first responsibility for the citizen of the Kingdom, then, is to understand historic Christian truth: to know Scripture and the classic fundamentals of the faith. This is not to say that Christians are to mindlessly accept whatever they are told is an orthodox creed. Honest inquiry and thoughtful examination of the evidence, I believe, are healthy and should be encouraged, for these invariably lead to firmer belief in the truth of God's revelation interpreted by the great theologians through the ages. As Chesterton said, "Dogma does not mean the absence of thought but the end [result] of thought."[5]

When Christians either lack knowledge or are insecure about what they believe, as is the case with many today, they forfeit their place in contending for theological truth, and secularism advances. This is why James Schall implores Christians "to regain their confidence in their own dogmas.... These are not idle speculations," he writes, "but the order of reality out of which a right order in human things alone can flow."[6] Such confidence is essential if Christians are to contend for values in culture and restore a sense of the transcendent to secular thought.

The problem is, as literary critic Harry Blamires states flatly, "there is no Christian mind."[7] By this he means that Christians have their own set of beliefs but, lacking confidence, keep them to themselves. As long as they are in a secular context, they act by secular values. When they return to the privacy of their religious enclaves where they can safely think and act in Christian terms, they do so. As a result their most fundamental beliefs never penetrate the culture. Jacques Ellul reminds us that the only way theological truth reaches the world is through the actions of laypeople in the marketplace.[8]

It is this first step of Christian citizenship in the Kingdom of God—knowledge and confidence in classical Christian truth—that enables the Christian to be a good citizen in the kingdoms of man. And it is in Scripture and classical doctrine that he or she finds the clearest expression of an individual's responsibility to both kingdoms.

On the one hand Scripture commands civil obedience—that individuals respect and live in subjection to governing authorities and pray for those in authority.[9] On the other it commands that Christians maintain their ultimate allegiance to the Kingdom of God. If there is a conflict, they are to obey God, not man.[10] That may mean holding the state to moral account through civil disobedience. This dual citizenship requires a delicate balance.

*　　*　　*

Christians who are faithful to Scripture should be patriots in the best sense of that word. They are "the salvation of the commonwealth," said Augustine, for they fulfill the highest role of citizenship.[11] Not because they are forced to or even choose to, not out of any chauvinistic motivations or allegiance to a political leader, but because they love and obey the King who is above all temporal leaders. Out of that love and obedience they live in subjection to governing authorities, love their neighbors, and promote justice. Since the state cannot legislate love, Christian citizens bring a humanizing element to civic life, helping to produce the spirit by which people do good out of compassion, not compulsion.

But Christians, at least in the United States, have all too often been confused about their biblical mandates and have therefore always had trouble with the concept of patriotism. They have vacillated between two extremes—the God-and-country, wrap-the-flag-around-the-cross mentality and the simply-passing-through mindset.

The former was illustrated a century ago by the president of Amherst College who said that the nation had achieved the "true American union, that sort of union which makes every patriot a Christian and every Christian a patriot."[12] This form of civil religion has endured as a peculiar American phenomenon supported by politicians who welcome it as a prop for the state and by Christians who see it enshrining the fulfillment of the vision of the early pilgrims.

The passing-through mindset is represented by those who believe they are simply sojourners with loyalties only in the Kingdom beyond. Patriotism has become a dirty word to them, particularly in the wake of Vietnam, and they believe it their real duty to oppose the United States in just about every endeavor on just about every front—from nuclear power to Nicaraguan policy to welfare for the homeless.

These two extremes miss the kind of patriotism Augustine had in mind. He believed that while as Christians we are commanded to love the whole world, practically speaking we cannot do so. Since we are placed as if by "divine lot" in a particular nation state, it is God's calling that we "pay special regard" to those around us in that state. We love the world by loving the specific community in which we live.[13]

C. S. Lewis likened love of country to our love for the home and community in which we were raised. It is a natural love of the place where we grew up, he said, "love of old acquaintances, of familiar sights, sounds and smells." He also pointed out, however, that in love of country, as in love of family, we don't love our spouses only when they are good. Similarly, a patriot sees the flaws of his country, acknowledges them, weeps for them, but remains faithful in love.[14]

Dr. Martin Luther King, Jr., spoke of love for his country even as he attempted to change its laws.

"Whom you would change, you must first love," he said.[15]

That's the kind of tough love Christians must have for their country. To love the land faithfully, but not at the expense of suspending moral judgment. Indeed, it is the addition of that moral judgment that makes Christian patriotism responsible. "Loyalty to the civitas can safely be nurtured only if the civitas is not the object of highest loyalty," is the way Richard Neuhaus expresses it.[16]

The basic principle from Scripture is straightforward: Civil authorities are to be obeyed unless they set themselves in opposition to divine law. As Augustine put it, "An unjust law is no law at all."[17] This is the other side of Caesar's coin and can lead to civil disobedience. Practical application of this principle, however, raises perplexing questions, as we have witnessed in recent decades.

Since the sixties, civil disobedience has become a preferred method of protest. As unlikely as it may seem to some, this is an area where the Christian church has a major contribution to make in public discussion. After all, we've wrestled with this matter for two thousand years.

If Scripture does give clear principles on the matter, as I believe it does, then when is civil disobedience justified? And how is it to be carried out?

Civil disobedience is clearly justified when government attempts to take over the role of the church or allegiance due only to God. Then the Christian has not just the right but the duty to resist. The Bible gives a dramatic example of this in its account of three young Jewish exiles who were drafted into the Babylonian civil service.[18]

All citizens of Babylon were required to worship the statue of Nebuchadnezzar, the king; those who disobeyed were incinerated. Like many political leaders, power and authority were not enough for King Nebuchadnezzar; he wanted spiritual submission as well. Shadrach, Meshach, and Abednego, the young Hebrews, refused. To worship an earthly king would be the ultimate offense against their holy God.

"Our God will deliver us," they told the king when they were condemned to death for their disobedience. "But if not, we will still not worship you."[19] (It is significant to note, a point we will address later, that they were willing to pay the price for their disobedience.) The three young men were thrown into a blazing furnace. God did miraculously deliver them—something we can't always count on—and as a result the king began to worship the one true God.

Civil disobedience is also mandated when the state restricts freedom of conscience, as in the case of Peter and John, two of Jesus' disciples.

Peter and John were arrested for disturbing the peace. They were taken before the Sanhedrin, a religious body holding authority from the government of Rome, and ordered to stop preaching about Jesus. Peter and John refused.

"Judge for yourselves whether it is right in God's sight to obey you rather than God," they said. "We cannot help speaking about what we have seen and heard."[20]

Their first allegiance was to the commandment

they had been given by the resurrected Christ: the Great Commission to preach the gospel first to Jerusalem, then to the rest of Judea, and then to the ends of the earth. They could not permit the authority of the government-backed Sanhedrin to usurp the authority of God Himself.

This is a very real conflict for many Christians around the world. For example, Christians in India are imprisoned for proselytizing; in Saudi Arabia and Afghanistan they are imprisoned for even preaching the gospel. During a recent visit to the United States, a pastor from Nepal told of his imprisonment in his own country for just this offense. In conclusion he gave an excellent summary of Christian duty. "Of course I must obey my Lord and spread His Word," he said. "But even though we are persecuted, we who are Christians in Nepal pride ourselves on being the best citizens our king has. We try to be faithful to the fullest extent we can. We love our country—but we love our God more."[21]

The third justification for civil disobedience is probably the most difficult to call. It is applied when the state flagrantly ignores its divinely mandated responsibilities to preserve life and maintain order and justice. Those last words are key for Christians in deciding to disobey civil authority. Civil disobedience is never undertaken lightly or merely to create disorder. Replacing one bad situation with another is no solution, but when the state becomes an instrument of the very thing God has ordained it to restrain, the Christian must resist.

Inadequate though it was, the resistance of the German church to Hitler was a clear modern example of this necessity. In the sixties we saw it in the Civil-Rights Movement, as we do today in the Right-to-Life Movement and nonviolent resistance to Apartheid in South Africa.

When civil disobedience is justified, how is that disobedience to be carried out? When all recourse to civic obedience has been exhausted and the evil of the state is so entrenched as to be impenetrable, then the Christian may be justified (as discussed in a later chapter) in organizing to overthrow the state. First recourse, however, is always minimum resistance. Good citizens always avoid breaking just laws to protest unjust laws.

Daniel in the Old Testament exemplifies the use of the least resistance necessary to accomplish the result.

Daniel was a contemporary of Shadrach, Meshach, and Abednego, another Jewish exile living in Babylon. King Nebuchadnezzar was impressed with Daniel and enlisted his service. As a member of the king's court, Daniel was required to eat from the king's table. While such delicacies were tempting, Daniel did not want to be "defiled"; that is, he did not want to break God's strict dietary laws for His people.[22] He quietly sought his superior's permission not to eat the food, and permission was granted. Daniel could have launched a hunger strike, but it was not necessary. He achieved his objectives with minimum resistance.

Where peaceful means are available, force should be avoided. Clearly, at least in a democratic society, this should be the path civil disobedience takes. A person who, for example, feels the state's action in war is immoral has the right to pursue the matter of conscientious objection (although technically our government allows that preference only to those who practice pacifism at all times, not just for what they may perceive to be right or wrong wars).

Another important principle related to civil disobedience is illustrated by the apostles Peter and John as well as the three young Hebrews: though they disobeyed authority, they showed the appropriate respect for that authority by a willingness to accept their punishment. Those who practice civil disobedience must be prepared to pay the consequences of civil disobedience.

These general principles from Scripture are clear enough; but it is often another thing to apply them to specific circumstances, as the case of a zealous and deeply devout young woman illustrates.

Joan Andrews is a slight, soft-spoken Roman Catholic who on March 26, 1986, entered an abortion clinic for a Pro-Life sit-in and attempted to damage a suction machine used to perform abortions. She was charged and convicted of criminal mischief, burglary, and resisting arrest without violence. The prosecution asked for a one-year sentence. The judge gave her five.

Miss Andrews announced to the court, "The only way I can protest for unborn children now is by noncooperation in jail." She then dropped to the courtroom floor and refused to cooperate with prison officials at any stage of her processing. Labeled a troublemaker, she was transferred to Broward Correctional Institute, a tough maximum-security wom-

en's prison where she was placed in solitary
confinement.

On one level, Joan Andrews's sentence was severe. For example, the same day she was sentenced,
two men convicted as accessories to murder were
sentenced by the same judge to four years. Five years
for Joan Andrews's crimes is disproportionately
harsh.

On the other hand, in her protest against abortion
Miss Andrews violated a trespassing law. Much like
the Civil-Rights Movement, today's Right-to-Life activists engage in sit-ins and deliberately violate trespassing laws as a means of attracting public attention.
In Joan Andrews's case, the fear of doing nothing, of
standing by while innocent lives were being taken,
was greater than the fear of prison. But even if the
cause is just, as I believe both Civil Rights and Right-
to-Life to be, are such means of opposition appropriate?

In a free or democratic society there are legal
means available to express political opposition: we
can picket, petition, vote, organize, advertise, or pressure political officials. Is it right to abandon our respect for the rule of law, the foundation for public
order, simply to make statements that could be made
legally in other forums? Can one break a just law in
the name of protesting an unjust law? Few biblical
precedents are set for us, and those that are clearly
deal with laws that were themselves unjust. In our
day, breaking laws to make a dramatic point is the
ultimate logic of terrorism, not civil disobedience.

There may be situations, however, in which one
has to respond to a higher law when life itself is at

stake. Many Jews and Christians during World War II refused to obey Nazi laws requiring registration of aliens. On the surface those might have seemed just laws, no different than alien registration laws on the books of most Western countries today. But the citizens disobeyed because they knew those laws were being used to identify individuals for extermination.

Rightly exercised, civil disobedience is divine obedience. But when Christians engage in such activities, it must always be to demonstrate their submissiveness to God, not their defiance of government.

Unfortunately, no neat formulas for civil disobedience exist. The citizen must seek wisdom in striking the fine balance between disobedience and respect for the law. The state, though ordained by God and thus deserving of respect, is not God. The true patriot, therefore, is not one who always obeys the law. If that were so, the sheriff enforcing Jim Crow laws or the Auschwitz guard would be the best of citizens. On the other hand, disobedience can never be undertaken lightly.

Many on both the political right and left seem all too eager to defy civil authority and disrupt order to make a point on the six o'clock news. Their causes range from preventing CIA recruiters from entering college campuses to sheltering illegal immigrants to saving California condors to censoring bookstores. Some seem temperamentally disposed to such protest, as if they get high on the thrill of civil disobedience. But as Harvard law professor Alexander Bickel warns, "Civil disobedience, like law itself, is habit-forming, and the habit it forms is destructive of law."

Good citizenship requires both discernment and courage—discernment to soberly assess the issues and to know when duty calls one to obey or disobey, and courage, in the case of the latter, to take a stand.

The citizens of the Kingdom of God should be patriots in the highest sense, loving the world by loving those in the nation in which they live because that government is ordained by God to preserve order and promote justice. Perhaps this is why John Adams wrote that a patriot must be "a religious man."[23] Christians understand the phrase "a nation under God" not as a license for blind nationalism or racial superiority but as a humbling acknowledgment that all people live under the judgment of God.

Christian patriots spend more time washing feet than waving flags. Ideally, flags should not even be thought of as symbols of military and economic might, but of the common good of the specific people a sovereign God has called them to serve.

Little Platoons

> The greatest thing is to be found at one's
> post as a child of God, living each day as
> though it were our last, but planning as
> though our world might last a hundred
> years.
>
> —C. S. Lewis

Ever since giving to the needy became chic in Hollywood, we've been treated to a billion-dollar bonanza of celebrity benefits. Band-Aid, the British concert to help starving children, started the aid wagons rolling. Then came 1985's Live Aid, a marathon rock concert simulcast from London and Philadelphia. This was followed by Fashion Aid, Farm Aid, and what could only be thought of as AIDS Aid. Hands Across America linked up from Los Angeles to New York to raise $100 million for domestic homelessness and hunger, while the Freedom Festival raised money for Vietnam veterans.

And then there's my favorite: Sport Aid, which began with a runner leaving Ethiopia with a torch lighted from a refugee's campfire. He jogged through several European cities. Then this tireless athlete flew to New York, torch in hand (I wonder what he did when the "no smoking" sign came on?), where he lighted a flame in Manhattan's United Nations Plaza, signaling the start of simultaneous 10-kilometer runs around the world. The plan, said organizer Bob Geldof, also the mastermind of Live Aid, was to raise money to fight disease and hunger in Africa.

While few of us would deny that helping starving, homeless, and needy people is a good thing, this sudden aid frenzy did raise some practical questions.

In an industry where publicity is the ticket to success, one may be excused for wondering if celebrity participation in such compassion extravaganzas is altogether altruistic. The "We Are the World" video, which has sold millions of copies, reminds us less of starving children than of the great humanitarianism of its showcase of rock idols. The goals may be worthy, but such slickly publicized charity certainly recalls biblical warnings against hiring trumpeters—or camera crews—to record one's good deeds.

We might put aside our suspicions as petty if only we knew that those in need were being helped. But are they?

The New Republic reports that while USA for Africa, the organization behind Live Aid, appeals for contributions to help the starving, 55 percent of its money is instead waiting to be spent on "recovery and long-term development projects," something celebrity efforts may be ill-equipped to pull off.[1]

As of early 1986, of the $92 million raised by Live Aid and Band Aid, according to Newsweek, only $7 million has gone to emergency relief. Another $6.5

million has been spent on trucks and ships to haul
supplies; $20 million has been earmarked for projects
like bridges in Chad. The rest sits in bank accounts
somewhere.[2]

Even noncontroversial goals such as feeding the
hungry can get bogged down in squabbles over how
money and food should be distributed, or stymied at
the Marxist-controlled ports of Ethiopia. Let's not kid
ourselves. Just because the fans in London or Philadelphia go home satisfied does not mean that the
hungry in Africa go home fed.

Rock promoter Bill Graham said of celebrity aid,
"It's an incredible power, knowing on any given day
you can raise a million dollars."[3] *Newsweek* observed: "Perhaps that is why Live Aid and Farm
Aid were such oddly upbeat exercises in self-
congratulation. An industry was celebrating its
power. Far from challenging the complacency of an
audience, such mega-events reinforce it. . . . Now by
watching a pop-music telethon and making a dona-
tion . . . fans can enjoy vicariously a sense of moral
commitment."[4]

Despite all the ballyhoo, feeding the hungry did
not originate with Live-Aid. Christians have been
doing it since the church began, not for T-shirts and
pop albums, but in obedience to Christ's command
to care for those in need. Organizations such as World
Vision, Catholic Relief Services, the Salvation Army,
and millions of local churches have for generations
been feeding the hungry, housing the homeless, and
clothing the needy without the glamorous carrot-and-
stick razzle-dazzle so recently discovered by the rich
and famous. This kind of Christian patriotism also

benefits society as a whole.

Jacques Ellul wrote that the answer to the big government illusion is small voluntary associations. As mentioned earlier, eighteenth-century statesman Edmund Burke described such voluntary groups as the "little platoons."[5] These are citizens—individuals or groups—who perform works of mercy and oppose injustice. They are the salt and light of which Jesus spoke.

Culture is most profoundly changed not by the efforts of huge institutions but by individual people being changed. In the process, these citizens provide the main bulwark against government's insatiable appetite for power and control, and a safeguard against the sense of impotence fostered by today's overwhelming social problems. One person can make a difference.

A few months after Bob Geldof announced the success of Live Aid, and while critics were still questioning whether food was actually arriving in the places of need, I went to Nairobi, Kenya, for a Prison Fellowship International conference. There I met a man who, though worthy of adulation, will never make the cover of *Rolling Stone*.

Pascal was a university professor when he was thrown into a Madagascar prison after a Marxist coup. While in prison he became a Christian.

After his release, Pascal began a small import-export company, but he kept returning to prison to preach the gospel to the men he had met there and others who had arrived since. During one such visit in early 1986, he walked past the infirmary and was shocked to see more than fifty naked corpses piled on the screened veranda, identification tags stuck between their toes.

Pascal went to the nurse. Had there been an epidemic, he asked. Of sorts, he was told. Prisoners were dying by the dozens of malnutrition.

Pascal left the prison in tears. He tried to get help to feed the starving inmates, but his own church was too poor, and there were no relief agencies to assist. So he began cooking food in his own kitchen and taking it to the prison.

Today, Pascal and his wife feed prisoners every week, paying for the food out of the earnings from their small business. Without benefit of a government agency or even a theme song, this little platoon makes all the difference for seven hundred prisoners in Madagascar.

There is no age limit for enlistment in the little platoons.

In December 1983, eleven-year-old Trevor Ferrell saw a television news report on Philadelphia's inner-city homeless. The young boy couldn't believe people actually lived on the streets. When he questioned his parents, Frank and Janet reluctantly agreed to broaden their son's sheltered horizons—and their own. They left their home in an exclusive suburb and drove downtown.

A block past city hall, they spotted an emaciated figure crumpled on a sidewalk grate. While his parents watched a bit apprehensively, Trevor got out of the car and approached the man.

"Sir," he said, "here's a blanket for you." The

man stared up at Trevor at first. Then, "Thank you," he said softly. "God bless you."

That encounter altered the Ferrells' lives forever. Night after night they drove downtown, trying in small ways to help the street people. They emptied their home of extra blankets, clothing, and dozens of peanut-butter sandwiches. When others learned what they were doing, someone donated a van and volunteers charted nightly food distribution routes. To the Ferrells' surprise, "Trevor's Campaign" had begun.

Young Trevor found himself explaining what they were doing to local media, then to the nation. Pat Robertson, Merv Griffin, Mother Teresa, Ronald Reagan—all wanted to meet the small boy with the big mission. He told them simply, "It's Jesus inside of me that makes me want to do this."

But Trevor is a reluctant celebrity. He endures interviews with one eye on the door. He doesn't know why people make such a fuss over him. Is it because helping the homeless is so unusual? In that case, says his father, the more who follow Trevor's example, the better.

"Our social life has changed a lot since the campaign began," Frank says. "Our church is behind us one hundred percent; but some of our old friends don't understand why we're messing with the homeless. They just tolerate our 'eccentricities.'"

Nightly now, the blue van travels the downtown streets of Philadelphia. It stops first to deliver food to the residents of Trevor's Place, a ramshackle rooming house where some of the formerly homeless now live. Then it proceeds to feed the hungry people gathered on sidewalk grates and street corners.

Asked how these handouts can make a difference in the complex business of helping the homeless, Frank Ferrell sighs. "We're trying to meet short-term needs and figure out ways to bring long-term changes to these people's lives. Sometimes it seems like just a band-aid. But this is how we build relationships. These people become our friends, and they trust us to help them in bigger ways."

Frank pauses for a moment, looking at the landscape of broken bottles and bodies. "There are plenty of struggles. But I know one thing: giving has made all the difference in my Christian life. I used to just read the Scriptures. Now I feel like I'm living them."

The little platoon that began with a small boy's concern makes a big difference to the homeless and hungry on the streets of Philadelphia—and to those who give as well.

Thousands of miles from the home of the Liberty Bell, a young Liberian woman operates her own little platoon in Monrovia.

Lorince Taylor had a future in management as a claims supervisor for an insurance company, but her passion was for telling people about Christ. She wanted to do it full-time. When her husband encouraged her to follow her vision, Lorince resigned her job and in September 1985 began preaching in the city marketplace and in prisons and hospitals.

Although a number of people became Christians, Lorince soon realized that their problems went beyond the spiritual. She had to do more than tell them about Jesus. This became particularly evident one day when she visited a local mental hospital and, inadvertently, arrived during a staff strike.

The halls were littered with trash and dirty food trays. No doctors or nurses were in sight. The patients lay naked on the floors in their own filth, abandoned not only by their families but by those paid to care for them.

Lorince Taylor left that building praying, "Lord, this is wrong. Help me do what I can to make it right."

Shortly thereafter Lorince went to the studios of ELTV, a national television station, and told them what she had found at the hospital. Reporters returned to the institution with her and filmed the shocking scenes of neglect. When the report aired, viewers were outraged. Public pressure not only got the hospital cleaned up, but brought forth donations of food and clothing for the patients.

Next Lorince went to the prostitutes of Monrovia. Many were receptive to her spiritual message; they became Christians and began studying the Bible with her. But sooner or later they returned to their old livelihood. Most had four or five children to support and had no other way to survive. Prostitution was all they had ever known.

"I believe," cried one young woman, "but I can't live the Christian life. I just can't climb out of the life I'm living."

It was then that Lorince envisioned a vocational center where the women could be trained in sewing, secretarial and other skills. When a friend of mine last saw Lorince Taylor, a Liberian Christian had just donated a brand-new building to her ministry, and she had begun her center where former prostitutes and others in need can learn vocational skills.

Lorince Taylor's little platoon offers a ladder of escape to women trapped in a lifestyle that usually has no escape.

Another one-woman platoon began when Frieda Weststeyn, in the course of her volunteer work in a California prison, noticed the number of pregnant inmates in the visiting room. Curious, she asked how the women would care for their babies. The answer jolted her. Most of the children would go into foster homes, be put up for adoption, or farmed out to the inmates' families. The mothers would rarely, if ever, see their babies once they were born.

Frieda went home, talked to her husband, prayed, and decided to do something practical to help these imprisoned mothers. Soon she was caring for five babies in her own home. (The state, which had no such program of its own, did enter at that point—ironically—to restrict Frieda to care for only three children at a time.)

At this writing, two-month-old Ryan, seventeen-month-old Petey, and eight-month-old Amber live at the Weststeyn home, where schedules revolve around bottles and diapers. Three days a week, Frieda takes the babies to see their mothers in the prison.

"I stepped out in faith," Frieda says. "I had no money to jump into a full-fledged ministry, but I knew this was a need I could help with." She does receive assistance from the Department of Human Services in the form of formula, milk, cheese, and other staples. Also, after Frieda was featured on the

NBC network news in 1986, people across the country sent donations to help with the babies.

There are hundreds of thousands of prisoners' children, one might respond. What difference can one person make? The answer is clear to Ryan, Petey, and Amber—and their mothers.

Frieda's little platoon fulfills Augustine's view of Christian citizenship; she is loving the world by loving her particular neighbors. In her case they happen to be in prison.

Robert Lavelle's neighborhood is one of the most isolated, forgotten, and helpless communities in America—the inner city.

"People tell me, 'You're crazy, man,'" says Lavelle, "but I have to do it." He is referring to his savings and loan and real estate operations in Pittsburgh's Hill District, an area where wrecking ball, drug dealer, and welfare check are a way of life. Many of Lavelle's bank loans go to people who would be unable to obtain credit elsewhere. Though federal regulators and others have urged him to move to a "better" location, Lavelle refuses.

Dwelling House Savings and Loan goes further than financial loans, however, for Lavelle takes a personal interest in his clients. If they fall behind in payments, he visits their homes to help them figure out budgets and challenges them to set an example of financial responsibility for their children. This appeal to self-respect and accountability is the key to helping needy people, he says. It is the only way to break the cycle of their poverty. Handouts enslave people. Teaching them how to manage and extend their resources helps set them free.

Lavelle doesn't have much faith in government programs. "Government is limited in what it can do," he says. "It primarily just perpetuates itself." But "when we provide the means for the poor and minorities, the economics of their neighborhoods change from dope, numbers, prostitution, pimping, and loan-sharking to home ownership, good city services, police and garbage collection, quality schools, viable businesses, and jobs."

Lavelle, who lives within walking distance of his office, is quick to tell his clients about spiritual freedom as well, but his faith is most evident by what he does, not by what he says. "For me," he says, "being a Christian is a matter of obedience—and that means helping people in need as the Holy Spirit leads."

Lavelle explains his little platoon of upside-down banking business in terms of the Good Samaritan: the people in the inner city are lying by the roadside, wounded by economic hardship; they don't even know how to help themselves. Meanwhile, he says, there are a lot of good church people passing by on the other side. "Someone needs to stop and take a risk," he says, "and who better to do that than a banker?"

John Perkins's little platoon dramatically illustrates a similar restoration of community.

John grew up picking cotton in Mendenhall, Mississippi, for eight cents an hour. Early on, he grew frustrated with the injustice and endless cycle of poverty that fettered generations of black families in the rural south. He determined to escape.

Eventually, John beat the system by making it work for him. He and his wife, Vera May, left Mendenhall far behind for a successful business and comfortable lifestyle in California. But in 1957 John became a Christian and could no longer ignore those he had left behind. So in 1960 John and Vera May returned to Mississippi with a vision of making the Kingdom of God visible there.

John had formulated a practical basis for change, what he now calls the three Rs of community development: relocation, reconciliation, and redistribution.

First, he saw that he couldn't help people from afar. Those who want to help the poor need to *relocate* and become part of their neighborhoods. Second, from his own experience, he realized that racial, social, and economic barriers created by racial hostility in the rural south of the sixties could be broken only by the forgiveness and healing that takes place through *reconciliation*; only the gospel of Christ truly provides this. And third, as he read his Bible, John saw that Christ presents a radical call for those who have, to share with those who do not. This means *redistribution* through sharing skills, technology, and educational resources.

As John, his family, and a growing platoon of individuals began to operate on these principles in Mendenhall, they formed what is now the Voice of Calvary Church. They soon began a store, a cooperative farm, nutritional and education programs. Meanwhile, the Christian community also came head to head with the injustice of racism dividing the

South. In 1970 John and several others were jailed
and nearly beaten to death by highway patrolmen
and county sheriffs for their Civil-Rights work. Once
again, John struggled with bitterness in his own life—
but he was able to forgive his tormentors.

Voice of Calvary expanded, adding organized tu-
toring and recreation programs, an adult education
program, and a health center. By 1978 the Mendenhall work had become a model of Christian development in a rural community. In keeping with
another of John's most passionate commitments, it
was led by those who had been trained to lead in
their own community.

In 1982 John and Vera May were ready for retirement. They returned to California, anticipating a
quiet life of writing and traveling. Instead, the Perkinses decided to move into a crime-and-drug-
infested neighborhood in otherwise peaceful and
affluent Pasadena.

John knew the same principles that had given
new life and dignity to people in rural Mendenhall
would apply as well in the inner city. The result is
the Harambee Center, a community of Christians
helping their neighbors through education, employment, nutrition, neighborhood pride, and leadership
training. Harambee, the Swahili word best translated
"let's get together and push," evokes the Perkinses'
commitment to working together with those who
need help to help themselves.

John Perkins's little platoons model the values
and hopes of the Kingdom of God for the kingdoms
of man. Like Lorince Taylor's work, they are based
in human dignity and a view of economics designed

to equip people to climb out of their condition rather than manacling them to their poverty.

Sometimes the work of the little platoons mushrooms into a movement.

One such movement began with Jerry Falwell, a man who often evokes controversy. But even those who disagree most violently with Dr. Falwell's political views have a hard time faulting his outreach ministries to women facing crisis pregnancies.

Several years ago during a press conference, a reporter asked Falwell, "What practical alternatives to abortion do pregnant girls have when they are facing an unwanted pregnancy?"

"They can have the baby," Falwell shot back.

"Do you really think it's that simple?" the young woman responded. "What are you doing for women who want to keep their babies but can't find any way to do it... who are young and poor and powerless? Is it enough to take a stand against abortion when you aren't doing anything to help the pregnant girls who have no other way?"[6]

Falwell couldn't forget the reporter's question, and the result was Liberty Godparent Ministries, formed in 1982. The Lynchburg, Virginia-based operation includes a crisis-pregnancy center where women can get confidential pregnancy tests and counseling; a national hotline that receives an average of 2000 calls a month; a home where thirteen-to-eighteen-year-olds can live during their pregnancy and receive health care, birth instruction, and continue their education; shepherding homes where older women can prepare for their baby's birth; and a licensed adoption agency.

Nearly 600 programs based on the Liberty God-parent concept have sprung up across the nation. Thousands of local churches and other ministries are also working in similar ways. With names like Bethany Christian Services, Samaritan Ministries, Salem Pregnancy Center, and Amnion, they mobilize Christians to speak out against abortion and to offer loving, viable alternatives that replicate Christ's care and compassion.

Another movement confronting widespread social evil is Mothers Against Drunk Driving (MADD). Started by a young mother whose teenage daughter was killed by a drunk driver, MADD has shattered complacency about alcohol and the carnage drunk drivers have created in our society. It offers services to victims through support groups and lobbies for legislatures to beef up drunk-driver laws. In a nation where a person is killed every twenty-seven minutes by a drunken driver, MADD has made a significant impact where government had made little progress.

Like the little platoons involved in MADD, who are committed to cracking down on a widespread social ill, millions of Americans have passionately campaigned against pornography. As one of the nation's least-regulated industries (earning $6 billion in 1985), pornography recognizes few standards except the increasingly perverse tastes of its clientele. Yet it prospers, despite the FBI Academy's report convincingly tracing pornography's role in fantasies prior to sex-related murders, and such statistics as those from the Michigan State Police directly linking pornography to 40 percent of its assault cases.[7]

Pornography was not an area the government had ignored. In 1984 the attorney general appointed a panel to report on the issue. A year later the Commission on Pornography surfaced from the murky world of smut, and antipornography campaigners pinned great hopes on the panel's recommendations. Working through the leverage of big government seemed the most effective way to destroy such a widespread social cancer.

The commission, which included Focus on the Family's Dr. James Dobson, strongly believed there was a connection between some pornography and violent crimes. It recommended tougher prosecution, stronger federal laws, and more vigorous enforcement of existing obscenity laws.

Even if the panel's laudable proposals make it through the tough legislative process, however, they can expect extended court challenges. As Barry Lynn of the American Civil Liberties Union boasted, "There are enough constitutional questions here [in the Meese report] to litigate for the next twenty years."[8]

As the commission was completing its report, the high-flying pornography industry suffered a major setback that caught everyone by surprise. It came from a little platoon.

When Jack Eckerd, founder of the Eckerd Drug chain, became a Christian in 1983, he called the company president and urged him to take *Playboy* and *Penthouse* magazines out of the Eckerd stores. The executive protested, telling him the magazines amounted to several million dollars a year in business. Jack Eckerd persisted. Eventually all 1,700 Eckerd drugstores stopped carrying *Playboy* and *Penthouse*. Eckerd then wrote to the directors of other retail stores and encouraged them to do the same. When his letters went unanswered, he wrote again.[9]

Meanwhile, the National Coalition Against Pornography was picketing and boycotting stores selling "adult" magazines. The pressure began to pay off. One by one Revco, People's, Rite-Aid, Dart Drug, Gray Drug, and High's Dairy Stores pulled pornography from their shelves. And finally 7–11 removed these magazines from its 4,500 stores and recommended that its 3,600 franchises do the same.

Thus, without one debate before Congress or one case entangled in the courts, the shelves of nearly 12,000 retail stores were cleared of pornography!

Playboy's lawyers, shocked at their declining circulation, charged that a letter from the Meese Commission had put coercive pressure on the stores. Maybe so. But the real impetus came from the little platoons—thousands of individuals and one courageous man who put his faith into practice in his own business.

One of my favorite little platoons is a group of prison volunteers whose names I don't even know.

It was a rainy, dismal day in February when we arrived at the Maryland prison at Jessup, but the entry area was filled with the bright lights of television cameras. Reporters scribbled notes while Maryland officials greeted us warmly. Governor Harry Hughes had even issued a proclamation for the occasion.

By the time we got to the prison chapel, it was on the verge of exploding with the excitement of more than 125 inmates and several dozen Prison Fellowship volunteers, all of whom had been participating in one of our in-prison seminars. With us was Wintley Phipps, the internationally known gospel singer who had sung only the day before for President Reagan at a prayer breakfast. When Wintley let loose in that cinder-block prison chapel, I thought the walls would come tumbling down.

Then Herman Heade gave his testimony. Herman had been converted while in a solitary-confinement cell. He had tremendous rapport with other inmates and his message was powerful, dramatic, and convicting.

The excitement continued as I challenged the men to accept Christ, then prayed with them. Afterward the inmates crowded around, hugging us and weeping.

The next day our instructor, Dick Robinson, was relieved to find all the inmates were back for the seminar's final session. He had thought the last day might be anticlimactic. Several inmates gave their impressions of the previous day.

"I really appreciated Chuck Colson's message," said one tall prisoner. "Wintley Phipps's singing stirred me beyond words, and Herman's testimony reached me right where I was at. But frankly, those things really didn't impress me as much as what happened later.

"When the celebrities and TV cameras left," he continued, "the ladies among the volunteers went into the dining hall, with all the noise and confusion, and sat at the table to have a meal with us. That's what really got to me," he concluded, his voice choked.

Wintley's singing and Herman's testimony and my sermon were all appreciated. But the most powerful message came from the volunteers who went into the crowded, dingy dining hall to share prison food with the inmates.

Celebrities don't make the difference in society. The little platoons of ordinary people living extraordinary lives do.

*   *   *

At the end of all the "feed the hungry" celebrity hoopla, when organizer Bob Geldof announced that his aid campaign's mission had been accomplished, he concluded, "It's like a shooting star . . . for once . . . something absolutely good and absolutely incorruptible came and went and worked."[10]

But shooting stars don't feed starving multitudes, and long after Hollywood has moved on to other causes, the hungry will remain.

Fortunately for the kingdoms of man, the little platoons march on.

NINETEEN

The Problems of Power

> *It is a magician's bargain: give up our*
> *souls, get power in return. But once our*
> *souls, that is, ourselves, have been given*
> *up, the power thus conferred will not*
> *belong to us. We shall in fact be slaves*
> *and puppets of that to which we have*
> *given our souls.*
>
> —*C. S. Lewis*

John Naisbitt observed in *Megatrends* that significant movements begin from the bottom up, not the top down.[1] Truly important changes in culture begin not from officials or celebrities, but through ordinary people: the little platoons. Every person can—and should—seek to make a difference in his or her corner of the world by personally helping those in need.

Beyond this, some people, like William Wilberforce, are called to work through government structures and by political means to bring Christian influence into the culture. Those who do, however, need to be forewarned: the everyday business of politics is power, and power, as I know so well from my own experience, can be perilous for anyone.

My purpose here is not to deal exhaustively with the complex issue of power, nor could I. Entire books have been written on the subject. Yet no discussion of Christianity and politics would be complete without at least examining the dynamics of power, particularly as it affects the political arena and those who enter it.

The history of the last fifty years has validated Nietzsche's argument that man's desire to control his own destiny and to impose his will on others is the most basic human motivation. While I reject Nietzsche's atheistic cynicism, I do agree with his diagnosis of human nature. So did Christian psychiatrist Paul Tournier, who wrote, "We are moved without knowing it by an imperious will to power, which brooks no obstacles."[2]

Nietzsche's prophecy that the "will to power" would fill the twentieth-century's vacuum of values has been fulfilled. We see it on an individual level in the quest for autonomy and the shedding of all restraints. On a corporate level, it is dramatically evident in the rise of gangster leaders like Hitler and Stalin, and evident as well in the bloated growth of Western governments.

The resultant illusion—that all power resides in large institutions—is the salient characteristic of modern politics. Since power is often measured by one's prominence and ability to influence others, in today's world, politics is the most visible means to both.

Hunger for political power lures men and women from the comfort of their homes and jobs in the private sector and drives them to spend months,

even years, traveling about their state or nation, sub-
sisting on stale sandwiches, greasy chicken, and little
sleep as they shout the same soul-stirring speech over
and over until they are hoarse. Candidates for Congress spend several million dollars to fight for a job
that pays $89,000 a year; others settle for lower-
paying bureaucratic positions. Still others give huge
political contributions in the hopes of acquiring even
an obscure embassy appointment.

Certainly in every generation there are statesmen
motivated by a genuine noblesse oblige, a sense of
high calling to serve humanity. For the most part,
though, it is Nietzsche's "will to power" that fuels
political passions in every culture.

I've seen it up close.

Even before I was invited to become part of the
White House staff in 1969, I felt a sense of guilt that
many of those I had worked with in the 1968 campaign were now in government at salaries far less
than my own lucrative law-practice income. And
duty to country had always weighed heavily with
me, the flag-waving, ex-Marine, conservative political activist.

So when the offer came, even as I made the perfunctory protests about sacrifice, interrupting my career and burdening my family, I was already packing
up my office files. More than duty called me, of
course. There was glamorous protocol, the possibility
of shaping headlines and history, the enticement of
being part of the inner circle surrounding the president of the United States. Deep down, though I
wouldn't admit it, the White House represented the
pinnacle of the power I had pursued all my life.

Joining the staff nine months into the new administration had some disadvantages. One of the first visible yardsticks of power is size and placement of office, and the best offices were already taken. I was given an inside suite a long way down the hall from the president's working office in the stately Old Executive Office Building. Also I reported not to the president, but to Bob Haldeman, his hard-nosed chief of staff. Not an auspicious beginning.

Within months, circumstances worked in my favor. An aide left, and everyone played musical offices. With a little fast footwork I maneuvered my way across the hall to an office commanding an impressive view of the South Lawn. From there I edged my way down the corridor toward the seat of power.

Within a short time my brusque get-it-done-at-all-costs approach won Nixon's favor, and I began to work directly with him. With that kind of clout I had little difficulty rearranging several secret-service agents and secretaries so I could occupy the office immediately next to the president's.

Though the evidence of my change in status was visible in the attitude of my visitors when they realized that the president himself was just on the other side of the wall, the move was symbolic of something much more important. It meant I had passed an invisible divide. I was now *inside*. A *Newsweek* feature article heralded my arrival with the news that I was now on the top of every Washington hostess's guest list (ironic, since I never attended parties) and that the mere mention of my name "makes the tensions come in like sheet rain."[3] In Washington that means power.

In the political arena one of the most important attributes of power is its visibility. So we went to great lengths to protect our territory or prerogatives.

One Sunday in June 1971 the White House faced a sudden crisis: the *New York Times* published the "Pentagon Papers," the highly classified documents stolen by Daniel Ellsberg, a one-time Johnson-administration official turned antiwar activist. Mr. Nixon feared that our secret negotiations with the North Vietnamese would be exposed. For two days meetings went on around the clock, with the president, egged on by Henry Kissinger, barking angry orders to the Pentagon, the Justice Department, and his staff. (One such order led to my involvement in smearing Ellsberg, for which I later pleaded guilty and went to prison.)

At 8:00 on Tuesday evening the president phoned me with his latest instructions. "Chuck, I want you to call Lyndon Johnson. You explain to him that I'm taking all the heat for this. These are *his* administration's papers—now, the least he can do is make some public statement supporting us. I mean, that will help us with the Democrats at least. You know what I mean? Now, just let Henry know and then you call Johnson. Understand?"

"Yes, sir," I replied.

"Good, good," said Nixon. "You get it done, and don't bother to call me back. I'm going to bed early."

Dutifully following orders, I called Kissinger first. The national security adviser, who admittedly had had a bad day, was outraged.

"If anyone is to call former President Johnson,

it is me," he insisted, his accent thickening with his resolve.

Nothing I said made any difference, so I played my trump. "But the president ordered *me*, Henry," I said.

"Then I will call the president, and he will reverse that order," Kissinger replied.

In our power game Kissinger had checked me. The president had been up most of the night before; he needed sleep. Besides, he shouldn't have to bother with such squabbles. Kissinger knew this and he knew that I knew it. I hesitated a moment, then folded.

"Okay, Henry. Let's agree that neither of us will call until morning. Then we'll ask the president when we see him at the eight o'clock meeting."

"Good, Chuck. That is very good," he answered.

"But now you promise me," I added quickly, "that you won't bother him about it tonight."

"You have my word, Chuck," Kissinger said somberly.

The heat of our exchange left no doubt in my mind that the call to Johnson was important to Kissinger. Perhaps he feared that my making the call would indicate he was losing his influence or that I was taking responsibility for national security affairs. Whatever his thinking, I wasn't surprised at the White House operator's reply when I called ten minutes later to ask if anyone had phoned the president. "Oh, yes, sir," she replied. "Dr. Kissinger called him ten minutes ago."

Later that night Kissinger placed the call to Lyndon Johnson. Maintaining the appearance of power is also paramount, even when the reality is inconsequential.

On Nixon's last presidential trip abroad, in June 1974, he was accompanied by two senior aides, Al Haig and Ron Ziegler, both of whom were vying for top position. The trip, begun in the Soviet Union and including stops in Iran and Israel, was a vain last-ditch effort to divert attention away from the president's political crisis. By that time everyone knew Mr. Nixon couldn't survive the public clamor more than another month or two; his entire administration was about to collapse. Even so, the advance team was equipped with tape measures and meticulous instructions to insure that in all sleeping accommodations Mr. Ziegler's bed and General Haig's bed would be equidistant from the president's.

The pursuit of power affects entire governments or regions, as well as individuals. Those in office use their power to keep themselves in office. This is an accepted tradition in most Western democracies. In every American election since the forties the party in power has used grants and federal aid programs for political advantage. Truman won his upset victory in 1948 by doling out federal funds to struggling farmers and openly courting special-interest groups. Eisenhower judiciously announced grants in key states during the 1956 campaign. In the Kennedy and Johnson years a special White House office monitored election-year grants, and party fund-raisers notified defense contractors of impending contracts. Administrations since have adopted similar practices.

We were certainly not to be outdone in the Nixon

years. I recall one incident from early 1972 when Bob Haldeman and I met with the president one morning to discuss reelection campaign strategy and schedules. We couldn't know at that point that Nixon would win in a record landslide. The polls showed him dead even with his expected opponent, Senator Edmund Muskie from Maine. Even though Nixon had only token primary opposition, I raised the question of visits to key primary states.

Haldeman chuckled. "No worry about the two big ones, New Hampshire and California. The Chinese and Russians will take care of those for us." Nixon laughed.

When I looked from one to the other in bewilderment, Haldeman delighted in detailing the tour de force he had arranged. Nixon's trip to China, he explained, was deliberately scheduled one week before the first primary in New Hampshire. Live coverage would dominate prime time for a week. Nixon would then receive a hero's welcome home, just days before New Hampshire voters went to the polls.

The summit in Moscow, Haldeman continued, would spotlight the first strategic-arms agreement ever signed on live television from inside the Kremlin. It was timed to transpire one week before the all-important California primary. The president would fly home on Air Force One, take a helicopter from Andrews Air Force base to the Capitol. There he would address a joint session of Congress—all televised live on prime time, just four days before millions of Californians cast their votes. Haldeman had arranged which network reporters would be included. History had been scheduled according to the Nielsen ratings.

Nixon leaned back in his chair, took a long, deliberate puff on his Meerschaum pipe, and grinned. "Not bad, is it, Chuck? The Democrats won't even be able to buy time on TV."

"No, sir, not bad," I replied with open admiration. Even foreign policy was fair game.

These are not isolated examples, of course. All governments use the reality as well as the façade of power to maintain their own power. In democratic structures the process is somewhat subtle, but in regimes where there are few moral restraints, power is wielded shamelessly. We call it totalitarianism. George Orwell captured this in one of the most riveting scenes of his classic 1984.

The book's central character, a hapless fellow named Winston, defies the state. He is eventually tracked down and tortured by the chief party functionary, O'Brien. As O'Brien administers massive electrical jolts to Winston's squirming body, he abandons all pretense and shrieks into Winston's ear, "The party seeks power entirely for its own sake... we are interested only in power... the object of power is power."[4]

Stalin rose to power by systematically murdering those who stood in his way; he then maintained his power by slaughtering millions. Hitler executed all potential threats to the Third Reich—even his own SA—then consolidated his power grip on Germany with a regime of terror. Recent tyrants, such as Idi Amin and the Cambodian Communists, have done the same.

One of the most startling commentaries on this century is the fact that millions more have died at the hands of their own governments than in wars with other nations—all to preserve someone's power.

*   *   *

In *The Masters*, British novelist C. P. Snow tells the story of a man who chooses not to be king but kingmaker, the ultimate achievement power affords.[5] Snow might well have been writing about me.

I entered government believing that public office was a trust, a duty. Gradually, imperceptibly, I began to view it as a holy crusade; the future of the republic, or so I rationalized, depended upon the president's continuation in office. But whether I acknowledged it or not, equally important was the fact that my own power depended on it.

While power may begin as a means to an end, it soon becomes, as O'Brien screamed in Winston's ear, the end itself. Having witnessed Watergate from the inside, I can attest to the wisdom of Lord Acton's well-known adage: Power corrupts; absolute power corrupts absolutely.

It is crucial to note, however, that it is power that corrupts, not power that is corrupt. It is like electricity. When properly handled, electricity provides light and energy; when mishandled it destroys. God has given power to the state to be used to restrain evil and maintain order. It is the use of power, whether for personal gain or for the state's ordained function, that is at issue.

The problem of power is not limited to public officials, of course. It affects all human relationships, from the domineering parent to the bullying boss to the manipulative spouse to the pastor who plays God. It is also wielded effectively by the seemingly weak who manipulate others to gain their own ends. The temptation to abuse power confronts everyone, including people in positions of spiritual authority.

The much-publicized corruption of some television evangelists can easily be traced to an inability to handle power. It's a heady business to run worldwide ministries, multimillion dollar television shows, or wealthy amphitheater churches. Leaders who rise to prominence in the religious world are placed on the precarious pedestal of Christian celebrity. When the celebrity is magnified a million times over by the electron tube, the dangers of falling increase dramatically.

Take the case of Jim and Tammy Bakker. When I first visited their ministry in 1976, their shoestring operation was housed in an old building. They were, I was convinced, sincerely concerned with reaching others with the Good News. A year later I was invited to their new, modern facilities and was immediately struck by the change in their demeanor. I did not return. I witnessed the same phenomenon with one of the country's most popular daytime interviewers. The first time I was a guest on his show, before he had begun to soar in the ratings game, the interviewer was humble, keenly interested in the subject, well-prepared, and congenial. Two years later, when this man had become the sensation of the television world, he breezed into the room flanked by obsequious aides, was woefully unconcerned with what his guests had to say, and was arrogant and rude on the air—to the delight of his audience.

It's ludicrous for any Christian to believe that he or she is the worthy object of public worship; it would be like the donkey carrying Jesus into Jerusalem believing the crowds were cheering and laying down their garments for him. But the perks and public adoration accompanying television exposure are enough to inflate nearly anyone's ego. This leads to the self-indulgent use of power some have dubbed the "Imelda Marcos syndrome," which reasons, "because I'm in this position, I have a right to do whatever I want," with total selfishness and disregard for others. Power is like saltwater; the more you drink the thirstier you get.

The lure of power can separate the most resolute of Christians from the true nature of Christian leadership, which is service to others. It's difficult to stand on a pedestal and wash the feet of those below.

It was this very temptation of power that led to the first sin. Eve was tempted to eat from the tree of knowledge to be like God and acquire power reserved for Him. "The sin of the Garden was the sin of power," says Quaker writer Richard Foster.[6]

Power has been one of Satan's most effective tools from the beginning, perhaps because he lusts for it so himself. Milton wrote of Lucifer in *Paradise Lost*, "To reign is worth ambition, though in hell. Better to reign in hell than serve in heaven."[7]

In the process of announcing the Kingdom and offering redemption from the Fall, Jesus Christ turned conventional views of power upside down. When His disciples argued over who was the greatest,

Jesus rebuked them. "The greatest among you should be like the youngest, and the one who rules like the one who serves," he said.[8] Imagine the impact His statement would make in the back rooms of American politicians or in the carpeted boardrooms of big business—or, sadly, in some religious councils.

Jesus was as good as His words. He washed His own followers' dusty feet, a chore reserved for the lowliest servant of first-century Palestine. A king serving the mundane physical needs of His subjects? Incomprehensible. Yet servant leadership is the heart of Christ's teaching. "Whoever wants to be first must be slave of all."[9]

His was a revolutionary message to the class-conscious culture of the first-century, where position and privilege were entrenched, evidenced by the Pharisees with their reserved seats in the synagogue, by masters ruling slaves, and by men dominating women. It is no less revolutionary today in the class-conscious cultures of the East and West where power, money, fame, and influence are idolized in various forms.

The Christian understanding of power is that it is found most often in weakness. This paradox has been a thorn in the flesh of tyrants. The Judeo-Christian teaching that man is vulnerable to the temptations of power has also caused democracies and free nations to build restraints and balances of power into their structures.

Clearly this is what motivated the revolutionaries in England to guarantee a Parliament independent of the monarchy. And in America the Founding Fathers, influenced by Judeo-Christian teaching about the vulnerability of man, wisely adopted the principle of the separation of powers. Within the government, power was diffused through a system of checks and balances so no one branch could dominate another. The Founders also assumed that the religious value system, evidenced through the separate institution of the church, would be the most powerful brake on the natural avarice of government. As Tocqueville observed, "Religion in America takes no direct part in the government or society but it must, nevertheless, be regarded as the foremost of the political institutions of that country."[10]

The most important restraint on power, however, is a healthy understanding of its true source. When power in the conventional sense is relinquished, one discovers a much deeper power.

Prisoners often discover this, as did Jerry Levin and Aleksandr Solzhenitsyn. In his memoirs of the gulag, Solzhenitsyn wrote that as long as he was trying to maintain some pitiful degree of worldly power in his situation—control of food, clothing, schedule—he was constantly under the heel of his captors. But after his conversion, when he accepted and surrendered to his utter powerlessness, then he became free of even his captors' power. Perhaps this is why Boris Pasternak once wrote that the only place one can be free in a communist society is in prison.

The apostle Paul said, "My power is made perfect in weakness," and concluded, "When I am weak, then I am strong."[11] And throughout Scripture God reveals a special compassion for the powerless: widows, orphans, prisoners, and aliens. Though the message of the Kingdom of God offers salvation for all who repent and believe, God does not conceal His disdain for those so enamored of their own power that they refuse to worship Him or to acknowledge His delight in the humble.

A culture that exalts power and celebrity, that worships success, dismisses such words as nonsense. Strong individuals rely on their own resources—which will never, ultimately speaking, be enough—but the so-called weak person knows his or her own limits and needs, and thus depends wholly on God. Perhaps this is why God so often confounds the wisdom of the world by accomplishing His purposes through the powerless and His most powerful work through human weakness.

I first learned this in prison. When the frustration of my helplessness seemed greatest, I discovered God's grace was more than sufficient. And after my imprisonment I could look back and see how God used my powerlessness for His purposes. What He has chosen for my most significant witness was not my triumphs or victories, but my defeat.

Similarly, Prison Fellowship's work in the prisons has been effective not because of any power we may have as an organization, but because of the powerlessness of those we serve. During an unforgettable trip to Peru in 1984, for example, I visited Lurigancho, the largest prison in the world. There seven thousand inmates, including a number of terrorists, were crowded in abysmal conditions; hatred, hostility, and despair seeped out of the cellblocks. Yet within the darkness of Lurigancho is a thriving Christian community—men who have found Christ and experienced renewed hearts and minds.

After visiting with these brothers, I went directly from the prison to meet with a number of government officials in downtown Lima. Covered with prison dust and marked with the sweaty embraces of Christian prisoners, I addressed these officials at the highest level of government—and they listened intently.

Had I gone to Peru specifically to meet with the key government leadership, I would have likely been stymied. They wanted to meet me not because of any power or influence I had, but because of our work in the prisons. They knew that in the chaos of Lurigancho, Prison Fellowship was doing something to bring healing and restoration. Therefore, they were eager to listen to our recommendations, ready to discuss a biblical view of justice and prison issues. Whatever authority I had in speaking to these powerful men came not from my power but from serving the powerless. I have experienced this in country after country. It is the paradox of real power.

*   *   *

Nothing distinguishes the kingdoms of man from the Kingdom of God more than their diametrically opposed views of the exercise of power. One seeks to control people, the other to serve people; one promotes self, the other prostrates self; one seeks prestige and position, the other lifts up the lowly and despised.

It is crucial for Christians to understand this difference. For through this upside-down view of power, the Kingdom of God can play a special role in the affairs of the world.

As citizens of the Kingdom today practice this

view of power, they are setting an example for their neighbors by modeling servanthood and exposing the illusions power creates.

But how does this paradoxical view of power apply to the Christian who is in a position of influence and control? Sociologist Tony Campolo, drawing on the classic work of Max Weber, offers helpful guidance through the distinctions he draws between power and authority. Power involves the use of coercive force to make others yield to one's wishes even against their own will. Authority is achieved—or is conferred upon one—by virtue of character that others are motivated to follow willingly.[12]

Therefore, the citizen of the Kingdom should seek authority that comes from his or her own spiritual strength. Never for self-advantage, but for the benefit of others.

This does not mean that the Christian can't use power. In positions of leadership, especially in government institutions to which God has specifically granted the power of the sword, the Christian can do so in good conscience. But the Christian uses power with a different motive and in different ways: not to impose his or her personal will over others but to preserve God's plan for order and justice for all.

Those who accept the biblical view of servant leadership treat power as a humbling delegation from God, not as a right to control others.

Moses offers a great role model. Though he had awesome power and responsibility as the leader of two million Israelites, he was described in Scripture as "a very humble man, more humble than anyone else on the face of the earth."[13] He led by serving—

intervening before God on his people's behalf, seeking God's forgiveness for their rebellion and caring for their needs above his own.

The challenge for the Christian in a position of influence is to follow the example of Moses rather than fulfill Nietzsche's prophecy concerning the will to power. In doing so the citizen of the Kingdom has an opportunity to offer light to a world often shrouded by the dark pretensions of a devastating succession of power-mad tyrants.

TWENTY

Christians in Politics

*Who's to say religion and politics
shouldn't mix? Whose Bible are they
reading anyway?*
—Archbishop Desmond Tutu

Frequently I'm asked whether I would have participated in Watergate if I had been a Christian when I worked in the White House. The implication is that Christians are immune to corruption.

I'm always tempted to say, "Of course not." But that's self-righteous nonsense. While Christians know that their faith requires high standards of righteousness, they are human and often capitulate to the same temptations as anyone else. In fact, Christians may well face more problems than others when they become involved in the political process.

How does a Christian deal with the inherent divided loyalties: duty to God and duty to the national interest? Can a Christian successfully avoid the subtle snares of power? Can a Christian make the compromises necessary for the everyday business of politics?

What about the question of candor, for example? At times national security may well require not only concealing the truth, but lying. When I was in the White House, we went to elaborate lengths to conceal essential secret negotiations. Henry Kissinger had a bad cold when he visited Pakistan in 1971—or so we told the press. Actually he had been flown to Bejing to conduct clandestine meetings in preparation for Mr. Nixon's historic visit to China.

Or take the day Nixon announced a major troop withdrawal in Vietnam. He immediately ordered Kissinger to bring Soviet Ambassador Dobrynin to a secret meeting room in the White House basement. "Henry," he roared, "You shake him up. Tell him not to believe these news stories. We're only pulling out a few troops—and if the Russians don't back off in sending supplies to Hanoi, we'll bomb the daylights out of that city. Tell him the president is uncontrollable, a madman—that he'll do anything. Let's keep them off balance." That such meetings took place was flatly denied in order to protect the lives of the withdrawing troops.

President Reagan did the same thing in 1983. When reporters asked about a rumored invasion of Grenada, official White House spokesmen dismissed such questions as "preposterous." Actually, troops were at that moment disembarking on the island's beaches. A "no comment" to the press, however, would have been tantamount to a "yes"—an admission that would have endangered lives.

In these days of delicate international tensions and the instant communications ability of an almost omnipresent press, such deceit is a common instrument of foreign policy. The press even accept it. In a 1987 *Newsweek* interview, crack ABC interviewer Ted Koppel acknowledged that government officials must be "prepared to mislead and . . . sometimes even to lie."[1]

Deliberate lies, the corruption of power, compromise with ideological opponents, temptations on all sides—these appear to be the mechanisms of modern government. Should the Christian circumvent the messy business of politics altogether?

The answer must be an emphatic no. As Robert L. Dabney wrote, "Every Christian . . . whether lawmaker or law executor or voter, should carry his Christian conscience, enlightened by God's Word, into his political duty. We must ask less what party caucuses and leaders dictate, and more what duty dictates."[2]

There are at least three compelling reasons Christians must be involved in politics and government. First, as citizens of the nation-state, Christians have the same civic duties all citizens have: to serve on juries, to pay taxes, to vote, to support candidates they think are best qualified. They are commanded to pray for and respect governing authorities. (For years many Christian fundamentalists shunned the "sinful" political process, even to the extent of not voting. Whatever else may be said about it, the Moral Majority performed a valuable public service in bringing these citizens back into the mainstream.)

Second, as citizens of the Kingdom of God they are to bring God's standards of righteousness and justice to bear on the kingdoms of this world. This is the cultural commission discussed earlier. As former Michigan state senator and college professor Stephen Monsma says, Christian political involvement has the "potential to move the political system away from . . . the brokering of the self-interest of powerful persons and groups into a renewed concern for the public interest."[3]

Third, Christians have an obligation to bring transcendent moral values into the public debate. All law implicitly involves morality; the popular idea that "you can't legislate morality" is a myth. Morality is legislated every day from the vantage point of one value system or another. The question is not whether we will legislate morality, but whose morality we will legislate.

Law is but a body of rules regulating human behavior; it establishes, from the view of the state, the rightness or wrongness of human behavior. Most laws, therefore, have moral implications. Statutes prohibiting murder, mandates for seat belts, or regulations for industrial safety are all designed to protect human life—a reflection of the particular moral view that values the dignity and worth of human life. And efficacy doesn't affect morality. If in America we have more homicides per capita than in any other country, it's not reason to repeal the laws making murder a crime.

The common argument against the legislation of morality is Prohibition, which conjures up such caricatures as Billy Sunday waving a chair over his head and Carrie Nation chopping up whiskey barrels. The church has taken an undeserved bad rap for this. No one entity imposed Prohibition; it was voted in by a clear majority after a lengthy national debate.

Admittedly, over the years of its existence Prohibition became increasingly difficult to enforce; it encouraged organized crime and ultimately led to widespread disrespect for the law. Eventually the costs outweighed the benefits.

But was it morally justified? Certainly one's personal decision to drink alcohol is a private matter. When millions do it to such excess that public safety is endangered, however, it becomes a public concern. That was the case in the pre-Prohibition era. Thousands reported to their factory jobs under the influence and were maimed or killed by the heavy industrial machines then being introduced in the American economy. The tavern trade spawned prostitution rings at a time when, like AIDS today, there was no cure for the raging epidemic of venereal disease.

Though many write off Prohibition as a complete failure, the facts are that industrial safety improved dramatically as per capita drinking, particularly among working people, dropped precipitously, and the VD epidemic slowed. Not until 1970 did per capita consumption of alcohol again reach pre-Prohibition levels.[4]

With one person being killed every twenty-seven minutes in the U.S. by a drunk driver and the majority of crimes being committed by people under the influence of drugs or alcohol, can anyone really argue realistically today that moral issues are not matters of public interest?

The real issue for Christians is not whether

they should by involved in politics or contend for laws that affect moral behavior. The question is how.

*   *   *

On an individual level, political involvement for the Christian entails not only voting and other basic responsibilities of citizenship, but dealing directly with political issues, particularly where justice and human dignity are at stake. A friend of mine, a prominent attorney in Ecuador, experienced this firsthand.

Dr. Jorge Crespo has always been an activist. For years he was an attorney for labor unions, fighting for justice and humane working conditions for Ecuador's laborers. Later he ran unsuccessfully for the presidency of his country. Then, after meeting with Prison Fellowship's South American regional director, Javier Bustamante, he agreed to consider prison ministry, even though he had always seen prisons as places where delinquents—and some clients—ended up.

But as soon as Dr. Crespo walked the cellblocks of a Quito prison, he felt "a deep sensation of pain, something like an echo of the pain of the prisoners. Since we are made in His image, we have been given His compassion toward our neighbor," he explained.

So Dr. Crespo became president of Prison Fellowship Ecuador. As he investigated prison conditions, he uncovered, to his horror, instances of cruelty, deprivation, and misery. In one prison twenty prisoners were wedged into a cell the size of a small bedroom. In another inmates received less care than animals; their food budget was less than that of the officers' guard dogs. In most women's prisons, children were incarcerated along with their mothers. In some cases they were being used as pawns in child prostitution rings to make profits for their parents, the prison guards, or both.

There were also reports of inhumane treatment. Some prisoners had confessed to crimes of which they were innocent in order to escape such measures.

Dr. Crespo and his colleagues documented their case, then began to educate the public through press, radio, and television. They sent letters to the prison wardens with copies to the minister of government; they met with ministers of social rehabilitation and justice. Their campaign was not without personal sacrifice and political risk.

Finally, they approached the tribunal overseeing constitutional enforcement, a governmental committee safeguarding Ecuador's provisions for human rights.

Crespo spent two hours testifying about the despicable prison conditions as well as the inhumane treatment of inmates and those who had been detained for crimes but not yet proven guilty.

The justices were shocked. Never before had such ugly topics been addressed in their ornate chambers. At the conclusion, the vice-president leaned forward to Dr. Crespo. "You have come here as Christians," he said, "and what you have done today is truly Christian."

As a result of Dr. Crespo's boldness, a series of

reforms have been adopted in Ecuador. He has also organized a group of Christian police officers who are working to assure humane police investigation that does not rely on brutality.

Dr. Crespo is seeing slow but deliberate progress in the prisons.

The political and personal risks have been worth it, he says. "To act as Christians we have to stand against injustice, and with prophetic voice talk courageously about truth, justice, fear, love. We ought not to bear infamy or atrocities. I believe a Christian who will remain silent is not a Christian."

Activist Christians like Jorge Crespo who work as private citizens to address problems within the structures of government do so, as Stephen Monsma has written, "not as moral busybodies who are seeking to foist their morals onto all of society by the force of law, but as those who have a passion for justice, as those who respect all persons as unique image bearers of God and who therefore seek to treat them with justice."[5]

*   *   *

But many others are called to make a Christian witness from positions within government itself. After all, as men like William Wilberforce or the great nineteenth-century social reformer, Lord Shaftesbury, clearly illustrate, Christians who are politicians can bear a biblical witness on political structures, just as they do in medicine, law, business, labor, education, the arts, or any other walk of life. Augustine called God-fearing rulers "blessings bestowed

. . . upon mankind.'"[6] They exhibit this in their moral witness and their willingness to stand up for unpopular causes, even if such causes benefit society more than their own political careers.

U.S. Senators Nunn of Georgia and Armstrong of Colorado attended a Bible study several years ago on the topic of restitution as a biblical means of punishment. The two leaders later examined the federal statutes and discovered that restitution was only vaguely mentioned. Even though "lock 'em up" legislation was in political vogue, the two men, both committed Christians, sponsored legislation to set new standards for sentencing: prison for dangerous offenders, but tax-dollar-saving alternative punishments, such as work and restitution programs, for nondangerous offenders. In 1983 the bill was adopted, after heated debate, as a resolution of the Congress and later was used as model legislation by several states.

Christians can also bring mercy, compassion, and friendship to those in the cutthroat business of politics.

After his resignation Mr. Nixon withdrew to isolation behind the walls of his San Clemente compound. For nearly a year, as he struggled to recover from both the deep emotional wounds of Watergate and life-threatening phlebitis, Mr. Nixon saw only his family and a few close friends. No one, other than gloating reporters, tried to visit him.

No one, that is, except one man who had opposed Mr. Nixon as vigorously as anyone in the Senate. Without fanfare, Mark Hatfield, an evangelical Christian, traveled twice to San Clemente. His reason? Simply, as he told me later, "to let Mr. Nixon know that someone loved him."

Sometimes even minor things can have a significant ripple effect in the everyday business of government. Concerned about the pressures government service puts on congressional families, Congressmen Frank Wolf and Dan Coats hosted a series of receptions to show James Dobson's excellent family-counseling films. More than a hundred members and their spouses attended; several later sought counseling help. Through Coats and Wolf the films were also shown to the Joint Chiefs of Staff and Pentagon officials, who have since made them available for use in military training programs.

Christians in public office are motivated by something more than popularity or self-interest, something that frees them from being held hostage to political expediency. Their motivation to pursue what is right, in obedience to God, also gives them a source of wisdom and confidence beyond their own abilities. Michael Alison, member of Parliament and Prime Minister Thatcher's senior parliamentary aide, offers a clear example.

After his Christian conversion at Oxford in the forties, Michael Alison initially planned to go into the ministry. But his keen interest in politics—and a desire to serve his nation—led him to change vocational directions. Elected to Parliament in 1964, he quietly earned his way from the back bench to leadership.

In 1979 Michael was named minister of state for Northern Ireland, a responsibility that included administration of Ulster's notorious prisons. Then, in the late fall of 1980, young Catholic terrorists in Belfast's Maze prison began to starve themselves to death in protest of British rule in Northern Ireland. By Christmas the first prisoner had gone nearly two months without food and was near death. Worldwide attention focused on Belfast. Would the British government allow this young inmate to die, or would they force-feed him once he slipped into a final coma?

The prison doctor came to Michael Alison for the decision. It was, of course, a Hobson's choice. To force-feed the protester would cause riots among the Irish Republican Army faithful; to let him die would be callous.

Michael had been praying for weeks for wisdom in the horrible situation. "Go to the prisoner's fellow hunger strikers," he told the doctor. "Ask them to make the decision." The other protesters could not have their brother's death on their consciences, but in the process of putting him on life-support equipment, they saw the inconsistency of their own position. The hunger strike ended, the crisis averted.*

But while being biblically motivated and informed may give wisdom, it does not necessarily assure political success. In this arena Christians in politics are often at a disadvantage.

In the self-aggrandizing world of politics, Michael Alison is an anomaly. He seems more comfortable helping his adversary to his feet than cutting

---

*By the time of a second IRA hunger strike several months later, the protesters hardened their resolve, and ten of their comrades starved to death.

him down in debate. Though one of the most powerful men in British government, he has the unpolitical knack of blending into the background of any crowded political gathering.

His unconventional attitude begins early in the day with his morning devotional. "If I was consumed with politics," he explains, "my first priority would be the morning newspapers, not the Bible." But Michael's first priority is not his political career; it is his relationship with God.

Because of that, though Michael is conscientious in his work, his first ambition is not for the continued pursuit of position. He spurns political infighting and places a higher premium on trust than power. Of his role as Prime Minister Thatcher's assistant, he says he is one of the few people she knows she can take for granted. "That's the highest compliment I could hope for in my role."

This servantlike attitude is so diametrically opposed to society's that it can easily be mistaken for weakness. In reality it gives a greater strength. The Christian in a position of power is not enslaved by that position—and thus the Christian has tremendous freedom to follow the dictates of conscience, not the fickle winds of self-interest.

But Christians are also exposed to greater struggles of conscience. They are honor bound to be the best statesmen they can be, as well as the best Christians they can be. These competing allegiances caused British writer Harry Blamires to conclude that perhaps "a good Christian [can] be a good politician... but it is probably quite impossible for a good Christian to be a highly successful politican."[7]

Blamires may well have been referring to some of the dilemmas mentioned at the beginning of this chapter. Foremost is the issue of divided allegiances between God and the state. When there is a conflict of loyalty, the sincere Christian must obey God. Yet the politician's oath of office is to uphold the laws of the state.

The prevailing American view that faith is something private with no effect on public responsibility was first put forth by John Kennedy in a dramatic speech to the Houston Ministerial Association in the 1960 campaign. Protestants feared that Kennedy, a Catholic, would be bound by the dictates of the Roman church. So Kennedy pulled off a political masterstroke when he told the Texas ministers, mostly Baptists, that "whatever issue may come before me as president, if I'm elected . . . I will make my decision in accordance . . . with what my conscience tells me to be in the national interest, and without regard to outside religious pressure or dictate. And no power or threat of punishment could cause me to decide otherwise."[8]

Kennedy's message, which brought the house down, was a key to his election. But it set a precedent that has now become part of established American political wisdom: One's religious convictions must have no effect on one's public decisions.

But consider Kennedy's words: "No power . . . could cause me to decide otherwise." Not God? Though Kennedy's approach was enormously popular, it was also a renunciation of any influence his religion might have. He subsumed his church responsibility under his patriotism—or his candidacy.*

What else can a public official do? you may ask. The officeholder in a free society cannot *impose* personal views on the electorate; the democratic process must be respected in a pluralistic society. That is true.

Some go on to conclude, however, that the Christian officeholder is thus free, in the name of political prudence, to support or accept the majority will when it is contrary to Christian teaching (a view eloquently espoused by Governor Mario Cuomo in his 1984 Notre Dame address). Religious conviction is thereby reduced to a private matter; the social implications of the gospel are simply ignored. And as we have seen, the results of such privatization can be dangerous to society as a whole.

Another position, often taken in reaction to the Kennedy-Cuomo view, is represented by the fictional President Hopkins of our prologue, who was prepared to thrust his own theological view on an unsuspecting nation. This view, articulated by some in political debate today, argues that a Christian politician should use his position to speak for God.

---

*By contrast, Hilaire Belloc stood for election in 1906 in the British Parliament. As a Roman Catholic, he knew he would have to struggle to overcome religious prejudices, so he decided to confront the issue head-on. In his first campaign speech, he stood at the rostrum with a rosary in his hand and said, "I am a Catholic. As far as possible I go to Mass every day. As far as possible I kneel down and tell these beads every day. If you reject me on account of my religion, I shall thank God that He has spared me the indignity of being your representative." He was elected. From *The Little, Brown Book of Anecdotes* (Boston: Little, Brown, 1985), 50.

But such reasoning has no place in a pluralistic society and would, if carried out, make the frightening conclusion of Hopkins's fictional scenario entirely plausible. In his case the issue was not a conflict between human rights or human life and state policy, areas where a Christian leader must take a stand. Rather, it was a question of biblical prophecy, whose fulfillment is the responsibility of God, not man. Hopkins presumptuously, if unconsciously, played God.

Hopkins was also confused about the duty of government. As God's servant, his sworn task was to preserve order, promote justice, and restrain evil, which in this case meant acting decisively to prevent war in a volatile international situation. Richard Neuhaus writes, "To gain public office and take an oath before God to maintain the constitutional order, and then to use that office as a tool for advancing one's reading of Bible prophecy is an act of hubris, treachery, treason and deceit."[9]

Both views—privatized faith and using political power to play God—are deeply flawed. This brings us full circle: Is it possible for a devout Christian to serve in public office without compromising either his or her conscience or constituency?

It is possible. But only if the Christian officeholder understands several key truths. First, a government official must not play God; one's duty is to facilitate government's ordained role of preserving order and justice, not to use government to accomplish the goals of the church. Second, the Christian must respect the rights of all religious groups and insure that government protects every citizen's freedom of conscience.

There is an alternative to the imposition of religious values or the passive acceptance of majority opinion, a principle that pays both pluralism and conscience their due. Christian politicians must do all in their power to make clear, public arguments on issues of moral and political importance, to persuade rather than coerce. A recent Vatican statement put it this way: "Politicians must commit themselves through their interventions upon public opinion, to securing in society the widest possible consensus on ...essential points (matters concerning human rights, human life, or the institution of the family)."[10]

A third concern brings us back to the question posed at the outset of this chapter. What about the Christian responsibility in an age where national leaders in the nuclear age do not—perhaps, cannot—be entirely candid in public pronouncements? Consider the dilemma posed by the Reagan administration's disinformation campaign designed to unsettle the government of Mohammar Khadaffi—a murderous tyrant imperiling any number of nations. Confronted with this question, Secretary of State George Shultz defended the government's actions by quoting Winston Churchill: "In times of war, the truth is so precious, it must be attended by a bodyguard of lies."[11]

The pressures of nuclear-age diplomacy create conscience-wrenching agony for sincere Christians in office. Yet the Bible offers some surprising principles, citing Rahab, a prostitute, as one of the great heroes of the faith. Why? Rahab's place in history was established by the fact that she lied to protect Hebrew spies. Similarly, concentration-camp survivor Corrie Ten Boom lied to the Nazis to protect the Jews she was hiding. Most Christians today would likely do the same, for in this cruel and complex world, a lesser evil may be required to prevent a greater one. A Christian in public office may be placed in a similar situation, say, to save the lives of hostages. If the situation forced the Christian to lie against his or her conscience, the Christian should resign.

*   *   *

So far we have considered only laymen. But what about priests or ministers in public office, a question made timely by the presidential candidacies of the Reverends Pat Robertson and Jesse Jackson?

Before Constantine's Christianizing of the Roman empire, all Christians were advised to avoid civil office because of the idolatrous emperor worship it demanded. (In some instances that concern is as relevant today as it was in ancient Rome.)

Even after Constantine, church policy restricted members of the clergy from holding office on the grounds that civil office would inevitably prevent their giving full attention to their ecclesiastical concerns.*

At one point in England's history, the govern-

---

*There were few exceptions over the centuries; when they were made, it was to protect religious liberty, as, for example, when anti-Catholic legislation was being enacted in Hungary; the priests were released to engage in politics "for the sake of safeguarding religion or promoting the common good."

ment prohibited ordained ministers from holding office. The American colonists wrote similar prohibitions into several state constitutions, which remained in effect until 1978, when the U.S. Supreme Court struck down the Tennessee restrictions as a violation of a minister's First Amendment right.[12]

Despite the Tennessee case and the fact that the U.S. Constitution contains no such prohibition, the tradition remains strong. Few clergy have held major offices in Western democracies.

In the Catholic church, Pope John Paul's rejection of the tiara of temporal authority was a clear signal: ecclesiastical goals would not be sought through political means. Thus it was consistent that John Paul II in 1980 ordered priests out of secular office entirely. Five-term Congressman Robert Drinan, a Jesuit priest and outspoken liberal, quietly resigned.

In Nicaragua, however, three priests defied the papal order. This has been a major cause of the rift not only within the church, but it has compromised the integrity of the church. Those priests may say they are acting in a civil capacity but can they really disavow responsibility for the expulsion of missionaries, restriction on the free press, including *Iglesia*, the official Catholic newspaper?

The cleric in public office can hardly avoid such double-mindedness. And presenting two faces to the world inevitably damages the work that should be of primary concern: the witness of the church.

Regardless of one's stand on abortion, for example, no one could seriously imagine Sister Agnes

Mary Mansour as commissioner of Health and Welfare in Michigan, supervising state-funded abortions while in conscience maintaining her vows to a church that forbids abortion. Definitions of integrity have been stretched in recent years, but not that far.

Any priest or minister who feels called to seek public office should, as a citizen, be free to undertake that vocation. But doing so means that he must leave the pulpit, resigning all ecclesiastical functions. He must make it clear that he is acting as a private citizen seeking office to fulfill civic, not spiritual, goals. (In many denominations, however, the priestly office cannot actually be resigned.)

But if the clergy should not hold office, should the institutional church be silent on political issues? This is perhaps the most sensitive question of all.

As we've noted earlier, the church acts as the conscience of society. Christopher Dawson notes that Christianity is "the soul of Western civilization. And when the soul is gone, the body putrefies."[13] So the church must address moral issues in society and measure public actions by biblical standards of justice and righteousness.

But there are pitfalls. One of the greatest is the tendency Christians have to believe that because the Bible is "on their side" they can speak with authority on every issue. Many church bureaucracies have succumbed to this temptation in recent decades, spewing out position papers on everything from public toilet facilities to nuclear war. The New Right has engaged in such excesses with its scorecards covering the gamut of issues from trade legislation to the Panama Canal. When Christians use the broad brush, they become simply another political interest group, pontificating on matters about which they are often woefully uninformed.

A case in point was the U.S. Catholic bishops' position paper on nuclear war. It hardly seems necessary to convene a conference to announce that it is a moral issue to unleash weapons that would annihilate millions. The bishops did, however, and they went on to conclude that the deterrent posture of the United States was unsatisfactory from a moral point of view.[14]

That could be true—particularly if one realizes that our missiles are aimed at Soviet cities, just as Soviet missiles are aimed at U.S. cities. But deterrence itself is not immoral by definition; deterrence is impeding another nation's hostile act. The existence of a nuclear weapon (as with a policeman's gun) may prevent a much greater evil.

Any moral analysis must take into account the complexity of modern nuclear strategy and the actual efficacy of deterrence. To determine this, one cannot simply consider just numbers of bombs or throw-weight, but targeting studies and the whole range of strategic options: what would remain after a surprise attack; what defenses neutralize attacking missiles; what would the communications capacity be, and the like. Ironically, the country that renounces a first strike (the more moral position, as the bishops would no doubt agree) has need for a much larger deterrent capability (which the bishops

decry as immoral). The logical consequences of
their paper is a Catch–22.

While the bishops certainly could have commented on the immorality of unleashing nuclear war,
they simply didn't have all the facts necessary to
render an authoritative judgment beyond that. This
was summed up by a University of Chicago professor
who agreed personally with the bishops' position,
but concluded that they could not determine whether
deterrence was immoral because such judgment
depended on facts "which are secret—and thus,
unknown to the bishops."[15]

Russell Kirk, a Catholic layman himself, has described the delegates to such conferences as "uto-
pians . . . wondrously unaware of the limits of
politics."[16] Certainly the heated controversy resulting from the bishops' attempt to formulate United
States defense policy called their own competence
into question far more than the government's. After
attending a conference in which religious leaders addressed issues on every imaginable question of policy, most about which the church demonstrably
lacked expertise, Kirk mused that he would "as soon
go to a bartender for medical advice as to a church
secretary for political wisdom."[17]

Poland's Catholic bishops seem to have understood the need to deal with issues within their particular competence better perhaps than their U.S.
counterparts. When the Polish government engaged
in one of its periodic purges of political dissidents
in 1985, the bishops quickly condemned the persecution. A clear issue of human rights was at stake,
and the moral question was unambiguous. They

added, however, that "the Church is not and does
not, want to be a political force [but it] has the right
to give moral assessments, even in questions of political affairs when the basic rights of the individual
or the salvation of the soul demands it."[18]

The Polish bishops understood the restraints imposed on the church when it speaks as the church.
This is a crucial distinction. It is one thing for an
individual Christian to address whatever issue his or
her conscience dictates, but the church as a body,
which purports to speak God's truth, should speak
only to those matters in which fidelity to holy Scripture itself makes it necessary to speak out: issues
where human life or dignity, religious liberty, or justice are involved. Even then, the church should claim
no superior wisdom except in those areas where it
is uniquely able to bring biblically informed truth to
the debate.* An excellent example, one that stands
in distinct contrast to the pastoral letter on nuclear
policy, was the 1987 Vatican statement on human
life and biomedical ethics. It spoke forthrightly to a

---

*Russell Kirk quotes Renee Divismay Williamson at length in Kirk's classic
article, "Promises and Perils of 'Christian Politics'," *Intercollegiate Review*
(Fall/Winter 1982), 13, to clarify these difficult questions.

There are controversial issues in which the principle is unmistakable and
the command of the hour comes through loud and clear. On these issues
the church must make pronouncements....

But there are other general issues in which facts and motives are mixed,
consequences contradict the principles involved and equally dedicated and
knowledgeable Christians disagree. In these cases the church should remain
silent, letting individual Christians and Christian groups decide for themselves what Christian witness means....For the church to sponsor a political party, engage in lobbying, form coalitions with secular pressure
groups and become entangled in the decisions of private business corpo-
rations, would be to take a position on precisely those issues in which the
religious significance is unclear, ambiguous or non-existent.

clear biblical issue on which the church has special competence and about which the secular world was grossly confused. It has been perhaps the single most useful document issued thus far to clarify moral questions in the growing debate over reproductive technology.

Politics is not the church's first calling. Evangelism, administering the sacraments, providing discipleship, fellowship, teaching the Word, and exhorting its members to holy living are the heartbeat of the church. When it addresses political issues, the church must not do so at the risk of weakening its primary mission. As mainline churches discovered in the sixties, the faster they churned out partisan statements, the faster they emptied their pews.

And while the Christian citizens can afford to be as partisan as they wish, Christian pastors cannot. If they are, they may soon discover they have compromised both their own witness and that of their church.

An extreme example was the case of the bishop who presided at the May 1987 funeral of former CIA Director William Casey. Because President Reagan, former President Nixon, and a host of other government officials were in the congregation, the bishop used the occasion to attack U.S. foreign policy in Central America, for which the deceased Mr. Casey was an outspoken proponent. It was in such deplorably bad taste that the incident, reported worldwide, resulted in an adverse reaction not against U.S. policy, but against the church. Grieving families should receive spiritual comfort, not a political harangue against their loved one's views.

Admittedly a fine line exists here. It is clearly partisan for a pastor to stand in a pulpit and endorse a particular candidate, as some clergymen endorsed Jimmy Carter in 1980, and others endorsed Ronald Reagan in 1984. But what about Cardinal O'Connor's statement in the same campaign that a Catholic could not in conscience vote for a candidate who supported abortion? His remarks were reported as a partisan rebuke of the views of two of his New York parishioners, Governor Mario Cuomo and vice-presidential candidate Geraldine Ferraro. Admittedly, the cardinal's timing made his remarks suspect, but they could also be regarded as no more than a statement of elementary logic. Since the Catholic church believes that the taking of unborn lives violates God's law, could a Catholic in conscience logically vote for one who willfully violated that law? While I believe an open pulpit endorsement of a candidate is improper, I also feel that—if made responsibly from the right motivations—a cleric's statement that Christians should not support candidates who reject basic human rights is justified.

Within these limits, then, we can conclude that Christians, both individually and institutionally, have a duty, for the good of society as a whole, to bring the values of the Kingdom of God to bear within the kingdoms of man.

It is fair to say, however, that Christians have not done a particularly good job at this task. Often they have terrified their secular neighbors, who see Christian political activists as either backwoods bigots or religious ayatollahs attempting to assault them with Bible verses or religious magisteriums. In a pluralistic society it is not only wrong but unwise for Christians to shake their Bibles and arrogantly assert that "God says . . ." That is the quickest way for Christians, a distinct minority in civil affairs, to lose their case altogether.

Instead, positions should be argued on their merits. If the case is sound, a majority can be persuaded; that's the way democracies and free nations are supposed to work.

I'm often asked to meet with government officials concerned with criminal-justice policies. They are frustrated. The more prisons are built—at great expense—the more the crime rate goes up. So whenever I suggest restitution as an inexpensive and effective alternative to prison for nonviolent offenders, politicians are receptive. But only after I have cited the facts of the position (for instance, only one tenth of the cost of incarceration is statistically effective in reducing recidivism) do I explain that the source of restitution was God's law prescribed to Moses at Sinai.[19]

Christians are to do their duty as best they can. But even when they feel that they are making no difference, that they are failing to bring Christian values to the public arena, success is not the criteria. Faithfulness is. For in the end, Christians have the assurance that even the most difficult political situations are in the hands of a sovereign God.

This assurance comes from the teaching of Christ. Jesus likened the Kingdom to the humble act of a farmer sowing seeds. The farmer tills the soil, but the seeds sprout and grow because of a power beyond the farmer's control.

What Jesus was saying is that Christians are to do their part, of course, as best as they are able, but the manifestation of the Kingdom comes through God's power, not theirs. I saw this firsthand over a six-year span in one of the toughest penitentiaries in America. It all began with one of the most frightening days I've spent in any prison.

TWENTY-ONE

Signs of the Kingdom

> He also said, "This is what the kingdom
> of God is like. A man scatters seed on the
> ground. Night and day, whether he sleeps
> or gets up, the seed sprouts and grows,
> though he does not know how ... The
> Kingdom of God is like ... a mustard seed,
> which is the smallest seed you plant in
> the ground. Yet when planted, it grows
> and becomes the largest of all garden
> plants."
>
> —Mark 4:26–27, 30–32

They called it the "Concrete Mama," the nearly one-hundred-year-old patchwork of brick and concrete surrounded by thirty-foot walls set amid the beautiful hilly country of Washington State. Mama wasn't beautiful inside, however—not on that October morning in 1979 when I first visited there.

The state penitentiary at Walla Walla, considered one of the toughest prisons in America, had been cited by an inspection report of the American Corrections Association as overcrowded, filthy, and out of control. The inmates carried knives; homosexuals and drug pushers in silk shirts roamed the cellblocks; an inmate biker gang ran roughshod over underpaid and ill-trained guards as well as the other inmates. Walla Walla was, in the words of a longtime California warden, "Simply the worst prison in the U.S."

Four months before our visit a guard had been killed, and Walla Walla had been locked down ever since. That meant the prisoners were confined to their cells for twenty-three out of every twenty-four hours. Fifty-eight guards had gone on strike during the lockdown; most had subsequently been fired. Morale was miserable.

"When were the men released from lockdown?" I asked the officer at the gate, privately wondering who in my office had managed this kind of scheduling.

"Yesterday," he said, straightening his visored cap and squinting into the sun. "But don't worry. Riot police are standing by."

As I was digesting that heartwarming piece of information, the assistant warden, a former Jesuit priest, arrived at the gatehouse. "Glad you're here, Mr. Colson," he said cheerily. (I wasn't sure I was.)

"What's it like inside?" I asked.

He shrugged. "Tense, I guess. I don't really know. I don't get into the yard much. Whatever you can do I'm sure will help, though."

Unaccompanied by guards, we toured the concrete prison yard, and the cellblocks confirmed that the ACA had not exaggerated the conditions. The filth and overcrowding were incredible, and the tension in the air was as palpable as the concrete. The two thousand men in Walla Walla were angry.

At the moment their anger was directed at something that had happened during lockdown, senior chaplain Jerry Jacobson told me. The one relief from the sterile cement world inside the walls had been a grass playing field in the center of the compound.

There, the inmates could lounge on the grass and play football. But when the men had been released from lockdown the day before, they discovered that their field had been covered by tons of concrete.

Officials said it had been done for security reasons; the men hid weapons in the grass. Valid or not, the fact was that the prison was now solid concrete. And to make it even worse, during the days the men had been locked in, the concrete pad had absorbed the heat of the hot autumn days. In every way Walla Walla was heated to the boiling point.

Chaplain Jacobson accompanied me on my tour, including a visit to the dungeonlike basement cellblock containing the more than ninety men in protective custody. These were inmates who could not be mixed with the rest of the prison population: informers, psychopaths, and sex offenders. As we completed the tour, a crackling loudspeaker invited all inmates to the auditorium to hear me speak immediately after lunch.

The auditorium was a cavernous room that seated a thousand men. The acoustics were terrible, but the only other meeting place was the chapel, and no one would attend if it was held there, since the chapel was used chiefly as a meeting place for homosexuals.

At 2:00 Jerry introduced me. In front of 850 empty chairs and 150 pairs of unresponsive eyes, I told how Prison Fellowship began, using lines that never failed to produce laughter. There was stony silence.

Two older inmates stared intently from the front row. Both sat erect, arms folded across their chests with an air of authority. I concentrated on them as I concluded my talk.

Later, as I walked across the yard to leave, consoling myself that at least there had been no trouble, I heard a gruff voice call my name. I turned and saw the two inmates from the front row. The first, a man in his forties with graying hair, stuck out his hand.

"I'm Don Dennis. We've been talking, and we believe you," he said without expression.

The other inmate slapped me on the back. "Yeah," he said, grinning, "you're one helluva guy."

"We'll do everything we can to help you guys," I said, grabbing their hands. I didn't realize then what that promise would mean.

The following week I asked George Soltau, Prison Fellowship's most experienced instructor, to conduct two Bible-study seminars at Walla Walla.

When George arrived at the penitentiary, the chief of security told him that he expected a bloodbath any day. So George didn't know what to expect as he went to the private meeting that inmate Don Dennis had requested. With Dennis were six young prisoners who had long sentences, nothing to lose, and were ready, as Don put it, to "blow this place." George's palms were moist as he shook hands with each of the men.

From them George learned what we had not known the week before. After my sermon, inmate leaders had called off a riot they had planned. Six guards had been targeted for murder; there had even been talk of taking me hostage. Instead, the inmates had decided they could trust us and would seek our help in working out their grievances.

George was face-to-face with the kind of hatred and anger that leads men to kill. People's lives were in his hands. One misstep and the pent-up fury of the four-month lockdown would be unleashed.

George conducted a series of intense meetings with convict groups. When he learned that there had been no communication between inmates and prison officials for eighteen months, he approached the warden, who promised he would consider meeting with inmate leaders.

That promise at least bought time. When George returned to Walla Walla a week later, there was a glimmer of hope. The inmate power bases—the lifers, the bikers, the native Americans, the Hispanics, and others—who were almost perpetually at war with each other were at least, for the moment, talking. Two men had become Christians in George's seminar, and they, along with Don Dennis, were gradually taking some leadership. Several guards who had been charged with brutality had been dismissed, and the warden was still promising to meet with the prisoners.

Over the next few months, George Soltau and Al Elliott, another Prison Fellowship staffer, shuttled in and out of Walla Walla, meeting with prison officials and convict leaders. Progress was slow, but violence was at a minimum. One night, however, frustrations erupted. Several men slashed their wrists and barricaded themselves in their cells to protest conditions.

Al Elliott was called to the scene. He stood alone outside the barricaded cells and pleaded with the men. Pools of blood gathered on the concrete floor.

As Al talked, one man surrendered, then another, and finally the whole group. Medics rushed in with gurneys and plasma.

Later Al was in the mess hall when a chant began at several corner tables. The noise grew louder, echoing off the high ceilings. Al climbed on top of his table and shouted, trying to make himself heard above the clamor. Gradually the voices subsided.

"Don't blow this thing," he begged. "The politicians are beginning to listen, finally. But you'll lose it all if there's bloodshed. Chuck Colson has been asked to address the state legislature about the situation." At that, there was a loud roar of approval.

Two Christian politicians, Bob Utter, chief justice of the Washington State Supreme Court, and Skeeter Ellis, a newly elected Republican representative, had proposed that I speak to the Republican caucus committee about the conditions at the prison. When I laid out the hard facts of what I had seen at Walla Walla and what needed to be done, the legislators seemed interested, even receptive.

Later that day I gave the same message to an equally responsive Democratic caucus, and shortly thereafter the House passed a resolution vowing to deal with conditions at Walla Walla. This had no legal effect but signaled to the inmates that those in power were listening.

Justice Utter then organized a committee of prominent Christians to work with the legislators who were developing model legislation. My associate, attorney Dan Van Ness, now president of Justice

Fellowship,* and a Christian attorney in Seattle named Skip Li proposed several significant amendments, which were incorporated in the reform package. After his election Governor John Spellman appointed Amos Reed, a committed Christian, to head the state corrections system. Amos immediately backed the proposed bill.

Meanwhile, a federal court was nearing a decision on an inmate lawsuit complaining of conditions at Walla Walla. Indications were that the case would go against the state.

These developments electrified the atmosphere at the prison. "Someone has finally heard us," an inmate told Al Elliott, choking back his tears.

During those months I also met with representatives from each of the ruling inmate gangs. Al warned me that they were a tough and unusual bunch of characters. *They can't be any more unusual than anyone else I've met in Walla Walla,* I thought. I was mistaken.

At the first meeting they were waiting for me, shoulder-to-shoulder in a tight semicircle, at the bikers' club headquarters, a small, bare-walled room with one barred window. One by one I greeted them, some of the toughest inmates I'd ever seen. Their leader, Bobby, had black hair hanging over a leather

_____

*Justice Fellowship was incorporated in 1983 as the criminal justice affiliate of Prison Fellowship Ministries. As a national volunteer organization, Justice Fellowship works to make federal and state criminal justice systems more consistent with biblical teaching on justice and righteousness. It promotes restorative punishments, such as restitution and community service, based on the conviction that crime is primarily an offense against a victim rather than the state. For further information contact Justice Fellowship, P.O. Box 17181, Washington, D.C., 20041.

headstrap adorned with badges; a bushy beard flowed down the front of his leather jacket.

"Bobby," I said as I gripped his tattooed hand, "I'm here to help you."

His response was a nod and a grunt.

The next inmate wore elaborate eye makeup and deep red lipstick. He took my hand limply and said in a high-pitched voice, "Thank you, Mr. Colson." My eyes widened with shock; this was Bobby's cellmate, a transvestite and leader of the "Queens." Walla Walla had its own rules, its own code for survival. The inmates' hard eyes defied me to pass judgment.

In May 1980 the U.S. District Court ruled that Walla Walla had violated the constitutional prohibition against "cruel and unusual punishment." Trial testimony had produced a litany of horrors: an inmate sodomized by a guard, another whose leg had to be amputated because gangrene was neglected, a third held naked in isolation for four days. But what proved decisive was the startlingly honest admission under oath of warden James Spaulding. His prison, he said, ought to be "closed down." It was simply beyond saving.

The inmates were jubilant. Help might finally be coming.

George and Al cut back their Walla Walla trips to once a month. Even the guards seemed to breathe easier as the court order transferred inmates to other prisons and relieved the overcrowding.

But the transferred inmates created dangerous overcrowding at the other prisons, and by the end of the year bloody riots erupted. One inmate was killed, twenty-five were injured, and there was $2 million in property damage. The tension affected the entire prison system, and officials imposed new restrictions at Walla Walla.

By early 1981, despite the best efforts of inmate leaders to prevent it, Walla Walla was again seething. A gang burned a prison office building. The warden threw the troublemakers, along with several inmate leaders who had had nothing to do with the riot, into segregation. The arbitrary order infuriated the inmates, who retaliated with a work strike. Their one demand was the removal of warden Jim Spaulding.

Spaulding ordered another lockdown, and I returned to Walla Walla.

"Visit the hole," one inmate whispered to me. "But don't announce it. Just walk in." I followed his advice.

When the guards grudgingly swung open the heavy steel gate of B tier of segregation, I immediately stepped back. A foul mist hung in the air, giving an eerie glow to the dim overhead lights. Piles of rotting food and human excrement littered the floor. I had to force myself forward.

At the first cell the inmate rubbed his eyes. "You Colson?" he asked. Not even waiting for a reply, he continued listlessly, "What can you do?" as if my answer couldn't matter anyway. *Maybe he's right*, I thought.

I asked his name. It sounded familiar I said.

"No." He shook his head. "You might have heard the name, but it's my brother. He hung himself in here last week. Just couldn't take no more after a year!"

"A year!" I exclaimed.

"Man, that ain't nothin'." He shook his head again. "Some dudes been in here like two and three years."

Once outside I bent over, my hands on my knees, almost retching as I gulped the cold air of the prison yard. My face was hot, flushed with anger. How could human beings be allowed to live in such degradation? I made my way to Warden Spaulding's office.

Jim Spaulding was a decent and intelligent man, seemingly unflappable. But like his predecessors he had wrestled with the beast of Walla Walla and lost.

"Jim," I said, "you have to clean up segregation. Today. Use fire hoses or whatever it takes, but that swill has got to go."

"Wait a minute," he snapped. "What can I do? They throw everything at the officers. I can't order my men to clean it up."

"Have you been in that place?" I asked.

He shook his head.

The next day I held a press conference at which I described Walla Walla's segregation unit in detail. Spaulding fired back in the press, saying that the inmates "wouldn't let the staff clean the building." But soon thereafter, after a state investigation, Jim Spaulding was transferred.

Amos Reed, the corrections chief, began courting the Washington legislature to overhaul the criminal-justice system in the state. Justice Utter's committee continued to mobilize public support, and the court ruled in the inmates' favor and appointed a liaison to oversee the situation.

In the spring of 1981, almost two years after the

Walla Walla lockdown began, the Washington state legislature passed the first in a series of reforms. A sentencing commission established a policy to put nonviolent offenders in alternative programs. Early-release plans relieved overcrowding, and several million dollars were allocated to clean up and refurbish Walla Walla.

*   *   *

Easter morning 1985 I returned to Walla Walla. From the road approaching the gatehouse, nothing seemed to have changed. Concrete Mama still loomed on the hilltop, as forbidding as it had looked nearly six years earlier.

The new warden, Larry Kinchloe, met us at the gate. "Wait until you see this place," he said enthusiastically.

Our first service was in the protective-custody wing. The floors were scrubbed clean, most of the cells newly painted, and recreation areas had been constructed in every block. It was still a prison, cold and sterile, but it had been miraculously—if that's a fair term to apply to a building—transformed. The prison population was stable, conditions were decent, and alternative programs were beginning. The reform legislation was working, and millions of state tax dollars were being saved.

The service for the maximum-security unit was held in the brand-new chapel, and I stood at the door greeting the men as they crowded in. I recognized some I had met years before as angry, hostile convicts; by their open faces and enthusiastic greetings, I realized they were now brothers in Christ.

Then came one vibrant, middle-aged inmate surrounded by a cluster of friends. "Remember me?" he grinned and grabbed my hand. I struggled for recognition. "Don't blame you," he laughed, stroking his clean-shaven chin. "I'm Bobby."

It was Bobby, the boss biker who had lived with the transvestite. He was a Christian now and sat through the service with a broad smile on his face, holding a well-worn Bible.

I watched in amazement, realizing that it was not just an institution that had been transformed. The story of Walla Walla was more than legislation and fresh prison paint, important as those changes were. It was the story of transformed lives.

Easter weekend at Walla Walla ended with a fitting postscript, yet another sign of the Kingdom at work. Fred, a young man with a heroin habit and a robbery record, had done time at Walla Walla. The family of one of his robbery victims had prayed for him for years, visited him in prison, and eventually led him to Christ. During a subsequent parole hearing, Fred had confessed to additional crimes of which he had not been convicted, explaining to the startled parole board that as a Christian, he felt he could not do otherwise.

Fred's original conviction was overturned; he was released from prison and began to rebuild his life. He became active in a local church and got involved in a Christian ex-prisoner fellowship while awaiting his retrial.

As it happened, Fred's case was scheduled to be heard on Easter Monday. The Seattle Superior Court was filled with friends, family, and supporters who had already testified on his behalf. Fred had freely confessed his guilt; and now he told Judge Francis Holman that he was prepared to accept whatever punishment the judge deemed appropriate. For in any event, said Fred, "I am ready to go back to prison and serve Jesus Christ in there."

The judge leaned back in his tall leather chair and ticked off a long list of possible sentences. There was an awkward, drawn-out silence.

Then Judge Holman pounded his gavel. Ten years on each count of robbery—suspended. Fred would be free on probation, providing he would continue in a drug-treatment program and make restitution to his victims at 150 percent of their loss, or $2,200. He looked down at Fred again, his face still solemn: "We send you on your way with best wishes."

For a moment no one moved. Then Fred's pastor jumped to his feet and gestured to the packed courtroom. "Let's sing it!" he shouted.

A reporter for the *Seattle Times* captured what came next: "Everyone stood up, little old ladies in spring dresses, ex-cons, girls in jeans, men in business suits, a biker with his motorcycle jacket and helmet, prison guards—and they began to sing: 'Praise God from whom all blessings flow....'"[1]

Officials later said that it was the first time a Seattle Superior Court case had ever closed with the Doxology.

As I flew back home after that glorious Easter weekend in Washington State, I was exuberant. I have to confess I was thrilled at Prison Fellowship's involvement in the changes at Walla Walla, in the transformed lives of men like Bobby and Fred. Sending out a puffy fund-raising letter about the story was a tempting idea; the first lines were already beginning to form in my mind.

But as I started to put words on paper I was stopped by the sudden realization that I couldn't definitively say how the changes had come about at Walla Walla or who was responsible. Certainly George Soltau and Al Elliott had risked their lives going in there in the early days when the situation was red hot. Don Dennis, Bobby the Biker, and others played a vital role in convincing angry cons to talk with bitter guards and exhausted administrators. And then there was the work of Christian lawyers, legislators, and politicians: men like Amos Reed, Bob Utter, Skip Li, Skeeter Ellis, Dan Van Ness.

But the real transforming miracle at Walla Walla had been accomplished not by the efforts of all these people, but by the unseen work of the hand of God. I suddenly saw on the page before me the words of Christ—that the signs of the Kingdom of God are like a man planting seed. We do our part; but then God makes the seed—or the prison reform—grow.

And so I threw away my fund-raising letter, and the words of the Doxology from that Seattle courtroom filled my mind: "Praise God, from whom all blessings flow." For it is God who produces the signs of His Kingdom on this earth. We are merely the instruments.

We need to constantly be reminded that our efforts, vital as they are, will never bring utopia to this earth. Walla Walla, after all, is still bleak; it is still a prison filled with the angry, desperate, broken lives of those who seem unable to live in society. But it *has* changed. Because of God's power, not ours, Walla Walla is a "concrete" example of the Kingdom of God transforming places of hopelessness in the kingdoms of man. Justice and hope can now be found where there was once only inequity and despair.

Should Christians get involved in political issues and social reform?

Can anyone look at the story of Walla Walla and believe otherwise?

TWENTY-TWO

Perils of Politics

*Christian faith may work wonders if it
moves the minds and hearts of an
increasing number of men and women.
But if professed Christians forsake heaven
as their destination and come to fancy
that the state... may be converted into the
terrestrial paradise—why they are less
wise men than Marx.*

—Russell Kirk

Christians in politics can make a difference—as
Justice Utter, Skeeter Ellis, and others in Washington
State illustrate. But these men were only part of the
Walla Walla story. Private citizens, church groups,
the courts, wardens, even inmates all had a hand in
the process. Man planted, and God, using many people, brought in the crop.

But in recent years many Christians have urged
a more direct approach for bringing needed social
change: simply elect Christians to political office.
One spokesman has even suggested a religious version of affirmative action; if, for example, 24 percent
of the people are born again, then at least 24 percent
of the officeholders should be born again. Others
have argued that Christians should "take dominion"
over government, with those in public office speak-

ing "for God as well as for the American people."[1]

On the surface this shortcut might seem to some an appealing answer to America's declining morality. It is, however, simplistic and dangerous triumphalism. To suggest that electing Christians to public office will solve all public ills is not only presumptuous and theologically questionable, it is also untrue.

Today's misspent enthusiasm for political solutions to the moral problems of our culture arises from a distorted view of both politics and spirituality—too low a view of the power of a sovereign God and too high a view of the ability of man. The idea that human systems, reformed by Christian influence, pave the road to the Kingdom—or at least, to revival—has the same utopian ring that one finds in Marxist literature. It also ignores the consistent lesson of history that shows that laws are most often reformed as a result of powerful spiritual movements. I know of no case where a spiritual movement was achieved by passing laws.

In addition, history puts the lie to the notion that just because one is devout one will be a just and wise ruler. Take the nineteenth-century leader who forged a unified Germany from a cluster of minor states. Otto von Bismarck-Schönhausen was a committed Christian who regularly read the Bible, spoke openly of his devotion to God, and claimed divine guidance in response to prayer. "If I were no longer a Christian, I would not serve the king another hour," he once declared.[2]

Yet Bismarck was also the ruthless architect of *Deutschland Uber Alles* (Germany Over All), a chauvinistic worldview that laid the foundation for two world wars. Historians describe Bismarck as a Machiavellian master of political duplicity who specialized in blood and iron.

As we have said earlier, power can be just as corrupting—or confusing—to the Christian as to the non-Christian. And the results in some ways are more horrible when power corrupts men or women who believe they have a divine mandate. Their injustices are then committed in God's name. This is why an eminent conservative historian has suggested that "religious claims in politics should vary inversely with the power or prospects for power one has."[3]

It's a fair distinction: Prophets should make religious claims. Political leaders should not—otherwise they can become ayatollahs.

So the first test for public office should not be a spiritual one. The celebrated claim that "the ability to hear from God should be the number one qualification for the U.S. presidency"[4] is dangerously misguided.

Politicians, like those in any other specialized field, should be selected on the basis of their qualifications and abilities *as well as* on their moral character. Even in Israel's theocracy, Jethro advised Moses to select "capable men ... who fear God" to help in governing the Jewish nation.[5]

Jethro's advice makes sense. If terrorists were to take control of an airport, would we want policemen who were merely devout Christians handling the situation, or would we choose those who had specialized training in hostage negotiations? Luther had it right when he said he would rather be ruled by a competent Turk than an incompetent Christian.

470 ===== Charles Colson

The triumphalist mindset also fails to make the crucial distinction between a Christian's function as a private citizen and as an officeholder. As private citizens, Christians are free to advocate their Christian view in any and every form. In America that is a fundamental constitutional right. Christian citizens should be activists about their faith, striving by their witness to "Christianize" their culture—not by the force of the sword, but by the force of their ideas.

But Christians elected to public office acquire a different set of responsibilities. Now they hold the power of the sword, which God has placed with government to preserve order and maintain justice. Now they act not for themselves but for all whom they serve. For this reason they cannot use their office to evangelistically "Christianize" their culture. Their duty is to ensure justice and religious liberty for all citizens of all beliefs.

This does not mean they can compromise their faith or their first allegiance to God; they should speak freely of their Christian faith and witness Christian values in their lives. But they cannot use their offices to seek a favored position for Christianity or the church.

A Christian writer has summed this up well: "The 'Christian state' is one that gives no special public privilege to Christian citizens but seeks justice for all as a matter of principle."[6]

At the turn of the century a towering Dutch theologian, Abraham Kuyper, was elected prime minister of the Netherlands. His opponents voiced fears of theocratic oppression. Instead, his administration was a model of tolerance and public pluralism as

Kuyper affirmed proportional representation, that the legitimate rights of all be fully represented.[7]

If Christians today understood this distinction between the role of the private Christian citizen and the Christian in government, they might sound less like medieval crusaders. If secularists understood correctly the nature of Christian public duty they would not fear, but welcome responsible Christian political involvement.

But Christians should not unwarily plunge into the political marshlands, thinking they will drain the swamp.

There are traps. I know; I used to set them.

My first assignment as President Nixon's special counsel was to develop strategies for his 1972 re-election. A tough task. He had been elected by only a small margin in the three-way 1968 election against Hubert Humphrey and George Wallace. Not only was the Republican party a minority, but Nixon had inherited an unpopular war and a hostile press. Added to this, he himself projected something less than a charismatic presence for the television image-makers just beginning to dominate politics.

I studied the political classics, particularly the strategy devised by Clark Clifford for Harry Truman in the 1948 election. I learned that Clifford had curried the favor of disparate special-interest groups, one by one, assembling voting blocks into a surprise majority.

My first memorandum to the president outlined a similar strategy: write off the minorities, but reach out to traditional supporters in business and farm groups; pick off some conservative labor unions; cultivate Southern evangelicals; build a new coalition among Catholic, blue-collar voters of the Northeast and Midwest. I labeled it the "Middle America Plan," later dubbed the "Silent Majority Strategy." It was cynical, pragmatic, and good politics, designed to exploit whatever allies would let us cultivate them.

Nixon loved it. The memo was returned a few days later with his markings all over the margins: "Right. . . . Do it. . . . I agree." It became one of the key documents for the political strategy of Mr. Nixon's presidency.

Setting out to put it into practice, I began by inviting key leaders to the White House, following a scenario staged for maximum benefit.

First, they dined with me in the executive dining room located in the basement of the West Wing. I would escort my guests past saluting guards, down a long corridor lined with dramatic photographs of the president in action, then pause at the door to the dining room, pointing to another door to the right. "That's the situation room," I'd say in hushed tones. They all knew of the legendary super-secret national-security nerve center. The very words conjured up images of map-covered walls, whirring computers, and a bevy of generals studying the movements of Soviet aircraft. (Actually, it was then nothing more than a large, crowded office with some communications equipment and old charts on the wall; the real command centers had been moved to the Pentagon after World War II.)

The executive dining room was paneled in rich, hand-rubbed mahogany, lined with a waiting row of red-jacketed Navy stewards. Seated at the dozen tables, huddled in conversation, would be most of the cabinet and senior staff.

The dramatic effect overwhelmed even the staunchest adversary. One union leader, a lifelong Democrat who had never been to the White House before, blurted out during our first lunch together that he'd be available to help in any campaign. A Chicago alderman strong in the Polish neighborhoods signed up on the spot.

Those who needed more prodding were treated to a walk upstairs after lunch. If the president was out, I'd usher them reverently through the Oval Office; if Mr. Nixon was there, I'd ask (always by prearrangement) if my visitor would like to meet the president. His chin would drop as I led him in the side door, cut almost unnoticeably into the wall, and remarked casually, "Oh, Mr. President. I was just having lunch with Jim here. Could we say hello?"

Nixon was a master at the game. He always gave his dazzled visitor gold-plated cuff links with the presidential seal. The person would be overwhelmed as he left, almost bowing, not more than sixty seconds later. It's not easy to resist the allure of the Oval Office.

I took all kinds of groups to see the president, from friendly cattlemen to sophisticated educators enraged over budget cuts or the Vietnam war. It was always the same. In the reception room they would rehearse their angry lines and reassure one another, "I'll tell him what's going on. He's got to do something."

When the aide came to escort us in, they'd set

their jaws and march toward the door. But once it swung open, the aide announcing, "The president will see you," it was as if they had suddenly sniffed some intoxicating fragrance. Most became almost self-conscious about even stepping on the plush blue carpet on which was sculpted the Great Seal of the United States. And Mr. Nixon's voice and presence— like any president's—filled the room.

Invariably, the lions of the waiting room became the lambs of the Oval Office. No one ever showed outward hostility. Most, except the labor leaders, forgot their best-rehearsed lines. They nodded when the president spoke, and in those rare instances when they disagreed, they did so apologetically, assuring the president that they personally respected his opinion.

Ironically, none were more compliant than the religious leaders. Of all people, they should have been the most aware of the sinful nature of man and the least overwhelmed by pomp and protocol. But theological knowledge sometimes wilts in the face of worldly power.

I frequently scheduled meetings for evangelical groups, denominational councils, and individual religious leaders. Henry Kissinger's briefings in the Roosevelt Room across the hall from the Oval Office were always a big hit.

The weekly church services Nixon scheduled most Sundays for the East Room provided great opportunities as well. To select the preacher, we determined who would give us the greatest impact— politically, that is, not spiritually. At the time I was a nominal Christian at best and had no way to judge the spiritual. And there were always two hundred or more seats to be filled, tickets that were like keys to the political kingdom.

Then there were invitations to social functions and state dinners. I was allowed a quota for every event and filled it with those whose support we coveted most. It is difficult to resist the allure of that most regal of events, the state dinner, held in honor of visiting world leaders. Each of the twelve tables seated ten of the most influential people in America—Supreme Court justices, senators, ambassadors, film stars, cabinet members—and my targets for political support.

One instance I recall illustrates just how well the system works. We needed several electoral-rich Northeastern and Midwestern states to win the 1972 election—or so we thought. So one spring day I called a prominent Christian leader whose influence was particularly great in that region and invited him for a private dinner cruise with the president.

As we arrived at the Washington Navy Yard, sailors in white dress uniforms lined the gangway at attention and saluted as the three of us boarded the presidential yacht, Sequoia. Its mahogany sides and brass fittings sparkled as the grand old vessel eased away from its dock.

The Washington skyline faded into the distance, and the president escorted us to dinner in the main salon. White House china, silver, and crystal appointed the starched white tablecloth; stewards scurried back and forth serving chateaubriand and the vintage La Fête Rothschild.

The dinner discussion was as impressive as the

food. When our guest mustered the courage to raise
points of concern to the religious community, Mr.
Nixon showed an amazing grasp of even the intricate
details of those issues (as a dutiful aide, I had briefed
him thoroughly that afternoon). Every now and then
he would stop and say, "Chuck, I want this done.
This man is right. You order the attorney general to
take care of that tomorrow morning." Then he would
resume the conversation.

It wasn't all sham, of course. The president
meant what he said, and we even thought some of
the things might be accomplished. But whatever else
happened, that religious leader was convinced that
Richard Nixon was on his side.

Before we arrived at Mount Vernon, the president led us to the foredeck and stood at attention as
the colors were retired, his hand over his heart. Our
guest did the same. When the bugle had faded, we
docked; a waiting Marine helicopter took our new
friend back to the airport, and another returned Mr.
Nixon and me to the White House lawn.

It would be wrong to suggest that this leader was
unduly influenced; but even such a wise, honorable,
and religious man could not help but be impressed
by the trappings of power. He got what he wanted—
the president's ear on certain key issues. And we got
what we wanted.

Nixon's prominent public friendship with this
leader sent a powerful signal to millions of voters.
That fall we carried more than 58 percent of the vote
in many Northeastern and Midwestern precincts that
had never before voted for a Republican.

This is not to suggest that the Nixon White House

was engaged in a sinister conspiracy to corrupt the church. It is simply the way political systems work. People in power use power to keep themselves in power. Even if they are genuinely interested in a special-interest group's agenda—or naturally disposed to their position—they will work that relationship for everything they can get out of it.

In totalitarian regimes some officials are so unscrupulous as to feign religious interest simply to ensnare Christians. In Nicaragua, Interior Minister Thomas Borge maintains two offices. When he is receiving churchmen or American visitors, he sits in a Bible-laden office adorned with crucifixes. When he meets with government officials or visitors from socialist nations, he occupies an office displaying Marxist slogans and pictures of such revolutionary heroes as Marx, Engels, and Lenin.

I'm not advocating that religious groups or leaders boycott the White House or the palaces and parliaments of the world. That's where the political action is, and Christians need to influence policies for justice and righteousness. That is in the best biblical tradition of Jeremiah, Amos, Micah, Daniel, and a host of others—though many prophets clearly preferred the desert to the palace.

But Christians (and others as well) need to do so with eyes open, aware of the snares. C. S. Lewis wrote that "the demon inherent in every [political] party is at all times ready enough to disguise himself as the Holy Ghost."[8] Tolstoy made a similar point: "Governments, to have a rational foundation for the control of the masses, are obliged to pretend that they are professing the highest religious teachings known to man."⁹

Consider several of the most dangerous pitfalls awaiting the unwary.

The first is that the church will become just another special-interest group.

When President Reagan was challenged by the press during the 1980 campaign for mixing religion and politics by attending a meeting of Religious Right activists, he responded that the church was like any other special-interest group, after all—like a union, for example.¹¹ Reagan was refreshingly candid, but dead wrong.

The church is not and must never allow itself to become just another special-interest group lined up at the public trough. For in doing so, as one contemporary scholar observes, it would "sacrifice its claim to objective ethical concern which [is the church's] chief political as well as moral resource."¹¹

Tocqueville warned that if the church were to become a mere interest group, it would then be measured and honored according to political and not moral criteria.¹² The great strength of the American church, he believed, was that it was not linked to a partisan cause. By way of contrast, he pointed out that in Europe people "reject the clergy less because they are representatives of God than because they are friends of authority."¹³

A second danger is that politics can be like the proverbial tar baby. Christian leaders who are courted by political forces may soon begin to overestimate their own importance. The head of one large international relief agency mistakenly came to believe that heads of state welcomed him because of who he was rather than what he represented. It wasn't long before his work and his personal life failed to measure up to his delusions of power. He left his family and was eventually removed from his position—after doing great harm to the cause he had served for much of his life.

A side effect of this delusion is that rather than lose their access to political influence, some church leaders have surrendered their independence. "If I speak out against this policy," they reason, "I won't get invited to dinner and my chances to minister will be cut off." While such rationalizing is understandable, the result is exactly the opposite; they keep their place but lose their voice and thus any possibility of holding government to moral account.

In this way the gospel becomes hostage to the political fortunes of a particular movement. This is the third and perhaps most dangerous snare. Both liberals and conservatives have made this mistake of aligning their spiritual goals with a particular political agenda.

One Christian New Right leader, when asked what would happen if the Democrats won the 1988 U.S election, said, "I don't know what will happen to us."[14] After the 1980 election, a Methodist bishop wrote, "The blame [for Reagan's victory] ought not to be placed on all the vigor of the Right, but maybe on the weakness of saints." A better day will come, he said, "If the people of faith will be strengthened by defeat and address themselves to the new agenda which is upon us."[15] The implication was clear: if you disagreed with the bishop's partisan politics, you were not among "the people of faith."

Several years ago a prominent leader of a large Christian mission visited a Third World nation ruled by an authoritarian leader. The leader was friendly to the U.S. and held a regal dinner party at the palace honoring the mission executive. The awestruck visitor publicly and effusively praised the head of state. Months later when that head of state was deposed, the Christian's mission work in that country was deposed right along with him.

Inevitably, this kind of political alignment compromises the gospel. James Schall writes, "All successful Christian social theory in the immediate future must be based on this truth: that religion be not made an instrument of political ideology."[16]

Because it tempts one to water down the truth of the gospel, ideological alignment, whether on the left or right, accelerates the church's secularization.[17] When the church aligns itself politically, it gives priority to the compromises and temporal successes of the political world rather than its Christian confession of eternal truth. And when the church gives up its rightful place as the conscience of the culture, the consequences for society can be horrific.

As we've seen, many German churches in the thirties allied themselves with the new nationalistic movement. One churchman even described the Nazis as a "gift and miracle of God."[18] It was the confessing church, not the politically-minded church, which retained its orthodoxy and thus resisted the evils of Hitler's state.

Today's liberation theologians have fallen into this trap, putting ideology ahead of orthodoxy. It began, as did many Christian political movements, with noble intentions. Righteously outraged at injustices to the poor in so-called Christian cultures, priests and church workers began to organize communities for action. So far, so good.

But as those organizations failed to solve problems, frustrations grew; attacks on structures became more strident.

When Christians put economic issues ahead of spiritual salvation, they are embracing economic determinism; it is then but a short step to revolutionary politics, Marxism, and the fatal mistake of believing the Kingdom of God can be ushered in by political means, as Father Ernesto Cardenal, a Nicaraguan government official, well illustrates: "A world of perfect communism is the Kingdom of God on earth."[19]

Does all of this mean that Christians cannot work with political groups? Certainly not. In fact, often Christians must work with coalitions of like-minded people who have different motivations. But as Donald Bloesch has pointed out, "In order to maintain their Christian identity they must inwardly detach themselves from the motivations and ultimate goals of their ideological colleagues."[20]

In World War II, for example, a devout Christian might have fought to stop the evil of Nazism and the Holocaust because he believed God commanded that the state is to restrain evil. Next to him in the same foxhole might have been a soldier fighting solely for national pride or honor. Both would have been shooting at the same enemy, but for different reasons.

Today Christians may find themselves suspect—

I have experienced this myself—to the very people on whose side they are fighting. But that is the price they must pay to preserve their independence and not be beholden to any political ideological alignment.

Only a church free of any outside domination can be the conscience of society and, as Washington pastor Myron Augsburger has written, "hold government morally accountable before God to live up to its own claims."[21] And as the amazing events in the next chapter demonstrate, when the church faithfully fulfills this role, even the most determined of tyrants topple.

TWENTY-THREE

People Power

*Justice without mercy is tyranny, and
mercy without justice is weakness. Justice
without love is pure socialism, and love
without justice is baloney.*
—Jaime Cardinal Sin, speaking at a
    Prison Fellowship International
    conference in Nairobi, Kenya, 1986

A small Filipino man with penetrating brown eyes stared, unbelievingly, at his prison door's cool, smooth surface. It was 1972. Moments before, the door had crashed shut on him with metallic finality. It felt like a bad dream. Never before had he been in a prison. In fact, until that day he had expected to become the next president of the Philippines.

It seemed impossible—ridiculous, really. Benigno Aquino was the boy wonder of Philippine politics—mayor of a large town at twenty-two, governor of a province at twenty-eight, at thirty-five elected senator, the youngest ever. Now he measured the entire extent of his freedom in two or three paces. He sat on his bunk and thought, and as the day passed into night he continued to sit there. For the first time in his life he had nothing else to do—nothing.

Son of a wealthy family, this charismatic, gre-

garious politician suddenly found himself stripped
of everything that had propped up his ego. All his
plans, his friends, his busy schedule, all his carefully
cultivated followers were gone, replaced by the sheer
loneliness and boredom of the prison cell and the
venomous hostility of his guards. He kept waiting
for Marcos to send for him, to offer a deal. Surely he
could not simply leave him to rot in prison!

Half a year went by before Aquino was even
questioned or confronted with any charges. Then a
trumped-up murder case was brought, and a rigged
military court condemned him to death. This too was
a bad dream, for the real reason for his imprisonment
was President Ferdinand Marcos's greed for power.
With his two-term limit as president due to expire
in 1973, Marcos had declared martial law, granting
himself almost unlimited powers. He had thrown
Aquino and other political opponents into prison.
Marcos intended never to leave office—and so was
determined never to let a popular Aquino out to challenge him.

Prison had, for Aquino, the same bewildering
effect it has held for so many others. He lost all sense
of direction and perspective. He became bitter not
only at Marcos, but at the world, even at God. He
hated everyone and his prison guards goaded him
on. They sometimes put his dinner plate on the
ground and let a mongrel dog wolf part of it down;
then, kicking the dog aside, they gave what was left
to Aquino. He lost forty pounds. He suffered two
heart attacks. When he was not longing for revenge,
he wanted to die.

His mother, deeply concerned, sent him a book,

the memoirs of another prisoner. It was my story—
Born Again.

At first Aquino looked at it with little appetite.
Watergate was poorly understood outside America.
Nonetheless, there were similarities in our careers.
So Aquino read the book—and it touched him.

He read how I too had lost everything and entered the disorienting, mocking maze of prison. But
God had shown me that such losses were not in vain
as I found my true life in Christ.

Aquino began to search for the meaning I had
found. A voracious reader, he poured over the Bible
and other Christian books. He found great inspiration
in a little classic, *The Imitation of Christ* by Thomas
à Kempis. He was surprised to discover in reading
the works of an early Filipino hero, José Rizal, that
the same book had motivated his life and struggle for
his country.

One night Aquino knelt in his jail cell and gave
his life to Jesus Christ. Overcome with grief for his
anger toward God, he begged forgiveness. His viewpoints, his life, most of all his bitterness—all
changed. He had a sense that his life had suddenly
moved into a different channel with another purpose.

As Jaime Cardinal Sin of the Philippines has
said, it is hard for our doubting hearts to believe that
spiritual power—which is peaceful, prayerful, humane, forgiving, willing to suffer on the side of the
poor and oppressed—can change society. We know
the gospel affects the lives of individuals, but can it
make an impact on institutions and governments,
where the heartless realities of power pierce like a
knife? It is hard to fathom this.[1]

Nevertheless, it can happen. It does happen. One can never quite calculate how one conversion like Benigno Aquino's in a lowly prison cell may set in motion a train of events to shake a nation.

I met Benigno Aquino in 1980—a chance encounter, seemingly, on an airplane. He reached out to grasp my arm as we boarded the plane. "You're Mr. Colson," he exclaimed. "I must talk with you." Since we were blocking the aisle I offered him the empty seat next to mine. "I can't believe I am meeting you," he said. "I wanted to die in prison until I read your book." I knew when we had completed our flight, I had another Christian brother.

After eight years in prison Aquino had been released by Marcos under then President Carter's prodding. The grounds were humanitarian—he needed triple-bypass surgery. Aquino survived the heart operation and took a fellowship at Harvard. Marcos would not let him return to his own country.

Robert Shaplen, a foreign correspondent who had known Aquino for many years, wrote for the *New Yorker* magazine, "At fifty, he seemed to have acquired a new maturity, and, though he also retained his natural ebullience, a relative serenity that he had never had before. Some of his friends felt he had undergone something like religious conversion as a result of his years in prison. . . ."[2]

Indeed he had. Yet that conversion took away none of his heartfelt concern for his nation. Ninoy, as his friends called him, vowed he would one day return to the Philippines. If he could run for office he believed he would be president. If Marcos threw him in prison, then he would be president of Prison Fellowship. "If I'm killed, I'll be with Jesus," he told me, smiling.

Marcos was using martial law as a cover while he raped the country. He and his business cronies were bleeding the nation dry, making huge profits through monopoly powers and putting the money into New York real estate and Swiss banks. Meanwhile, half the working population could not find jobs. The ugly scabs of slums, many without running water or flush toilets, spread across Manila and other cities.

Marxist guerrillas were quickly gaining ground, and the military, riven by corruption, seemed unable to stop them. They found it easier to savage poor peasants than to fight the Communists. Things had reached the point where anyone who helped the poor was under suspicion. Filipino army units arrested, killed, and tortured even Catholic priests and nuns who had chosen to work with the desperately poor. A few Catholics had, it is true, taken the side of the Marxists, but the vast majority simply ministered in the name of Jesus to those in need. Between the Marxist insurgency and the Marcos dictatorship, there was little room in the middle.

Aquino knew Marcos's ruthless side—he had, after all, suffered in solitary confinement. He also thought he knew of a better side; he believed he might reason with him to restore free elections. So in the summer of 1983 he decided, after much soul searching, to leave comfortable Cambridge and return home.

Shortly before leaving, Aquino testified at a

congressional subcommittee: "It is true, one can fight hatred with a greater hatred, but . . . it is more effective to fight hatred with greater Christian love. . . . I have decided to pursue my freedom struggle through the path of nonviolence, fully cognizant that this may be the longer and the more arduous road. . . . Only I will suffer solitary confinement once again, and possibly death. . . . But by taking the road of revolution, how many lives, other than mine, will have to be sacrificed?"[3]

It was August 21, 1983. Benigno Aquino rose in Taiwan at 5:00 A.M. after only four hours of sleep. His first act was prayer. He then called his wife Cory, still in Massachusetts. She read the Bible to him over the phone. He spoke briefly to each of his five children, and tears spilled down his cheeks. After hanging up he sat down and wrote each child a letter. "The one regret I have," he told his brother-in-law who was traveling with him, "is that Cory has had to suffer so much."

Though Aquino had tried to keep his flight to Manila a mystery to the government, the plane was jammed with journalists. Filipino passengers, startled to find themselves flying with a celebrity, mobbed him. One woman repeatedly kissed him while news cameras clicked and Aquino squirmed uncomfortably. He gave a series of interviews to the journalists on board. The mood was celebration. Aquino hoped to lead a march of 20,000 supporters to Marcos's lush Malacalang Palace.

Eventually, when the plane began its descent, the cabin sobered. Aquino went into the bathroom, removed the shirt to his cream-colored safari suit, and grimly put on a bulletproof vest.

Back in his seat he thoughtfully removed his watch and handed it to his brother-in-law. "I just want you to have it," he said. Then he sat quietly as the plane landed. His lips moved in silent prayer.

The airliner eased to a stop at the gate and the jetway crawled out to clamp its mouth to the door. Journalists and passengers pressed their foreheads to the windows, watching for signs of trouble. Suddenly they saw a blue van pull up, and a contingent of uniformed soldiers carrying automatic weapons leaped out and circled the plane. Some of the passengers had stood up ready to deplane, but now a voice over the intercom asked them to be seated. "They're coming!" someone sang out from a window seat.

Three khaki-clad soldiers entered the cabin. Blinded by television lights and the commotion of photographers fighting for a good angle, they pushed down the aisle looking about them. The first soldier missed Aquino altogether, walking past his seat. But the second soldier, wearing sunglasses, recognized him and stopped. The third soldier leaned over, and Aquino smilingly took his hand. They exchanged a few words in Tagalog.

The soldiers slowly led Aquino through the crush to the front of the plane. Behind them came a sea of journalists, pushing, shouting. The jetway was jammed; no one could hear or see over the crush of bodies and the noisy confusion.

The soldiers escorted Aquino out of the plane door. But as soon as they turned the corner into the jetway, one of them opened the service door leading to a set of stairs descending to the tarmac below. The soldiers pushed Aquino through and slammed the door shut behind them. A soldier's body blocked the door window. Left inside, cameramen shouted, pushing and banging against the door. Nine seconds later, above the frantic noise, a shot rang out. People screamed, cursed. Then three more shots. Then a burst of automatic rifle fire.

At the foot of the stairs, sprawled on the pavement face down, his arms akimbo and blood oozing from his mouth, lay Aquino. He was dead, shot in the back of the head.

Two million people walked in the rain to his funeral. Soft warm drops from a gray sky glazed their faces, but they seemed not to notice. For hours they streamed through Manila streets, a seemingly endless mass of dazed people, moving as if by memory. Some wept. Some carried banners. But on the whole they were frighteningly silent.

Few Filipinos gave any credence to the military's story that a Communist-hired gunman had penetrated the tight airport security and shot Aquino, then died himself in a hail of soldier's bullets. They believed that their government had reached a new low; it had murdered, in cold blood and in front of the world, a man who had come in peace. It was an act so callous that it shocked many into action who had until then accepted corruption and violence with a cynical shrug.

Cardinal Sin gave an eloquent, moving sermon to those who found space in the crowded Santo Domingo Church. Among them was the frail-looking, grave woman who had read the Bible to Aquino on the day of his death: Cory Aquino. Privately Sin predicted, "This is the beginning, when people will be opening their eyes."

A few weeks later the government organized a rally in the affluent Makati district of Manila. No one quite knew why Marcos staged these affairs; the organizers sometimes slept through the speeches, and the crowds had to be bussed in from distant suburbs where ward leaders could round up, at ten to twenty pesos a head, enough people with nothing to do. But this time the utterly unexpected happened. From the glass and chrome skyscrapers of the Philippines Wall Street poured tens of thousands of office workers. They had not been paid to attend, but then they were not cheering for Marcos. They carried hurriedly scrawled banners: "I love Ninoy," "Ninoy our Hero," "Justice for Aquino—Justice for All," "Who Killed our Hero?" The air rained colored paper and computer tapes. It was an unprecedented, spontaneous outburst of outrage and—yes, unmistakably—of joy. No one had ever seen anything like it in the Philippines—People Power. Aquino's death had awakened them.

Jaime Sin is a heavy-set, jovial man with a face as round as a wheel, a deep infectious laugh, and a rich sense of humor. He was appointed cardinal in 1983, the same year that Aquino died.

In 1984 the *New York Times* referred to Sin as the most popular man in the Philippines. He is certainly a lovable character and a remarkable preacher, but his popularity was due to more than that. The Philippines was disintegrating, its deep tradition of democracy degraded by a government that made less and less pretense of justice. Aquino's murder brought a wave of grief and revulsion.

Marcos himself was rumored to be desperately sick; it was not clear who ran the government on any given day. Communist guerrillas grew in strength. Yet the moderate opposition was a rat's nest of infighting. Among this confusion only Sin and the Christian church he represented had credibility and moral authority.

Sin refused to serve on the official government commission investigating Aquino's murder, for he felt sure the commission would be a tool in the hands of the government. Instead he poured his energies into preaching the demands and privileges of the Kingdom of God. He sent pastoral letters criticizing the government for human-rights abuses; these were read in every Roman Catholic church in the Philippines. Yet Sin made clear that he did not speak for opposition politicians. He spoke for God.

He saw his role as a spiritual, not a political leader. Sin had been studying the Book of Chronicles. He saw in the account of Israel's corrupt leaders a parallel with the grief his own nation was enduring. *When God wants to punish a people*, he reasoned, *He gives them unjust rulers. Like Marcos.* So the answer is for the people to repent, turn from their ways, be converted, and seek God.

Among the lush green islands Sin preached to legions of poor farmers as well as the stylishly dressed elite. His simple message took root. His battle cry was "Cor," which means "heart"—an acronym: C for conversion, the changed life created through repentance and forgiveness from God. O stood for the offering of obedient lives to God—for true conversion had to make a difference in behavior. R stood for reparation—for the "making right" required of true repentance. Sin called Filipinos to prayer and fasting. Bible studies and prayer groups spread, even in the military. As Sin told one visiting reporter, "You will see our churches filled up. There is no space even on weekdays. . . . They are complaining to God. They are bringing their sadness before the altar of God."

Throughout the Philippines people felt that change was coming. But along with hope there was much fear. People did not know how change would come or with how much blood.

Cardinal Sin walked through the familiar halls of Malacalang Palace wondering just what he would say to Marcos. A glance at the velvet upholstery, the mahogany paneling, the rich heavy curtains reminded Sin that this world was well insulated from the climate of change he sensed throughout the Philippines. The ostentatious style smelled of money and privilege. What words would cut through the confidence of Marcos's political and business cronies?

Sin had talked to Marcos many times, to no avail. Marcos often promised to change or to investigate abuses. Then he would proceed to do the opposite of what he had promised. A crisis was coming for the Philippines. Sin felt it.

Marcos stood respectfully in welcome, though

he seemed to totter slightly on his feet. His handshake was weak; his face looked gray and puffy. Nonetheless he was the familiar man: shrewd, genial, talkative, sidestepping questions when it suited him. Marcos was known even by those who hated him as the smartest, shrewdest politician in Philippine history. It was very difficult to be sure where truth ended and fiction began with Marcos. It was not certain Marcos knew or cared.

"The reason I have come," Cardinal Sin said when the pleasantries were done, "is this, Mr. President. Your term of office is due to end next year. Why are you calling for a snap election?"

Marcos had announced elections to be held early in February, just two months away. It was not clear why. The U.S. had been pressing him, but why do it on such short notice? Did he realize how unpopular he had become? Why run when he was so sick? Sin had come to try to understand what he was up to.

Marcos smiled at Sin. "I want to have a fresh mandate from the people," he said.

"It is very dangerous for you to call a snap election," Sin said. "You may lose. You will be forced to step down."

Marcos kept a smile stuck on his mouth, but his bland, puffy face looked as warm as a cobra's. "You think that you understand politics, which they never taught you in seminary. So you interfere. When you should support your government in its struggle against Communists, you instead disturb the peace by criticizing. But you do not understand the way things are done. I cannot lose an election to an op-

position that is hopelessly divided. They will tear
each other to pieces.''

The two men stared frostily at each other. Sin
was angry—at Marcos's insolent words and at his
disregard for his own people's needs. He only cared
about power, not the good he could have done with
power. And he was so seemingly confident that he
could control, through political maneuvers, the people's will.

Sin spoke slowly: "Sir, I will unite the opposition in order that there may be a fair election.''

The two maintained a fierce stare. Did Marcos
feel a slight pull of panic underneath his expressionless mask? Did he have a hint of what Sin could
unleash? He gave no sign of it.

Sin stood. "Good-bye," he said. "And may the
Lord come down to protect our people." Without a
handshake he turned and left, his red robe swirling
behind him, Marcos still in his chair.

Sin, in anger, had crossed a line. Until that time
he had been very careful not to marry the church to
the opposition. He had maintained the careful role
of a church leader in the political realm: that of conscience, of reconciliation, of proclaiming God's good
promises. But part of the risk of politics is that emo-
tions become involved.

Sin was convinced only one person could unite
the squabbling opposition: Cory Aquino, the quiet,
self-effacing widow of the slain Ninoy. Sin knew her
well. He knew of her deep Christian faith. She alone
could raise the level of opposition above mere politics to a moral plane. She alone could ride on the

wave of emotion that her husband's assassination had begun two and a half years before.

But she claimed no political aspirations. Sin met with her several times, urging her to stand for the presidency. She always said no. Then one day, after a huge worship service celebrated in Manila's Luneta Park, which six million people attended, Sin returned home to find Cory Aquino waiting for him.

She was the opposite of Marcos; disinterested in appearances, she wore no makeup, and her simple dress was yellow, her husband's favorite color. Yellow had become the symbol of those seeking to carry out the work he had begun.

"Why are you here?" Sin asked mildly.

"I have decided to run," she said quietly.

"Cory, under what political party? Who will be your running mate?"

"I will run alone," she said.

Sin knew that without a political organization her campaign would be hopeless. "Don't do that," he said. "You cannot organize a political party now. There is too little time. You run under UNIDO, with Laurel as your vice-president. Will you do that?"

"But Laurel is planning to run himself."

"I will get him to agree if you accept him first."

After a few moments of quiet reflection, Aquino said simply, "Yes, yes, I will run with him."

Sin's face broke into a wide and sunny smile. "God bless you. Out of your weakness this great man will come down. He has been insulting you, saying that women are only good for the bedroom. So you will win."

She fell to her knees in front of him, her hands

clasped together, and Sin leaned down slightly to place his hand on her head and give his blessing. "I bless you and you will win." Cardinal Sin had now consciously crossed the line—to stay.

The Philippine election was remarkable for two reasons. The first was the outpouring of emotion that accompanied Cory Aquino wherever she went. Her motorcade was perpetually late because of the chanting crowds jamming the roads, the people swarming alongside her begging for a scrap of conversation or a handshake. She did not seem to care about the schedule: she always took time to talk to the lowliest person. Her campaign soon stood for more than a political faction; it became a festival of democracy. And it was accompanied by a great deal of prayer. Sin's preaching of repentance and conversion had made a deep impact on the nation, and now it bore fruit.

Democracy is not prescribed in the Bible, and Christians can and do live under other political systems. But Christians can hardly fail to love democracy, because of all systems it best assures human dignity, the essence of our creation in God's image.

Such a love for democracy was plain in the Philippines: in the cordons of nuns wrapping their arms around the aluminum ballot boxes as though they were protecting human life; in the crowds of fervent poll watchers, often from church groups; in the computer operators who walked off their vote-counting jobs because they saw the discrepancy between their count and the officially released results, and who were rushed to a nearby church for protection from the police. The enthusiasm, the tears, the confrontations all reflected a tremendous will for government of the people and for the people. Cory Aquino, in her calm, firm, common-sense manner—just the opposite of a glib, polished professional politician—seemed to embody democracy. She was a housewife pressed into politics by the need of her nation.

The other exceptional aspect of the election was the sheer cynicism and brutality of Marcos's party. They made very little attempt to hide what they were doing from foreign reporters, so American television audiences were shocked to witness ballot boxes stolen at gunpoint, votes purchased like potatoes, thousands of voters driven away from polling places by armed thugs. Filipinos were unable to see such reports; the state-controlled news calmly reported that everything was normal, that there were only scattered reports of fraud. But millions of Filipinos personally witnessed the election being stolen.

Sin had seen it coming and had issued a statement two weeks before:"If a candidate wins by cheating, he can only be forgiven by God if he renounces the office he has obtained by fraud. There will be no divine forgiveness for this act of injustice without a previous decision to repay the damage done."[4]

But apparently God's forgiveness was unimportant to those ruling the Philippines. They rigged the vote. All the passion for democracy and all the prayers of the people had not stopped them.

On February 14, one week after the election, the Marcos dominated National Assembly laid all doubts about their objectivity to rest by proclaiming Ferdinand Marcos the electoral winner. Public anger and frustration was mounting and the danger of it erupting grew more likely each day. Aquino called a protesting political rally for the sixteenth, a Sunday. Small knots of marchers gathered at different points in the vast city of Manila, converging from all directions on Manila's downtown Luneta Park.

Many wore yellow T-shirts in memory of the slain Benigno Aquino. Yellow headbands proclaimed, "I love Ninoy." Marchers carried signs and banners and chanted, "Cory, Cory." The procession gradually grew as it entered the main city arteries. Supporters poured out of apartments, slums, churches. They did not stroll; they dog-trotted along, swinging their elbows. Mothers, children, old wizened men—it seemed as though half of Manila was marching, singing, chanting. The air of celebration that had marked Aquino's campaign had hardened into a tougher sense of determination.

Well over a million people reached the park together. Elbow to elbow they sang "Bayan Ko," the haunting, emotive melody of Philippine independence:

> Even birds who freely fly
> When caged will struggle to escape.
> What more of a country endowed with nobility,
> Would she not strive to break free?
> The Philippines, my cherished land,
> My home of sorrow and tears,
> Always I dream to see you truly free.

Now, with such a mass of humanity together, the cry "Cory, Cory" seemed to saturate the air, the ground. Many wept.

This was the kind of crowd a politician might dream of. They would march anywhere, do anything, on command.

Yet Cory Aquino stood in front of the vast assemblage spread like a colored mosaic at her feet and spoke in her calm, rational, head-librarian manner. She did not send them to storm Malacalang Palace—though they would have gone. She asked them for a day of prayer.

She also called for a series of nonviolent protests—boycotting certain banks and businesses owned by Marcos cronies and setting up a "noise barrage" every evening after she spoke on the Catholic radio station. They were to do this patiently until the government conceded. "You have given a lot to the country," she said, "but in the coming days you will have to give more. We thought election day was the day of our redemption, but it proved the start of our further struggle."

A young Catholic bishop read a statement issued by the bishops two days before: "The people have spoken. Or tried to. Despite the obstacles thrown in the way of their speaking freely, we the bishops believe what they attempted to say is clear enough. In our considered judgment the polls were unparalleled in the fraudulence of their conduct."

The church leaders supported nonviolent civil disobedience. "A government that assumes or maintains power through fraudulent means has no moral basis," they said. "If it does not of itself freely correct the evil it has inflicted on the people, then it is our serious moral obligation as a people to make it do so." Nonetheless they warned against "the enormous sin of fratricidal strife."

Some American reporters left the rally shaking their heads. How could this nonviolent, prayerful approach make a revolution?

During that tense, rumor-filled week, it seemed the reporters might be correct. Marcos might ride it out. He controlled the guns, after all.

Marcos did not, however, entirely control the men who carried the guns. Secret meetings were held, mainly by younger officers. They discussed the possibility of announcing their loyalty to Aquino whom they considered the duly elected president. A plan was hurriedly formed in consultation with the minister of defense, Juan Ponce Enrile.

The officers were a group who, years before, had begun questioning orders to make arrests without legal evidence or to use torture in interrogations. Their military training had given them no basis for judging how to respond to such orders. When was it right, if ever, for a military officer to refuse to obey?

The search for answers had led them to Christ. They began holding Bible classes and prayer meetings. As they studied the Bible their sense of moral outrage grew. They began demanding change and became known as the Reform Group.

Benigno Aquino's murder heightened their awareness that more than politics was at stake. Perhaps they intuitively grasped that the dignity of the individual, created in the image of God, was on trial.

Now, with the election stolen, they felt it impossible to remain loyal to Marcos.

But Marcos discovered their plans to desert him and late Friday began to move loyal military units into position. By Saturday morning a watchful Enrile knew something was going on; he had reports of troops ferried into Manila. While eating a late breakfast with his daughter, Enrile received a warning telephone call from another cabinet minister. He suddenly realized that he would be arrested soon along with many others. He had to react within hours or face possible death.

They could flee the city. Or they could take a stand within Manila and appeal for popular support. There was no time to think through all the implications of the choices. Enrile elected to stay and at about 3:00 P.M. helicoptered into the ministry of defense headquarters at Camp Aguinaldo on the edge of town. Only a few hundred troops were on duty. It was virtually defenseless.

Enril's first action was to call his wife. He asked her to reach Cardinal Sin and appeal to him for help.

At 6:30 that night, as darkness settled over Manila, Enrile and a much-respected general, Fidel Ramos, held a press conference in Camp Aguinaldo. Radio Veritas, the Catholic station, covered it live. Enrile explained their decision: "We can no longer support Marcos as our commander-in-chief—because of our honest belief that he did not receive the people's mandate in the election. I believe in my heart and mind that Mrs. Aquino was duly elected president of the Philippines. . . . We will never sur-

render, and if we are assaulted, we will all die together."

Death seemed a real possibility. Though they
had stretched a thin defense force around the camp's
perimeter, they were sitting ducks. As military men,
they knew that they could be quickly overwhelmed
by superior forces. They could only hope that somehow, something would turn in their favor.

At 9:00 that night it did. Sin's familiar warm
voice suddenly came on Radio Veritas. He ordered
all nuns into their chapels where they were to pray
continuously until God delivered the Philippines.
Then he spoke to *all* Christians. "Go to Camp Crame
and Camp Aguinaldo. Lend your support to Enrile
and Ramos. Protect them and bring them food; they
have nothing to eat."

Within thirty minutes two million people were
on the streets. Unarmed, often gathered as church
groups, they simply waited, listening to their radios,
praying, and singing through the long night. No one
had told them how to carry out their unprecedented
assignment to protect soldiers.

Catholic believers provided the impetus for this
mass movement; but they were joined in the streets
by Protestants. CONFES, and evangelical Protestant
group formed to push for an honest election, was one
of the earliest groups to make its way to the gates of
the military camps. There, with barbed-wire fences
for their backdrop, they organized into shifts for the
vigil. They read Scripture, sang hymns, made signs.
Everyone felt the tension. This was a protest that
could end in blood.

The next day Marcos's troops began to come.

One long column of tanks and trucks carried a regiment of marines, headed by a muscular, bronzed general, one of Marcos's strongest supporters. In the midday heat the tanks ground noisily over the Manila streets toward the camps. Thousands of civilians crowded around, shouting, beckoning. Some of the crowd began hurriedly pushing cars and buses into a major intersection ahead of the tanks. A barricade of dozens of vehicles forced the convoy to a temporary halt.

Groups of marines armed with automatic rifles leaped out of the trucks and jogged to the front. They took up menacing positions, guns ready. The general came forward with his bullhorn and ordered the people to disperse. The huge milling crowd, composed largely of women and children, instead moved closer. Some held out crosses; others offered flowers. Still others were praying. An old woman in a wheelchair cried out for the soldiers; kill her if they must, but not their own people.

The soldiers did not know what to do. None of these rebels threw anything at them or even insulted them. Apparently they had no fear. Could they shoot?

"We're all Filipinos!" shouted one woman. "What are you doing? Don't kill us!"

One slender, brave woman pushed her way between two bewildered soldiers right up to the general. She threw her arms around him, calling his name. "You have a wife and children too! Don't do it! Don't kill us in the name of a dictator."

The general gently pushed her away. For some time he nervously surveyed the masses of people in front of him. Finally, he ceremoniously took off his bulletproof vest. "We don't want to kill civilians," he told one of his aides. "Our quarrel is with Enrile and Ramos."

He climbed on top of a tank and with his bullhorn told the people that the tanks would have to pass. "We will not hurt you. We have orders to enter Camp Aguinaldo."

"No, no!" people cried. Many threw themselves to their knees and began praying out loud. The general ordered his men to start the tanks. The people prayed louder above the roaring engines. The tanks jerked forward, their treads creaking and clattering. There were high screams of horror; men held their heads, anticipating the moment when the first bodies would be crushed. But just as the lead tank reached the first kneeling bodies—many of them priests and nuns—it stopped. For just a moment there was virtual silence. Then the crowd let out a prolonged cheer.

The top of the tank opened and a helmeted, bemused soldier poked his head out, looked around at the masses of happy people, and shrugged his shoulders, as though to say, "What can we do about this?"

By Monday morning there were dozens of such tanks on the streets all around the military camps, stopped not by antitank missiles but by the bodies of praying Filipinos. Young soldiers sprawled on top of their beached vehicles eating food offered by the people who had stopped them.

On Tuesday Marcos fled the country, defeated.

*   *   *

Benigno Aquino was felled by an assassin's bullet. But what he represented could not be destroyed. In two and one half years Marcos was gone and Aquino's wife was president. Miraculously it was a bloodless transition.

The problems of the Philippines were not solved overnight—and its political future remains clouded. Communist insurgents continue to try to achieve with bullets what the Filipino people have rejected with their ballots. And Cory Aquino's first year in office was shaky at best; this simple housewife with faith of iron, narrowly survived several coup attempts while she grappled to get control of a government that had been almost wholly corrupt.

I met with Cory Aquino in her office on the very weekend in November 1986 that she was to depart for her first trip to Japan. The press worldwide was speculating that her now defiant defense minister, Juan Enrile, would take over in her absence. Manila was abuzz with rumors. The young man who met me at the airport to drive me to Mrs. Aquino's office suggested I also visit Enrile: "He'll be president next week."

But Cory Aquino was at perfect peace. "I didn't seek this," she told me, "and I only want to serve my people. I simply have to put my trust in the Lord." Then she explained that she had given Cardinal Sin full instructions on what to say to the people if she were "unable to do so myself." I had the impression she could face death as resolutely as had her husband.

The next morning I went to Cardinal Sin's residence. We had met earlier when he addressed our International Conference in Nairobi—and we had become fast friends. I was delighted to discover at the chancery that the bishop had several months earlier instructed his entire staff to read *Born Again*. Several told me they had.

The cardinal, wearing a huge smile, swung open his door. "Welcome to the House of Sin, dear brother," he chuckled, enveloping me in a massive embrace.

During our conversation I expressed concern over the expected coup. Sin leaned back in his chair, rolled his eyes upward, and put both hands up, palms out. "There will be no coup, praise God," he said. Then with a mischievous expression he told me that he had met with Enrile the night before. "I've taken care of that, now you can do your part," he said, grinning. "You preach to those businessmen tonight from the Scripture." I was that evening to address a thousand conservative evangelicals at a major dinner. Many of them had been Enrile sympathizers. "You tell them to be born again—and pray for those in authority, for their Christian president."

There was no coup. Nearly a year after the revolution Jaime Cardinal Sin remained the most powerful individual in the Philippines.

*   *   *

Regardless of the future of Philippine politics, the February revolution will be remembered as the most remarkable church-state confrontation in this century. The contrast with Nazi Germany in the thirties is striking. In Germany the church was institutionalized and lacked evangelical fervor and the emotional support of the populace; so Hitler could strike fast and dismember it before it could collect itself for opposition. In the Philippines, on the other hand, the church was strong, the masses were powerful, conversions were sweeping the islands, Benigno Aquino was a powerful martyr, and there was never any doubt that the remarkable Cardinal Sin was in charge. So in the Philippines the church prevailed, withdrawing its moral legitimization for a corrupt, repressive regime; it succeeded in holding the state "morally accountable before God to live up to its own claims," as one prominent pastor put it.[5]

But the church went further than simply withdrawing its support. It was the chief instrument in the overthrow of Marcos. In an earlier chapter we discussed an individual's right to disobey the state, but this story raises even more difficult questions as to the role of Christians as a body—the church. What are the grounds for disobedience? What form may it take? And what about the role of the clergy, which, as discussed in previous chapters, is called to preach the Good News, minister to the church, not form opposition political parties. And in the light of Scripture, can Christians actively advocate and participate in political revolutions? The apostle Paul does not equivocate in his instructions to the Romans. God has ordained government to preserve order; Paul offers no exception because even a bad government is a better alternative than no government—which results in chaos.

But Paul also says that government's authority

is from God; it is a delegation. Therefore, governments—all governments—whether they acknowledge it or not, rule under God. But does God give an unrestricted delegation? Certainly not. As Jesus made clear with the coin, there are two realms—and Caesar is not to usurp what belongs to God. Any government that violates the law that is higher than its own is exceeding the legitimate authority God has granted.* As Dietrich Bonhoeffer put it, "If government persistently and arbitrarily violates its assigned task, then the divine mandate lapses."[6]

In that case the state becomes evil incarnate, as in Nazi Germany. Instead of acting as God's instrument for preserving life and order, it does the reverse, destroying life and order.

Then the church must resist. Though as argued earlier, the church's primary function is evangelization and ministering to spiritual needs; as the principal visible manifestation of the Kingdom of God, it must be the conscience of society, the instrument of moral accountability. Richard Neuhaus eloquently wrote that "the church can and should subject to moral questioning every political agenda or cause, thus keeping the entirety of human politics under the transcendent judgment of God."[7]

The real question then is not whether to resist,

---

*One eminent authority cautions that in interpreting Paul's word in Romans, a distinction must be made between government and nation. Government must always be respected, otherwise anarchy results; but the nation may attempt to venerate a culture or race. Donald Bloesch writes, "When the state is made to serve the aspirations of race or nation instead of the cause of justice for all, it becomes a demonic state warranting resistance and rejection by the Christian faith." Donald Bloesch, *Crumbling Foundations* (Grand Rapids, Mich.: Zondervan, 1984), 183.

but how. The same principle applies with the individual Christian. Earlier I cited the example of Daniel's refusing the king's choice food: Use the minimum resistance necessary to achieve the result.

The church's first duty then would be to publicly expose the state's immorality. Though I have argued that the clergy should avoid partisanship, it is not partisan to speak against unjust war—as the British bishops did against their own government bombing of civilian targets in World War II—corruption, oppression, the deprivation of civil liberties, or the taking of innocent lives.

As a second step the church should refuse to have any part in the state's immorality. When New York barred discrimination against hiring active homosexuals by private agencies that had city contracts, the church faced a serious dilemma: Lose vital financial support or violate clear, biblical teaching. To their everlasting credit the Salvation Army forfeited $4.5 million in state contracts; Augdath Israel Temple, $513,000; and the Catholic Archdiocese of New York, $72 million.

But what if speeches and sermons and noncooperation fail to deter the state? The church must take the next more severe measure of resistance lest its words be rendered hollow. In the abolition campaign the church used internal discipline and external pressure. The great evangelist Charles Finney refused communion to slave-holders. Others organized the underground railroad and rescued fugitive slaves from prison. Many ministers broke the law, were arrested, and some imprisoned.

But the state's evil, even as egregious as slavery,

does not give an unrestricted license to disobey any law; only the unjust law can properly be disobeyed. While active resistance may succeed, as it did with slavery and the Civil-Rights Movement, it may not, however, be enough in the face of the raw power modern totalitarian states have achieved. So what does the Christian do when all peaceable means fail? Is revolution ever justified?

Scottish reformation theologians like John Knox and Samuel Rutherford believed they could be, advocating the right of Christians to rise up against ungodly rulers. Many ministers in the colonies agreed as well; when they preached that the people had the authority to resist the king when the king violated God's commands, they were setting the stage for the American Revolution. After dumping tea in Boston Harbor the next step of resistance was the musket. A Boston preacher said that for a people to "arise unanimously and resist their prince, even to dethrone him, is not criminal but a reasonable way of vindicating their liberties and just rights."[8] John Adams observed, "The revolution was in the minds and hearts of the people, a change in their religious sentiments of their duties and obligations."[9]

Some Christian activists today loosely call for a new American Revolution just as the young radical youth movements did in the sixties. But as history reveals, revolution most often results, after the bodies are buried, in one form of tyranny replacing another. G. K. Chesterton summed it up well: "The real case against revolution is this: That there always seems to be much more to be said against the old regime than in favor of the new regime."[10]

So for the Christian, revolution is never to be lightly regarded. It is the most extreme form of disobedience. It could only be contemplated on the same justification as a just war; that is, that there must be a better alternative as a result of the revolution. Its advantages must outweigh the suffering, and the evil employed in the revolution must prevent a far greater evil than the status quo. This was the reasoning that caused Albert Einstein to abandon his pacifism in the face of Hitler's rise to power. "To prevent the greater evil, it is necessary that the lesser—the hated military—be accepted for the time being," Einstein contended.[11] It was this reasoning that caused Bonhoeffer to participate in the plot to assassinate Hitler.

For Christians to justify participation in revolution, therefore, they would have to be convinced that the state had become totally opposed to the purposes of God for the state and there was no other recourse to prevent massive evil.*

In the light of this, then, what about the Philippines? What lessons are to be drawn from it?

Though commonly called the February Revolution, it is, I believe, a misnomer. It was not the overthrow of an existing order, rather the replacement of a corrupt ruler, one who was clinging to power, in fact, by fraud and deceit, having reversed the outcome of a legitimate election. And the anti-

---

*The Exodus from Egypt is often cited as a model for political action by liberation theologians, but they ignore the fact that in the Exodus, God did not overthrow the political system in Egypt. He extracted His own people from that system, taking them to Mount Sinai that they might worship Him.

Marcos forces were unarmed, engaging throughout in peaceful protest.

So what happened in the Philippines was more like a coup, removing an unlawful leader. Mrs. Aquino was following the will of a democratic electorate that had been thwarted by Marcos's tyranny. She was not overthrowing, but rather restoring and fulfilling a system that had been in place since 1946.

But regardless of whether it was properly labeled a revolution, did the church have grounds to take the leadership it did? When I was in Manila in late 1986 I talked with businessmen and politicians, both conservative and liberal. The conclusion was unanimous: If Marcos had remained in power the Philippines would have collapsed and fallen into the hands of Communist insurgents. Those I talked to believed that justified the revolution; but that alone would not be a basis for the church to act.

Nor would Mrs. Marcos's 3,500 pairs of shoes or the incredible greed of Marcos, who stashed away billions in U.S. and Swiss banks while half the populace was unemployed and starving.

While no one could ever develop a rigid formula, it seems to me that the combination of the Marcos regime's refusal to allow free elections, the suspension of civil liberties, the massive corruption of the governmental process, the trampling of human rights, and Marcos's own blasphemous, at times messianic pretensions, gave the church a mandate to act. Cardinal Sin acted heroically in mobilizing the church to say no to evil.

And in the first stage his approach was entirely biblical. By preaching repentance and conversion, he encouraged outbreaks of spiritual revival all across the Philippine islands. He called people to pray for their country.

But when Sin stared down Marcos, in the passion of the moment, he crossed an invisible divide. He did not just denounce raw injustice. He married the church to an opposition political movement. And when he created the UNIDO ticket, convincing Salvador Laurel to run with Cory Aquino, he momentarily left the sanctuary and entered the back rooms of power-brokering politics. For this he was immediately chastised by the Vatican and disciplined again in early 1987.

Sin later acknowledged his excess, issuing orders that all clergy would remain out of partisan, political camps. He also announced he would stay "in the background." I know Cardinal Sin; and I can only hope that while he will keep his word not to step over the line, he will not fail to keep the church a vital instrument for holding government to moral account.

A courageous cardinal, the Philippine church, and two million ordinary citizens opened a crack of light in the dark canopy that envelops so much of planet earth. Through their civil disobedience and resistance to evil, the Kingdom of God has been made visible.

The late Francis Schaeffer once wrote, "If there is no place for civil disobedience, then the government has been made autonomous, and as such, it has been put in the place of the living God."[12]

The belief that government is autonomous, the ultimate repository of power, the solution to all of society's ills, is the greatest imposter of the twentieth century. As the next chapter demonstrates, Christians and the church have no higher calling than to expose it by every legitimate means.

TWENTY-FOUR

The Political Illusion

*Governments are composed of persons
who meet occasionally in a hall to make
speeches and to write resolutions; of men
studying papers at desks, receiving and
answering letters and memoranda,
listening to advice and giving it, hearing
complaints and claims and replying to
them; of clerks manipulating more papers;
of inspectors, tax collectors, policemen,
and soldiers. These officials have to be
fed, and often they overeat. They would
often rather go fishing, or make love, or do
anything than shuffle their papers. They
have to sleep. They suffer from
indigestion and asthma, bile and
palpitation, become bored, tired, careless,
and have nervous headaches. They know
what they happen to learn, they are aware
of what they happen to observe, they can
imagine what they happen to be interested
in, they can accomplish only what they
can command or persuade an unseen
multitude to do.*

—Walter Lippmann

What is so remarkable about the story of the Philippines is that millions of people believed more in the power of prayer than in the power of politics; they believed that the message "repent, be converted, and trust in Jesus" could topple even an authoritarian leader. They believed their deliverance was spiritual.

Such belief runs counter to the myth that all human problems are political and solvable by all-powerful human institutions. An extreme example was the prominent New Right leader who declared in 1985, after Congress failed to pass his legislative agenda, "The only way to have a genuine spiritual revival is to have legislative reform.... I think we have been legislated out of the possibility of a spiritual revival."[1] Evidently, the work of the Kingdom of God had been defeated by a majority vote in the kingdoms of man.

I'm sure that individual didn't mean to deny the sovereignty of God, but his statement insinuates that nothing can be accomplished except through government. Jacques Ellul could well have been describing this leader when he wrote that politics has become "the supreme religion of the age."[2]

This political illusion springs from a diminishing belief in God and the growth of big government. What people once expected from the Almighty, they now expect from the almighty bureaucracy. That's a bad trade for anyone; but for the Christian, it's rank idolatry.

The media encourage the illusion. Stories of spiritual conversion, growth, and revival don't make good thirty-second news spots. While the everyday actions of ordinary citizens lack headline punch, pol-

itics offers confrontation, controversy, and scandal.*
News coverage gravitates to political power centers,
exalting the momentary, assuring suspense. The public waits expectantly for the next installment in the
unfolding political soap opera.

On one level media and government are natural
antagonists; on another they are natural allies, depending on each other for their influence. News organizations concentrate their resources in political
capitals; governments gear their policies and decisions for prime-time audiences. The media spotlight
politics and politics feeds the media. Because the
illusion serves those with the power to perpetuate it,
neither side cares to expose it.

The 1972 summit meetings between the Soviet
Union and the United States provide a good illustration. All agreements had been reached before Mr.
Nixon's arrival in Moscow; there was nothing further
to be negotiated or discussed. The president, in fact,
was so bored that he resorted to calling me in Washington every night to discuss domestic affairs—at
length.

Though all the summit events were ceremonial,
television cameras covered every one. Anchormen
gave breathless blow-by-blow accounts of the five-
day proceedings. To the viewer back home, world
peace hung in the balance. (White House officials did
everything possible to encourage that impression.)
So as the world watched anxiously, the two leaders

---

*When religion does make the cover of *Time* or a spot on the network news,
it is usually the result of scandal, as with the extraordinary coverage of Jim
and Tammy Bakker. That's not a complaint; it's simply the way the news
business works, which in turn is merely satisfying the public appetite.

met, discussed the weather in Moscow, and signed already confirmed documents.

The 1985 Reagan-Gorbachev summit in Geneva followed an identical format—except there were no prearranged agreements to be signed. More than three thousand journalists pounded the pavements of the beautiful Swiss city, desperate for something to film. Some, in a daring exposure of East-West competition, compared the fashions of Mrs. Gorbachev and Mrs. Reagan. Others analyzed Mrs. Reagan's antidrug campaigns and Mrs. Gorbachev's interest in schoolchildren. Some cameramen shot footage of each other. A few gave up and went out for fondue.

In a rare moment, one network anchorman questioned whether the Geneva meetings actually warranted such coverage. Such a question treads perilously close to heresy. News is big business, after all, with hundreds of millions of dollars riding on Nielsen ratings. Network personalities hold multimillion dollar contracts, and they, as well as many print journalists, enjoy the handsome rewards of celebrity. Even in nations with public-owned media, the illusion guarantees power, privilege, and access to the elite. These are not willingly surrendered.

This unwavering focus heightens both the promise and expectation of what government can do. Political rhetoric, therefore, must offer panaceas to all human ills. Can anyone recall a major candidate who did not claim he could solve any problem if elected?

President Gerald Ford and his opponent Jimmy Carter, for example, devoted an entire debate in the 1976 campaign to the question of who would balance the budget first. Ford insisted he would do so by

1979; the best Carter could promise was 1981.[3] In reality, of course, both men must have known that more than 80 percent of the federal budget—entitlement programs and other congressionally mandated outlays—was beyond their control. Neither candidate could have balanced the budget.

But politicians have little choice. Modern technology has reduced all issues to their lowest common denominator. Since there is no time to explain the complexities of the budget process, and since instant perceptions shape voter attitudes, politicians can do no more than create appealing visual impressions.

In his memoirs, former Budget Director David Stockman chided Reagan aides Baker and Meese for being more interested in the evening network news than in government policy. But perhaps they were more realistic. Policy has no meaning apart from how it is perceived, and that perception is heavily influenced by newscasters.

That is why Lyndon Johnson obsessively watched three evening news programs simultaneously on a three-console television set. He knew public reaction to the televised portrayal of Vietnam would influence opinion far more than battlefield strategies. He was right: the outcome of that war was decided in American living rooms.

To maintain the illusion, government attempts to shape, even manipulate public perceptions. One of my White House assignments was to do just that. I chaired a committee of White House staff who worked full time studying daily news briefings, monitoring public reactions to presidential speeches, taking daily polls, and feeding positive information to friendly reporters. Often we aggressively tried to manipulate public opinion.

For example, immediately after every presidential speech, I would unleash a small army of assistants who would call key leaders in every walk of life. We might make five hundred calls, each following the same script: "The president asked me to call to find out what you thought of his announced policy...." The reactions would be collated, typed, and within hours a report surveying the opinions of hundreds of leaders would be in the president's hands. We got helpful information, but we also influenced public reactions toward acceptance of our policy. To be told that the president wanted one's opinion flattered even the cynics. Those called rarely offered a critical reply; most could hardly wait to call their friends and casually mention that "by the way, the president just called" to ask their opinion.

Our efforts were at times singularly successful. During the weekend of August 15, 1971, President Nixon was closeted at Camp David with his key economic advisors. The economy was sluggish, the trade deficit rising, and both unemployment and inflation were approaching what were then unacceptable levels of 5 percent. Something had to be done. Nixon was trailing in the polls with only fifteen months until the election.

On Sunday morning the president decided on a bold stroke recommended by Treasury Secretary John Connally: wage and price controls, and closing the gold window, thus allowing the dollar to float in world markets.

I was stunned—but at the same time impressed

with Mr. Nixon's boldness. For his entire political career the president had opposed economic controls; to make them work would require a massive bureaucracy. Other advisors were equally shocked, some predicting that the stock market would plummet. On one thing we all agreed: Mr. Nixon was taking the biggest gamble of his presidency. The policy's success would depend entirely on the public reaction— especially the stock market.

At 8:00 that evening the president announced his "new economic policy" on national television.* Even the news commentators were caught off guard. But before the president's speech was over, I was on the phone to the heads of the ten largest brokerage firms in the country. I knew most of them, and I knew how the pack mentality worked.

The first call was to an old friend. He thought the bottom might drop out of the market. I assured him he was wrong, that I had talked to five other brokerage firm heads and all were bullish.

Each call followed the same pattern, and by 9:30 I had spoken with the opinion leaders of Wall Street. Though most were unenthusiastic at the outset, they were quickly converted when told that everyone else expected the market to soar.

The next day it did—up 32.93 points, the largest single one-day rise in its history to that point. The media immediately declared the president's policy "the Nixon Rally," and as public support grew, the controls, mostly voluntary, succeeded—at least well

---

*We didn't discover until later—and to our considerable embarrassment— that the term *new economic policy* was not original. Lenin had first coined the phrase for his 1921 Plan.

enough to perk up the flagging economy just ahead of the 1972 election. It would have failed disastrously had the market turned down. (If I had not gone to prison for my part in Watergate, perhaps I should have for manipulating the stock market—not for personal but political profit. Such maneuvers, unfortunately, are not uncommon in the age of the political illusion.)

This manipulation of public attitudes by politicians is not a peculiarly American phenomenon. In the seventies President Nicolae Ceausescu of Romania, though a pragmatic and often ruthless ruler, was frequently photographed at the scene of fires or disasters. In deference to the media age, other Communist leaders, most recently Gorbachev and Castro, have carefully cultivated favorable public images. Castro even agreed to extensive interviews with compliant American broadcasters to clean up his image in the U.S. Even in totalitarian societies the illusion has power.

With government policy so dependent on public reaction, it's little wonder that the celebrity syndrome has become such a major force in Western politics. During the debate on the farm bill of 1985, for example, a parade of farm groups, agricultural experts, and government officials appeared before the House committee. The press found little to cover. No one was excited and the bill was mired in committee.

So the committee chairman scheduled actresses Jane Fonda, Sissy Spacek, and Jessica Lange to testify. All three networks covered the hearings. The chairman later gushed, "I knew everyone would pay attention when they came."[4] The bill was whisked through committee and was passed by the House.

What were the qualifications of these stars? None had agricultural expertise. But in a fitting tribute to the media age, all three had *played* farm women in recent films. Celebrities, as *Time* film critic Richard Schickel has observed, have become "the chief agents of moral change in America."[5]

The subtle danger of all this manipulation is that people no longer view their own circumstances as reality. Only what appears in print and on the screen is real. As Ellul puts it, "The man of the present day does not believe in his own experiences, his own judgment and his own thought. . . . In his eyes, a fact becomes true when he has read an account of it in the paper and he measures the importance by the size of the headlines."[6]

The individual gradually loses all sense of continuity. Whether a policy is good or bad, a success or failure, is of no account; all that matters is the emotion its instant image induces. No one remembers from one day to the next. On a Monday a president can say that "the Russians blinked." Everyone is happy. The next day it is disclosed the Russians didn't blink—we did—but no one remembers. So on to the next night.

The process is mesmerizing. Images pile on images, day after day, anesthetizing the public so they feel individually impotent and that all power resides in images they see on their television screens.* This eventually erodes their own sense of political re-

---

*This point is developed at length by Neil Postman in his masterful book *Amusing Ourselves to Death: Public Discourse in the Age of Show Business* (New York: Viking, 1985).

sponsibility and makes them easy prey to the appetite of an authoritarian state. Ellul believes that that consequence is irresistible. Jewish philosopher Hannah Arendt would agree, writing that the chief characteristic of tyranny is isolation of the individual, denying him access to the public realm "where he would show himself, see and be seen, hear and be heard."[7]

"Even democracies need institutions and agencies through which the individual can resist the tendency of all central governments to grow larger, stronger, and more domineering."[8] For the only thing that stands between the multitudes and totalitarianism, says Ellul, are the mediating structures of society: families, small groups of citizens, churches, voluntary associations that are independent of and resistant to the collective state.

Long before the age of instant media, Tocqueville made the same point that if the American experiment were to succeed, it would require the continued help of voluntary associations.[9]

Of all these independent institutions, the church should be the one best able to expose the political illusion. For the message of a transcendent reality is a resounding warning against the futility of seeking immortality from the instruments and institutions of this life. Mastery of nature through technology has given modern man the illusion that he has mastered life itself. The message of the Kingdom is that only God is master of life, and attempts to create alternatives to His rule are futile.

Hannah Arendt, who spent much of her life studying man's attempts to construct his social and political environment, has pointed out how Western society first learned this painful lesson: "The fall of the Roman Empire plainly demonstrated that no work of mortal hands can be immortal, and it was accompanied by the rise of the Christian gospel of an everlasting individual life to its position as the exclusive religion of Western mankind. Both together made any striving for an earthly immortality futile and unnecessary."[10]

My own experiences have repeatedly confirmed this truth; one incident in particular left an indelible impression. It happened in Colombia, South America, in the spring of 1984 while I was visiting Prison Fellowship ministry leaders there.

Immediately after speaking to the inmates in the central prison in Bogotá, I was taken to meet the minister of justice. Several Prison Fellowship Colombia board members were with me. It was late in the day, and the minister had a packed schedule. His announced crackdown on drug traffickers was all over the front pages that day. His aide suggested that I be brief, and I assured him we would confine our visit to five minutes.

Minister Rodrigo Lara Bonilla was a handsome young man with intense, penetrating eyes. He bounded up from his chair to shake our hands and invited me to describe Prison Fellowship's ministry. His English was flawless, so I spoke rapidly. Five minutes into the meeting I thanked him for his courtesy, particularly for allowing me to visit his country's prisons, and I prepared to leave.

He leaned forward. "You've been in the prisons?" he asked. "What do you think of them?"

Did he not know what rat holes his prisons were? I wondered. *Should I be politic or tell him the truth?*

I blurted out, "They're dreadful, sir."

"Hah!" He slammed his palm on the polished table. "You are right; they are pigsties, unfit for humans. Corrupt too. The inmates pay more for food than people on the street."

I was startled. Bonilla had a reputation as a reformer; he was leading a massive assault on the biggest industry in Colombia, the drug traffic. But never had I heard an official be so critical of his own department.

"What do you think we should do?" he asked.

I outlined the reforms Prison Fellowship has advocated in many countries. Bonilla's mind was razor sharp, and he frequently interrupted with questions. Our discussion went on for about a half hour.

Then he leaned back in his chair. "Finally," he sighed, "I've met people who understand the problem. Will Prison Fellowship work with me, Mr. Colson? Send me someone who can help straighten out these holes."

I promised to send an expert to Colombia the next month.

Bonilla then summoned an aide, instructing him that the ministry was to extend full cooperation to Prison Fellowship. We would have open access to the prisons.

After we had photographs taken together, Bonilla embraced me. It was spontaneous, as if to seal our covenant to join together to clean up the horrors of Colombia's prisons. I gave him a Spanish edition of my book, *Life Sentence*, which he said he would read.

Outside the office, our Colombian directors were jubilant. "This man is the second most powerful man in the government, expected to be elected president in the next election," one said enthusiastically. Another exclaimed, "With his backing Prison Fellowship will be able to do anything!"

Two hours later I arrived at the penthouse apartment of one of Bogota's leading businessmen, where I was to speak at a dinner gathering of business leaders and government officials. My host greeted me at the door, ashen faced. "Have you heard the news?" he asked. I shook my head.

He told me Rodrigo Lara Bonilla had been assassinated, shot to death by two gunmen—agents of the drug lords—as he was driven home from his office. I had been the minister's last appointment.

That night the president of Colombia declared the country in a state of siege. We were fortunate to get to the airport the next morning to catch our scheduled flight to the U.S. On the front page of the Bogotá newspaper was a grisly picture of the blood-spattered interior of Bonilla's Mercedes. On the seat, covered with shattered glass, was the copy of *Life Sentence*.

I was horrified at the death of this vigorous and brilliant young leader, saddened by the loss of a new friend. I was also sobered as I remembered our enthusiasm the day before. We had talked as if Bonilla's endorsement would assure Prison Fellowship's success.

A year later, in spite of the loss of this dynamic leader, we found that the ministry was actually flourishing, with more seminars going on in Colombian prisons than ever before. Though we had lost a friend and ally in a position of influence, the work of the Kingdom of God is not dependent on power in the kingdoms of man. "It is better to take refuge in the Lord than to trust in princes," wrote the psalmist.[11] Political kingdoms may rise and fall—but the Kingdom of God goes on forever.

Modern history is replete with similar lessons about the futility of putting ultimate trust in much-vaunted political systems. A greedy tyrant is over-thrown in Nicaragua; the idealist replacing him promises liberation and hope for the oppressed. The people are jubilant. But in a short time the liberator becomes the oppressor himself, resplendent in his $3,500 designer glasses. When autocracy is replaced by bureaucracy, only the icons change.

Ideology, which in so many parts of the world has replaced true religion, is powerless as well. As Ellul points out, the promised utopias of the twentieth century, either Marxist or Facist, are doomed because they accept the essential premises of current civilization and move with its lines of internal development: "Thus, utilizing what this world itself offers them, they become its slaves, although they think they are transforming it."[12] Even massive weapons of destruction fail to assure anything for today's mightiest governments. Wars reach no permanent solutions; there is no such thing as a lasting peace or, as Americans so fondly believed, "a war to end all wars." Terrorists stalk the globe, and governments can do little to stop them.

Wars proliferate; political solutions fail; frustrations rise. Yet we continue to look to governments to resolve problems beyond their capability. The illusion persists.

Nowhere is that more evident than in one troubled corner of the world. But even there, in the midst of carnage, violence, and hatred, the example of a few people offers hope, pointing the way for civilization to emerge from its darkness.

TWENTY-FIVE

The Indestructible Kingdom

That which man builds man destroys, but the city of God is built by God and cannot be destroyed by man.

—Augustine

Before my first visit to Northern Ireland in 1977 I stopped in England. Perhaps I could gain insight into Ulster by discussing her problems with British politicians.[1]

In London my friend Michael Alison arranged a dinner for us with a number of the members of Parliament. As we convened in an elegant Westminster dining room, a page stepped through a side door, formally announcing, "Gentlemen, the Speaker."

With that, George Thomas strode into the room. He was a short, feisty Welshman, bubbling over with enthusiastic good humor. In his black knickers, white

---

This chapter is based on accounts of actual events in the day-to-day struggle of Northern Ireland; all the participants are real people, and the stories are told with their permission. In a few instances, however, events have been consolidated and chronology reconstructed somewhat for purposes of clarity.

lace shirt, and powdered wig, he looked like he had emerged straight from the pages of Punch.

The beef Wellington matched the excellence of the conversation; seated next to George Thomas, I enjoyed myself immensely. After dessert I was asked to speak. I told the MPs about my conversion and responded to a number of questions. As the evening drew to a close, I said, "I've been answering questions all evening, gentlemen. Now I think it's only fair that we do a turnabout and I ask you one.

"I'm going to Belfast tomorrow for a series of meetings. Perhaps you could give me some insights into government policy and Ulster's political solutions." I paused. "What are the answers to the struggles in Northern Ireland?"

Several MPs glanced at each other; others toyed with their silverware. George Thomas grinned and then spoke for the group.

"That's easy," he said. "There is no answer in Northern Ireland."

*   *   *

Northern Ireland. A small nation with less than two million people. Yet scarcely a week goes by without a bombing, a shooting, or a riot. Between 1969 and 1987 several thousand people were killed and more than 26,000 injured in what the people of Northern Ireland euphemistically call "the Troubles."

The Troubles are centuries old and result from the clash between two deeply rooted traditions: the Roman Catholics who make up 40 percent of the population, and the Protestants who make up the other 60 percent. The Catholics tend to be Republicans who want Northern Ireland's six counties united with the Republic of Ireland and free of Great Britain's control. Protestants tend to be Loyalists, determined to keep their British allegiance.

The struggle is more political—a contest for power—than religious, however. As one wag put it, the combatants are Catholic atheists on one side and Protestant atheists on the other. And so deep is the conflict that it cannot be resolved by new political parties, British troops, or even the impassioned pleas of those who have suffered the most—the families of the slain.

Belfast, Northern Ireland's capital, lies between the chill waters of Belfast Lough and Lough Neagh. It is a gray industrial city of crowded nineteenth-century houses. Viewed from the air, the great ship-building cranes on the River Lagan stand like giant croquet wickets in the sea of gray and brick-red roofs. Smoke rises from tall chimneys nearby and blends with the low-hanging clouds that so often blanket the city.

In downtown Belfast nearly every block contains bomb-blackened, boarded-up buildings. Police stations of the Royal Ulster Constabulary are fortresses rolled in barbed wire, their thick, high walls tented with steel mesh to guard against the terrorists' habit of lobbing homemade bombs over the walls. Army vans filled with British soldiers are everywhere.

Yet the wartime setting is incongruous. Belfast is still a place of laughter, and the people are hospitable, friendly, and a bit apologetic about their country's reputation.

"Surely we're not as bad as you've heard we are?" a shopkeeper inquires anxiously. "We don't shoot strangers—just each other."

"Well, what do you think of the Troubles?" a cab driver asks. And when you apologize for not really understanding the complexity of the conflict, he responds cheerfully, "We don't understand it either."

Most would agree, however, that the modern struggle began in August 1969 when British troops marched onto the streets of Belfast and Londonderry, or Derry, as Republicans call the ancient walled city in the north of Ulster.

At that time unrest over civil rights and bottled-up bitterness had exploded into widespread rioting that the British government believed could be quelled only by a military presence. The soldiers' presence added to the tension. Sectarian shootings dominated the headlines, and the troops were targets of booby traps, ambushes, and bombings. The Protestant-controlled government, meeting at Stormont, the official government chambers, could do nothing.

Then came Bloody Sunday: January 30, 1972. British soldiers, attempting to break up a civil-rights rally in Londonderry, shot and killed thirteen demonstrators.

By mid-February retaliatory bombs were exploding in Northern Ireland at the rate of four a day. Those who survived each new blast lived in terror of the next. Citizens sometimes paid dearly just by going about their daily business, as did the six shoppers who died—and the 147 who were wounded—the day the Irish Republican Army, or IRA, left a gelignite bomb in a parked car in a busy Belfast shopping district.

Fifty-four days after Bloody Sunday, the Stormont government fell. British Prime Minister Heath declared Northern Ireland incapable of handling its own affairs and imposed direct rule from Westminster.

Since then there have been more than 2,600 bloody deaths in Ulster. One out of every twenty households has felt the pain of either death or injury from the incessant shootings and bombings.

It isn't the grim statistics that tell the story of Northern Ireland, however. It is the lives of those who live, work, and survive there.

Pearl and Karen...

It was a Saturday evening in Belfast, September 25, 1982. As twenty-year-old Karen McKeown drove her mother, Pearl, home from a special service at their Protestant church, she was still humming the song the choir had sung: "I will enter into His courts with praise." Mother and daughter talked about Karen's classes at Queen's University, Pearl's early shift the next morning at the hospital, the contact lens Karen had lost.

Pearl watched Karen, thinking her daughter had never looked prettier. Her dark hair was glossy and thick with a determined curl that Karen spent much of her energy trying to tame. Her new white sweater and skirt set off her dark eyes and pale complexion beautifully. *She has so much ahead of her*, Pearl thought proudly.

Karen dropped off her mother at home, waved good-bye, and headed back to the church to help clean up for Sunday services. She pulled into the church parking lot, got out, and was locking the car when a young man appeared by her side.

"I want you to know that I'm going to shoot you," he said, placing a heavy pistol against the base of Karen's neck.

He pulled the trigger.

The bullet ripped into Karen's neck and tore through her spinal column. She collapsed to the concrete, bleeding and paralyzed, unable to breathe. Her assailant ran away into the night.

Friends in the church heard the crack of the gun and called the ambulance, which took Karen to the Royal Victoria Hospital. By the time Pearl and John McKeown arrived, their daughter was fighting for her life in intensive care.

Pearl refused to believe that Karen was the latest victim in Belfast's endless violence. Only as she sat day after day by her daughter's bedside did the full implication dawn.

Karen could still communicate, and Pearl would lean close to her face as she mouthed her words. It was through those words that Pearl learned the answers to the bloody bitterness of Northern Ireland.

One afternoon when she arrived to visit, she found Karen propped up on several crisp white hospital pillows with tubes coming out of her throat, nose, and arms. Machines, screens, and dials monitored her every breath.

Karen's eyes brightened when she saw her

mother. "Mum," she mouthed, "could you squeeze my hands?"

Pearl gripped the slender fingers.

Karen's eyes fell. "I can't feel anything," she said. After a pause she continued, "But it doesn't matter. The only thing that matters is that we trust the Lord and never give the Devil a victory."

The inverted glass container of an intravenous tube was dripping a solution into Karen's veins, and the drug made her sleepy. Her eyelids batted a few times; then she drifted into sleep.

Pearl sat down in the armchair next to the bed, bowed her head, and wept. A few minutes later she looked up and discovered Karen awake again. "Mum," she whispered, "you think you have troubles. But just think about the troubles *his* mum has.

"When he said he was going to shoot me, I thought he was one of the boys from church, and I laughed," Karen continued. "It was as if the Lord put His arms around me. When I hit the ground I was still laughing."

Late that evening at home Pearl went into Karen's cluttered room and picked up her thick leather Bible. It had been a Christmas gift a year and a half earlier and was already worn, its pages marked with Karen's notes and underlinings. Pearl looked at the inside cover page where Karen had written, "To be a brave disciple is to be a bondslave to Jesus Christ, and to find that His service is perfect freedom."

In the Book of Job she found more notes. "This is not an explanation but an inspiration. Job's soul was a battleground without his knowledge. Could this be the reason for suffering today? In all cases,

God is supreme and just. The Devil functions within God's purpose." Karen's underlining clotted the chapters of the short book. "Though he slay me, yet will I hope in Him. . . . You will lie down, and no one will make you afraid."

Pearl's eyes filled with tears. Here in her daughter's strong, square script were notes that clearly prefigured what had happened. *If this is how Karen views suffering,* Pearl thought, *then this is how I must see what has happened to her.*

Meanwhile, the forensic results came back from the crime lab; the bullet taken from Karen's neck was from the same gun used to assassinate a prominent attorney. The gun could be traced to the INLA, the Irish National Liberation Army, a Catholic terrorist organization.

The next day Pearl went home, tired and frustrated, to pick up the mail before returning to Karen's bedside. A thin white envelope fell out of the stack of get-well cards and letters. The handwriting was unfamiliar. Her eyes went to the return address: Her Majesty's Prison, Magilligan.

She slit the envelope and unfolded the sheet inside. The writer explained that he had heard about Karen's attack through a Bible study in his prison. He was, he said, an ex-INLA prisoner who had become a Christian. He was no longer a member of the organization responsible for Karen's attack, but he wanted to ask Mrs. McKeown's forgiveness and permission to pray for Karen. Would she mind?

Pearl stared at the letter in her hand. The signature read "Liam McCloskey." She thought about her daughter's peaceful face, about the underlined

verses in her Bible, and about her forgiving spirit and
absolute trust in Christ. She realized Karen would
welcome this man's request.

Pearl jotted a quick note to Liam McCloskey,
enclosing an old photograph of Karen and telling him
a little about her daughter and her faith.

Liam...

Liam McCloskey had not always been part of a
Bible-study group praying for Protestant victims of
terrorism. For much of his violent young life he had
been a member of the Irish National Liberation Army,
an impatient, Marxist offshoot of the IRA—the same
INLA that would later shoot Karen McKeown. But
he had been changed unalterably during one of the
most notorious chapters of Northern Ireland's troubled history.

In December 1977 Liam had been convicted of
armed hijacking and robbery offenses. At the time he
was in his early twenties—a freckled young man
with reddish brown hair and a quick, whimsical
laugh.

Liam began his ten-year sentence at Belfast's
Maze Prison, the highest-security prison in the
world, where the immense perimeter was rolled with
huge coils of razor wire that could slit a man's skin
in an instant. Its eight steel and concrete H-blocks
were a forbidding reminder of both the desperation
of those in the Maze and the determination of their
captors. Though a good part of the prison population
were deemed "ODCs"—Ordinary Decent Crimi-

nals—the Maze was packed with those convicted of terrorist offenses.

Liam shared a cell with Kevin Lynch, a childhood friend who now shared the same political goals. Inmates like Liam and Kevin had at one time been given a political-prisoner status, but in 1976 the British government had rescinded that designation, preferring not to allow paramilitaries—Protestant or Catholic—special privileges. Ever since, the paramilitaries had been trying to get the status reinstated.

They had started with blanket protests, during which the inmates refused to wear prison clothes. When this failed, they began what was called the dirty protest.

Prisoners on dirty protest refused to wash, refused to wear clothing, refused to leave their cells. They sat on the concrete floor, covered only by a blanket with a ragged hole cut out for the head. They smeared their excrement on the walls and rinsed their hands in their own urine. Their hair and beards grew long and knotted, streaked with filth. Uneaten food molded in the corners of their cells.

Though the men inside grew accustomed to the incredible stench, officers often vomited and fainted. Visitors were nonexistent. Periodically the inmates were forcibly washed down with firehoses and moved to new cells while the old ones were cleansed and repainted. Then the cycle began again.

As the level of filth increased in the cellblock, so did the level of frustration. The inmates had broken the glass out of the narrow cell windows so they could smear excrement on the walls outside their cells. Orderlies used high-powered firehoses to clean the walls.

Liam would wait until they had rolled up the hoses; then he would put his waste out. One morning as he was about to do so, an orderly came past his window. On an impulse Liam threw the filth at him. The man turned his face away just in time, but it struck his shoulder, hair, and the side of his head.

Liam got down from the window and waited for the warders. It wasn't long before he heard the sound of heavy boots. The door opened, and he was told to put on a pair of pants. Then he was marched down the hall.

He was told to face the wall, then instructed to turn around. As he did so, an orderly hit him in the face. When he fell to the ground in a ball, a sea of fists and boots punched and kicked him. He was then taken to the punishment block where orderlies washed him down with scrubbing brushes. A bristle from one of the brushes entered his ear, opening an old wound from childhood.

Liam continued on the dirty protest for years, with periodic washings. By Christmas Eve 1980 the protest had accomplished nothing. Liam began to pray for inner strength and to read the Bible. Yet outwardly he seemed as deeply committed to his political cause as ever. "I was trying to walk with God and Republicanism at the same time," he says. "But there appeared to be more and more contradictions between the two."

Gladys . . .

While Liam McCloskey sat in his own filth on Christmas Eve 1980, Miss Gladys Blackburne was having her tea in a small Belfast flat and preparing to visit the Maze Prison. A retired schoolteacher in her midsixties, Miss Blackburne was an inch shy of five feet, with gently curled gray hair, sensible shoes, and a determined way about her.

In August 1969, when civil unrest erupted in Northern Ireland, Gladys Blackburne took her country's situation personally.

"I was desperately ashamed," she says. "The whole world was watching, and here in our land the name of Jesus was being dragged in the gutter. I wept and asked God to show me what I could do to honor His name."

Since then, Gladys had been doing what she believed God told her to do: to be the best citizen she could in her small troubled nation and to show the love of Christ to soldiers, as she was already doing with children, students, and other groups. That love was desperately needed. The soldiers were rotated out of Northern Ireland every few months; service there was too stressful for them to last much longer than that.

Whether they accepted her message or not, the soldiers loved Miss Blackburne. She had access to every army post in Northern Ireland, and when she wanted to visit soldiers in the field or injured men in the hospital, the army gladly gave her a lift. It was not unusual for Gladys to step out of a helicopter or an army lorry, handbag firmly in her grasp, and march off for a day of visiting soldiers.

She was also approved for a position on the Maze Prison Board of Visitors, a citizens' group set up to monitor the prison and report any irregularities or abuses. As such, she had access to any part of the prison, day or night.

On this Christmas Eve Miss Blackburne prayed about how God would have her celebrate the birth of His Son. *I must do something as near as possible to what Jesus did when He left His home in glory and was born in a Bethlehem stable*, she thought.

A stable, she repeated to herself. *Does God want me to go to the dirty protest where the cells smell like stables? I can't do that.* But Gladys Blackburne was not a person to take God's direction lightly. So she put on her coat and gloves, and prayed for the grace to be able to handle what she would find at the Maze.

She hitched a ride to the prison and cleared the laborious security checks at the main gate. Before she went to the cells of the dirty protesters, however, a prison officer took her aside.

"There's a Protestant lad in a different wing asking a lot of questions about Christianity," he said. "Why don't you visit him first?"

Chips...

Chips McCurry was sitting on the edge of his bunk, head down, when his heavy cell door swung open. A Protestant paramilitary, Chips had been committed to terrorism since he was twelve years old—when the IRA murdered his father.

When he was sixteen he had joined the Ulster Volunteer Force, an illegal paramilitary organization passionately opposed to Republican attempts to bring about a unified Ireland. He was bent on inflicting as much pain as his family had suffered. But on February 19, 1976, when he carried out his first order, it was to assassinate a fellow Protestant suspected of spying within UVF ranks. Chips was convicted of murder and sent to the Maze.

He was by then a thin, solemn young man with wire-rimmed glasses and thick curly hair already flecked with gray. After several months in prison his exposure to Catholic inmates made him realize that families on both sides had been fractured by the violence. *There has to be an answer*, he thought. *It's a political situation. There must be a political solution.*

Chips began reading everything he could get his hands on—first a flirtation with fascism, then a stint as a Marxist. He studied smuggled guerrilla-warfare manuals, hoping to start a full-scale revolution when he got out.

His political search ended in disillusionment. Politics didn't offer any real answers. Perhaps religion did. *If there is a God*, he thought, *and if there is a hell, then I'm surely heading toward it. But there are so many different religions. These Christians can't have a monopoly on truth. If I ever come across the truth, then I'll follow it.*

So Chips began a new search, questioning both inmates and officers he knew were Christians. They, in turn, began to pray for him. Tracts arrived mysteriously in his cell. He threw them all away. His search for truth was philosophical and abstract. He wasn't looking for any kind of personal faith.

When Gladys Blackburne entered his cell on Christmas Eve, Chips recognized her. He had often seen her in the prison and knew, like most of the other inmates, that "if you don't want to hear the gospel, then you'd better run when you see Miss Blackburne coming."

But there was nowhere to run. Miss Blackburne took the chair at the small desk directly opposite Chip's cot and asked if she could read some Scriptures. Chips prepared himself for a recitation of the Christmas story. Instead, Miss Blackburne opened her Bible to Luke 23, the account of the Crucifixion. She stopped when she came to the words of the thief on the cross: " 'Lord, remember me when you come into your kingdom.' "

"Now who was this thief calling 'Lord?' " Miss Blackburne asked Chips, her pale blue eyes looking intently into his. "Here was a man who had had a crown of thorns thrust into His head. Here was a man who was spat upon, stripped, beaten, whipped, and so disfigured He was unrecognizable. Does that look like a Lord to you? But this thief called Him 'Lord'—because Jesus was still Lord on the cross."

Chip's eyes fell. He didn't know quite why, but Gladys Blackburne's words made him aware of all the hatred and bitterness that had consumed him for years. For the first time he caught a glimpse of a connection between Christ's death and himself. *Christ was perfect*, Chips thought. *And I am full of evil—the sin He had to die for.*

He looked at the small woman. "How do I become a Christian?" he asked.

"You need to accept Christ as Lord, just like the thief on the cross," she said. "You need to turn away from your sins and believe that He died for them. And you need to confess Him as Lord to others."

Confess Christ as Lord? Chips hesitated. He had taunted enough Christians himself to know how hard that was in prison.

Miss Blackburne didn't push it. "Let me show you one more verse," she said. "Then I need to go visit some other friends." She flipped the pages of her worn New Testament and read him John 6:37: " 'He who comes to me I will in no wise cast out.' "

"If you come to Christ," she said, "He will never let you go."

After Miss Blackburne left, Chips McCurry sat in his cell thinking. Finally, late that night, he knelt by his cot and committed his life to Jesus Christ. He had seen the self-perpetuating emptiness of violence and the impotence of political philosophy. He realized he had finally met the Truth.

The next morning, Christmas Day 1980, Chips woke early. A cold gray light pierced the thick concrete slates of his cell. His first thought was, *I'm not really a Christian.*

Then he remembered Miss Blackburne's words: "If you come to Christ, He will never let you go."

At the usual time Chips was released from his cell to go to the canteen for breakfast; there he smiled broadly as he stirred sugar into his tea. The man across the small table glared at him.

"What're you smilin' about?" he growled. "No

one smiles in prison on Christmas morning."

Here I go, Chips thought. Aloud he said, "I've become a Christian."

The man exploded, his kindest incrimination being to call Chips a phony.

"Just wait and see," Chips told the man.

Liam ...

That same Christmas morning, the Catholic prisoners in the Maze were preparing for their final protest. The dirty protests had achieved nothing; paramilitaries were still denied political status. In pursuit of their objectives, the IRA leaders determined to turn the violence upon themselves.

Hunger strikes had been a revered form of protest for IRA faithful since the turn of the century. To threaten death by starvation was an act of defiance that could not be ignored—or so the IRA leaders thought.

A hunger strike held that fall had already ended in failure, however; no one died and no demands were met. So the IRA asked for volunteers to begin a new strike—to the death. One hundred of the Maze's seven hundred Catholic paramilitaries volunteered.

Liam McCloskey was one of those men.

At first Liam had wanted nothing to do with the hunger strikes, since he was questioning his political allegiance anyway. Then Liam's cellmate, Kevin, signed up for the strike. In spite of a knot of fear within him, Liam signed up as well.

Bobby Sands, leader of the Catholic inmates, was

to begin the fast in early March. Shouting through his cell door to the others on the wing, he said there was a strong possibility he would die. But if he did, Sands said, it could be enough to "light the flame of freedom in the Irish people's hearts that would lead to British withdrawal and a Socialist Ireland."

Though attention to the hunger strike grew slowly, a county election in which Bobby Sands was elected to Parliament on April 9, 1981, gave it the boost it needed to capture the interest of the world press. Liam hoped the publicity would save Bobby's life, but it was not to be.

Death [came] at last to convicted IRA Terrorist and Hunger Striker Robert (Bobby) Gerard Sands, 27, by virtue of his own will. His earthly remains were little more than a husk after a 66-day fast in the H-block section of Northern Ireland's Maze Prison. . . .

As the clanging of garbage can lids announced the news of Sands' death, gangs of Catholic youths once again rampaged through the streets, despite calls from the IRA itself for calm as the organization prepared its martyr's farewell. . . . One youngster blew himself up as he tried to plant a crudely made bomb . . . a Belfast policeman was shot to death. . . . Heavy police protection was given to scores of British Members of Parliament.

Sands' fatal hunger strike now appears to be only the prelude to a sustained movement by other Maze prisoners. . . . One senior Whitehall official repeated the government's refusal to compromise with the prisoners or to propose any solutions to the deeper problems in the near term. The situation was, he said, evoking centuries of bitterness, "a classic Irish tragedy from which at the moment

there seems no escape." The desperate death of Bobby
Sands appears to be the start of a new chapter in just such a
prolonged and dangerous tragedy.[2]

Then came Kevin's turn to strike. Liam was
racked with doubts and questions. He refused to believe that his cellmate would die. Yet it had become
apparent that the British government was digging in
on the issue and that there was little hope of a solution. Liam also wrestled with the fact that he was
next on the list. His fear of death made him hesitant,
along with his own changing views and growing
faith. *Since I have doubts about the rights and wrongs
of killing,* he thought, *I won't be any good to Republicanism. And since I haven't fully accepted the
Word of God, I'm no good to Him either. Better that
I die than someone who would be of use to the movement.*

Kevin died. *My own hunger strike,* Liam thought,
*will be my last act as a Republican, one way or an-
other. Live or die.*

Even when the end is not far off, there are some lighter
moments. Only days before he died, Kevin Lynch asked his
family to bring him some cigars. He lay there, his body
emaciated, his voice a whisper, blowing smoke toward the
ceiling.[3]

Liam began the strike on August 3, 1981, a Monday morning.

Hundreds of families . . . live in dread of the sudden
news that their sons have volunteered to starve. When the

name of the latest hunger volunteer, Liam McCloskey, 25, was announced last week, his [family] protested to the IRA that their son had a chronic ear infection that could cause early death. They dared to express their indignation.[4]

During the first two weeks of the strike, Liam's main problems were coldness and an almost over-whelming desire to eat one last pea, chip, or bean just to taste food again. Food was blown out of pro-portion in his mind.

But after two weeks, the war of nerves becomes irrelevant. The trays kept arriving, but by now the prisoners have lost their craving for food. The stomach cramps and pains recede and eventually disappear. The prisoners concentrate instead on their daily five pints of water. Now their only concern is whether they can hold down the water without retching. A small bowl of salt is provided for each prisoner, and he can sprinkle in as much as he wants. When the hunger strikes are far along, the prisoners ask for carbonated water and the British grant the request.

This is the world of the zealots, where Irish youth are willing to starve themselves for their cause of driving the British out of Northern Ireland. It is an astounding kind of sacrifice—a brutal, lingering death, full of hatred and martyrdom, so fanatical and Irish. The moment one striker dies, 50 volunteer to take his place.[5]

After four weeks, Liam was moved to the prison hospital. On his forty-second day of the strike, August 14, 1981, his eyes began to roll uncontrollably back and forth and he began to vomit green digestive fluid. Within a few days the vomiting eased, but August 17 Liam was totally blind.

At 42 days, almost exactly, a nightmarish experience occurs. . . . They are struck by something called nystagmus, a loss of muscular control due to severe vitamin deficiency. If they look sideways, their eyes begin to gyrate wildly and uncontrollably, first horizontally and then vertically. The prisoners struggle to stare straight forward, even cupping their hands against the sides of their heads, but they cannot help themselves. . . .

Now the end is not far off. Their speech is slurred, and they try not to talk because the sound of their own voices echoes in their heads. Their hearing is failing and visitors have to shout during normal conversations. They are slowly going blind. Even their sense of smell is failing.[6]

Liam began to pray. *There has to be a God,* he thought. *Life makes no sense without one.* He thought back on twenty-five years of life with nothing to show for it. *Can I go before God with nothing but a self-centered life of striving after sex, drink, and good times? And what about my involvement in Republicanism?*

If I had continued as I was outside of prison, he thought, *I would have taken life for that cause. Who was I that I should appoint myself judge, jury, and executioner of any man?*

Will my life even show up as a dot on eternity? he wondered. *Here I am, about to throw it all away for Ireland, like countless others who are prepared to do evil for Ireland or Ulster or Britain.*

By this time the hunger strike was falling apart.

Ten men had died; one protester was taken off the strike by his mother, another by his wife. Liam's resolve weakened. Yet he felt he had to keep going for the sake of his fellow prisoners. He also decided it would be better to die than to live blind. Still, he prayed the prayer that had haunted him since he began the strike: "Not mine, but Thy will be done."

By August 26, his fifty-fourth day on the strike, Liam knew he would be in a final coma in a day or two. How great it would be to walk through a field of grass, to smell flowers, to see the waves lapping on the seashore. His thoughts were hazy and dream-like.

David...

While Liam McCloskey lay dying in the Maze, a Protestant inmate in a prison on the other side of Belfast knelt in prayer for him. Yet anyone who knew David Hamilton would have said it most unlikely that he would pray for the recovery of a Catholic terrorist, for David had spent most of his life trying to eliminate enemies like Liam. His hatred of Catholics had started young.

David had grown up in Rathcoole, the largest government housing project in Europe, a product of a late-fifties Belfast slum-clearance program that moved the urban working class into the suburbs. Yet even with its bare concrete row houses and its maze of high-rise flats, Rathcoole was still a place where children played together happily.

David was one of those children, a sturdy Protestant boy with thick dark hair and startling blue eyes. He thrived on being "one of the boys," and in those days that meant playing football every afternoon with a gang his own age, including Catholic boys like Bobby Sands who lived just down the block—the same Bobby Sands who would later starve himself to death in the Maze.

But after the summer of 1969, when David was twelve years old, being one of the boys meant something else entirely. Suddenly the difference in religious beliefs mattered, and the Protestants, who made up roughly 60 percent of Rathcoole, let their unwanted neighbors know. Within months, thousands of Catholic families had fled to the Falls or Divas Flats or other places in the city where the Catholics were in control and the Protestants had moved out.

One afternoon David stole a ride into Belfast on the back of a lorry. On a downtown corner he spied Tom, an old friend he used to play with in Rathcoole every Sunday after Tom came home from Mass. Tom's family had moved away from Rathcoole some months ago and this was the first time David had seen his friend since then.

David raised his arm and yelled, "Hello, Tom."

Tom, who was standing with several other lads, looked at David like he had never seen him before. "Get away from me, you Orange bastard," he screamed, shaking his fist and letting loose a string of profanity. The other boys joined in.

David stared for a moment, then turned away, his heart pumping with anger and shame. From that moment on, his lighthearted spirit was replaced by a growing bitterness. Soon all Catholics were suspect;

they were all probably members of the IRA, David thought.

We aren't doing enough to fight back, he thought. He had no faith in the British security forces, but he had observed the power of the street gangs in Rathcoole. Security came in aggression and numbers. So when the Ulster Volunteer Force came recruiting, David was one of the first of the boys in his gang to enlist. He was fifteen.

So David went from football to automatic weapons. He became an expert at robbing banks and post offices.

When he was seventeen, David was arrested for his paramilitary activities. While awaiting trial and sentencing, he was held at Long Kesh, an old airforce base near Belfast where prisoners lived in wartime Nissen huts grouped into compounds. Long Kesh was a graduate school in terrorism for David.

One evening several of the prisoners, agitated by the home brew they were drinking (made by fermenting bits of fruit kept hidden from the officers), seized a man they suspected of being an informer. It was Charlie, a likable fellow David had just been talking to that afternoon. As Charlie pleaded his innocence, they held a mock courtmartial, found him guilty, and pronounced sentence. Death.

Later that night, Charlie was murdered.

Despite his terrorist involvement, David had never seen murder before. He was scared. He had never been religious, but he began to pray desperately. He hated prison. He hated being separated from his family and his girlfriend. And now he was frightened of the violence. He promised God he would

attend church every Sunday—the ultimate sacrifice—if God would just get him out of Long Kesh.

Shortly thereafter, his case came before the court
and he was sentenced to five years in prison.

So much for praying, David thought.

But late that night as he lay in the solitary-
confinement cell where just-sentenced prisoners
were held, he spotted a bit of writing high in the
corner of the white concrete wall next to his bunk.
It was a name, written in precise block letters: Charlie—his friend who had been murdered.

There are worse fates than prison, David
thought. *Charlie would gladly trade places with me
now. Maybe God hasn't given me such a bad deal
after all.*

But David wasn't ready to think much about
God. If God did exist, He had nothing to do with the
flesh-and-blood struggles of Northern Ireland. *All
that church stuff's no use to me,* he thought. *I'm just
a bad egg, and if I go to hell, I go to hell.*

So when he was unexpectedly released from
prison, with a warning from the judge to stay out of
paramilitary organizations, David ignored the warning. He married his girlfriend Roberta and promised
her he wouldn't get involved with UVF again, though
he had no intention of keeping his word.

One Friday evening David was showing a few of
his mates how to assemble automatic weapons while
Roberta was out shopping with her mother. They had
gun parts spread all over the kitchen table, when
suddenly the back door creaked open, and his wife
and mother-in-law stood in the doorway.

His wife's eyes filled with tears of rage. "You

promised!'' she screamed. She turned and ran out the door, her mother close behind her. David didn't see her for a week. When she returned, nothing was said about the UVF. It had become an acknowledged reality but a closed subject.

Sometimes, however, his involvement could not be ignored. Like the night David and Roberta were sitting in a Chinese restaurant in Belfast eating chicken chow mein and three hooded IRA men stormed in the front door. In the sudden silence that followed their entrance, David threw down his tea cup and told Roberta to take cover under the table.

"It's me they want," he said.

He slid out of the booth, crashed past tables of terrified diners and through the double doors to the kitchen, shoving cooks and waiters aside in his effort to reach the back door. Behind him, he could hear people screaming as the gunmen followed.

David cursed when he reached the back door, a fortress of bolts and chains. He ripped them apart, tore the door open, and fled. As he scrambled up an outside wall and over the top, the gunmen began firing. The last thing he heard was his would-be assassins cursing their aim.

Then in 1978 the reality of David's paramilitary involvement burst into their lives again. David and dozens of other UVF men were arrested in their homes at 4:00 one morning in a police sweep. David ended up in the Crumlin Road Prison where he had spent the thoughtful night after Charlie's death several years earlier.

Months later an utterly alien thought entered David's mind: *Become a Christian.* David had been working in the prison laundry with a man named Trevor who was an outspoken Christian. David knew from listening to Trevor that becoming a Christian meant making a lot of changes. For starters, it would mean giving up the UVF, drinking, violence, and chasing women—the things that made his life meaningful.

He discarded the thought, but it kept returning. The next morning in the laundry he said, "Trevor, I'm thinking about becoming a Christian."

All that day while Trevor worked double time, David sat on a pile of towels reading gospel tracts. The other inmates taunted him.

"Thinkin' about becoming a member of the God squad?" they shouted.

By suppertime, David had made his decision. He returned to his cell and knelt to pray for the first time since childhood.

"If you want this life," he told God simply, "it's yours."

The next day he approached an IRA prisoner. The two men had never spoken but had come to blows one day in the laundry.

"I've become a Christian," David told the man.

"What are you tellin' me for?" the inmate sneered.

David looked him in the eye. "I figure that's as good a reason as any to start talkin' to you," he said.

In the days that followed David was shocked to find that God had taken away his hatred of IRA men. He joined a prayer group, and several of the members were former Catholic paramilitaries, now Christians. David still considered himself "a good Prod," but he found himself accepting Catholics as people, not faceless enemies.

Seeing years of hatred eradicated gave David new vigor and certainty about God's miraculous power in situations humanly impossible to resolve.

An IRA man serving time for three murders spoke to him one day. "I've been watchin' you," he said. "You must be the happiest man in this prison."

"That I am," David said. "I know God."

"How can you say that?" the other man sputtered.

David told how he had seen God work in his life and explained the gospel. The IRA man prayed to receive Christ, and he and David hugged there in the prison cell.

*　　*　　*

While such reconciliation was taking place between Protestants and Catholics within prison walls, the violence on the streets of Belfast was reaching spectacular proportions. It even extended across the Irish Sea to the British Parliament.

Airey M. S. Neave had been a Tory member of Parliament for twenty-five years. In 1976 Margaret Thatcher had appointed Neave to her shadow cabinet as spokesman for the affairs of Northern Ireland. Though he was consequently a natural target for terrorist violence, Neave had always firmly stated that British troops should remain in the strife-torn land.

Northern Ireland was not much on Neave's mind on the chill afternoon of March 30, 1979, as he prepared to leave the Parliament buildings in London. Mrs. Thatcher was to formally open her campaign the next day, and Neave had been planning election strategy for months. He was tired.

As usual, he had left his blue Vauxhall in the five-story underground parking garage beneath the heavily guarded government buildings. He got into the car and slowly accelerated up the long ramp leading to the street with its famous silhouettes.

Less than fifty yards from Big Ben, Neave's car exploded. In the deadly stillness that followed, staff and members of Parliament came running from the House of Commons. A British reporter was one of the first to arrive. He wrote:

> The car was swollen like a balloon by the force of the blast. There was glass everywhere. The driver was still in his seat—almost standing—his face bloody and blackened. He was unrecognizable. His gray pinstripe trousers and black jacket were torn and ragged. I thought he looked dead, but a policeman who felt his pulse shouted, "He's still alive." Blood was running from the car and there was glass and mangled pieces of metal thrown up above the ramp into the yard."[7]

Airey Neave died forty minutes later.

That evening, telephones rang at Dublin newspaper offices. "We have a message for the British government," said a husky Irish voice. "Before you decide to have a general election, you had better state that you have decided not to stay in Ireland."

The next day Scotland Yard announced that both the Provisional IRA and the Irish National Liberation Army had claimed responsibility for the killing. Both claims were under investigation.

*   *   *

Protestant terrorists were not to be outdone by Catholic terrorists, as one of Belfast's most shocking murders proved.

Mervyn and Rosaleen McDonald, a young Catholic couple, lived on a Belfast street called Longlands Road. Though not politically active, the McDonalds had Republican ties. Rosaleen's father was a member of the political wing of the official faction of the IRA; Mervyn drank in a Republican bar. Those were reasons enough for them to be on a Protestant paramilitary death list.

One warm, hazy evening Mervyn was sitting at the kitchen table having dinner while Rosaleen watched the local television news in the main room. She held baby Margaret in her arms; two-and-a-half-year-old Seamus sat next to her on the sofa.

A white Austin pulled slowly up to the curb outside beyond the McDonalds' tall hedge. One man remained at the wheel; the other two got out. One had on a long overcoat.

The men knocked on the door and Rosaleen answered. "We're from the New Lodge. Is your husband in?" said one of the men. Thinking they were friends of her husband's family, who had connections on New Lodge Road, Rosaleen motioned them in.

Hearing strange voices, Mervyn got up from the dinner table and came to the doorway. As he did so, the man with the overcoat ripped a submachine gun from behind his back and fired at Mervyn, blowing off part of his face.

Clutching her baby, Rosaleen screamed, "Why us?"

The gunman turned toward her, tore the baby from her arms, pushed Rosaleen toward the sofa, and fired into her back. She fell in a pool of blood, while her children cried hysterically on the sofa.

The assassins left the house nonchalantly, climbed into the white Austin, and drove back to their base in Rathcoole. They agreed that their mission had been a success.

A neighbor found the McDonalds. Mervyn had been killed instantly; Rosaleen died four hours later—two more statistics in Northern Ireland's bitter toll.[8]

* * *

Liam . . .

When Liam McCloskey woke on Saturday morning, August 27, 1981, the fifty-fifth day of his hunger strike, he was considerably weaker. He was blind; his hearing was going.

His mother arrived. As soon as Liam went into a coma, she told him tearfully, she would have him fed intravenously. But by then it would be too late; his blindness would be permanent. She pleaded with him to end the strike before it was too late, since she was going to take him off it anyway.

Even in his weakened state, Liam was coherent enough to understand how supremely unfair he was being. His mother could not carry the responsibility for his death—or his blindness—on her conscience. He was trapped. He decided to end the strike.

"As I made that decision," he said later, "tears

streamed out of my eyes. Tears of relief, tears of frustration, tears of sadness, tears of joy. I received a vitamin injection almost immediately and soon after some milk to drink.

"Waves of guilt washed over me as I sat eating, thinking about the men still on the hunger strike. So when the strike ended the Saturday of that week, I was a happy man. Even though it had ended in failure, no more would die that slow, lingering death."

Sectarian tensions were at their highest level since the early 1970s, when the region hovered on the verge of civil war. At the source of Ulster's new troubles is an apparent shift in IRA tactics. Having failed to win political concessions with hunger strikes, which disintegrated in the face of Prime Minister Margaret Thatcher's unyielding resistance and an erosion of support from families of participating prisoners (ten of whom died this year), the IRA has returned to the gun and stepped up its campaign of terror.

During the past three weeks, twelve people have been killed in Northern Ireland, including the 17-year-old son of an Ulster Defense Regiment soldier, and an 18-year-old Catholic youth who was shot as he walked home on the night of Bradford's murder. [The Rev. Robert Bradford, a Protestant member of Parliament and an evangelical Christian, was assassinated by IRA gunmen on November 17, 1981.] The IRA has also launched a series of bomb attacks in Britain. Four bombs have exploded in London during the past six weeks, killing three people.[9]

Liam's eyesight began to return, then his equilibrium. In the prison hospital he learned to walk again, rebuilding leg muscles deteriorated by the fast.

He also began to think about resigning from the INLA.

"I was ripping myself apart inside," he says, "thinking about the men who had died, thinking about God, and the truths I had begun to discover on hunger strike.

"The first decision was to stop walking the way of Republicanism and the way of Jesus at the same time. It was impossible to walk both; one must override the other. I had to choose.

"I had reached the crossroads of life, and I took the way of Jesus. I found the rest I had long sought. Things became clearer in my mind. The Bible was no longer a book, but the way to God. I began to realize that God loved me and I loved God."

After Liam left the hospital, he was moved to a special H-block in the Maze for former protesters. He kept putting off his letter of resignation to the INLA, until one night he saw a television interview with the father of a young boy killed by an IRA bomb. The man said he forgave those who had planted the bomb and asked that no one retaliate.

There is a truly Christian man, thought Liam. *A beam of light in the darkness that engulfs this land. With people like that here, we are not beyond hope.*

He requested a transfer to Magilligan Prison, and it was granted. The night before he left he wrote his resignation to the INLA.

"As I left the Maze," says Liam, "it felt like a cloud lifting from me. I had left behind much of my old self in that place." He was finally ready to submit entirely to God, to pray with conviction, "Thy will be done."

As he was taken by van to Magilligan, he noticed

the beauty of the countryside, and a wave of sadness swept over him. *People are dying together rather than living together to enjoy the land that God has given us all.*

Ready to be a force for reconciliation, Liam sought bold ways to show it. He decided to begin by breaking the stark lines of segregation between Protestants and Catholics in Magilligan Prison.

One place that segregation was already broken was in the Monday afternoon Bible study of Dr. Bill Holley, who later became one of Prison Fellowship's most faithful volunteers. His study was a proving ground for the unity to be found in Christ. Muscled inmates sporting "God & Ulster" tattoos up and down both arms shared Bibles with prisoners tattooed with "God & Ireland."

Several members of Dr. Holley's study had spent time in the Maze. Liam even became friends with UVF men and with Gerry, a former IRA man and now an outspoken Christian.

Jimmy...

Another man who ended up in Dr. Holley's Bible study had traveled many of the same roads as the other prisoners. Short and muscular, with even white teeth and fine brown hair, Jimmy Gibson had gotten involved with the Protestant paramilitaries and was now in prison for attempted murder.

When he arrived at Magilligan, Jimmy wanted nothing to do with Christianity. He thought there probably was a God, but he certainly wanted nothing to do with Him. Certainly not with the things he was planning to do when he got out of prison. Retaliation against Catholic paramilitaries headed his list.

Jimmy respected the Christians at Magilligan, however. They weren't wishy-washy about their faith. He watched several of them closely—not only fellow Protestants, but Catholics like Gerry and Liam McCloskey, the slight, freckled prisoner who walked with a limp. Jimmy knew Liam had spent fifty-five days on a hunger strike; he also knew Liam had resigned from the INLA and become some sort of religious fanatic.

One day as Jimmy and two other Loyalist prisoners sat down for dinner, Liam limped toward their table, tray in hand. Jimmy's cellmate nodded at Liam.

"That's okay," he said. "You can sit here."

Jimmy kicked his mate under the table and felt his face grow hot. Liam sat down, said his grace, and took a forkful of beans. Excluding the prayer, the rest of the table followed suit.

The invisible line segregating Catholics from Protestants had been crossed.

Jimmy wasn't prepared to start a hunger strike of his own, so he continued to come to meals, despite the fact that Liam McCloskey did too—and his usual place was right next to Jimmy.

Slowly, as months went by, Jimmy began to see Liam as a person, not just a former hunger striker turned religious fanatic. Finally, one day Jimmy addressed him for the first time.

"What are you going to do to the other side when you get out?"

"Nothing," Liam responded.

I don't believe it, Jimmy thought to himself. He

knew he couldn't give up the revenge he was plotting against his enemies.

Jimmy's inner turmoil continued to build until he knew he had to become a Christian. To tell God, "I reject You," would only mean God would reject him.

Finally Jimmy glumly told God he would give his life to Him. Later he went to Dr. Holley's Bible study. Liam, Gerry, and his other sworn enemies were jubilant, slapping him on the back and laughing. Jimmy was quiet—embarrassed—possibly the most miserable convert in Northern Ireland.

But the misery of his conversion didn't alter its veracity. Jimmy had thought it all through; he was ready to obey God's Word whatever it took. He hadn't come to Christianity to feel good; he came because it was true. He began speaking to Catholics and prison guards, whom he had hated equally. He began reading his Bible and telling others about his faith. He began learning how to forgive and seek reconciliation rather than plot revenge.

Liam and Jimmy . . .

One autumn evening as the men in the Magilligan Bible study met for prayer, a young girl named Karen McKeown headed their list. Dr. Holley had told them the week before about the young Protestant girl who had been shot by the INLA. Their prayer list always contained victims of the Troubles, but Liam had felt a special responsibility for Karen's suffering. He had written to her mother.

"I heard from Mrs. McKeown," Liam said, passing Karen's picture around the circle. "I haven't been able to stop thinking about her."

The group bowed their heads and joined hands. Then, one by one, the former terrorists—Catholic and Protestant—prayed for Karen McKeown and her family, asking that God heal this latest young victim of Belfast's violence.

Liam closed the prayer with the words he had first prayed during his months on the hunger strike. "Not ours, Lord, but Thy will be done."

Pearl and Karen...

By the end of her second week in the hospital, Karen slept a little more each day. Pearl treasured the moments she was awake. By the third week, meningitis set in, and Karen slipped into a coma.

Then, early one morning while the rain fell outside the hospital windows, Pearl watched her daughter die.

Shortly after that, another letter arrived from Liam McCloskey.

"Pearl, we make strange friends in this troubled land. It is to the glory of God and He who makes it possible. Remember John 8:51, 'And I tell you most solemnly. Whoever keeps My Word will never see death.' Karen has left us, and even though it was no choice of mine, yet you can make a conscious decision in your own mind to see it as a gift of God. Your beautiful daughter to our beautiful Father who knows best. Surely the peace of Christ will be yours."

*   *   *

In the summer of 1983 Prison Fellowship conducted its first international conference in Belfast, Northern Ireland. At a time when travelers were passing up the troubled country, we decided it was a fitting backdrop for the theme of our conference: "In Christ, Reconciliation."

The work of Christians like Dr. Bill Holley and Gladys Blackburne and the reality of Christ in the lives of former terrorists clearly portrayed the power of God to bring unity. The struggles of Belfast represented the unresolved conflicts throughout our world. Northern Ireland illustrated both the hope and the desperate needs.

The highlight of the conference came one evening during a meeting open to the public. Hundreds of townspeople—both Protestant and Catholic—streamed into Queen's University's elegant Whitlow Hall, donated for the occasion. Clearly our ministry in Northern Ireland's prisons had captured the interest of many of Ulster's citizens.

Liam McCloskey and Jimmy Gibson had been furloughed from prison to be with us for the week. Their presence, more than anything else, evidenced the reconciling nature of the gospel. That evening, each told how he had come to know Christ. Liam concluded by putting his thin arm around Jimmy's muscular shoulders.

"My hope is to believe that God is changing the hearts of men like myself and Jimmy," Liam said. "That's the only hope I have for peace in Northern Ireland. Before, if I had seen Jimmy on the street, I would have shot him. Now he's my brother in Christ. I would die for him."

As members of the audience murmured in disbelief, James McIlroy, director of Prison Fellowship for Northern Ireland, took the microphone.

"There's a woman I'd like you to meet," he said, motioning to someone in the back row. A lithe, energetic woman began to thread her way toward the front.

As she did, James briefly told the story of Pearl and Karen McKeown; of Karen's death at the hands of an INLA gunman; of Pearl's friendship through the mail with Liam, the former INLA terrorist; how Pearl and Liam had grown to love one another as mother and son, though they had never met.

Pearl climbed the stage steps and walked slowly toward Liam, arms outstretched. They hugged. Then Pearl held Liam's hand as she tearfully explained how Karen's death had been to God's glory.

"Liam told me his prayer is now that of St. Francis," she said." 'Lord, make me an instrument of your peace. Where there is hatred, let me sow love. Where there is injury, pardon. Where there is death, life. Where despair, hope. Where there is darkness, light. Where there is sadness, joy.'

"And Liam *has* been God's instrument of peace to me," she concluded in a choked voice. "For he is the one who has showed me how to love God again."

By now tears glistened in many eyes as the audience strained to capture the incredible tableau: the two former terrorists, Catholic and Protestant, once sworn enemies, now standing together as brothers in Christ; the bereaved Protestant mother and the Catholic terrorist, holding hands.

Such is the reconciling power of God in Northern Ireland.

*   *   *

But widespread peace in Northern Ireland is as remote as ever. Bombs and bullets continue to fly. Political solutions continue to fail. And death tolls of civilians, paramilitaries, soldiers, and police continue to mount. Yet this seemingly endless cycle is weakened a little every time someone seeks peace rather than war, forgiveness rather than retribution, love rather than hate.

What is the answer to the troubles of Northern Ireland? Nothing in its chaotic history suggests there are political answers. George Thomas was right that night at our dinner in London: politically speaking, "There is no answer in Northern Ireland." But when every political effort of men and their institutions has been frustrated, when the kingdoms of man are utterly impotent, it is then that the power of the Kingdom of God, in all its glory, breaks into the dark stream of history. And it is the citizens of the Kingdom of God who carry that light into the darkness—which cannot overcome it. Thus these Christians of Northern Ireland—and many others—continue the witness of the indestructible Kingdom in the midst of their nation's chaos.

Pearl McKeown works as a nursing assistant and serves as a Prison Fellowship volunteer, sharing her message of forgiveness and reconciliation with those who are imprisoned as well as those bound up in hatred outside prison walls.

Liam McCloskey was released from prison in late 1983 and now lives quietly in Derry near his family. He works on a farm owned by Columba House, a Catholic outreach to those in need.

Gladys Blackburne has now passed the age of seventy and is thus no longer eligible to serve as a member of the Maze Prison Board of Visitors. She contents herself with visits to British soldiers at their Northern Ireland outposts. She has confided to friends that she would like the following epitaph on her tombstone: "She did what she could—Mark 14:8."

David Hamilton, released from prison in 1983, is now assistant director for Prison Fellowship of Northern Ireland. He spends much of his time counseling ex-prisoners and urging young men to seek Christ rather than drift into violence as "one of the boys."

Jimmy Gibson, released in late 1983, works at a Belfast YMCA, teaching teenage boys carpentry skills. He also occasionally speaks to community groups, telling about the Carpenter who changed his life from one of revenge to reconciliation.

Chips McCurry, released from prison in 1985, is now studying at Baptist College in conjunction with Queen's University. When a BBC radio program interviewed Chips and an ex-IRA man together, Chips told the story of his conversion. Gladys Blackburne happened to hear the broadcast and was thrilled; until then, she had not known the results of her Christmas Eve visit with him in 1980.

Perhaps it is Chips who best articulates the problems—and the solution—for Northern Ireland.

"I spent almost ten years in prison. I saw guys fighting, dying for God and Ulster. Or for God and Ireland. What would happen if either side got what they wanted? You see that politics can't bring any lasting solutions.

"The only thing that will make any lasting peace, the only things that will bridge the gulf between the Catholics and the Protestants here is for people to give up violence and learn forgiveness. The only way that can possibly happen is through Jesus Christ."

Epilogue

The light shines in the darkness, and the darkness has not overcome it.
—John 1:5 [RSV]

It is said that as Winston Churchill lay critically ill, he reflected on conditions in the world he had so heroically helped rescue. "There is no hope," he sighed. "There is no hope." And with that despairing observation, the great leader died.

Churchill's words might well have been describing the tragedy of Northern Ireland; though on the surface a religious war, it is in reality a long-standing struggle for political and economic power. Indeed, political and economic solutions there have failed.

But Ireland is only one of the seemingly hopeless political situations of our world today. Consider Lebanon. Once a beautiful seaside land of pine trees and fragrant flowers, today it reeks of death. The blood of Jews and Christians and Muslims runs together through the gutters of Beirut.

Or Sri Lanka, an island paradise once called the place where people always smile. Few smile there today amid the terror of Tamil bombs. Or the peasants of Nicaragua, caught in a crossfire of ideology, money, helicopters, and guns. Their chickens and produce are taken one day by pillaging Sandinista soldiers, stolen the next by marauding Contras. Or consider the fact that hardly a Cambodian has not lost a son or brother, wife or mother, in the most massive genocide since the Holocaust: Three million people murdered by their own government.

Millions live under the repression of South Africa's Apartheid, which strips black, colored, and white of their dignity. Political options promise only more chaos, and when the seething cauldron of bitterness boils over, Communist revolutionaries will be standing by, ready to offer collectivist salvation for a tired and turbulent land.

Over half the world lives under the ultimate result of such "salvation." Millions in this century have been condemned to live—bound, gagged, and tortured—and die in the gulag. And today's much-heralded *glasnost* is little more than a public-relations campaign; the deadly face of Communism remains the same.

But in the other half of the world, which lives ostensibly in freedom, millions are enslaved by more subtle rulers. In the inner cities of America, a generation is in bondage to the rule of drugs and poverty; many see crime as their only way out and end up in the wasteland of America's prisons. Meanwhile more affluent Americans embrace the false gods of materialism, hedonism, egoism. And man's basest passions have unleashed a plague called AIDS, which now holds millions hostage.

And hovering over all of planet earth is the mushroom cloud, the same gray ghost that Douglas MacArthur saw that day in 1945 when he warned the world it had but one last chance. The cloud seems darker and more ominous when tanks roll in Eastern Europe or Central America, in Southeast Asia or Africa, when vessels in the Persian Gulf patrol at full alert. At other times it seems to recede. Yet it is always a heartbeat away.

In this latter part of the twentieth century, a great irony persists. Technology has given man power he has never known before; giant institutions offer panaceas for all human ills. But never has man seemed less able to devise political strategies to produce order and harmony among people. The more powerful the institution appears, the more impotent it is. The proudest pretensions of the strongest nations are mocked by a single bomb-laden terrorist truck. Belfast, Beirut, Central America, South Africa, Cambodia, Korea, Chad, and forty other places like them are but open sores on the body politic, reminding us that even in this age of technological wonders, modern governments have devised nothing to cure the unbridled passions of man.

Is there no hope? Were Churchill's dying words the epitaph for our age?

Like any author, I would like to end this book on a triumphant note, announcing that ultimate peace and harmony can be achieved through human efforts. But that utopian illusion is shattered by the splintered history of the human race. Governments rise; even the most powerful fall. The battle for people's hearts and minds will continue.

Where then is hope? It is in the fact that the Kingdom of God has come to earth—the Kingdom announced by Jesus Christ in that obscure Nazareth synagogue two thousand years ago. It is a Kingdom that comes not in a temporary takeover of political structures, but in the lasting takeover of the human heart by the rule of a holy God.

Certainly, as I hope this book has shown, the fact that God reigns can be manifest through political means, whenever the citizens of the Kingdom of God bring His light to bear on the institutions of the kingdoms of man. But His rule is even more powerfully evident in ordinary, individual lives, in the breaking of cycles of violence and evil, in the paradoxical power of forgiveness, in the actions of those little platoons who live by the transcendent values of the Kingdom of God in the midst of the kingdoms of this world, loving their God and loving their neighbor.

Thus in the midst of the dark and habitual chaos of earth, a light penetrates the darkness. It cannot be extinguished; it is the light of the Kingdom of God. His Kingdom *has* come, in His people today, and it is yet to come as well, in the great consummation of human history. While the battle rages on planet earth, we can take heart—not in the fleeting fortunes of men or nations, but rather in the promise so beautifully captured in Handel's *Messiah*.

Stop. Listen. Over the din of the conflict, if you

listen carefully, you will hear the chorus echoing in the distance: "The kingdom of this world has become the kingdom of our Lord and of His Christ."

Listen. For in that glorious refrain is man's one hope.

Let us then ... rejoice that we see around us at every hand the decay of the institutions and instruments of power, see intimations of empires falling to pieces, money in total disarray, dictators and parliamentarians alike nonplussed by the confusion and conflicts which encompass them. For it is precisely when every earthly hope has been explored and found wanting, when every possibility of help from earthly sources has been sought and is not forthcoming, when every recourse this world offers, moral as well as material, has been explored to no effect, when in the shivering cold the last faggot has been thrown on the fire and in the gathering darkness every glimmer of light has finally flickered out, it's then that Christ's hand reaches out, sure and firm. Then Christ's words bring their inexpressible comfort, then His light shines brightest, abolishing the darkness forever. So finding in everything only deception and nothingness, the soul is constrained to have recourse to God Himself and to rest content with Him.[1]

WITH GRATITUDE

If this book accomplishes nothing more than to cause readers to turn to Richard John Neuhaus's *Naked Public Square*, I shall consider my labors well rewarded. Of the thirty or more books I studied in preparation for writing *Kingdoms in Conflict*, Neuhaus's work was second only to Augustine's classic *The City of God*. I am thus deeply indebted to Richard. My prayer is that what I have written will in some way contribute to his heroic struggle to defend religious values in Western culture.

I'm also indebted to esteemed theologian Dr. Carl F. H. Henry, my beloved friend, for both his various writings on church and state issues and for his critique of this manuscript. When I asked Carl for his counsel, the publisher's deadline was imminent and he was leaving in twelve hours for an extended teaching trip. I was astonished to discover the entire manuscript in my office the next day, thoroughly reviewed. With characteristic generosity and devotion, he had simply stayed up all night to read it.

I'm also profoundly grateful to Jacques Ellul, the French sociologist and critic, for his many prophetic works, most significantly *The Political Illusion* and *The Presence of the Kingdom*. These are classic commentaries on our times and, in what is in itself a sad commentary on our times, are out of print. Also of tremendous importance was Donald Bloesch's *Crumbling Foundations*.

Paul Johnson's *Modern Times* was a great inspiration as well. If my writing has aroused in the reader's mind a desire to know more of the philosophical undercurrents of this century, I could recommend nothing more highly than this insightful, provocative critique.

In the "For Further Reading" section, I've listed other contemporary writers and their works that greatly assisted me in the reference section to follow, in the hope that readers will go deeper into the complex and crucial issues of church, state, and the Kingdom of God.

As with *Loving God*, this book was the result of a team effort: My wonderfully gifted editorial associate, Ellen Santilli Vaughn, who assisted with certain chapters of *Loving God*, was this time my colleague in the fullest sense, as the title page properly acknowledges. It is a joy to work closely with one who combines keen editorial skills with such an uplifting Christian spirit.

Kenneth Myers, editor of *This World: A Journal of Religion and Public Life*, provided research help with early drafts and wise theological counsel throughout. So did David Coffin, a doctoral candidate at Westminster Theological Seminary and head of Berea Ministries.

Tim Stafford, another *Loving God* collaborator, provided tremendous assistance with the Prologue, the material on the Philippines, and particularly with his fascinating research and reporting of the events leading up to World War II.

My very talented friend Jim Manney, editor of *New Covenant Magazine*, provided outstanding research for the Christianity and Marxism material. My research assistant, Michael Gerson, did a brilliant job, providing provocative research and well-reasoned drafts. Elizabeth Leahy, director of the Prison Fellowship Information Center, gave invaluable and exhaustive help, excavating mounds of obscure sources and cities—without ever losing her smile.

But the most important member of the team was my editor, Judith Markham. Judith edited *Loving God*; and, in spite of the pain an editor's surgery causes any writer, we ended up good friends. I also gained enormous admiration for Judith's ability—her availability was the deciding factor in my selection of a publisher. She did not disappoint me. Judith Markham is, in my opinion, the master craftsman of her trade.

I was enormously helped as well by my extremely competent executive secretary, Grace McCrane, who tamed this manuscript through, in some cases, ten or more drafts, offering important suggestions and helpful additions throughout. She was assisted with typing of early drafts by Patti Perkins. I am grateful as well to Margaret Shannon, who provided the idea and initial research for the Clivedon material, as well as to Jim Park, Prison Fellowship Oklahoma area director, for his research into Collinsville.

In addition to Carl Henry, Richard Neuhaus, and

theologian Arthur Lindsley, several of my Prison Fellowship colleagues read and critiqued the manuscript. I'm particularly grateful to Dan Van Ness, president of Justice Fellowship, and his colleague David Coolidge, who as a church-state student himself, offered excellent and insightful suggestions throughout. I'm indebted as well to Prison Fellowship president Gordon Loux, who from the beginning of our ministry has been my closest confidant and friend. A word of thanks is also due to Ron Nikkel, executive director of Prison Fellowship International, for his consistent encouragement, and to Fellowship Communications president Nelson Keener and my executive assistant, Jim Jewell, for their help with contract matters and book promotion.

The support of my family, especially Patty, the helpmate God has given me, proved indispensable to this book. Five months before the deadline I was hospitalized for major surgery. Patty and my daughter, Emily Colson Boehme, were faithfully at my side during the month I spent in the hospital; my sons Wendell and Chris also came from great distance to offer encouragement, as did my mother and stepfather. I wonder if I would have made it without them.

Patty then nursed me through the two months of recovery only to lose me to long days—and nights—as I labored over this manuscript. There are far easier callings than to be married to those who periodically feel compelled to take pen in hand; but without Patty's consistent encouragement, *Kingdoms in Conflict* could not have been written.

Finally, my gratitude to all those in Prison Fellowship who encourage and support me; to the teachers who have given so unstintingly of their time; and to the readers of my books who frequently encourage me with their letters. And of course most important, my eternal gratitude goes to the One who guides my hand across the page. May this book glorify Him in every way.

Charles W. Colson
June 20, 1987
P.O. Box 17500
Washington, D.C. 20041

NOTES

Chapter 1

1. Paul Vitz, *Psychology as Religion: The Cult of Self-Worship* (Grand Rapids, Mich.: Eerdmans, 1977), 114. Quoted in Donald G. Bloesch, *Crumbling Foundations* (Grand Rapids, Mich.: Zondervan, 1984), 67.

2. Justice William O. Douglas's opinion in *Zorach v. Clauson*, 343 U.S. 306 (April 28, 1952) is cited in Robert T. Miller and Ronald B. Flowers, *Toward Benevolent Neutrality: Church, State, and the Supreme Court*, rev. ed. (Waco, Texas: Markham Press Fund, 1977), 327.

3. Jack Kroll, "The Most Famous Artist," *Newsweek* (March 9, 1987), 64.

4. Justice Goldberg's dissenting opinion in *Abington Township School District v. Schempp*, 374 U.S. 203 (June 17, 1963) is cited in Miller and Flowers, *Toward Benevolent Neutrality*, 372.

5. Walter Shapiro, "Politics and the Pulpit," *Newsweek* (September 17, 1984), 24.

6. Ronald Reagan speech at an ecumenical prayer breakfast in Dallas, Texas, is quoted in Jeremiah O'Leary, "Reagan Declares that Faith Has Key Role in Political Life," *Washington Times* (August 24, 1984).

7. Shapiro, "Politics and the Pulpit," 24.

8. Mario M. Cuomo, "Religious Belief and Public Morality: A Catholic Governor's Perspective," a paper presented to the Department of Theology at the University of Notre Dame (September 13, 1984), 12.

9. *New York Times* (April 10, 1983). Quoted in a speech given by Stephen V. Monsma, "The Promises and Pitfalls of Evangelical Political Involvement," (October 17, 1986).

10. Will Durant, *Caesar and Christ: A History of Roman Civilization from Its Beginnings to* A.D. *337* (New York: Simon and Schuster, 1944), 164.

11. St. Augustine, *The City of God* (Garden City, N.Y.: Image/Doubleday, 1958), 88.

12. *London Times* editorial: "Evil in the Air," (May 12, 1983), 15A.

13. Quoted in Richard John Neuhaus, *The Naked Public Square* (Grand Rapids, Mich.: Eerdmans, 1984), 95.

14. Quoted in Neuhaus, *Naked Public Square*, 115.

15. Adam Michnik, *Letters from Prison and Other Essays* (Berkeley, Calif.: University of California Press, 1986). Quoted in Norman Davies, "True to Himself and His Homeland," *New York Times Book Review* (October 5, 1986).

16. Vernon J. Bourke, "Introduction," in St. Augustine, *City of God*, 9–10.

17. "Indian Leader Urges Gandhi to 'Stamp Out' Missionaries," *Presbyterian Journal* (November 20, 1985), 6.

Chapter 2

1. This chapter is based on several studies of Hemingway's life, the most helpful of which were John Killinger, *Hemingway and the Dead Gods* (Lexington, Ky.: The University of Kentucky Press, 1960), and A. E. Hotchner, *Papa Hemingway: The Ecstasy and Sorrow* (New York: Quill, 1983).

2. "Hero of the Code," *Time* (July 14, 1961), 87.

3. Killinger, *Hemingway and the Dead Gods*, 69.

4. Maurice Natanson, "Jean-Paul Sartre's Philosophy of Freedom," *Social Research*, XIX (September 1952), 378.

5. E. L. Allen, *The Self and Its Hazards: A Guide to the Thought of Karl Jaspers* (London: Hodder and Stoughton, 1953), 7.

Chapter 3

1. The information in this chapter is based on news reports and an interview with Jerry and Sis Levin conducted by Ellen Santilli Vaughn (April 9, 1987).

Chapter 4

1. Quoted in R. C. Sproul, *If There Is a God, Why Are There Atheists?* (Minneapolis: Dimension Books, 1978), 48.

2. Harry Blamires, *The Christian Mind* (Ann Arbor, Mich.: Servant Books, 1963), 44.

3. Carl Sagan, *Cosmos* (New York: Random House, 1980), 4.

4. Eugene Mallove, "Gravity: Is the Force that Makes the Apple Fall the Clue to Creation?" *Washington Post* (March 3, 1985), C–1-a.

5. Bertrand Russell, *The Autobiography of Bertrand Russell*, a letter to Lady Ottoline Morrell dated August 11, 1918 (Boston: Little, Brown, 1968), 121.

6. Quoted in Joseph Frank, *Dostoyevsky: Years of Ordeal* (Princeton, N.J.: Princeton University Press, 1983), 159.

7. Jeremiah 22:16

8. Paul Johnson, "A Historian Looks at Jesus," unpublished speech (1986).

9. "Conversation with an Author: Mortimer J. Adler, Author of *How to Think About God*," *Book Digest Magazine*, (September 1980).

Chapter 5

1. Aleksandr Solzhenitsyn, *The Cancer Ward* (New York: Dell, 1968).

2. Paul Johnson, "The Necessity for Christianity," *Truth*, 1:1 (1985), 2.

3. Peter Singer, "Sanctity of Life or Quality of Life?" *Pediatrics* (July 1983), 129.

4. Quoted Thomas Molnar, *Utopia: The Perennial Heresy* (London: Tom Stacey, 1972), 4.

5. William Golding, *The Lord of the Flies* (New York: Wide View/Paragrees Books, 1954).

6. E. L. Epstein, "Notes on *Lord of the Flies*," in Golding, *Lord of the Flies*, 186.

7. Armando Valladares, *Against All Hope* (New York: Knopf, 1986), 4.

8. Valladares, *Against All Hope*, 135.

9. Paul Johnson, *Modern Times: The World from the Twenties to the Eighties* (New York: Harper & Row, 1983), 11.

10. Charles Murray, "No, Welfare Really Isn't the Problem," *Public Interest* (Summer 1986), 10.

11. Leszek Kolakowski, "The Idolatry of Politics," *New*

Republic (June 16, 1986), 29–36.
12. Quoted in James V. Schall, *Christianity and Politics* (Boston: St. Paul Editions, 1981), 295.
13. Molnar, *Utopia*, 7.

Chapter 6

1. Luke 4:18, in which Jesus quotes Isaiah 61:1–2. The story that follows is related in Luke 4:20–30.
2. Matthew 6:33.
3. St. Augustine, *The Confessions of St. Augustine*, translated and edited by J. G. Pilkington (New York: Liveright, 1943), 1.
4. Acts 16:30.
5. Edmund Clowney, "The Politics of the Kingdom," *Westminster Theological Journal* 41 (Spring 1979), 302.

Chapter 7

1. Paul Johnson, "The Family as an Emblem of Freedom," *Emblem of Freedom: The American Family in the 1980s*, edited by Carl A. Anderson and William J. Gribbon (Durham, N.C.: Carolina Academic Press, 1981), 23.
2. Beth Brophy, "Children Under Stress," *U.S. News and World Report* (October 27, 1986), 58.
3. Paul C. Vitz, *Censorship: Evidence of Bias in Our Children's Textbooks* (Ann Arbor, Mich.: Servant Books, 1986), 37–38.
4. Stanton E. Samenow, *Inside the Criminal Mind* (New York: New York Times Book Co., 1984).
5. James Q. Wilson and Richard J. Herrnstein, *Crime and Human Nature* (New York: Simon and Schuster, 1985).
6. Carl F. H. Henry: "The Modern Flight from the Family," *The Emblem of Freedom, the American Family in the 1980s*, edited by Carl A. Anderson and William J. Gribbon (Durham, N.C.: North Carolina Academic Press, 1981), 46.
7. Romans 13:4.
8. 1 Peter 2:14.
9. Quoted in Michael Harrington, *The Politics at God's Funeral* (New York: Penguin, 1983), 107.

10. Jay Marcellus Kik, *Church and State in the New Testament* (Grand Rapids, Mich.: Baker, 1962), 20.

11. Exodus 18:13.

12. Exodus 18:15–16.

13. 1 Timothy 2:2.

14. Robert Nisbet, *The Quest for Community* (New York: Oxford University Press, 1953).

15. Robert L. Saucy, *The Church in God's Program* (Chicago: Moody Press, 1972), 91.

16. Floyd Filson, *Jesus Christ the Risen Lord* (Nashville: Abingdon Press, 1956), 253.

17. Jacques Ellul, *The Presence of the Kingdom* (New York: Seabury Press, 1948/1967), 47.

18. Pope John Paul II, "Opening Address at Puebla," (1979). In *The Pope and Revolution: John Paul II Confronts Liberation Theology*, edited by Quintin L. Quade (Washington, D.C.: Ethics and Public Policy Center, 1982).

19. Edmund Clowney, "The Politics of the Kingdom," *Westminster Theological Journal* 41:2 (Spring 1979), 306.

20. Clowney, "Politics of the Kingdom," 307.

Chapter 8

1. This chapter was based on a number of studies of Wilberforce's life and the fight for the abolition of the slave trade in England. Several of the most helpful sources were: Robin Furneaux, *William Wilberforce* (London: Hamilton, 1974); John Pollock, *Wilberforce* (New York: St. Martin's Press, 1978); William Wilberforce, *Real Christianity*, a modern edition edited by James Houston (Portland: Multnomah, 1982); Ernest Marshall Howse, *Saints in Politics: The Clapham Sect* (Unwin, 1974); Garth Lean, *God's Politician: William Wilberforce's Struggle* (London: Darton, Longman and Todd, 1980).

Chapter 9

1. Acts 17:6–7.

2. F. F. Bruce, *The Spreading Flame: The Rise and Progress of Christianity from Its First Beginnings to the Con-*

version of the English (Grand Rapids, Mich.: Eerdmans, 1958), 293.

3. Etienne Gilson's "Foreword," quoting Fustel de Coulanges, in St. Augustine, *The City of God* (New York: Image/Doubleday, 1958), 15.

4. Alexis de Tocqueville, *The Old Regime and the French Revolution*, translated by Stuart Gilbert (Garden City: Doubleday/Anchor Books, 1955), 149.

5. Tocqueville, *The Old Regime and the French Revolution*, 149.

6. Romans 13:5, 7.

7. Edmund Clowney, "The Politics of the Kingdom," *Westminster Theological Journal* (Spring 1979), 306.

8. Harold J. Berman, "Atheism and Christianity in the Soviet Union," in *Freedom and Faith: The Impact of Law on Religious Liberty*, edited by Lynn R. Buzzard (Westchester, Ill.: Crossway Books, 1982), 127–43.

9. William Blake, "And Did Those Feet," *The Norton Anthology of Poetry*, 3d ed. (New York: W. W. Norton, 1983), 266.

10. Richard John Neuhaus, *The Naked Public Square* (Grand Rapids, Mich.: Eerdmans, 1984), 231.

11. Patricia Hynds, a Maryknoll lay missionary, was quoted in an article by Juan Tamayo, *Miami Herald* (March 6, 1983).

12. Oscar Cullman, *The State in the New Testament* (New York: Scribner's, 1956), 91.

13. Hugh T. Kerr, ed., *Compendium of Luther's Theology* (Philadelphia: Westminster Press, 1966), 218.

14. Carl F. H. Henry, "The Gospel for the Rest of Our Century," *Christianity Today* (January 17, 1986), 25-I.

15. Quoted in Neuhaus, *Naked Public Square*, 61.

16. "James Madison's Memorial and Remonstrance, 1785," in Edwin S. Gaustad, ed., *A Documentary History of Religion in America: Vol. I* (Grand Rapids, Mich.: Eerdmans, 1982), 262–63.

17. Quoted in A. James Reichley, *Religion in American*

Public Life (Washington, D.C.: The Brookings Institute, 1985), 105.
18. Reichley, *Religion in American Public Life*, 360.

Chapter 10

1. The following sources were particularly useful in the research of this chapter: Eberhard Bethge, *Dietrich Bonhoeffer* (New York: Harper & Row, 1977); John Conway, *The Nazi Persecution of the Churches* (New York: Basic Books, 1968); Arthur C. Cochrane, *The Church's Confession Under Hitler* (Allison Park, Penn.: Pickwick, 1977); Richard Gutteridge, *Open Thy Mouth for the Dumb! The German Evangelical Church and the Jews* (New York: Barnes and Noble, 1976); Dietmar Schmidt, *Pastor Niemoller* (New York: Doubleday, 1959); William Shirer, *A Berlin Diary* (New York: Knopf, 1941).

Chapter 11

1. This chapter is based on a number of studies on England and the thirties, including: Neville Chamberlain, *In Search of Peace* (Salem, N.H.: Ayer, facsimile of 1939 edition); Keith Middlemas, *The Strategy of Appeasement: The British Government and Germany, 1937–1939* (New York: Times Books, 1972); John W. Wheeler-Bennett, *Munich: Prologue to Tragedy* (Duell, 1962); David Dilks, *Neville Chamberlain* (New York: Cambridge University Press, 1984); Martin Gilbert and Richard Gott, *The Appeasers* (Boston: Houghton Mifflin, 1963).

Chapter 12

1. Many of the historical details in this chapter are taken from William Manchester, *American Caesar: Douglas MacArthur 1880–1964* (Boston: Little, Brown, 1978). See especially chapter 7, "At High Port," for additional information.
2. Quoted in John Lukacs, *1945: Year Zero* (Garden City: Doubleday, 1978), 239.

3. Paul Johnson, *Modern Times: The World from the Twenties to the Eighties* (New York: Harper & Row, 1983), 430.

4. Friedrich Nietzsche, *The Gay Science*, as quoted in Michael Harrington, *The Politics at God's Funeral* (New York: Penguin Books, 1983), 85.

5. Quoted in Robert Byrne, *The Other 637 Best Things Anybody Ever Said* (New York: Fawcett Crest, 1984), 6.

6. James V. Schall, *Christianity and Politics* (Boston: St. Paul Editions, 1981), 102.

7. Harrington, *The Politics at God's Funeral* 85.

Chapter 13

1. Walter Kaufmann, ed. and trans., *The Portable Nietzsche* (New York: Penguin Books, 1954), 95.

2. Paul Johnson, *Modern Times: The World of Christianity from the Twenties to the Eighties* (New York: Harper & Row, 1983), 50.

3. Patrick Egan, "Christians Under Communism," *Pastoral Renewal* (January 1984), 72–74.

4. Evangelical Press News Service (September 26, 1986).

5. Egan, "Christians Under Communism."

6. Richard N. Ostling, "The Definitive Reinhold Niebuhr," *Time* (January 20, 1986), 71.

7. Aleksandr I. Solzhenitsyn, *The Gulag Archipelago: Book II* (New York: Harper & Row, 1974), 374.

8. Joseph Mindszenty, *Mindszenty* (New York: Macmillan, 1974).

9. Quoted in George Seldes, *Great Thoughts* (New York: Ballantine, 1985), 241.

10. Evangelical Press News Service (December 19, 1986), 13, quoting a speech made in Tashkent, USSR, on November 24, 1986.

11. Seldes, *Great Thoughts*, 397.

12. "Christ Would Never Approve that Man Be Considered Merely as a Means of Production," *New York Times* (June 10, 1979), 1:6.

13. "Urged the Government to Honor the Cause of Fundamental Human Rights, Including the Right to Religious

Liberty," *New York Times* (June 6, 1979), 1:3.

14. "Told Poles to Set a Christian Example Even If It Means Risking Danger," *New York Times* (June 7, 1979), 8:1.

15. Evangelical Press News Service (November 21, 1981).

16. Stefan Wyszynski, *The Freedom Within: The Prison Notes of Stefan Cardinal Wyszynski* (New York: Harcourt Brace Jovanovich, 1982), 12.

17. Jacques Ellul, "Lech Walesa and the Social Force of Christianity," *Kattalagete* (June 1982), 5.

18. Ellul, "Lech Walesa and the Social Force of Christianity," 6.

19. Wyszynski, *The Freedom Within*, 26.

20. Beth Spring, "Campus Crusade Director Describes Government Harassment of Evangelicals," *Christianity Today* (February 7, 1986), 52–53. Most of the details concerning Jimmy Hassan were drawn from this article.

21. The information on Nicaragua was drawn from Humberto Belli, *Breaking Faith: The Sandinista Revolution and Its Impact on Freedom and Christian Faith in Nicaragua* (Westchester, Ill.: Crossway Books, 1985).

22. Benjamin Cortes quoted in Belli, *Breaking Faith*, 158.

23. Belli, *Breaking Faith*, 212.

24. Belli, *Breaking Faith*, 156.

25. Belli, *Breaking Faith*, 152.

26. Belli, *Breaking Faith*, 161.

27. Belli, *Breaking Faith*, 162.

28. Belli, *Breaking Faith*, 161.

29. José Felipe Corneado, quoted in "Cuba: A New Attitude," *Christianity Today* (September 5, 1986), 4, International News Section.

30. The story of Poland's school children and the crucifixes was gathered from articles in the following issues of the *New York Times*: (March 8, 1984), I, 15:1; (March 9, 1984), I, 1:3; (March 10, 1984), I, 24:1; (March 11, 1984), I, 3:4; (March 14, 1984), I, 1:1; (March 15, 1984), I, 4:3.

Chapter 14

1. *Stone v. Graham*, 449 U.S. 39 (1980), cited in Robert T. Miller and Ronald B. Flowers, *Toward Benevolent Neu-*

trality: Church, State, and the Supreme Court, rev. ed. (Waco, Tex.: Markham Press Fund, 1977), 327.

2. Material regarding the Marian Guinn case was taken from a wide variety of news stories and wire reports, a transcript of a CBS "60 Minutes" interview (April 22, 1984), and a number of articles, including Lynn Buzzard, "Is Church Discipline an Invasion of Privacy?" Christianity Today (November 9, 1984), 37–39; and "Marian and the Elders," Time (March 26, 1984).

3. 1 Corinthians 5:9.

4. 1 Timothy 5:20.

5. Richard John Neuhaus, The Naked Public Square, (Grand Rapids, Mich.: Eerdmans, 1984), 142.

6. Nat Hentoff, "Religion on School Property," Washington Post (November 1, 1984), A–25.

7. The information from the Dayton Christian School case was taken from William Bentley, "Secularism: Tidal Wave of Repression," in Freedom and Faith, edited by Lynn L. Buzzard (Westchester, Ill.: Crossway Books, 1982).

8. Dorothy Korber, "No Adverse Reaction to Prayer Ban," from an undated California newspaper clipping.

9. Jonathan Kalstrom, "Fire and Brimstone: An Atheist Takes on Small Town America," Liberty (January/February 1987), 22–25; and NFD Journal (August 1986), 14.

10. New York Times (March 6, 1984), II, 6:1.

11. Zorach v. Clauson, 343 U.S. 306 (April 28, 1952). Cited in Miller and Flowers, Toward Benevolent Neutrality, 327.

12. Abington Township School District v. Schempp, 374 U.S. 203 (June 17, 1963). Cited in Miller and Flowers, Toward Benevolent Neutrality, 372.

13. United States v. Seeger (no. 50); United States v. Jakobson (no. 51); Peter v. United States (no. 29) 380 U.S. 163 (March 8, 1965). Cited in Miller and Flowers, Toward Benevolent Neutrality, 177.

14. Richard John Neuhaus, "Moral Leadership in Post-Secular America," Imprimis, 2:7 (July 1982), 3.

15. Will Herberg, Protestant, Catholic, Jew: An Essay in American Religious Sociology (Chicago: University of Chicago Press, 1983), 269.

16. John F. Kennedy, "For the Freedom of Man," inaugural address, Washington, D.C., January 20, 1961. Quoted in *Vital Speeches of the Day*, February 1, 1961.

17. Daniel Bell, *The Cultural Contradictions of Capitalism* (New York: Basic Books, 1978), 77.

18. Quoted in James Hitchcock, *What Is Secular Humanism?* (Ann Arbor, Mich.: Servant Books, 1982), 66.

19. Hitchcock, *What Is Secular Humanism?*, 66.

20. Jack Kroll, "The Most Famous Artist," *Newsweek* (March 9, 1987), 64.

21. Kroll, "The Most Famous Artist," 64.

22. Quoted in David Brock, "A Philosopher Hurls Down a Stinging Moral Gauntlet," *Insight* (May 11, 1987), 12.

23. Robert N. Bellah, et al., *Habits of the Heart: Individualism and Commitment in American Life* (New York: Harper & Row, 1985), 281.

24. Meg Greenfield, "The Grinches vs. the Creche," *Newsweek* (December 24, 1984), 72.

25. "Creation Trial: Less Circus, More Law," *Washington Post* (December 21, 1981), A-3-b.

26. Carl Sagan, *Cosmos* (New York: Random House, 1980), 4.

27. "The Week," *National Review* (May 8, 1987), 16.

28. G. K. Chesterton, *The End of the Armistice* (New York: Sheed and Ward, 1936), 121–22.

29. Quoted in Martin E. Marty, "A Profile of Norman Lear: Another Pilgrim's Progress," *Christian Century* (January 21, 1987), 57.

30. Paul C. Vitz, *Censorship: Evidence of Bias in Our Children's Textbooks* (Ann Arbor, Mich.: Servant Books, 1986).

31. Vitz, *Censorship*, 15.

32. Vitz, *Censorship*, 16.

33. Vitz, *Censorship*, 3.

34. Vitz, *Censorship*, 16.

35. Joseph Sobran, "Pensees: Notes for the Reactionary of Tomorrow," *National Review* (December 31, 1985), 48.

36. Richard John Neuhaus, "The Naked Public Square," *Christianity Today* (October 5, 1984), 32.

37. Henry Hyde, *For Every Idle Silence* (Ann Arbor, Mich.: Servant Books, 1985), 12–13.

38. Donald G. Bloesch, *Crumbling Foundations* (Grand Rapids, Mich.: Zondervan, 1984), 83–84.

39. Bloesch, *Crumbling Foundations*, 57.

40. Quoted in Neuhaus, *Naked Public Square*, 260.

41. Bloesch, *Crumbling Foundations*, 19.

42. "Persecution Next Step—Roberts," *Washington Times* (April 6, 1987).

43. Quoted in Sydney E. Ahlstrom, *A Religious History of the American People* (New Haven, Conn.: Yale University Press, 1972), 954.

44. Walter Shapiro, "Politics and the Pulpit," *Newsweek* (September 17, 1984), 24.

45. *New York Times* (August 14, 1984), A-21.

46. *New York Times* (August 14, 1984), A-21.

47. Mario M. Cuomo, "Religious Belief and Public Morality: A Catholic Governor's Perspective," a paper presented to the Dept. of Theology at the University of Notre Dame (September 13, 1984).

48. The infromation and citations concerning St. John the Divine Cathedral are drawn from Kenneth L. Woodward and Deborah Witherspoon, "The Awakening of a Cathedral," *Newsweek* (June 16, 1986), 59–60.

Chapter 15

1. Walter Shapiro, "Ethics: What's Wrong?" *Time* (May 25, 1987), 14.

2. Ezra Bowen, "Ethics: Looking to Its Roots," *Time* (May 25, 1987), 26.

3. Elwood McQuaid, "Lying as a Lifestyle," *Moody Monthly* (July/August 1987), 8.

4. C. S. Lewis, *The Abolition of Man* (New York: Macmillan, 1974), 35.

5. Richard John Neuhaus, *The Naked Public Square* (Grand Rapids, Mich.: Eerdmans, 1984), 86.

6. Neuhaus, *Naked Public Square*, 89.

7. Neuhaus, *Naked Public Square*, 153.

8. Arthur Schlesinger, *The Vital Center* (New York:

Houghton Mifflin, 1962), 188. Quoted in Neuhaus, *Naked Public Square*, 91.

9. Peter L. Berger, "Religion in Post-Protestant America," *Commentary* 81:5 (May 1986), 44.

10. Russell Kirk, *The Roots of American Order* (LaSalle, Ill.: Open Court, 1974), 81.

11. Will Durant, *Caesar and Christ: A History of Roman Civilization from Its Beginnings to A.D. 337* (New York: Simon and Schuster, 1944), 164.

12. Etienne Gilson, "Foreword," in St. Augustine, *The City of God* (New York: Image/Doubleday, 1958), 19.

13. Edmund Burke, *Reflections on the Revolution in France*. Quoted in *The Portable Conservative Reader* (New York: Penguin, 1982), 27.

14. A. James Reichley, *Religion in American Public Life* (Washington, D. C.: Brookings Institute, 1986), 9.

15. Kirk, *Roots of American Order*, 17.

16. Quoted in Sydney E. Ahlstrom, *A Religious History of the American People* (New Haven, Conn.: Yale University Press, 1972), 386.

17. Will and Ariel Durant, *The Lessons of History* (New York: Simon and Schuster, 1968), 50.

18. Boris Rumer, "Soviet Writers Decry Loss of Spiritual Values in Society," *Christian Science Monitor* (October 7, 1986), 1.

19. Rumer, "Soviet Writers Decry Loss of Spiritual Values in Society," 1.

20. Walter Lippmann, *A Preface to Morals* (New York: Time, 1929), 134.

21. Aleksandr I. Solzhenitsyn, *A World Split Apart: Commencement Address Delivered at Harvard University, June 8, 1978* (New York: Harper & Row, 1978), 49.

Chapter 16

1. *Westminster Confession of Faith*, XX, 2.

2. John 13:34.

3. Quoted in Richard John Neuhaus, *The Naked Public Square* (Grand Rapids, Mich.: Eerdmans, 1984), 178.

4. *The Religion and Society Report*, 3:9 (September 1986), 5.

5. Matthew 5:13–14.

6. Quoted in George F. Will, *Statecraft as Soulcraft: What Government Does* (New York: Simon and Schuster, 1983), 129.

7. See Matthew 25:14–30 and Luke 16:10–31 for discussion of this issue.

8. James Q. Wilson, "Crime and American Culture," *The Public Interest* 70 (Winter 1983), 22.

9. Paul Johnson, *Modern Times: The World from the Twenties to the Eighties* (New York: Harper & Row, 1983), 246–47.

10. Edwin J. Orr, *The Flaming Tongue: The Impact of 20th Century Revivals* (Chicago, Ill.: Moody Press, 1973), 17–18.

11. Etienne Gilson, "Foreword," in St. Augustine, *The City of God* (New York: Image/Doubleday, 1958), 32.

12. Neuhaus, *Naked Public Square*.

Chapter 17

1. "Jesus Christ in the Lives of Americans Today," a poll conducted by the Gallup Organization, Inc., for the Robert H. Schuller Ministries (February 1983), 12.

2. Joseph Sobran, "Pensees: Notes for the Reactionary of Tomorrow," *National Review* (December 31, 1985), 50.

3. Donald Bloesch, *Crumbling Foundations*, (Grand Rapids, Mich.: Zondervan, 1984), 38.

4. Bloesch, *Crumbling Foundations*, 73.

5. G. K. Chesterton, *The Victorian Age in English Literature* (New York: Holt, 1913), 43.

6. James V. Schall, "The Altar as the Throne," in Stanley Atkins and Theodore McConnell, eds., *Churches on the Wrong Road* (Chicago: Regnery, 1986), 231–32.

7. Harry Blamires, *The Christian Mind* (Ann Arbor, Mich.: Servant Books, 1963/1978), 3.

8. Jacques Ellul, *Presence in the Kingdom* (New York: Seabury Press, 1948/1967), 119.

9. Romans 13:1; 1 Timothy 2:2.

10. Acts 5:29.
11. St. Augustine, *The City of God* (Garden City, N.Y.: Image/Doubleday, 1958).
12. Quoted in Richard John Neuhaus, *The Naked Public Square* (Grand Rapids, Mich.: Eerdmans, 1984), 209.
13. St. Augustine, *City of God*.
14. C. S Lewis, *The Four Loves* (New York: Harcourt, Brace, World, 1960), 41.
15. Quoted in Neuhaus, *Naked Public Square*, 237.
16. Neuhaus, *Naked Public Square*, 75.
17. Quoted in Lynn Buzzard and Paula Campbell, *Holy Disobedience: When Christians Must Resist the State* (Ann Arbor, Mich.: Servant Books, 1984), 123.
18. Daniel 1–3.
19. Paraphrase of Daniel 3:16–18.
20. Acts 4:19–20.
21. Charles Mendies, in an interview with Ellen Santilli Vaughn (September 1986).
22. Daniel 1:8.
23. Quoted in A. James Reichley, *Religion in American Public Life* (Washington, D.C.: Brookings Institute, 1986), 104.

Chapter 18

1. Mickey Kaus, *New Republic* (February 24, 1986), 16.
2. *Newsweek* (February 10, 1986), 7, graph.
3. "Brother Can You Spare a Song?" *Newsweek* (October 28, 1985), 95.
4. "Brother Can You Spare a Song?" 95.
5. Quoted in George F. Will, *Statecraft as Soulcraft: What Government Does* (New York: Simon and Schuster, 1983), 129.
6. Jerry Falwell, *If I Should Die Before I Wake* (Nashville: Thomas Nelson, 1986), 10–11.
7. Cited in March Bell, "A Justice Department Commission is Escalating the War Over Pornography," *Eternity* (May 1986), 15–21.
8. "ACLU Reports, Deplores Antipornography Drive," *Washington Post* (February 24, 1986), A–12.

9. This story is told in more detail in Jack Eckerd, *Finding the Right Prescription* (Old Tappan, N.J.: Revell, 1987).
10. Quoted in "Personalities" section of *Philadelphia Inquirer*.

Chapter 19

1. John Naisbitt, *Megatrends: Ten New Directions Transforming Our Lives* (New York: Warner Books, 1983).
2. Paul Tournier, *The Violence Within*. Quoted in Cheryl Forbes, *The Religion of Power* (Grand Rapids, Mich.: Zondervan, 1983), 17.
3. *Newsweek* (September 6, 1971), 16.
4. George Orwell, *1984* (New York: New American Library, 1961), 217.
5. C. P. Snow, *The Masters* (New York: Scribner's, 1982).
6. Richard J. Foster, *Money, Sex and Power* (New York: Harper & Row, 1985), 175.
7. John Milton, *Paradise Lost and Paradise Regained* (New York: New American Library, 1968), 54.
8. Luke 22:26.
9. Mark 10:44.
10. Quoted in Sydney E. Ahlstrom, *A Religious History of the American People* (New Haven, Conn.: Yale University Press, 1972), 386.
11. 2 Corinthians 12:9–10.
12. Anthony Campolo, *The Power Delusion* (Wheaton, Ill.: Victor Books, 1984).
13. Numbers 12:3.

Chapter 20

1. "America's Question and Answer Man," *Newsweek* (June 15, 1987), 56.
2. Robert L. Dabney, *Discussions*, vol. 2, edited by C. R. Vaughan (Harrisburg, Virginia: Sprinkle Publications, 1982), 408.
3. Stephen Monsma, "The Promises and Pitfalls of Evangelical Political Involvement," a speech (October 17, 1986), 9.

4. Andrew Sinclair, *Prohibition: The Era of Excess* (Boston: Little, Brown, 1962).

5. Monsma, "The Promises and Pitfalls of Evangelical Political Involvement," 15–16.

6. St. Augustine, *The City of God* (Garden City, N.Y.: Image/Doubleday, 1958), 88.

7. Harry Blamires, *The Christian Mind* (London: S. P. C. K., 1963), 25.

8. Vernon Grounds, "Crosscurrents," *Moody Monthly* (July/August 1986), 80.

9. Personal letter from Richard John Neuhaus (June 8, 1987).

10. "Vatican Statement on Respect for Human Life in Its Origins and on the Dignity of Procreation: A Reply to Certain Questions of the Day" (1987), 37.

11. Quoted in Joseph Laitin, "Web of Lies," *Washington Post* (October 5, 1986), C-6.

12. *McDaniel vs. Paty*, 435 U.S. 618.

13. "Christopher Dawson: His Interpretation of History," *Modern Age* (Summer 1979), 263.

14. U.S. Bishops' paper on nuclear war, *The Challenge of Peace: God's Promise and Our Response* (May 3, 1983), from the National Conference of Catholic Bishops is discussed in William McNeal, *New York Times* (December 26, 1982), E-3.

15. McNeal, *New York Times* (December 26, 1982), E-3.

16. Russell Kirk, "Promises and Perils of 'Christian Politics'," *Intercollegiate Review* (Fall/Winter 1982), 15.

17. Kirk "Promises and Perils of 'Christian Politics'," 23.

18. Roman Catholic Polish bishops' statement (June 23, 1985).

19. Exodus 21–22.

Chapter 21

1. Richard W. Larsen, "A One-Eyed Angel," *Seattle Times* (April 14, 1985).

Chapter 22

1. Quoted in *Christianity Today* (September 5, 1986), 54.
2. Vernon Grounds, "Authentic Piety," *The Other Side* 21:7 (October 1985), 56–57.
3. George Marsden, *Reformed Journal* (November 1986), 3.
4. Quoted in *Christianity Today* (September 5, 1986), 54.
5. Exodus 18:21.
6. James Skillen, "The Bible, Politics and Democracy," a speech delivered at Wheaton College (November 7–8, 1985), 5.
7. McKendree Langley, *The Practice of Political Spirituality* (Jordan Station, Ontario, Canada: Paideia Press, 1984).
8. C. S. Lewis, *God in the Dock* (Grand Rapids, Mich.: Eerdmans, 1970), 198.
9. Quoted by Colman McCarthy, "For Bennett, A Failing Grade in History," *Washington Post* (September 22, 1985), G-8.
10. Interviews with Ronald Reagan after his meeting with the Religious Roundtable in Dallas (August 22, 1980).
11. A. James Reichley, *Wall Street Journal* (November 25, 1985), 28.
12. Quoted in *Journal of Law and Religion*, 2:1 (1984), 71.
13. "Keeping the Church Doors Open," *Christianity Today* (March 21, 1986), 14.
14. *Time* (September 2, 1985), 58.
15. Kent R. Hill, "Religion and the Common Good: In Defense of Pluralism," *This World 83* (Spring 1987), 83.
16. James V. Schall, "The Altar as the Throne," in Stanley Atkins and Theodore McConnell, eds., *Churches on the Wrong Road* (Chicago: Regnery, 1986), 233.
17. Donald Bloesch, *Crumbling Foundations* (Grand Rapids, Mich.: Zondervan, 1984), 39.
18. Bloesch, *Crumbling Foundations*, 40.
19. Richard Wurmbrand, *Marx and Satan* (Chicago: Crossway, 1986), appendix.
20. Bloesch, *Crumbling Foundations*, 39.
21. Myron Augsburger, *Christianity Today* (January 17, 1986), 21-I.

Chapter 23

1. Jaime Cardinal Sin, from a press conference of the Prison Fellowship International Triennial Symposium in Nairobi, Kenya (August 3, 1986).

2. Robert Shaplan, "Letter from the Philippines," *New Yorker* (February 2, 1985), 61.

3. Benigno Aquino, testimony before the House Foreign Affairs Committee (June 20, 1983).

4. Jaime Cardinal Sin, "A Call to Conscience," a pastoral letter (January 1986).

5. Myron Augsburger, *Christianity Today* (January 17, 1986), 21-I.

6. Quoted in Lynn Buzzard and Paula Campbell, *Holy Disobedience: When Christians Must Resist the State* (Ann Arbor, Mich.: Servant Books, 1984), 142.

7. Richard John Neuhaus, *Religion and Society Report* 3:6 (June 1986), 2.

8. Jonathan Mayhew, *A Discourse Concerning Limited Resistance and Non-Resistance* (Boston, 1750).

9. Buzzard and Campbell, *Holy Disobedience*, 58–59.

10. G. K. Chesterton, *Sidelights on New London and Newer New York,* (New York: Dodd and Mead, 1932), 191.

11. Quoted in David R. Weber, *Civil Disobedience in American History* (Ithaca, N.Y.: Cornell University Press, 1978), 244.

12. Francis Schaeffer, *The Complete Works of Francis A. Schaeffer: A Christian Worldview,* vol. 5 (Westchester, Ill.: Crossway, 1981), 491.

Chapter 24

1. "Leaders of the Christian Right Announce Their Next Step," *Christianity Today* (December 13, 1985), 65.

2. Jacques Ellul, *The New Demons* (New York: Seabury Press, 1975), 167.

3. *Time* (November 1, 1976), 20.

4. "The Farm Act," *Washington Post* (May 7, 1985), B-1; and "Actresses Appeal for Aid to Farmers," *New York Times* (May 7, 1985), 8.

5. Richard Schickel, *Intimate Strangers: The Culture of Celebrity* (New York: Doubleday, 1985).

6. Jacques Ellul, *The Presence of the Kingdom* (New York: Seabury Press, 1948/1967), 100.

7. Quoted in Parker J. Palmer, *Company of Strangers: Christians and the Renewal of America's Public Life* (New York: Crossroads Publishing, 1981), 80.

8. Alexis de Tocqueville, quoted in Palmer, *Company of Strangers*.

9. Tocqueville, *Democracy in America*. Cited in Arendt, *Company of Strangers*, 80.

10. Quoted in Palmer, *Company of Strangers*.

11. Psalm 118:9.

12. Ellul, *Presence of the Kingdom*, 35.

Chapter 25

1. The information in this chapter is based on interviews conducted by Ellen Santilli Vaughn (April 1986).

2. George Russell, "Shadow of a Gunman" *Time* (May 18, 1981), 52–54.

3. Robert Ajemian, "Ready to Die in the Maze," *Time* (August 17, 1981), 48.

4. Ajemian, "Ready to Die in the Maze," 47.

5. Ajemian, "Ready to Die in the Maze," 46.

6. Ajemian, "Ready to Die in the Maze," 47.

7. *New York Times* (March 31, 1979), 1.

8. Based on an account in Jack Holland, *Too Long a Sacrifice* (New York: Dodd and Mead, 1981), 84–89.

9. Guy Garcia, "Edging Toward the Abyss," *Time* (November 30, 1981), 58.

Epilogue

1. Malcolm Muggeridge, *The End of Christendom* (Grand Rapids, Mich.: Eerdmans, 1980), 56.

FOR FURTHER READING

I would like to acknowledge the following works, which were especially useful in the research and preparation of this book. This is by no means intended to be an exhaustive bibliography on the issues of church and state, religion and politics—but readers will find these sources useful in their own further study.

St. Augustine. *The Confessions, The City of God, and On Christian Doctrine.* Chicago: University of Chicago, Great Books Series, Encyclopedia Brittanica, 1952.

Belli, Humberto. *Breaking Faith: The Sandinista Revolution and Its Impact on Freedom and Christian Faith in Nicaragua.* Westchester, Ill.: Crossway, 1985.

Berger, Peter. "Religion in Post-Protestant America." *Commentary* 81:5 (May 1986).

——. *The Sacred Canopy.* Garden City, N.Y.: Anchor, 1968.

Blamires, Harry. *The Christian Mind.* Ann Arbor, Mich.: Servant, 1963.

Bloesch, Donald. *Crumbling Foundations.* Grand Rapids, Mich.: Zondervan, 1984.

Bright, John. *The Kingdom of God.* Nashville: Abingdon, 1953.

Buzzard, Lynn, and Paula Campbell. *Holy Disobedience: When Christians Must Resist the State.* Ann Arbor: Servant, 1984.

Campolo, Anthony. *The Power Delusion.* Wheaton, Ill.: Victor, 1983.

Christianity Today Institute. For its extraordinarily useful summary of *The Christian as Citizen.* Christianity Today, 1985.

Clowney, Edmund. "The Politics of the Kingdom." *Westminster Theological Journal* 41 (Spring 1979).

Cullman, Oscar. *The State in the New Testament.* New York: Scribner's, 1956.

Durant, Will, and Ariel Durant. *The Lessons of History.* New York: Simon and Schuster, 1968.

Ellul, Jacques. *The Presence of the Kingdom.* New York: Seabury, 1948/1967.

———. *The New Demons.* New York: Seabury, 1975.

———. *The Political Illusion.* Translated by Konrad Keller. New York: Vintage, 1972.

Forbes, Cheryl. *The Religion of Power.* Grand Rapids, Mich.: Zondervan, 1983.

Herberg, Will. *Protestant, Catholic, Jew: An Essay in American Religious Sociology.* Chicago: University of Chicago, 1983.

Johnson, Paul. *Modern Times: The World from the Twenties to the Eighties.* New York: Harper & Row, 1983.

Jones, E. Stanley. *The Unshakable Kingdom and the Unchanging Person.* Nashville: Abingdon, 1972.

Kik, J. Marcellus. *The Story of Two Kingdoms.* New York: Nelson, 1963.

Kirk, Russell. "Promises and Perils of 'Christian Politics'." *Intercollegiate Review* (Fall/Winter 1982).

———. "Religion in the Civil Social Order." *Modern Age* (Fall 1984).

———. *The Roots of American Order.* LaSalle, Ill.: Open Court, 1974.

Mott, Stephen. *Biblical Ethics and Social Change.* New York: Oxford University, 1982.

Neuhaus, Richard John. *The Naked Public Square.* Grand Rapids, Mich.: Eerdmans, 1984.

———. *Unsecular America.* Grand Rapids, Mich.: Eerdmans, 1986.

Reichley, A. James. *Religion in American Public Life.* Washington, D.C.: Brookings Institute, 1985.

Runner, Evan. Especially his "Preface" to McKendree R. Langley, *The Practice of Political Spirituality.* Jordan Station, Ontario: Paideia, 1984.

Schaeffer, Francis. *How Should We Then Live?* Old Tappan, N.J.: Revell, 1976.

Schall, James V. "The Altar as the Throne." *Churches on the Wrong Road.* Chicago: Regnery, 1986.

——. *Christianity and Politics.* Boston: St. Paul Editions, 1981.

Skillen, James. "The Bible, Politics and Democracy: What Does Biblical Obedience Entail for American Political Thought?" In *The Bible, Politics and Democracy.* Edited by Richard John Neuhaus. Grand Rapids: Eerdmans, 1987.

Sproul, R. C. *If There Is a God, Why Are There Atheists?* Minneapolis: Dimension, 1978.

——. *Classical Apologetics.* Grand Rapids, Mich.: Zondervan, 1984.

Valladares, Armando. *Against All Hope.* New York: Knopf, 1986.

Vos, Gerhardus. *Biblical Theology: Old and New Testaments.* Grand Rapids, Mich.: Eerdmans, 1984.

Wood, James E., Jr. *Nationhood and the Kingdom.* Nashville: Broadman, 1977.

Index

Charles W. Colson received his bachelor's degree from Brown University and his law degree from George Washington University. From 1969 to 1973 he served as special counsel to President Richard M. Nixon. He pleaded guilty to offenses related to Watergate in 1974 and served seven months in prison. He is now Chairman of Prison Fellowship, a Washington, D.C.–based organization that he founded in 1976. Colson is the author of three best-sellers, *Born Again*, *Life Sentence*, and *Loving God*, and is also a frequent contributor to magazines and journals. All Mr. Colson's speaking fees and book royalties are donated to further the work of Prison Fellowship Ministries.

Ellen Santilli Vaughn, a native of Washington, D.C., received her bachelor's degree from the University of Richmond and her master's in English literature from Georgetown University. She serves as Editorial Director for Prison Fellowship Ministries and has worked as an editor and writer with Charles Colson since 1980. She and her husband, Lee, live in Wayne, Pennsylvania.